Transnasal Endoscopic Skull Base and Brain Surgery

Tips and Pearls

Thieme

Transnasal Endoscopic Skull Base and Brain Surgery

Tips and Pearls

Aldo Cassol Stamm, MD, PhD
Affiliated Professor
Department of Otolaryngology-Head and Neck Surgery
Federal University of São Paulo
Director
Department of Otolaryngology
Hospital Professor Edmundo Vasconcelos
São Paulo, Brazil

Foreword by

Albert L. Rhoton, Jr., MD
Department of Neurosurgery
University of Florida
Gainesville, Florida

Thieme
New York · Stuttgart

Thieme Medical Publishers, Inc.
333 Seventh Ave.
New York, NY 10001

Executive Editor: Timothy Y. Hiscock
Managing Editor: J. Owen Zurhellen
Editorial Assistant: Tess Timoshin
Editorial Director: Michael Wachinger
Production Editor: Barbara A. Chernow
International Production Director: Andreas Schabert
Vice President, International Marketing and Sales: Cornelia Schulze
Chief Financial Officer: Sarah Vanderbilt
President: Brian D. Scanlan
Compositor: Agnew's, Inc.
Printer: Asia Pacific Offset

Library of Congress Cataloging-in-Publication Data

Endoscopic skull base and brain surgery : tips and pearls / Aldo Cassol Stamm, MD, PhD, Editor.
p. ; cm.
Includes bibliographical references and index.
Summary: "The diagnosis and treatment of the diseases of the skull base have changed dramatically in the past few years, transforming the fields of neurosurgery and otolaryngology-head and neck surgery. The increasing advances in these fields have addressed the ENT physicians and neurosurgeons to keep up with the expanding information in the exciting area of skull base. By publishing this book, we are presenting a multidisciplinary approach to the lesions of the skull base. We bring chapters written by the most experienced groups around the world with both, basic information and the latest advances in macro and surgical anatomy, radiology, anesthesia, endocrinology, and all modalities of transnasal endoscopic assisted surgical approaches to the anterior, middle, posterior, zygomatic and infra temporal fossae. In addition, the extended approaches such as to the craniocervical junction and petrous apex are also addressed. Especial emphasis is also given to the reconstruction techniques"—Provided by publisher.
ISBN 978-1-60406-310-3 (hardback : alk. paper)
1. Skull base—Endoscopic surgery. 2. Brain—Endoscopic surgery. I. Stamm, Aldo Cassol, 1953– editor.
[DNLM: 1. Skull Base—surgery. 2. Brain—surgery. 3. Brain Diseases—surgery. 4. Endoscopy—methods. WE 705]
RD529.E53—2011
617.5'140597—dc22 2010049361

Printed in China

5 4 3 2

ISBN 978-1-60406-310-3

I dedicate this book to my family: my lovely and devoted wife, Dagmar, and my two children, Raquel and Guilherme, who have been endlessly supportive and patient during the development of this book. In honor of my mother, Ada, and in memory of my father, Arno, who provided me with my education.

Contents

Foreword

Professor Aldo Cassol Stamm has proven to be one of the world's truly great endoscopic surgeons. This book, *Transnasal Endoscopic Skull Base and Brain Surgery*, highlights his passion for perfection and is peppered with pioneering and novel insights presented under the label "Tips and Pearls." Leonardo da Vinci, Michelangelo, and many other great artists pursued human dissection as a way of achieving perfection in their art. Professor Stamm and a number of the contributors to this volume have spent time in our microsurgery laboratory where they created precise and accurate dissections of skull base anatomy as a way of improving the lives of their patients. We were fortunate to have had Professor Stamm, as he worked night and day for months to achieve the excellence in skull base anatomy that is reflected in many of these chapters. In addition, a number of the dissections shown in this book were performed in our laboratory by some of the world's leading neurosurgical anatomists. The work is further strengthened by contributions for many of the leading otorhinolaryngologists–head and neck surgeons and neurosurgeons in the world.

This book stands as a tribute to the accuracy, precision, and safety that surgeons like Professor Stamm can achieve in their endoscopic approaches to the skull base and brain. His book's focus on safe and accurate endoscopic surgical approaches is integrated with information on all of the modern technological advances, like three-dimensional reconstruction and navigation, which have improved the safety of endoscopic surgery. This volume deals with the full spectrum of endoscopic approaches to the sella and skull base and the pathologies one will encounter in the skull base, while providing guidelines for dealing with the complications encountered in such complex surgery. It deals with not only history and current practice but points to the future of skull base surgery. Overall, it represents a step forward in Professor Stamm's quest for perfection and is further enhanced by his tips and pearls based on years of experience in endoscopic skull base surgery. This magnificent and pioneering work reflects his passion for perfection in endoscopic approaches to the base of the skull and brain. It is a wonderful gift to all physicians dealing in this complicated area.

Albert L. Rhoton, Jr., MD
R.D. Keene Family Professor and Chairman Emeritus
Department of Neurosurgery
University of Florida

Preface

The diagnosis and treatment of diseases of the skull base have changed dramatically in the past few years, transforming the fields of neurosurgery and otolaryngology–head and neck surgery. The increasing advances in these fields have challenged ENT physicians and neurosurgeons to keep up with the expanding information in this exciting area. In this book, we are presenting a multidisciplinary approach to the lesions of the skull base. The chapters, written by the most experienced medical groups around the world, include both basic information and the latest advances in macrosurgical and surgical anatomy, radiology, anesthesia, endocrinology, and all modalities of transnasal endoscopic-assisted surgical approaches to the anterior, middle, posterior, zygomatic, and infratemporal fossae. In addition, the extended approaches, such as those to the craniocervical junction and petrous apex, are also addressed. Special emphasis is also given to the reconstruction techniques.

Although is not our intention to state that all skull bases diseases will benefit from these transnasal endoscopic surgical approaches, we cannot not deny the importance and contribution of such surgical techniques to patients with sellar and parasellar diseases, CSF leaks, and malignant tumors.

These chapters will serve as a consulting textbook for the new generation of neurosurgeons and otolaryngologists. We hope this comprehensive reflection on skull base and rhinology may serve as a guide and stimulus for the surgeon's daily practice, building inter- and multidisciplinary international scientific links.

Acknowledgments

Although it is not possible to list all the formidable individuals who contributed to this project, I would like to express my gratitude to everyone involved in the creation of this book. Special recognition must be given to those who made this work possible:

Many thanks to all the contributors for dedicating their time and enriching this book with wonderful manuscripts and suggestions.

Without the direction and organization of J. Owen Zurhellen and Timothy Y. Hiscock of Thieme Publishers, this project would have never become a reality.

My eternal gratitude to Professor Albert Rhoton will always exist for his generosity in sharing his wonderful pictures and work of many years. It is a privilege to have him listed as a contributor.

Thanks to Dr. Daniel Timperley, Dr. João Nogueira, Dr. Leonardo Balsalobre, and Dr. Eduardo Vellutini for their collaboration and manuscript preparation.

Also, I want to thank Ms. Suely Knoll for the elegant drawings.

Finally, my very special thanks to the marvelous Professor Shirley Pignatari for her continuous collaboration and friendship in every step of my work.

Contributors

Ilaria Acchiardi
Neurosurgical Department I
Policlinico di Monza
Monza, Italy

Luiz Carlos de Alencastro, MD, PhD
Department of Neurosurgery
Hospital Mae de Deus
Porto Alegre, Brazil

Luiz Felipe de Alencastro, MD
Department of Neurosurgery
Hospital Mae de Deus
Porto Alegre, Brazil

Vijay K. Anand, MD
Department of Otolaryngology
Weill Cornell Medical College
New York Presbyterian Hospital
New York, New York

Beng Ti Ang, MBBS
Duke-National University of Singapore Graduate Medical School
Department of Neurosurgery
National Neuroscience Institute
Singapore

Fernando Oto Balieiro, MD
Department of Otolaryngology
Hospital Professor Edmundo Vasconcelos
São Paulo, Brazil

Leonardo Balsalobre Filho, MD
Department of Otolaryngology and Head and Neck
Federal University of São Paulo
Department of Otolaryngology
Hospital Professor Edmundo Vasconcelos
São Paulo, Brazil

Iulo Barauna, MD
Department of Otolaryngology
Hospital Professor Edmundo Vasconcelos
São Paulo, Brazil

Luis Bassagaisteguy, MD
Catedra of Otolaryngology-Head and Neck Surgery
National University of Rosario
Hospital Provincial del Contenario
Rosario, Santa Fe
Argentina

Paolo Battaglia, MD
ENT Department
University of Insubria
Department of Otorhinolaryngology
Ospedale di Circolo e Fondazione Macchi
Varese, Italy

Maurizio Bignami, MD
ENT Department
University of Insubria
Department of Otorhinolaryngology
Ospedale di Circolo e Fondazione Macchi
Varese, Italy

Benjamin Bleier, MD
Harvard Medical School
Department of Otolaryngology-Head and Neck Surgery
Massachusetts Eye and Ear Infirmary
Boston, Massachusetts

Andrea Bolzoni Villaret, MD
Department of Otorhinolaryngology
University of Brescia
Spedali Civili
Brescia, Italy

Hans Rudolf Briner, MD
University of Zurich
Department of Otorhinolaryngology
Zentrum Klinik Hirslanden
Zurich, Switzerland

Roger S. Brock, MD
Department of Neurology
Clinics Hospital
São Paulo University Medical School
Department of DFVneuro
Hospital Israelita Albert Einstein
Hospital Sirio Libanês
São Paulo, Brazil

Marcelo D. Bronstein, MD
Department of Endocrinology
Neuroendocrine Unit
University of São Paulo
São Paulo, Brazil

Zachary M. Bush, MD
Division of Endocrinology
Department of Medicine
University of Virginia
Charlottesville, Virginia

Emiro F. Caicedo, MD
Department of Otolaryngology-Head and Neck Surgery
University of Minnesota
University of Minnesota Medical Center
Minneapolis, Minnesota

Alvaro Campero, MD
Department of Anatomy
School of Medicine
National University of Tucumán
Department of Neurosurgery
Angel Padilla Hospital
San Miguel de Tucumán, Argentina

Frank Rikki Canevari, MD
Department of ORL
University of Pavia
ORL Clinic
Foundation IRCCS Policinico San Matteo
Pavia, Italy

Paolo Cappabianca, MD
Department of Neurological Surgery
Università degli Studi di Napoli Federico II
Naples, Italy

Alberto Carlos Capel Cardoso, MD, PhD
Department of Neurology
Clinics Hospital
São Paulo University Medical School
Department of DFVneuro
Hospital Israelita Albert Einstein
Hospital Sirio Libanês
São Paulo, Brazil

Ricardo L. Carrau, MD
Department of Otolaryngology-Head and Neck Surgery
Ohio State University Medical Center
Columbus, Ohio

Paolo Castelnuovo, MD
ENT Department
University of Insubria
Department of Otorhinolaryngology
Ospedale di Circolo e Fondazione Macchi
Varese, Italy

Luigi Maria Cavallo, MD, PhD
Università degli studi di Napoli Federico II
School of Medicine
Division of Neurosurgery
Il Policlinico
Naples, Italy

Matteo De Notaris, MD
Department of Obstetrics and Gynecology, Pediatrics, Radiology, and Anatomy
Faculty of Medicine
School University of Barcelona
Clinical Department of Neurosurgery
Hospital Clinic
Barcelona, Spain

Wolfgang Draf, Dr. med
International Neuroscience Institute (INI) at the University of Magdeburg
Hannover, Germany

Ignazio Ermoli, MD
ENT Department
University of Insubria
Department of Otorhinolaryngology
Ospedale di Circolo e Fondazione Macchi
Varese, Italy

Felice Esposito, MD, PhD
Department of Neurological Sciences
Division of Neurosurgery and Department of Dentistry and Maxillo-Facial Sciences
Division of Maxillo-Facial Surgery
Università degli Studi di Napoli Federico II
Federico II University Hospital
Naples, Italy

Isabella Esposito, MD
Division of Neurosurgery
Università degli Studi di Napoli Federico II
Naples, Italy

Mario Faria, MD
Department of Neurosurgery
Hospital Mae de Deus
Porto Alegre, Brazil

Giovanni Farneti, MD
ENT Department
Azienda Ospedaliera
Bologna Nord, Italy

Juan C. Fernandez-Miranda, MD
School of Medicine
University of Pittsburgh
Department of Neurological Surgery
University of Pittsburgh Medical Center
Pittsburgh, Pennsylvania

Giorgio Frank, MD
Neurochirurgia
Ospedale Bellaria
Bologna, Italy

Paul A. Gardner, MD
Department of Neurological Surgery
University of Pittsburgh Medical Center
UPMC Presbyterian
Pittsburgh, Pennsylvania

Parul Goyal, MD
Department of Otolaryngology
SUNY Upstate Medical University
Syracuse, New York

Gustavo Hadad, MD
Cátedra de Otorrinolaringologia, Cátedra de Anatomia
Museo de Anatomia y Ciencias Morfológicas
Facultad de Medicina de la Universidad Nactional de Rosario
Provincial del Centanrio Hospital
Rosario, Argentina

Rainer Guilherme Haetinger, MD, PhD
Department of Anatomy
Institute of Biologic Sciences
University of São Paulo
Department of Radiology
Hospital Beneficencia Portuguese São Paulo
São Paulo, Brazil

Richard J. Harvey, MD
School of Medicine
University of New South Wales/Macquarie University
Department of Rhinology and Skull Case Surgery
St Vincent's Hospital
Sydney, New South Wales, Australia

Diego Hermann, MD
Department of Otolaryngology
Hospital Professor Edmundo Vasconcelos
São Paulo, Brazil

Alfredo Herrera, MD
Rhinology and Skull Base Division
Department of Otorhinolaryngology
Hospital San Ignacio Universidad Javeriana
Hospital Militar Central
Bogota, Colombia

David J. Howard, BSc, MBBS
Imperial College, London
Departmentt of Neurosciences
Charing Cross Hospital
London, UK

Peter H. Hwang, MD
Division of Rhinology
Department of Otolaryngology-Head & Neck Surgery
Stanford University School of Medicine
Stanford, California

Kohei Inoue, MD, PhD
Saga University
Department of Neurosurgery
Saga Univesity Hospital
Saga, Japan

John A. Jane Jr., MD
Department of Neurosurgery
University of Virginia
Charlottesville, Virginia

Nick Jones, MD
Department of Otorhinolaryngology, Head and Neck Surgery
Queens Medical Centre
University Hospital
Nottingham, UK

Larry H. Kalish, MBBS(Hons I), MS, MMed(Clin Epi)
University of Sydney
Department of ENT and Skull Base Surgery
Concord Hospital
Sydney, New South Wales, Australia

Amin B. Kassam, MD
Department of Neurosurgery
University of Ottawa
Ottawa, Ontario, Canada

David W. Kennedy, MD
Department of Otorhinolaryngology
University of Pennsylvania Medical Center
Philadelphia, Pennsylvania

Devyani Lal, MD
Department of Otolaryngology
Mayo Clinic
Phoenix, Arizona

John M. Lee, MD
Department of Otolaryngology-Head & Neck Surgery
University of Toronto
St. Michael's Hospital
Toronto, Ontario, Canada

W. Derek Leight, MD
Department of Otolaryngology/Head and Neck Surgery
University of North Carolina
Chapel Hill, North Carolina

Davide Locatelli, MD
Institute of Neurosurgery
Neurosurgical Clinical
Policlinico San Matteo
University of Pavia
Pavia, Italy

Ademir Lodetti, MD
Department of Neurosurgery
Hospital Mae de Deus
Porto Alegre, Brazil

Valerie J. Lund, CBE
Department of Rhinology
University College London
Royal National Throat, Nose and Ear Hospital
London, United Kingdom

Carolina Martins, MD, PhD
Department of Anatomy
Medical School of Pernambuco (IMIP)
Recife, Brazil

Diego Mazzatenta, MD
Center of Surgery for Pituitary Tumors and Endoscopic Skull Base Surgery
Bellaria Hospital
Bologna, Italy

María Chávez Méndez, MD
Otorrinolaringología
Cirugía Endoscópica de Nariz, Senos Paranasales y Base de Cráneo
Cirugía Funcional y Estética Nasal
Veracruz, Mexico

Nelson Mizumoto, MD
Department of Anesthesiology
University of São Paulo
São Paulo, Brazil

Hiroshi Moriyama, MD
Department of Otorhinolaryngology
Jikei University Hospital
Tokyo, Japan

Victor Morera, MD
Department of Neurosurgery
Javeriana University
Department of Neurosurgery
Palermo Clinic
Bogotà, Colombia

Piero Nicolai, MD
Department of Otorhinolaryngology
University of Brescia
Brescia, Italy

João Flávio Nogueira, MD
Sinus Centro
Hospital Geral de Fortaleza
Fortaleza, Brazil

Gurston G. Nyquist, MD
Department of Otolaryngology
Hofstra North Shore/LIJ School of Medicine
Department of Otolaryngology
North Shore University Hospital/Long Island Jewish Medical Center
New Hyde Park, New York

Shegeyuki Osawa, MD
College of Medicine
Kitsato University School of Medicine
Department of Neurosurgery
Kitsato University Hospital
Sasamihara, Japan

Nobuyoshi Otori, MD
Department of Otorhinolaryngology
Jikei University Hospital
Tokyo, Japan

Harshita Pant, MD
Department of Otolaryngology-Head and Neck Surgery
University of Adelaide
Adelaide, Australia

Ernesto Pasquini, MD
ENT Department
Sant'Orsola-Malpighi Hospital-University of Bologna
Bologna, Italy

Shirley S.N. Pignatari, MD, PhD
Department of Otolaryngolic Head and Neck Surgery
Paediatric Otolryngologic Division
Federal University of Sao Paulo (UNIFESP)
São Paulo, Brazil

Fábio Pires Santos, MD
Department of Otolaryngology
Hospital Professor Edmundo Vasconcelos
São Paulo, Brazil

Andrea Pistochini, MD
ENT Department
University of Insubria
Department of Otorhinolaryngology
Ospedale di Circolo e Fondazione Macchi
Varese, Italy

Daniel M. Prevedello, MD
Department of Neurological Surgery
The Ohio State University Medical Center
Columbus, Ohio

Albert L. Rhoton, Jr., MD
Department of Neurosurgery
University of Florida
Gainesville, Florida

Raymond Sacks, MD, MBBCh
Department Otorhinolaryngology
ASAM, Macquarie University
Sydney Medical School
University of Sydney
Department of Otorhinolaryngology-Head and Neck Surgery
Concord General and Macquarie University Hospitals
Sydney, New South Wales, Australia

Juan Eugenio Salas Galicia, MD
Otorrinolaringología
Cirugía Endoscópica de Nariz, Senos Paranasales y Base de Cráneo
Cirugía Funcional y Estética Nasal
Veracruz, Mexico

Rodney J. Schlosser, MD
Department of Otolaryngology
Medical University of South Carolina
Charleston, South Carolina

Theodore H. Schwartz, MD
Department of Neurological Surgery
Weill Cornell Medical College
New York Presbyterian Hospital
New York, New York

Vittorio Sciarretta, MD
ENT Consultant
Department of Otorhinolaryngology
University of Bologna
Department of Otorhinolaryngology
Az. Ospedaliera Sant'Orsola-Malpighi
Bologna, Italy

Brent A. Senior, MD
Rhinology, Allergy, and Sinus Surgery
Department of Otolaryngology/Head and Neck Surgery
University of North Carolina
Chapel Hill, North Carolina

Dharmbir S. Sethi, MD
Department of Otolaryngology
Singapore General Hospital
Singapore

Kristen Seiberling, MD
Department of Otolaryngology
Loma Linda University
Loma Linda Medical Center
Loma Linda, California

Francesca Simoncello, MD
Department of Otorhinolaryngology
Azienda Ospedaliera G. Salvini
Bollate (Milan), Italy

Daniel B. Simmen, MD
Center for Rhinology and Skull Base Surgery
The Hirslanden Clinic
Zürich, Switzerland

Ameet Singh, MD
Department of Surgery and Neurosurgery
Rhinology, Sinus, and Skull Base Surgery
George Washington University
Washington, DC

Carl H. Snyderman, MD
Department of Otolaryngology
University of Pittsburgh
Center for Cranial Base Surgery
University of Pittsburgh Medical Center
Pittsburgh, Pennsylvania

Aldo Cassol Stamm, MD, PhD
Affiliated Professor
Department of Otolaryngology-Head and Neck Surgery
Federal University of São Paulo
Director
Department of Otolaryngology
Hospital Professor Edmundo Vasconcelos
São Paulo, Brazil

Helder Tedeschi, MD
Department of Neurosurgery
State University of Campinas
São Paulo, Brazil

Marc A. Tewfik, MDCM, MSc
Department of Otolaryngology-Head and Neck Surgery
McGill University
Royal Victoria Hospital
Montreal, Quebec, Canada

Daniel Timperley, MD
Caloundra Hospital
Dicky Beach
Queensland, Australia

Raúl Omar Cadena Torrero, MD
Medicine II, Department of Otolaryngology Head and Neck Surgery
Villarica University
Medica Sante Centro de Cirugia Externa S.A. de C.V.
Veracruz, Mexico

Manfred Tschabitscher, MD
Department of Systematic Anatomy
Center of Anatomy and Cell Biology
University of Vienna
Vienna, Austria

Mary Lee Vance, MD
Department of Medicine
University of Virginia
Charlottesville, Virginia

Eduardo Vellutini, MD, PhD
São Paulo Skull Base Center-DFVneuro
São Paulo, Brazil

Matteo Vitali, MD
Division of Neurosurgery
SS Antonio e Biagio e C.
Arrigo, Alessandria, Italy

Jian Wang, MD, PhD
Institute of Neuroscience
Department of Neurosurgery
Second Affiliated Hospital of Guangzhou Medical College
Guangzhou, P.R. China

Arkadi Yakirevitch, MD
Sackler School of Medicine
Tel Aviv University
Department of Otolaryngology-Head and Neck Surgery
Sheba Medical Center
Tel-Hashomer, Israel

Kiyoshi Yanagi, MD
Department of Otolaryngology
Jikei University Hospital
Tokyo, Japan

Peter-John Wormald, MD
Department of Otorhinolaryngology and Head & Neck Surgery
The Queen Elizabeth Hospital
Woodville, South Australia
Australia

Alexandre Yasuda, MD, PhD
Department of Neurosurgery
Hospital Israelita Albert Einstein
São Paulo, Brazil

Matteo Zoli, MD
Department of Neurosurgery
Bellaria Hospital
Bologna, Italy

I Tips and Pearls: Understanding the Paranasal Sinus and Skull Base

1 Anatomical Basis of Skull Base Surgery: Skull Osteology

Carolina Martins, Alvaro Campero, Alexandre Yasuda, Luiz Felipe de Alencastro, Shigeyuki Osawa, and Albert L. Rhoton, Jr.

Tips and Pearls

- Each skull base area has a center, or midline portion, and two lateral parts.
- The center areas are lined up as a corridor, whereas the lateral parts radiate from the skull base center.
- On the exocranial side, the center surgical corridor comprises, from anterior to posterior, (1) the cribriform area, (2) planum, (3) sellae, (4) clivus, and (5) craniovertebral junction.
- On the exocranial side, the center surgical corridor comprises (1) the nasal cavity, (2) the sphenoid sinus, and (3) the pharynx, which enable surgical access to the corresponding endocranial areas.
- In the center surgical corridor, the anterior, middle, and posterior skull base areas are close together and bridged by the sphenoid body.

Introduction

Understanding the osteology of the skull base is a fundamental step in skull base surgery. It enables accurate topographic location and helps tailoring surgical routes to specific skull base areas. This chapter reviews the bony architecture of the anterior, middle, and posterior skull base.

General Anatomy

The skull is divided into the cranium and facial skeleton. The cranium in its turn is divided into calvaria, which is the domelike superior portion of the cranium, formed by the frontal, parietal, and squamous parts of the occipital and temporal bones and greater sphenoid wings, and the cranial base. The cranial base is formed by the occipital, temporal, ethmoid, and frontal bones arranged around, and connected by, a center element—the sphenoid bone.

The cranial base has an endocranial surface, which faces the brain and is naturally divided into anterior, middle, and posterior fossae (**Fig. 1.1**) and an exocranial surface (**Fig. 1.2**),

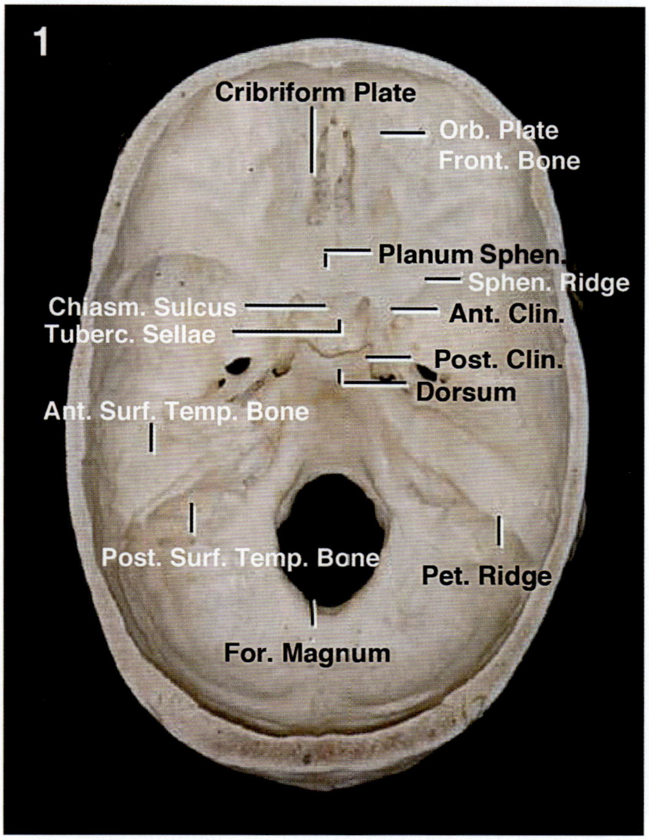

Fig. 1.1 Cranial base: endocranial surface. The upper surface of the anterior cranial base is formed by the frontal bone, which roofs the orbit; the ethmoid bone, which is interposed between the frontal bones and is the site of the cribriform plate; and the lesser wing and the anterior part of the body of the sphenoid, which form the posterior part of the floor of the anterior fossa. The upper surface of the middle cranial base is formed by the greater sphenoid wing and the sphenoid body anteriorly and the upper surface of the temporal bone posteriorly. The posterior part of the cranial base is formed by the temporal and occipital bones. Ant.: anterior; Clin.: clinoid; Chiasm.: chiasmatic; For.: foramen; Front.: frontal; Orb.: orbital; Pet.: petrous; Post.: posterior; Sphen.: sphenoid, sphenoidale; Surf.: surface; Temp.: temporal; Tuberc.: tubercle.

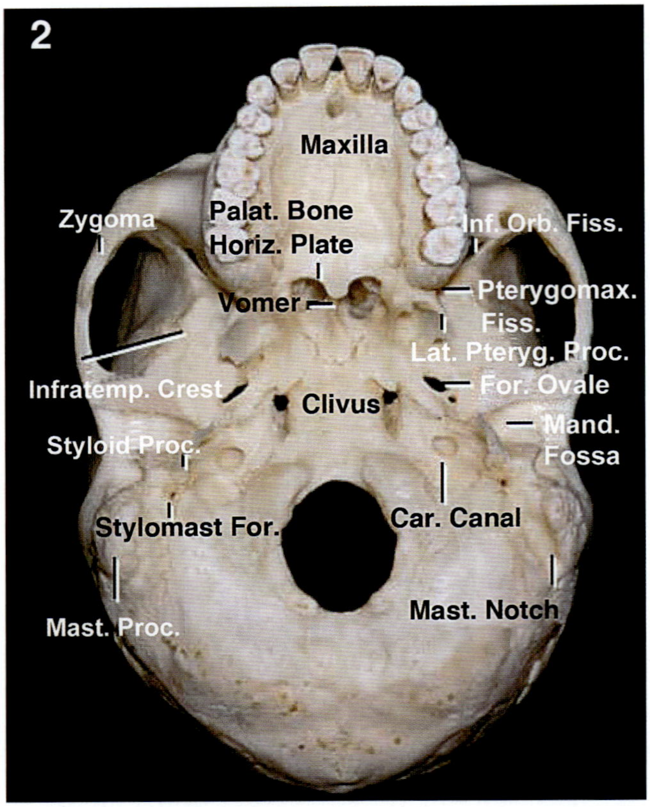

Fig. 1.2 Cranial base: exocranial surface. The exocranial surface is formed mainly by the maxillae, zygomatic, palatine, sphenoid, temporal and occipital bones, and vomer. The maxillae, the orbits, and the nasal cavity are located below the anterior fossa. The anterior part of the hard palate is formed by the maxillae, and the posterior part is formed by the palatine bone. The vomer attaches to the lower part of the body of the sphenoid and forms the posterior part of the nasal septum. The anterior part of the zygomatic arch is formed by the zygoma and the posterior part by the squamosal part of the temporal bones. The mandibular fossa is located below the posterior part of the middle fossa. The infratemporal fossa is located below the greater sphenoid wing and is limited anteriorly by the infratemporal crest. Car.: carotid; Fiss.: fissure; For.: foramen; Horiz.: horizontal; Inf.: inferior; Infratemp.: infratemporal; Lat.: lateral; Mand.: mandibular; Mast.: mastoid; Orb.: orbital; Palat.: palatine; Proc.: process; Pteryg.: pterygoid; Pterygomax.: pterygomaxillary; Stylomast.: stylomastoid.

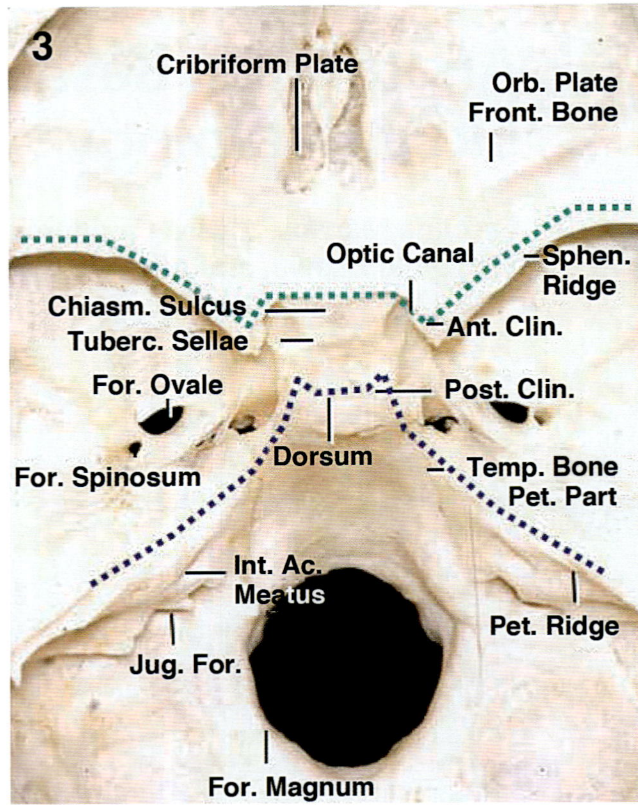

Fig. 1.3 On the endocranial side of the skull base, the border between the anterior and middle fossa is marked by the sphenoid ridge, joined medially by the chiasmatic sulcus (*dotted light blue line*), and the border between the middle and posterior fossae is formed by the petrous ridges joined by the dorsum sellae and posterior clinoid processes (*dotted dark blue line*). Ac.: acoustic; Ant.: anterior; Chiasm.: chiasmatic; Clin.: clinoid; For.: foramen; Front.: frontal; Int.: internal; Jug.: jugular; Orb.: orbital; Pet.: petrous; Post.: posterior; Sphen.: sphenoid; Temp.: temporal; Tuberc.: tubercle.

which faces the nasal cavity, sinuses, orbits, pharynx, infratemporal fossae, and pterygopalatine, parapharyngeal, and infrapetrosal spaces.[1,2]

On the endocranial side of the skull base, the border between the anterior and middle fossa is marked by the sphenoid ridge, joined medially by the chiasmatic sulcus. The border between the middle and posterior fossae is formed by the petrous ridges joined by the dorsum sellae and posterior clinoid processes (**Fig. 1.3**).

On the exocranial side, the anterior and middle fossae are divided by a transverse line, extending through the pterygomaxillary fissures and pterygopalatine fossae at the upper level, and the posterior edge of the alveolar processes of the maxillae at a lower level. Medially, this corresponds to the attachment of the vomer to the sphenoid bone. The middle and posterior cranial fossae are separated on each side by a transverse line crossing near the posterior border of the vomer-sphenoid junction, foramen lacerum, carotid canal, jugular foramen, styloid process, and mastoid tip (**Fig. 1.4**).

Each of the three skull base areas has a center and two lateral parts. The center parts are arranged as a midline corridor and comprise, on the endocranial side, the cribriform area, planum, sellae, clivus, and craniovertebral junction. On the exocranial side, this center corridor encompasses the nasal cavity, sphenoid sinus, and the pharynx.

In the center corridor, the anterior, middle, and posterior skull base areas are close together and bridged by the body of the sphenoid.

Anatomy of the Anterior Skull Base

The anterior endocranial surface is formed by the combination of three bones—frontal, ethmoid, and sphenoid (**Fig. 1.5**). The orbital plates of the frontal bones form most of the lateral parts of this fossa, are the roof of the orbital cavities, and give support to the dura and orbital gyri of the frontal lobe. The medial gap between the orbital plates is filled by the cerebral surface of the ethmoid bone, presenting the crista galli and cribriform plates. The crista galli gives attachment to the falx, whereas the cribriform plates give support to the olfactory bulbs and are traversed by the olfactory fila. Posteriorly, the anterior fossa is closed by the lesser wings of the sphenoid laterally and the sphenoid body medially. In this way, the medial portion of the anterior fossa is formed by three bones, whereas the lateral part which covers the orbit and optic canals, is formed only by two, the orbital plate of frontal bone and the lesser sphenoid wings, on each side.

On the exocranial side, the lateral portion of the anterior skull base is on the top of the orbit and maxillary sinus. Medially, it corresponds to the sphenoid sinus of sphenoid body and the ethmoid sinuses, on top of the nasal cavity (**Fig. 1.6**).

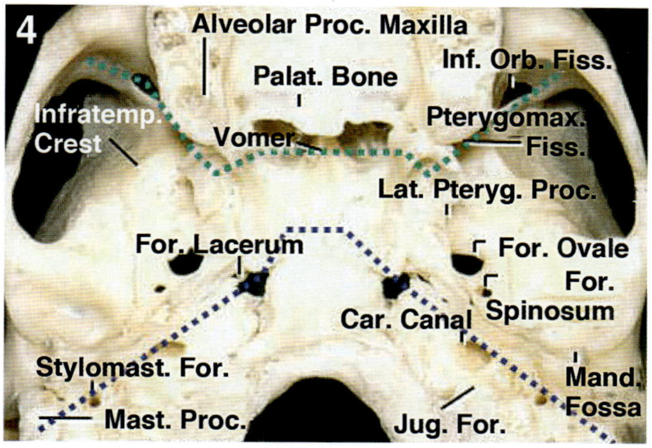

Fig. 1.4 On the exocranial side, the anterior and middle fossae are divided by a transverse line, extending through the pterygomaxillary fissures and pterygopalatine fossae at the upper level, and the posterior edge of the alveolar processes of maxillae at a lower level. Medially, this corresponds to the attachment of vomer to the sphenoid bone (*dotted light blue line*). The middle and posterior cranial fossae are separated on each side, by a transverse line crossing near the posterior border of vomer–sphenoid junction, foramen lacerum, carotid canal, jugular foramen, styloid process, and mastoid tip (*dotted dark blue line*). Car.: carotid; Fiss.: fissure; For.: foramen; Inf.: inferior; Infratemp.: infratemporal; Jug.: jugular; Lat.: lateral; Mand.: mandibular; Mast.: mastoid; Orb.: orbital; Palat.: palatine; Proc.: process; Pteryg.: pterygoid; Pterygomax.: pterygomaxillary; Stylomast.: stylomastoid.

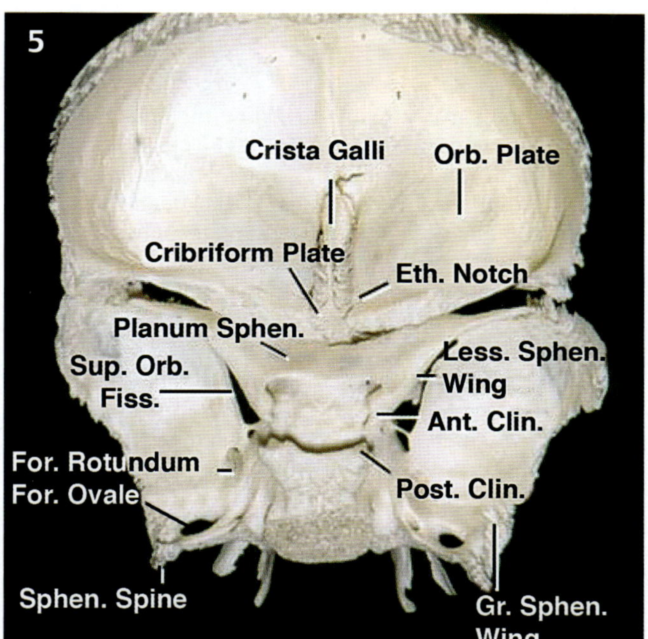

Fig. 1.5 The frontal, ethmoid, and sphenoid bones combine to form the anterior fossa, which is divided into medial and lateral portions. The medial part, covering the upper nasal cavity and sphenoid sinus, is formed by the crista galli and the cribriform plate of the ethmoid bone anteriorly and the planum of the sphenoid body posteriorly. The lateral part, which covers the orbit and the optic canal, is formed by the frontal bone and the lesser wing of the sphenoid bone, which blends medially into the anterior clinoid processes and points toward the middle fossa. Ant.: anterior; Clin.: clinoid; Eth.: ethmoid; Fiss.: fissure; For.: foramen; Gr.: greater; Less.: lesser; Orb.: orbital; Post.: posterior; Sphen.: sphenoid; Sup.: superior.

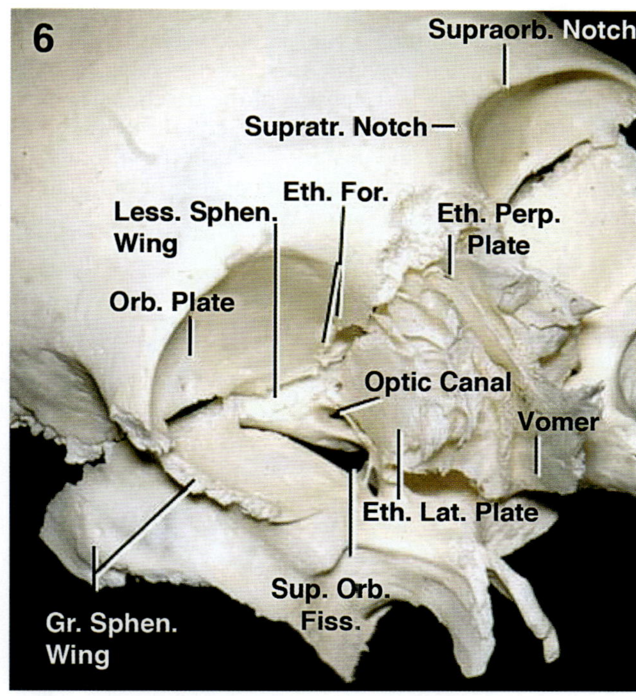

Fig. 1.6 On the exocranial side, the anterior cranial base is divided into a medial part related to the ethmoidal and sphenoidal sinuses and nasal cavity below, and a lateral part that corresponds to the orbit and maxilla. The ethmoid bone forms the anterior and middle thirds of the exocranial surface, and the sphenoid body forms the posterior third of the medial part. The ethmoid presents the perpendicular plate that joins the vomer in forming the nasal septum and two lateral plates located in the medial wall of the orbits. The lateral plates separate the lateral wall of the nasal cavity and the orbit. The main foramina of the region are the anterior and posterior ethmoidal foramina located in the superomedial orbital wall, along the frontoethmoidal suture, which transmit the ethmoidal nerves and arteries; the supraorbital and supratrochlear notches or foramina, transmitting the arteries and nerves of the same name; and the optic canal, which transmits the optic nerve and ophthalmic artery. The superior orbital fissure is located between the lesser and greater sphenoidal wings on the lateral side of the optic canal. It transmits the oculomotor, trochlear, ophthalmic, and abducens nerves, a recurrent meningeal artery, and the superior and inferior ophthalmic veins. Eth.: ethmoid; Fiss.: fissure; For.: foramen; Gr.: greater; Lat.: lateral; Less.: lesser; Orb.: orbital; Perp.: perpendicular; Sphen.: sphenoid; Sup.: superior; Supraorb.: supraorbital; Supratr.: supratrochlear.

The most posterior portion of the medial exocranial anterior surface is related to the sphenoid, whereas the medial and anterior thirds are related to the ethmoid bone.

The bony nasal septum, which is formed by the vomer and perpendicular plate of the ethmoid and attached to the sphenoid crest and rostrum, divides the nasal cavity along the midline, whereas the lateral plates of the ethmoid bones separate the nasal cavity from each orbit (**Figs. 1.7** and **1.8**).

Some foramina and grooves connect the endocranial and exocranial surfaces and transmit vascular and neural structures in this area. The foramen cecum in the midline serves as the site of passage of an emissary vein; the cribriform plate is pierced by the filaments of the olfactory nerve; the supraorbital grooves, on the superior orbital limits, are related to the frontal branch of the first trigeminal division; the anterior and posterior ethmoidal canals, located along the suture line formed by the frontal and ethmoid bones, transmit the anterior and posterior ethmoidal nerves and arteries; the superior orbital fissure, located between the lesser and greater sphenoidal wings, transmit the superior ophthalmic vein and the first division of the trigeminal, oculomotor, trochlear, and abducens nerves; and the optic canals between the anterior and posterior roots of the anterior clinoid processes transmit the optic nerve and the ophthalmic artery.

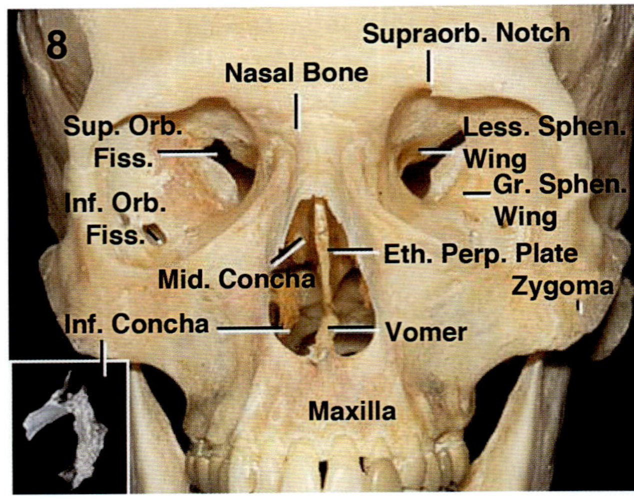

Fig. 1.8 Anterior norma. The orbital rim is formed by the frontal bone, zygoma, and maxilla. The nasal bone is interposed above the anterior nasal aperture, between the maxillae. The nasal cavity is located between the ethmoid bone above and the maxillae, palatine bones, and pterygoid processes of the sphenoid below. It is roofed by the frontal and ethmoid bones, and the floor is formed by the maxillae and palatine bones. The nasal septum forms the medial wall of the nasal cavities. The nasal conchae are located on the lateral walls of the nasal cavity. The inferior concha (*inset*) is a separate bone, and the middle and superior concha are appendages of the ethmoid bone. Eth.: ethmoid; Fiss.: fissure; Gr.: greater; Inf.: inferior; Less.: lesser; Mid.: middle; Orb.: orbital; Perp.: perpendicular; Sphen.: sphenoid; Sup.: superior; Supraorb.: supraorbital.

Anatomy of the Middle Skull Base

The endocranial surface of the middle fossa is formed by the sphenoid and temporal bones. The division between these bones usually is not easy to see unless one is focusing on the sphenoid spine, the most posterior prominence of the sphenoid bone, just posterolateral to the foramen spinosum.

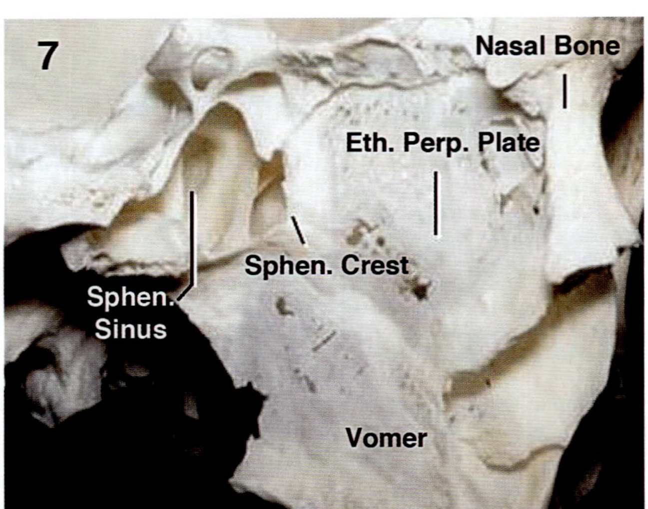

Fig. 1.7 The osseous nasal septum is formed by the attachment of the perpendicular plate of the ethmoid and vomer at the sphenoidal crest. Eth.: ethmoid; Perp.: perpendicular; Sphen.: sphenoid.

From this point it is possible to follow the sphenopetrosal and sphenosquamosal sutures (**Fig. 1.9**). The middle cranial base has medial and lateral parts. The medial part is formed by the body of the sphenoid, whereas the lateral parts result from the combination of lesser and greater sphenoid wings and squamous and petrous parts of the temporal bone. The medial portion of the middle cranial base is the sellae, whereas the most lateral portions are the temporal fossae. Between these two areas, on each side, are the parasellar regions. The parasellar regions are probably the smallest areas of the skull base with the highest concentration of important neural and vascular structures, as they house the cavernous sinuses.

The sphenoid contributes to the middle fossa mainly with its body, the greater and lesser wings. Laterally, the lesser sphenoid wings form the sphenoid ridges. Medially, the lesser wings are connected to the sphenoid body through the anterior root, and they form the roof of the optic canal and are continuous with the sphenoid planum. At the center of the planum is the sphenoid jugum, a faint ridge, which is the remnant of the fusion of the ossification centers. The posterior root of the anterior clinoid process, also called the optic strut, separates the optic canals above from the superior orbital fissure below. The chiasmatic sulcus is located posterior to the planum. On each side of the chiasmatic sulcus are the endocranial openings of the optic canals. Posteriorly, the chiasmatic sulcus is separated from the sellar cavity by the

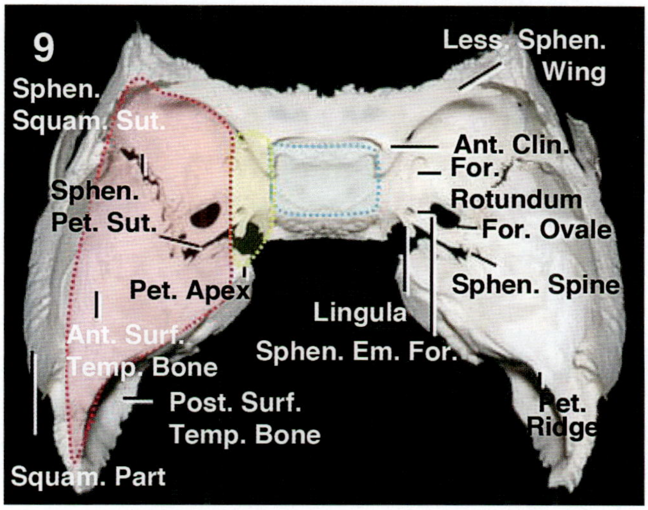

Fig. 1.9 The endocranial surface of the middle cranial base is formed by the sphenoid and temporal bones and can be divided into three regions: a medial part, the sellar region (*blue shaded area*), formed by the sphenoid body; a lateral part, the temporal fossa (*pink shaded area*), formed by the sphenoidal wings and the cerebral surface of the squamosal and petrous parts of the temporal bone; and an intermediate part, the parasellar area (*yellow shaded area*), formed by the transitional part of the sphenoid bone between the greater wing and body and receiving posteriorly a small contribution of the petrous apex of the temporal bone. The greater wing forms the largest part of the endocranial surface of the middle fossa, with the squamosal and the petrosal parts of the temporal bone completing this surface. Ant.: anterior; Clin.: clinoid; Em.: emissary; For.: foramen; Less.: lesser; Pet.: petrous; Post.: posterior; Sphen.: spheno, sphenoid, sphenoidal; Surf.: surface; Sut.: suture; Temp.: temporal.

tuberculum sellae. The posterior limit of the sellae is composed of the dorsum and posterior clinoid processes, which are the medial boundaries between the middle and posterior cranial fossae (**Fig. 1.10**).

The greater sphenoid wings contribute to the temporal fossae. Anteriorly it forms the lateral limit of the superior orbital fissure. The foramen rotundum, which transmits the maxillary division of the trigeminal nerve, is separated from the superior orbital fissure by a bridge of bone, the maxillary strut. The largest opening at the greater sphenoid wing is the foramen ovale, which transmits the third trigeminal division and, in most cases, the accessory meningeal artery. Lateral to this opening is the foramen spinosum for the middle meningeal artery. Occasionally there may be an opening medial to the foramen ovale—the emissary sphenoid foramen (foramen of Vesalius), which transmits a vein connecting the pterygoid venous plexus and the cavernous sinus and, in some cases, might transmit the accessory meningeal artery. The lingula is a protrusion of the sphenoid bone located at the junction of the body and the greater wing. As soon as the carotid artery leaves its canal on the petrous portion of the temporal bone it is embraced by the lingula, which holds the artery in place and enables it to run along the carotid sulcus on each side of sellae. Anteriorly, the carotid artery rests against the optic strut, in close relationship with the anterior clinoid. The lingula gives attachment to the petrolingual ligament, which divides the petroulingual carotid from the vertical cavernous carotid segment (**Fig. 1.11**).

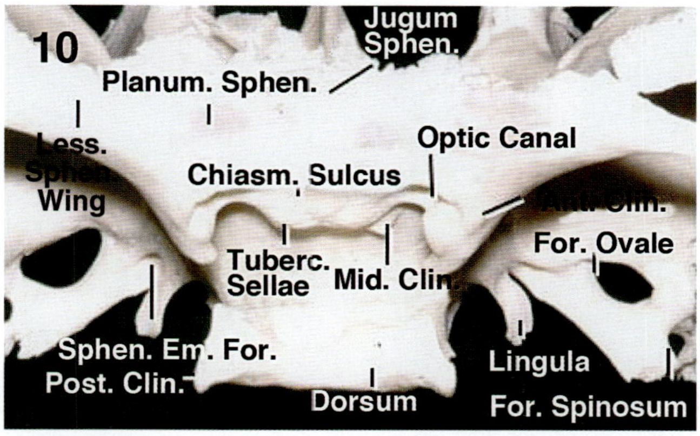

Fig. 1.10 Enlarged view of the medial part of the middle fossa, formed by the body of the sphenoid bone. Ant.: anterior; Chiasm.: chiasmatic; Clin.: clinoid; Em.: emissary; For.: foramen; Less.: lesser; Post.: posterior; Mid.: middle; Sphen.: sphenoid, sphenoidale; Tuberc.: tubercle.

The endocranial surfaces of the petrolingual and squamosal parts of the temporal bone also form the middle fossa (**Figs. 1.12** and **1.13**). In this area, the greater petrosal nerve runs into the facial hiatus just medial to the tensor tympani muscle and lateral to the carotid canal. The trigeminal impression, which houses the trigeminal ganglion, is lateral to the petrous apex and posterosuperior to the superior opening of the carotid canal.

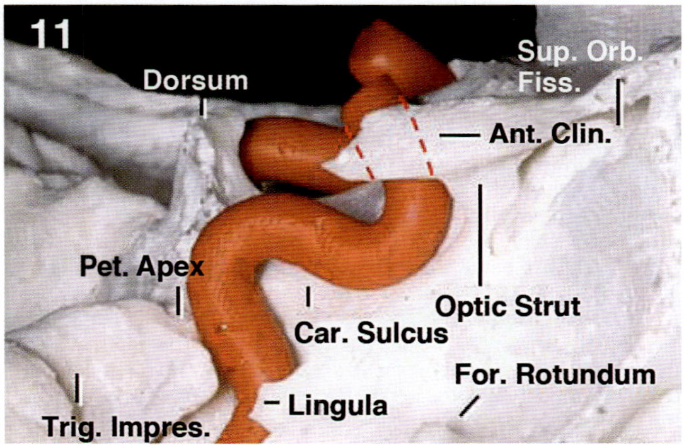

Fig. 1.11 Lateral view of the parasellar region. The course of the petrous, cavernous, and supraclinoid carotid have been represented. The cavernous sinus sits on the lateral aspect of the body of the sphenoid bone. The carotid sulcus is the shallow groove on the lateral aspect of the body of the sphenoid bone along which the cavernous carotid courses. The cavernous carotid sits against and is separated from the carotid sulcus by the dura of the medial sinus wall. The carotid sulcus starts on a position inferior and lateral to the dorsum sellae at the intracranial end of the carotid canal, turns forward to groove the body of the sphenoid immediately below the lateral edge of the floor of the sella, and turns upward to end on a position medial to the anterior clinoid process. Ant.: anterior; Car.: carotid; Clin.: clinoid; Fiss.: fissure; For.: foramen; Impres.: impression; Orb.: orbital; Pet.: petrous; Sup.: superior; Trig.: trigeminal.

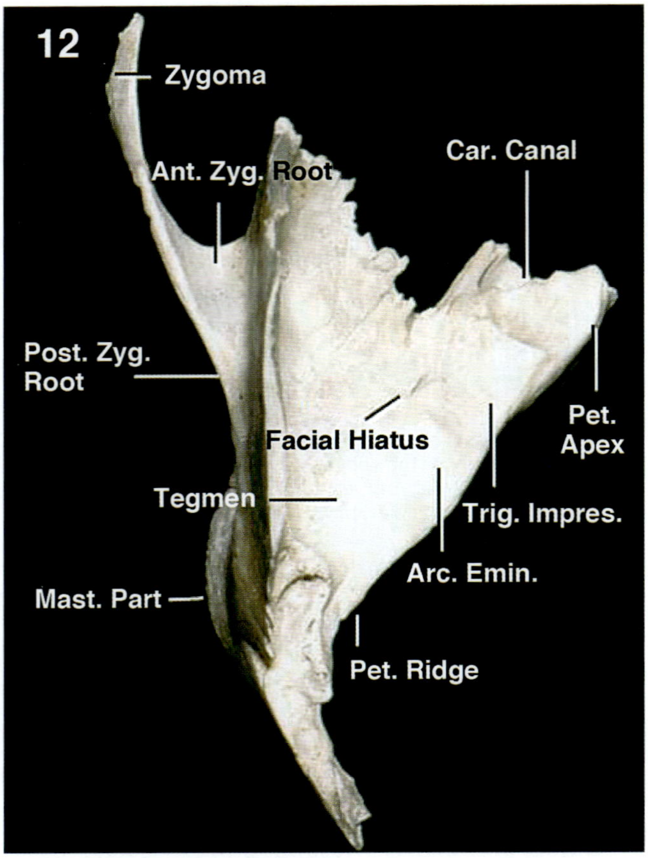

Fig. 1.12 The upper surface of the petrous bone is grooved along the course of the greater and lesser petrosal nerves. The lesser petrosal nerve, from the tympanic plexus, passes through the tympanic canaliculus, which is located anterior to the facial hiatus and courses in an anteromedial direction parallel to the greater petrosal nerve, which courses along the facial hiatus. The carotid canal extends upward and medially and provides passage to the internal carotid artery and carotid sympathetic nerves in their course to the cavernous sinus. The posterior trigeminal root, the semilunar ganglion, and Meckel's cave occupy the middle fossa on the upper surface of the petrous bone at the site of the trigeminal impression. The arcuate eminence approximates the position of the semicircular canals. The internal auditory canal can be identified below the floor of the middle fossa by drilling along a line approximately 60 degrees medial to the arcuate eminence, near the middle portion of the angle between the greater petrosal nerve and arcuate eminence. The petrous apex, medial to the internal acoustic meatus, is free of important structures. A thin lamina of bone, the tegmen tympani, extends laterally from the arcuate eminence and roofs the mastoid antrum, the tympanic cavities, and the canal for the tensor tympani muscle. Opening the tegmen from above exposes the heads of the malleus, incus, the tympanic segment of the facial nerve, and the superior and lateral semicircular canals. Ant.: anterior; Arc.: arcuate; Car.: carotid; Emin.: eminence; Impres: impression; Mast.: mastoid; Pet.: petrous; Post.: posterior; Trig.: trigeminal; Zyg.: zygomatic.

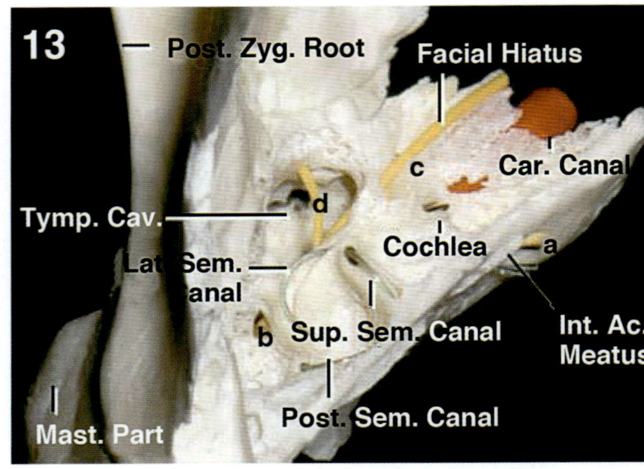

Fig. 1.13 The anterior surface of the temporal bone has been drilled to expose the internal structure of the temporal bone. The carotid artery is represented in red, the facial nerve in yellow, the cochlear nerve in black, and the vestibular nerves in green. The arcuate eminence approximates the position of the superior semicircular canal; however, the relationship between these two structures is greater at their anterior end, from which their main axis diverges. From the brainstem to its peripheral branches, the facial nerve can be divided into six portions: cisternal, meatal (a), labyrinthine, tympanic, mastoid (b), and extracranial. The labyrinthine segment, which is located in the petrous part, extends from the meatal fundus to the geniculate ganglion and is situated between the cochlea anteromedially and the semicircular canals posterolaterally. The labyrinthine segment ends at the site at which the greater superficial petrosal nerve arises from the facial nerve at the level of the geniculate ganglion. From there, the nerve turns laterally and posteriorly along the medial surface of the tympanic cavity, thus giving the name *tympanic segment* to that part of the nerve. The tympanic segment runs between the lateral semicircular canal above and the oval window below. As the nerve passes below the midpoint of the lateral semicircular canal, it turns vertically downward and courses through the petrous part adjacent to the mastoid part of the temporal bone. Thus the third segment, which ends at the stylomastoid foramen, is called the mastoid or vertical segment. Into the temporal bone the facial nerve gives off the greater petrosal (c) and chorda tympani (d) nerves. The chorda tympani nerve, which arises from the mastoid part, runs upwards, passes along the roof of the tympanic cavity, and exits the cavity through the anterior canaliculus. The greater petrosal nerve runs initially along the facial hiatus and beneath the dura of the middle fossa, reaches the sphenopetrosal groove formed by the junction of the petrous and sphenoid bones, immediately superior and anterolateral to the horizontal segment of the petrous carotid, and joins the sympathetic carotid nerves to help form the vidian nerve into the pterygoid canal. The cochlea lies below the floor of the middle fossa in the angle between the labyrinthine segment of the facial nerve and the greater petrosal nerve, just medial to the geniculate ganglion, anterior to the fundus of the internal acoustic meatus, and posterosuperior to the lateral genu of the petrous carotid artery. Ac.: acoustic; Car.: carotid; Cav.: cavity; Int.: internal; Lat.: lateral; Mast.: mastoid; Post.: posterior; Sem.: semicircular; Sup.: superior; Tymp.: tympanic; Zyg.: zygomatic.

The exocranial surface of the middle cranial base is also divided into medial and lateral parts (**Figs. 1.14** and **1.15**). The medial part encompasses the sphenoid body and the upper portion of the basal part of the occipital bone and corresponds to the sphenoid sinus and the nasopharynx. The lateral part is formed by the greater sphenoid wing and the lateral pterygoid plate; the petrous, tympanic, squamous, and styloid parts of the temporal bone; and the zygomatic, palatine, and maxillary bones. Between the lateral and medial parts of the middle cranial base, an intermediate part corresponds to the area between the pterygoid plates. This area is inferior to each cavernous sinus and extends from the pterygopalatine fossa anteriorly to the pterygoid fossa posteriorly. The pterygopalatine fossa is located between the pos-

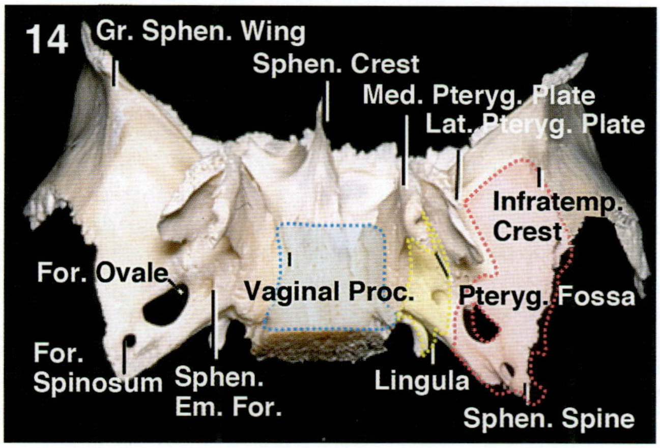

Fig. 1.14 The exocranial surface of the middle cranial base is also divided into medial (*blue shaded area*), intermediate (*yellow shaded area*), and lateral (*pink shaded area*) parts. Em.: emissary; For.: foramen; Gr.: greater; Infratemp.: infratemporal; Lat.: lateral; Med.: medial; Proc.: process; Pteryg.: pterygoid; Sphen.: sphenoid.

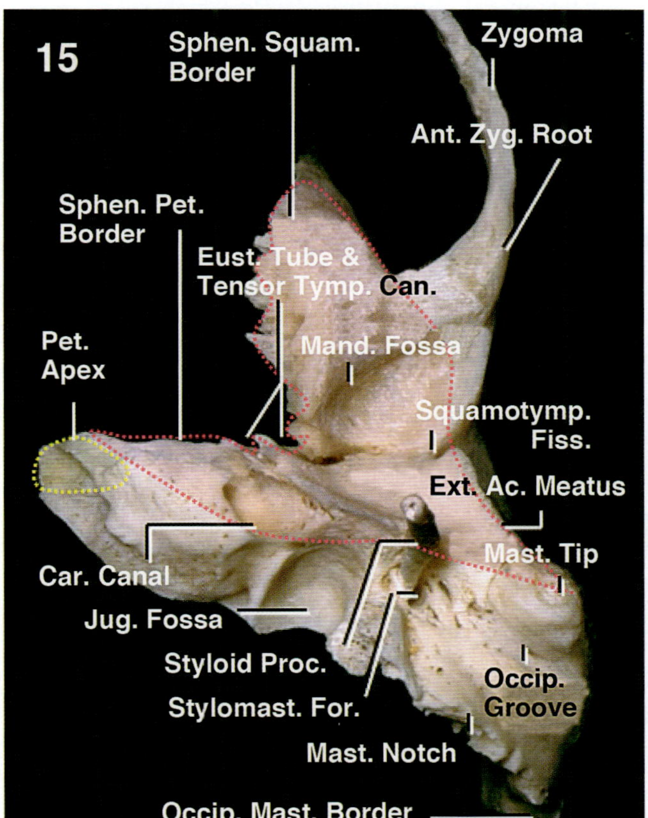

Fig. 1.15 Temporal bone: exocranial surface. The temporal bone is divided into squamosal, petrous, mastoid, tympanic, and styloid parts. The tympanic and squamosal parts, which form the roof of the mandibular fossa, are located anteriorly to the styloid part, the mastoid part is posterolateral, radially grooved by the occipital groove and mastoid notch, and the petrous part is located medial to the styloid part. Ac.: acoustic; Ant.: anterior; Can.: canaliculus; Car.: carotid; Eust.: eustachian; Ext.: external; Fiss.: fissure; For.: foramen; Jug.: jugular; Mand.: mandibular; Mast.: mastoid; Occip.: occipital; Pet.: petrous; Proc.: process; Sphen.: sphenoid; Squam.: squamous; Squamotymp.: squamotympanic; Stylomast.: stylomastoid; Tymp.: tympanic; Zyg.: zygomatic.

terior wall of the maxillary sinus in the front, the pterygoid process behind, the palatine bone medially, and the body of the sphenoid bone above. The fossa opens laterally through the pterygomaxillary fissure into the infratemporal fossa and medially through the sphenopalatine foramen to the nasal cavity. Both the foramen rotundum for the maxillary nerve and the pterygoid canal for the vidian nerve open through the posterior wall of the fossae formed by the pterygoid process of the sphenoid bone. The palatovaginal canal carrying the pharyngeal nerve and artery and the greater and lesser palatine canals conveying the greater and lesser palatine arteries also open into the pterygopalatine fossa. The inferior orbital fissure, across which the orbital muscle stretches, lies in front of the pterygopalatine fossa.

The lateral part of the middle cranial base that corresponds endocranially to the temporal fossa includes the infratemporal fossa, mandibular fossa, and the parapharyngeal space (**Fig. 1.16**). The infratemporal fossa is bounded anteriorly by the posterolateral surface of the maxilla and the infratemporal crest, which separates the infratemporal from the superolaterally located temporal fossa. The infratemporal fossa is bounded anteromedially by the lateral pterygoid plate, laterally by the

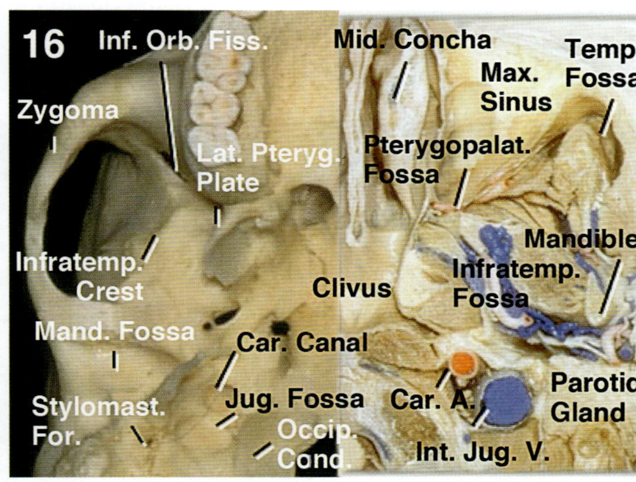

Fig. 1.16 Exocranial view of the articulated middle fossa. The components of the several compartments of this surface are seen on the right, and the bony limits of the compartments can be seen on the left. The lateral part of the middle cranial base that corresponds endocranially to the temporal fossa includes the infratemporal fossa, mandibular fossa, and the parapharyngeal space. The pterygopalatine fossa is located between the posterior wall of the maxillary sinus in front, the pterygoid process behind, the palatine bone medially, and the body of the sphenoid bone above. The fossa opens medially, through the sphenopalatine foramen, to the nasal cavity and laterally, through the pterygomaxillary fissure, into the infratemporal fossa. The parapharyngeal space is divided by the styloid diaphragm formed by the anterior part of the carotid sheath into pre-styloid and post-styloid parts. The prestyloid compartment, a narrow, fat-filled space, separates the infratemporal fossa from the medially located parapharyngeal space in which the eustachian tube is situated. A.: artery; Car.: carotid; Cond.: condyle; Fiss.: fissure; For.: foramen; Inf.: inferior; Infratemp.: infratemporal; Int.: internal; Jug.: jugular; Lat.: lateral; Mand.: mandibular; Max.: maxillary; Mid.: middle; Occip.: occipital; Orb.: orbital; Pteryg.: pterygoid; Pterygopalat.: pterygopalatine; Stylomast.: stylomastoid; Temp.: temporal; V.: vein.

mandibular ramus, and posteriorly by the tympanic part of the temporal bone and styloid process. The pterygomaxillary and inferior orbital fissures, the alveolar canals, the foramen spinosum, the ovale, and the emissary sphenoid foramen open into the infratemporal fossa. The mandibular fossa harbors the mandibular condyle. The roof of this fossa is divided into anterior and posterior parts by the squamotympanic fissure, along which the chorda tympani nerve passes. The parapharyngeal space lies between the structures in the pharynx wall medially, the medial pterygoid muscle and the parotid fascia laterally, and the styloid fascia investing the styloglossus, stylopharyngeal, and stylohyoid muscles posteriorly. The parapharyngeal space is divided by the styloid diaphragm into pre-styloid and post-styloid parts. The post-styloid part of the parapharyngeal space is also referred to as the infrapetrosal space. It is located behind the styloid fascia, below the petrous bone, and medial to the mastoid process. Among the foramina in the area connecting the intra- and extracranial spaces is the jugular foramen and carotid canal. The jugular foramen contains the jugular bulb and the lower end of the inferior petrosal sinus. It transmits branches of the ascending pharyngeal artery, the glossopharyngeal, the vagus, and the accessory nerves. The carotid canal transmits the carotid branch of the ascending pharyngeal artery, the sympathetic nerves, and the carotid artery. It is anterior to the jugular foramen and medial to the external auditory meatus.

Anatomy of the Posterior Skull Base

The posterior cranial base is formed by three bones—the sphenoid, temporal, and occipital (**Fig. 1.17**). The occipital bone is the major osseous component of the posterior fossa. It is formed of squamosal, condylar, and basal parts. The basal part fuses with the sphenoid to form the clivus. Laterally, it articulates with the temporal bone at the petroclival fissures. The squamosal part forms the posterior boundary of the fossae and has three angles. The superior angle fills the gap between the parietals along the lambdoid suture. The lateral paired angles mark the most lateral extension of the lambdoid sutures and the ending point of the transverse sinus. It joins the occipitomastoid and parietomastoid sutures at the asterion. The condylar part of the occipital bone forms a bridge between the squamosal and basal parts (**Figs. 1.18** and **1.19**).

The endocranial surface of the posterior fossa can be divided into medial and lateral parts. The medial part is formed by union of the sphenoid and the basal portion of the occipital bone. The endocranial surface of the basal part is concave from side to side and presents the sulcus for the inferior petrosal sinus. The condylar part of the occipital bone comprises a quadrilateral plate of bone—the jugular process. The anterior

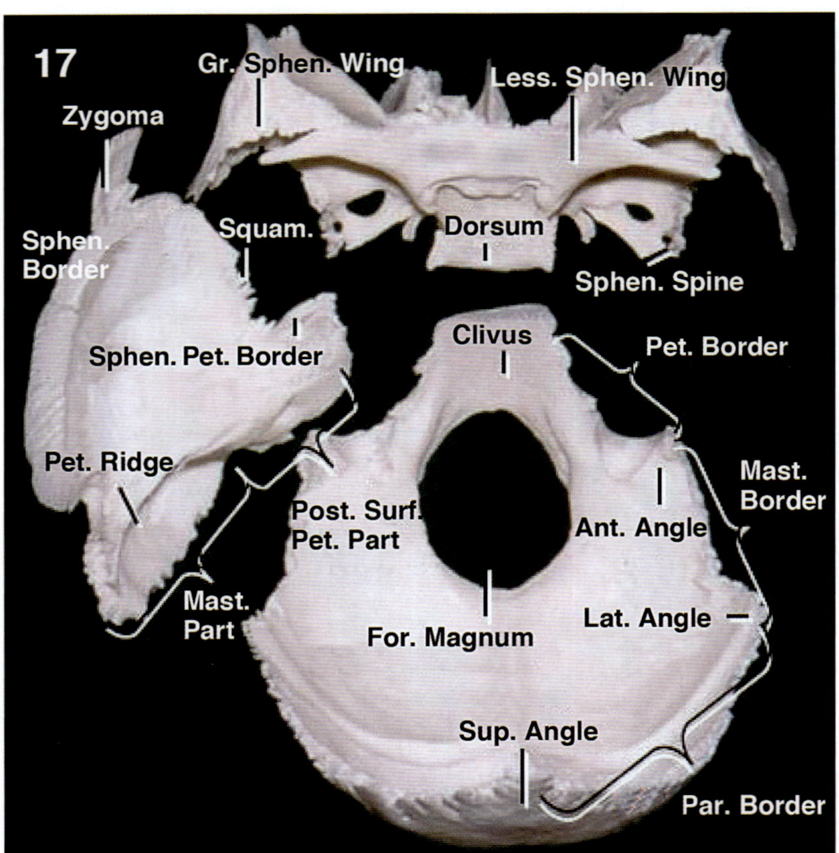

Fig. 1.17 The posterior cranial base is formed by three bones—sphenoid, temporal and occipital. The posterior fossa can be divided into medial and lateral portions. Medially, the sphenoid and the basal (clival) portion of occipital bone fuse at the sphenoclival synchondrosis. Laterally, the posterior fossa is composed by the apposition of the mastoid and the posterior surface of the petrous portion of the temporal bone with the condylar and basal portions of the occipital bone. The occipital bone is the main component of the posterior cranial fossa. It has three parts—basal (or clival), condylar, and squamosal; three borders—petrous, mastoid and parietal; and three angles—paired anterior and lateral angles, and an unpaired superior angle. The anterior angle marks the combination of the different parts of the temporal and occipital bones: medial to the anterior angle, the petrous border of the occipital bone meets the petrosal part of the temporal bone at the petroclival fissure, and the jugular fossa of the temporal bone combines with the jugular notch of the occipital bone to form the jugular foramen. Lateral to the anterior angle, the mastoid border of the occipital bone meets the mastoid part of the temporal bone to form the occipitomastoid suture. The parietal border, between the lateral and superior angle, combines with the parietal bone, forming the lambdoid suture. Ant.: anterior; For.: foramen; Gr.: greater; Lat.: lateral; Less.: lesser; Mast.: mastoid; Par.: parietal; Pet.: petrous; Post.: posterior; Sphen.: sphenoid; Squam.: squamous; Sup.: superior; Surf.: surface.

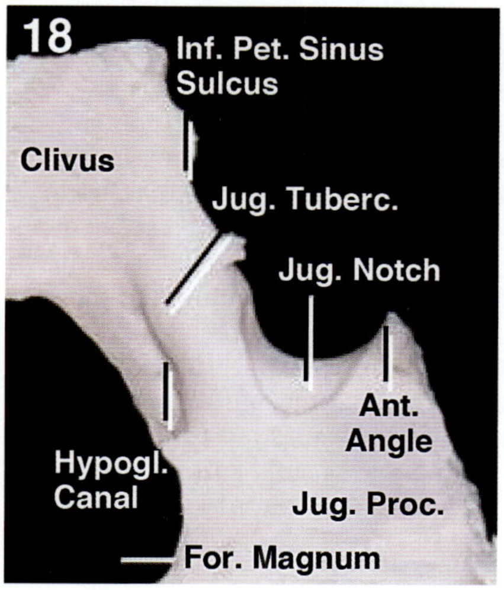

Fig. 1.18 Superior view of the endocranial side of the condylar and basal (clival) parts of the occipital bone. The condylar part can be considered a bridge connecting the basal (clival) and squamosal parts of the occipital bone. The basal (clival) part is concave from side to side and presents the sulcus for the inferior petrosal sinus. The inferior petrosal sinus links the cavernous sinus to the medial part of the jugular foramen. On the exocranial side, there is a similar sulcus for the inferior petrosal vein. The condylar part comprises a quadrilateral plate of bone, the jugular process, whose anterior border presents the jugular notch and the anterior angle of the occipital bone. Medial to the jugular notch, on the endocranial surface, is the jugular tubercle, a protrusion related to the course of the lower cranial nerves. Ant.: anterior; For.: foramen; Hypogl.: hypoglossal; Inf.: inferior; Jug.: jugular; Pet.: petrous; Proc.: process; Tuberc.: tubercle.

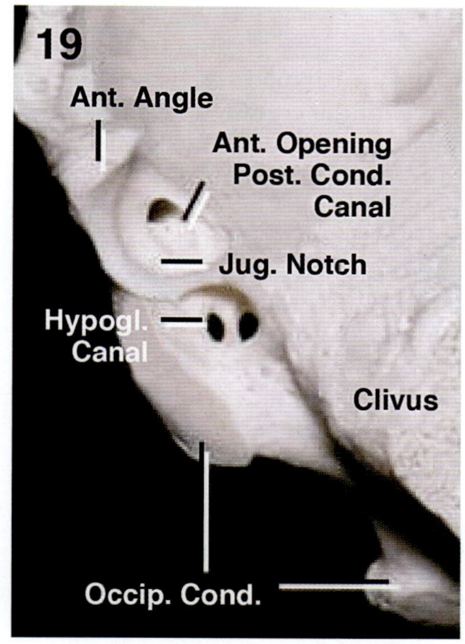

Fig. 1.19 The exocranial surface of the condylar part of the occipital bone. The jugular notch is located superolateral to the hypoglossal canal and occipital condyle. On its posterior wall there is the opening of the posterior condylar canal, which transmits an emissary vein connecting the vertebral plexus to the sigmoid sinus. The hypoglossal canal can be divided by a fibrous or a bony septum. Ant.: anterior; Cond.: condyle; Hypogl.: hypoglossal; Jug.: jugular; Occip.: occipital; Post.: posterior.

lip of the jugular process presents the jugular notch. Medial to the jugular notch and just superior to the intracranial opening of the hypoglossal canals are the jugular tubercles, two rounded elevations on the endocranial surface. The lower cranial nerves pass in close contact with the jugular tubercle on their course toward the jugular foramen, and in some cases can leave faint grooves on it.

The lateral part of the endocranial surface is composed by the apposition of the mastoid and the posterior surface of the petrous portion of the temporal bone with the condylar and basal portions of the occipital bone. The posterior surface of the temporal bone extends from the petrous apex medially to the sulcus for the sigmoid sinus laterally (**Fig. 1.20**). In this area, the internal acoustic meatus, the subarcuate

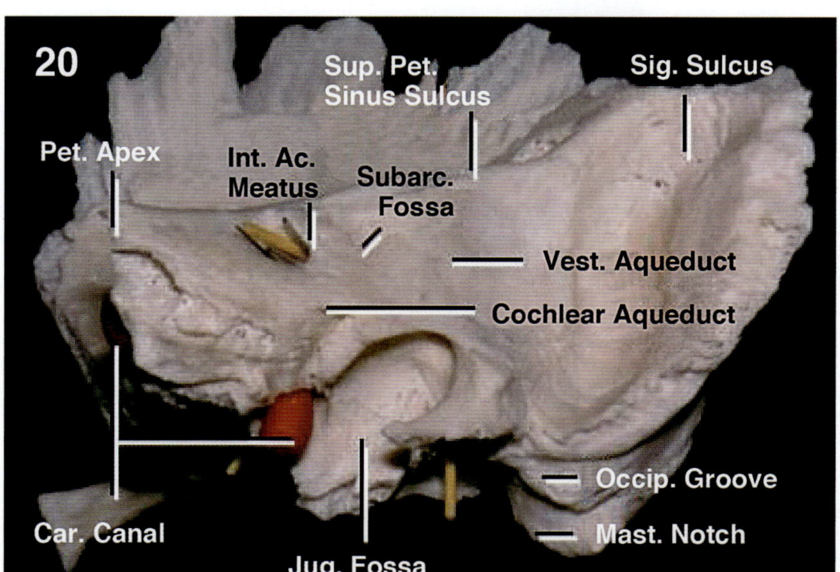

Fig. 1.20 The posterior surface of the temporal bone forms the anterolateral limit of the posterior fossa. It extends from the petrous apex medially to the sigmoid sulcus laterally and from the sulcus for the superior petrosal sinus and petrous ridge superiorly, to the sulcus for the inferior petrosal sinus and jugular fossa inferiorly. The nerves passing through the internal acoustic meatus have been represented with colored material: the facial nerve (*yellow*) is located anterosuperior, the cochlear nerve (*black*) is anteroinferior, and the vestibular nerves are located posterolaterally. The petrous carotid (*red*) is represented in the carotid canal. Ac.: acoustic; Car.: carotid; Int.: internal; Jug.: jugular; Mast.: mastoid; Occip.: occipital; Pet.: petrous; Sig.: sigmoid; Subarc.: subarcuate; Sup.: superior; Vest.: vestibular.

fossa, and the vestibular aqueduct are separated by a thin bony lamina from the sigmoid sinus. The meatus is located above the jugular fossa and jugular bulb. Its posterior lip has an intimate relationship with the crura of the semicircular canals, a fact that has implications during surgical removal of the posterior meatal lip. The meatus transmits the VII/VIII neural complex and the labyrinthine branches of the anterior inferior cerebellar artery (AICA). The anatomical understanding about the labyrinth, the sigmoid sinus, the jugular bulb, and the dura on Trautmann's triangle is also important when working through the mastoid, in a presigmoid and combined retrosigmoid approach to the posterior fossa.

The basilar and condylar parts of the occipital bone combine with different areas of the temporal bone. The basilar portion of the occipital bone meets the petrous apex, the jugular notch meets the jugular fossa, and the mastoid part of the temporal bone meets the occipital bone lateral to the jugular notch. In the articulated bone, the union between the jugular fossa and notch forms the jugular foramen; the combination of the clivus and the petrous apex forms the petroclival fissure (**Fig. 1.21**). Lateral to the jugular foramen, the anterior angle of the occipital bone, located at the quadrilateral plate of the jugular process, adapts to the temporal bone lateral to the jugular fossa, determining the meeting of the mastoid part and the squamous occiput and the formation of the occipitomastoid suture. In this lateral portion of the posterior fossa, the parietal meets the occipital bone (above the lateral angle) and the mastoid to form, respectively, the lambdoid and parietomastoid sutures. The meeting point of these three sutures—occipitomastoid, lambdoid,

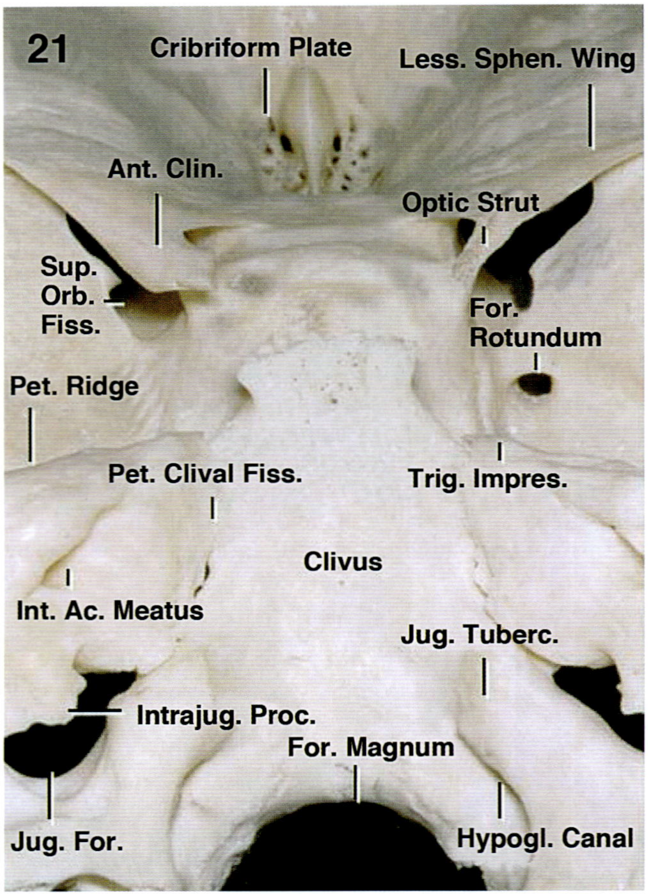

Fig. 1.21 Petroclival area. The combination of the basal (clival) part of the occipital bone and petrosal part of the temporal forms the petroclival fissure. The combination of the jugular notch of the occipital bone and the jugular fossa of the temporal forms the jugular foramen. The intrajugular processes of the temporal and occipital bones project into the jugular foramen and divide this area into petrosal and sigmoid parts. The intrajugular process of the temporal bone is usually more prominent. Ac.: acoustic; Fiss.: fissure; For.: foramen; Hypogl.: hypoglossal; Impres.: impression; Int.: internal; Intrajug.: intrajugular; Jug.: jugular; Less.: lesser; Orb.: orbital; Pet.: petrous; Proc.: process; Sphen.: sphenoid; Sup.: superior; Trig.: trigeminal; Tuberc.: tubercle.

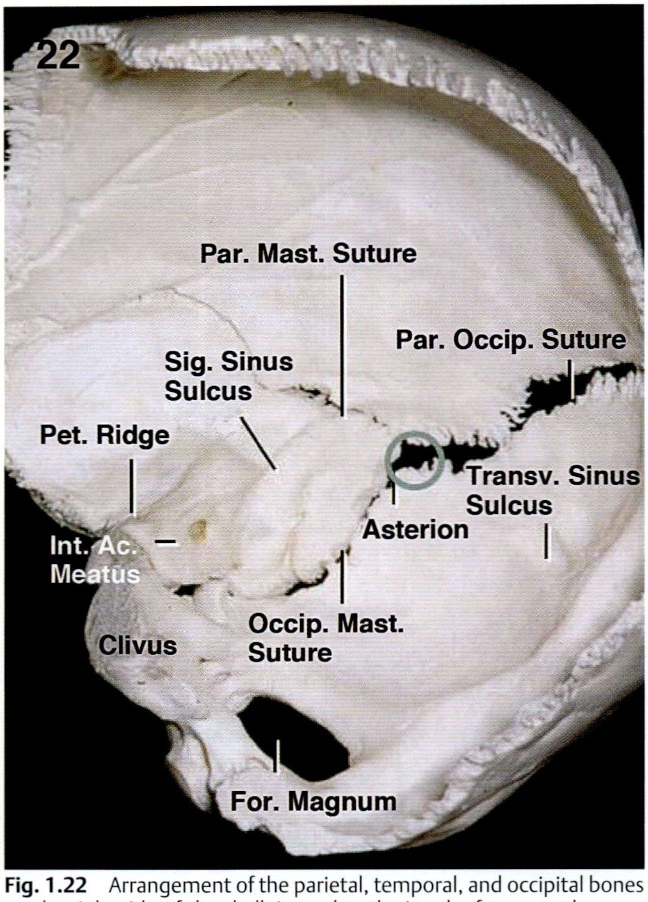

Fig. 1.22 Arrangement of the parietal, temporal, and occipital bones on the right side of the skull. Lateral to the jugular foramen, the mastoid border of the occipital bone meets the mastoid part of the temporal bone, forming the occipitomastoid suture. The parietal bone meets the mastoid part of the temporal bone at the parietomastoid fissure, and the parietal border of the occipital bone combines with the parietal bone at the parieto-occipital or lambdoid suture. The meeting point of the occipitomastoid, parietomastoid, and lambdoid sutures forms the asterion. The asterion is related to the lateral angle of the occipital bone and marks the transition between the transverse and sigmoid sinuses at the most lateral part of the posterior cranial fossa. Ac.: acoustic; For.: foramen; Int.: internal; Mast.: mastoid; Occip.: occipital; Par.: parietal; Pet.: petrous; Sig.: sigmoid; Transv.: transverse.

and parietomastoid—forms the asterion (**Fig. 1.22**), which is an important landmark for the junction of the transverse and sigmoid sinuses.

The occipital condyles are located on the exocranial surface of the condylar part of the occipital bone at each side of foramen magnum (**Figs. 1.23** and **1.24**). The basion is the most anterior point at the anterior arch of the foramen magnum, and the opisthion is the most posterior point at the posterior arch of the foramen. If the basion is considered to be in the 12 o'clock position and the opisthion in the 6 o'clock position, then the occipital condyles can be understood as projecting in a position between 1 o'clock and 3 o'clock and between 9 o'clock and 11 o'clock. Posteriorly, on top of the condyles, are the supracondylar fossae and the posterior opening of the posterior condylar canals. These canals transmit the posterior condylar veins, which connect the vertebral venous plexus to the jugular bulb. The anterior condylar veins, also called hypoglossal veins, course through the hypoglossal canals, which can at times be divided by fibrous or bony septa.

The posterior fossa can be considered to have an anterior limit, composed by the clivus, the posterior surface of the temporal bone, and the condylar part of the occipital bone on each side, and a posterior limit, mostly composed by the squamosal part of the occipital bone.

The anterior limit of the posterior fossa, composed by the clivus, the posterior surface of the temporal bone, and the condylar part of the occipital bone on each side and its endocranial and exocranial surfaces, is part of the so-called ventral skull base and can be approached endoscopically by working through the sphenoid sinus, nasopharynx, and adjacent compartments.

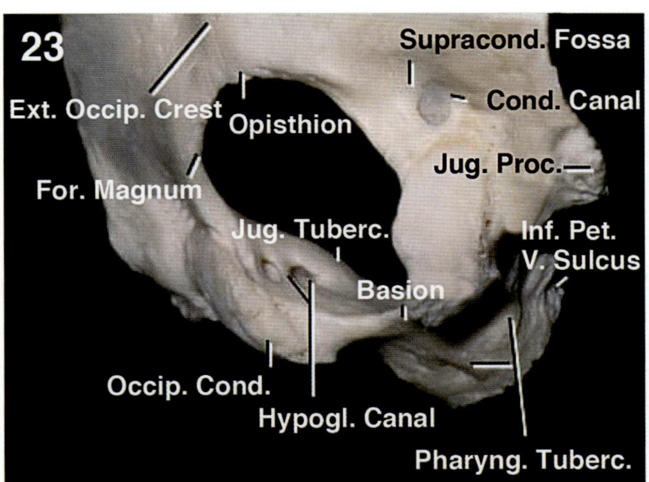

Fig. 1.23 The occipital bone surrounds the foramen magnum. The occipital bone is divided into a squamosal part located above and behind the foramen magnum, a basal (clival) part situated in front of the foramen magnum, and paired condylar parts located lateral to the foramen magnum. The basion is the most anterior part of the anterior edge of the foramen magnum. The opisthion is the most posterior point along the posterior edge of the foramen magnum. Cond.: condyle, condylar; Ext.: external; For.: foramen; Hypogl.: hypoglossal; Inf.: inferior; Jug.: jugular; Occip.: occipital; Pet.: petrous; Pharyng.: pharyngeal; Proc.: process; Supracond.: supracondylar; Tuberc.: tubercle; V.: vein.

The exocranial surface of the squamosal part of the occipital bone comprises most of the dorsal skull base, which is approached through the suboccipital approaches or its extensions. It is marked by four paired transverse ridges and one vertical crest that radiate from the external occipital protuberance (**Fig. 1.24**). The supreme nuchal lines are the highest ones and give attachment to the occipital aponeurosis. The superior nuchal line is just inferior to the supreme nuchal lines, and usually more marked. From medial to lateral, they give attachment to the trapezius, splenius capitis, and sternocleidomastoid muscles. The superior nuchal lines have a transverse part, close to the external occipital protuberance. Laterally, close to the mastoid, they describe an arched course, related to the mastoid emissary foramina. The transverse part of the superior nuchal line marks externally the position of the transverse sinuses and the transition level between the supratentorial and infratentorial compartments. The external occipital crest radiates vertically from the external occipital protuberance close to the midline. It affords attachment to the ligamentum nuchae. From the midpoint of the external occipital crest, an arched paired ridge, the inferior nuchal line, radiates just above the posterior edge of foramen magnum.

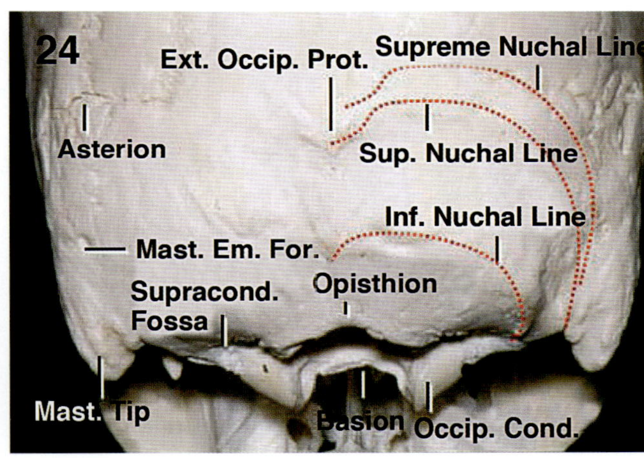

Fig. 1.24 The exocranial surface of the squamosal part of the occipital bone. The exocranial surface of the occipital bone forms most of the dorsal skull base. It is marked by four paired transverse ridges and one vertical crest that radiate from the external occipital protuberance. The supreme nuchal lines are the highest ones and give attachment to the occipital aponeurosis. The superior nuchal line is just inferior to the supreme nuchal lines, and usually more marked. From medial to lateral, they give attachment to the trapezius, splenius capitis, and sternocleidomastoid muscles. The superior nuchal lines have a transverse part, close to the external occipital protuberance. Laterally, close to the mastoid, they describe an arched course, related to the mastoid emissary foramina. The transverse part of the superior nuchal line marks externally the position of the transverse sinuses and the transition between the supratentorial and infratentorial compartments. The external occipital crest radiates vertically from the external occipital protuberance close to the midline. It affords attachment to the ligamentum nuchae. From the midpoint of the external occipital crest, an arched paired ridge, the inferior nuchal line, radiates just above the posterior edge of foramen magnum. The inferior nuchal line on each side gives attachment to the superior oblique and rectus capitis posterior major and minor. Cond.: condyle; Em.: emissary; Ext.: external; For.: foramen; Inf.: inferior; Mast.: mastoid; Occip.: occipital; Sup.: superior.

The inferior nuchal line on each side gives attachment to the superior oblique and rectus capitis posterior major and minor.

The occipital bones sit over the atlas by adapting the convex occipital condyles over the concavity of the lateral masses of atlas and piling on top of the cervical spine.

References

1. Rhoton AL Jr. The posterior cranial fossa. Microsurgical anatomy and surgical approaches. Neurosurgery 2000;47(3 suppl.):S1–S298
2. Rhoton AL Jr. The supratentorial cranial space. Microsurgical anatomy and surgical approaches. Neurosurgery 2002;51(4 suppl.):S1–S410

2 Anatomy of the Nasal Cavity and Paranasal Sinuses

Carolina Martins, Luiz Felipe de Alencastro, Alberto Carlos Capel Cardoso, Alvaro Campero, Alexandre Yasuda, Jian Wang, Luiz Carlos de Alencastro, and Albert L. Rhoton, Jr.

Tips and Pearls

- The nasal cavity is a natural pathway to the anterior cranial fossae, orbit, pterygopalatine and infratemporal fossae, as well as the frontal, maxillary, ethmoidal, and sphenoidal sinuses.
- Adjacent compartments, such as the maxillary and sphenoid sinuses and the pharynx, extend the reach of this natural pathway further to the sellae, cavernous sinus, petrous bone, clivus, middle and posterior cranial fossae, craniovertebral junction, and parapharyngeal and infrapetrosal spaces.

Introduction

The nasal cavity is the space between the nares and the choanae, separated along the midline by the nasal septum. It extends inferiorly from the palate up to the inferior surface of the cribriform plate, being on top of the oral cavity and anterior to the pharynx. The air space medial to the conchae and lateral to the septum is the common nasal meatus, which communicates at the lower edge of each concha with the superior, middle, and inferior meatus (**Figs. 2.1, 2.2, 2.3,** and **2.4**).

From a surgical point of view, this space is a natural pathway to and from several adjacent compartments. The compartments that can be reached through the superior part of the nasal cavity are, from anterior to posterior, the frontal sinus cavity; the ethmoidal sinuses and the center of the anterior cranial base; and the sphenoid sinus cavity and sellar region. Laterally, the compartments related to the nasal cavity can be separated at the level of the middle meatus. Above this level, the nasal cavity can lead to the orbit and its contents; below, there is a two-way route to and from the maxillary sinus. At the level of the choanae, the lateral relationship of the nasal cavity includes also the pterygopalatine and infratemporal fossae.

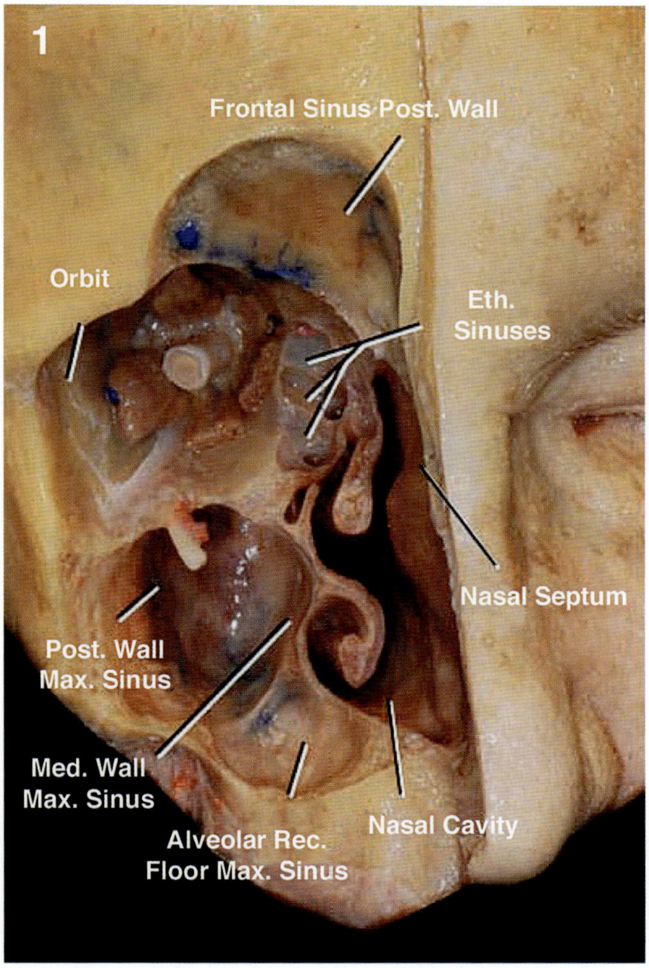

Fig. 2.1 The right side of the face has been dissected to expose the nasal cavity and its topographical relationships. Eth.: ethmoid, ethmoidal; Max.: maxillary; Med.: medial; Post.: posterior; Rec.: recess.

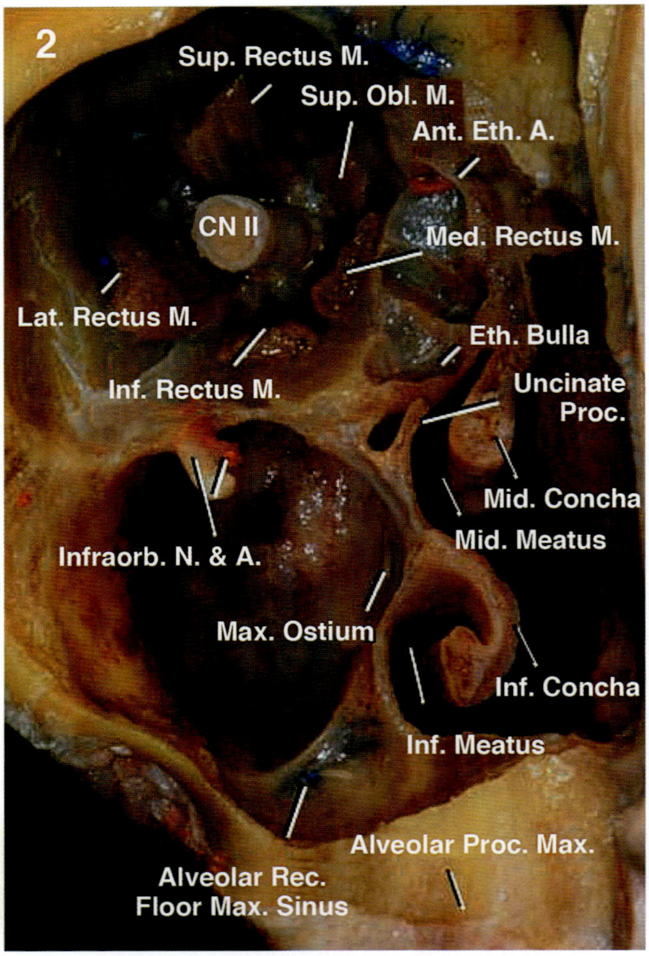

Fig. 2.2 Enlarged view of Fig. 2.1. The air space medial to the conchae and lateral to the septum is the common nasal meatus, which communicates at the lower edge of each concha with the superior, middle, and inferior meatus. The arrangement of the extraocular muscles, which attach posteriorly at the annulus of Zinn, helps divide the orbit into an intraconal and extraconal spaces. The optic nerve, the most important intraconal structure, is used as a reference to describe lesions located into this space. The maxillary sinus is a pyramidal cavity in the body of the maxilla. Its apex points laterally and extends into the zygomatic process. The base is the lateral wall of the nasal cavity below the middle meatus and presents the maxillary ostium. Its floor is the alveolar process of the maxilla. The alveolar canals transmit the posterior-superior alveolar nerves to the molar teeth and can protrude on the posterior wall of the sinus. The roof separates the sinus from the floor of orbit and presents the infraorbital canal for the infraorbital nerve and vessels. The anterior wall of the sinus forms the anterior surface of the body of the maxilla, faces the oral vestibule, and has been removed in this dissection. The uncinate process is a curved projection from the orbital plate of ethmoid at the medial wall of the maxillary sinus. A.: artery; Ant.: anterior; CN: cranial nerve; Eth.: ethmoid, ethmoidal; Inf.: inferior; Infraorb.: infraorbital; Lat.: lateral; M.: muscle; Max.: maxillary; Med.: medial; Mid.: middle; N.: nerve; Obl.: oblique; Proc.: process; Rec.: recess; Sup.: superior.

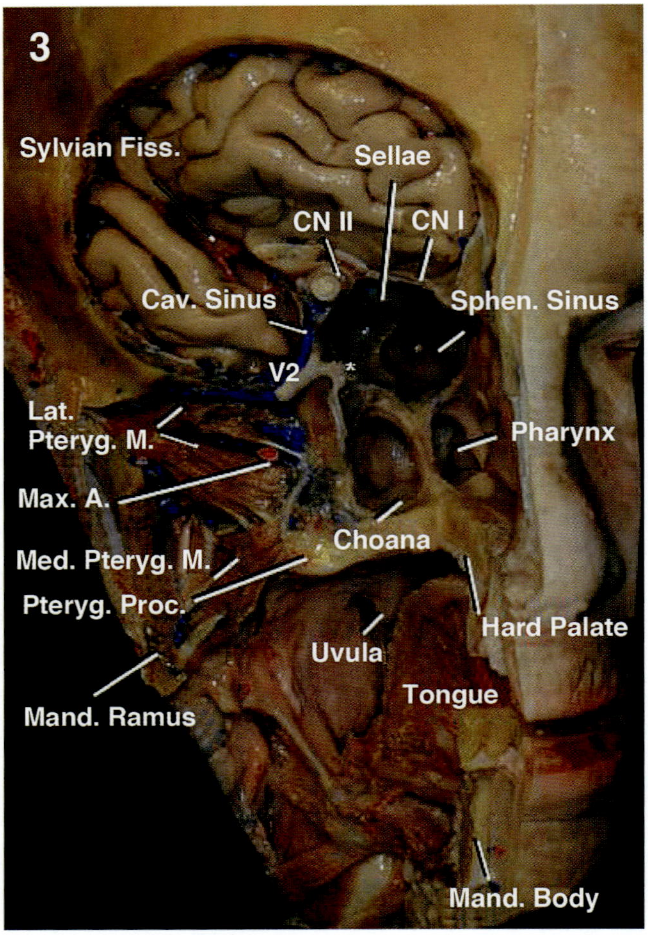

Fig. 2.3 The dissection has proceeded to the posterior limit of the nasal cavity. The orbit has been resected up to the apex, and the walls of the maxillary sinus, the nasal septum, and part of the palate have been removed. The pterygopalatine fossa, containing the pterygopalatine ganglion (*) and the infratemporal fossa, with structures related to the posterior wall of the maxillary sinus, have been exposed. The sphenoid sinus has been opened. The anterior and middle fossae have been exposed, and part of the tongue, the ramus, and the body of the mandible have been removed. At the level of the choanae, the lateral relationship of the nasal cavity includes the pterygopalatine and infratemporal fossae. Some of the adjacent compartments should be thought of as nasal cavity "amplifiers," because, when working through them, several other areas can be reached. This is especially true for the maxillary and sphenoid sinus and the pharynx. The maxillary sinus expands the reach, particularly to the infratemporal and pterygopalatine fossae, as well as the orbit. The sphenoid sinus offers the possibility to reach the anterior fossa, the cavernous sinus, the petrous part of the temporal bone, and the middle and posterior fossae, besides the well-known path it provides to the sellae. The nasopharynx offers a path to the inferior clivus and the foramen magnum area, the craniovertebral junction, as well as the contents of the parapharyngeal and infrapetrosal spaces. A.: artery; Cav.: cavernous; CN: cranial nerve; Fiss.: fissure; Lat.: lateral; M.: muscle; Mand.: mandibular; Max.: maxillary; Med.: medial; Proc.: process; Pteryg.: pterygoid; Sphen.: sphenoidal.

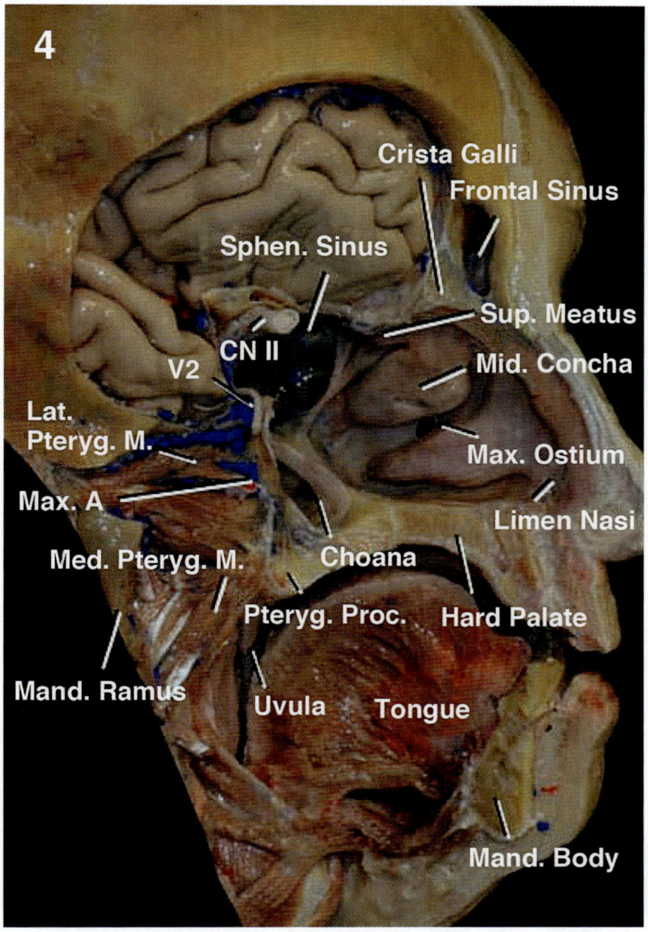

Fig. 2.4 The view along the lateral wall of the left nasal cavity. The nasal cavity proper extends from the limen nasi to the choana. The concha protrudes along this wall, delimiting the superior, middle, and inferior meatus. The frontal, anterior ethmoidal, and maxillary sinuses open into the middle meatus. A.: artery; CN: cranial nerve; Lat.: lateral; M.: muscle; Mand.: mandibular; Max.: maxillary; Med.: medial; Mid.: middle; Proc.: process; Pteryg.: pterygoid; Sphen.: sphenoidal; Sup.: superior; V2: second division trigeminal nerve.

Some of the adjacent compartments should be thought of as nasal cavity "amplifiers." When working through these compartments, several other areas can be reached. This is especially true for the maxillary and sphenoid sinuses and the pharynx. The maxillary sinus expands the reach particularly to the infratemporal and pterygopalatine fossae, as well as the orbit. The sphenoid sinus offers the possibility of reaching the anterior fossa, cavernous sinus, petrous part of the temporal bone, and middle and posterior fossae, in addition to the well-known path it provides to the sellae. The nasopharynx offers a path to the inferior clivus and foramen magnum area, the craniovertebral junction, and the contents of the parapharyngeal and infrapetrosal spaces.

Anatomy of the Nasal Cavity

The nasal cavity has a vestibule, which extends from the naris to the limen nasi and is related to the external nose. Posterior to the vestibule is the nasal cavity proper, extending from the limen nasi and piriform aperture to the choana (**Fig. 2.4**).

The piriform aperture is the anterior bony opening of the nasal cavity. It is formed by the nasal bones and frontal processes of the maxilla above and the alveolar processes of the maxilla below and laterally (**Figs. 2.5** and **2.6**). The anterior nasal spine is found at the inferior edge of the piriform aperture, at the meeting point of both maxillae. It relates superiorly to the free end of the septal cartilage, at the point that it unites with columella. The average superior width of the piriform aperture in adults is 16 mm; its breadth, 24 mm; and the height of the aperture, 29 mm.[1] The cartilages of the external nose are arranged along the margins of the piriform opening and delimit the anterior openings of the nose—the nares.

The choana is the posterior limit of the nasal cavity and opens the nasal cavity proper to the nasopharynx (**Figs. 2.3** and **2.4**). Acting as a door, each choana is delimited superiorly by the sphenoid rostrum, superolaterally by the sphenoid process of the palatine bone, and laterally by the medial pterygoid plate and the perpendicular plate of the palatine bone. The inferolateral angle of the choana is smooth and formed by the meeting point between the perpendicular and horizontal plates of the palatine. Superomedially the choana is delimited by the ala of vomer and medially by the bony septum, formed by sphenoid rostrum and the crest united with the vomer. Inferomedially the choana is delimited by the nasal surface of the horizontal plate of the palatine bone at the level of the nasal crest (**Figs. 2.7** and **2.8**). The posterior nasal spine is the midline protrusion on the nasal surface of the horizontal plate of the palatine at the posteriormost point of the nasal crest. In adults, each choana has an average height of 25.5 mm and a width of 13.5 mm.[1]

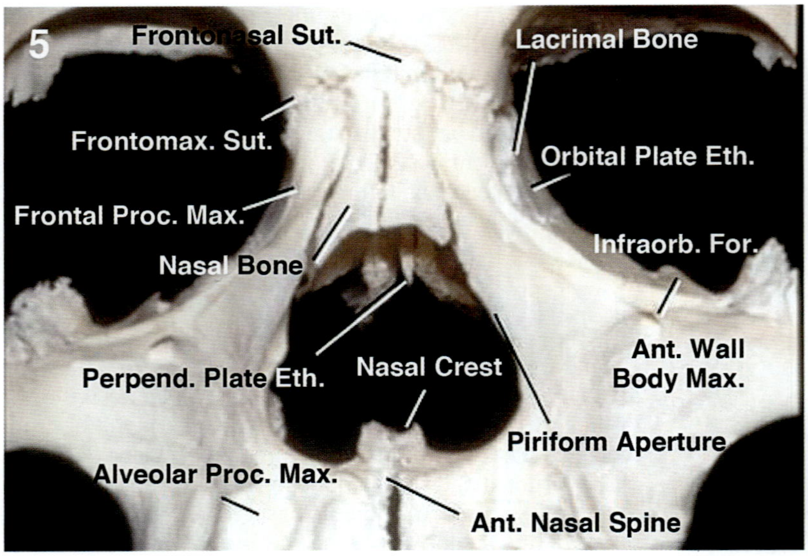

Fig. 2.5 The piriform aperture is the anterior bony opening of the nasal cavity. It is formed by the nasal bones and frontal processes of the maxilla above and the alveolar processes of the maxilla below and laterally. The nasal bones unite above with the frontal bone at the nasofrontal suture, and laterally with the frontal process of the maxilla at the nasomaxillary suture. The anterior nasal spine is found at the inferior edge of the piriform aperture, at the meeting point of both maxillae. Ant.: anterior; Eth.: ethmoid, ethmoidal; For.: foramen; Frontomax.: frontomaxillary; Infraorb.: infraorbital; Max.: maxillary; Perpend.: perpendicular; Proc.: process; Sut.: suture.

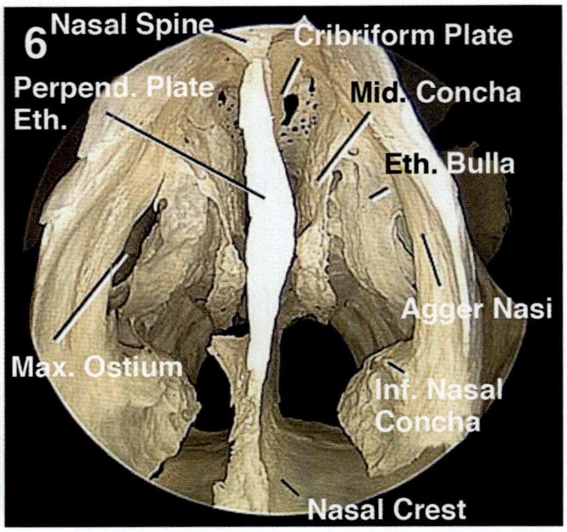

Fig. 2.6 Dry, articulated skull. Endoscopic view within the nasal cavity. The nasal spine of the frontal bone projects inferiorly and anteriorly. With the perpendicular plate of the ethmoid, the spine of the frontal bone supports the nasal bones, which lie upon them. Eth.: ethmoid, ethmoidal; Inf.: inferior; Max.: maxillary; Mid.: middle; Perpend.: perpendicular.

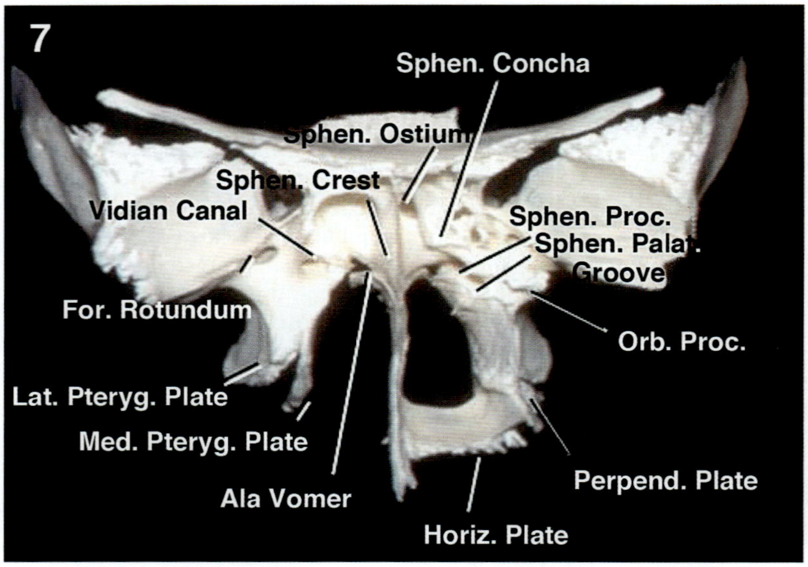

Fig. 2.7 The choanae are formed by the apposition of the sphenoid, vomer, and palatine bones. For.: foramen; Lat.: lateral; Horiz.: horizontal; Med.: medial; Orb.: orbital; Palat.: palatine; Perpend.: perpendicular; Proc.: process; Pteryg.: pterygoid; Sphen.: sphenoidal.

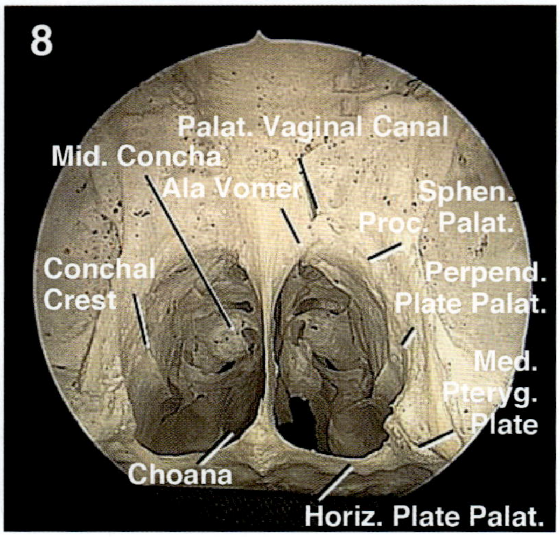

Fig. 2.8 A dry, articulated skull. Posterior endoscopic view of the choanae. Horiz.: horizontal; Med.: medial; Mid.: middle; Palat.: palatine; Perpend.: perpendicular; Proc.: process; Sphen.: sphenoidal.

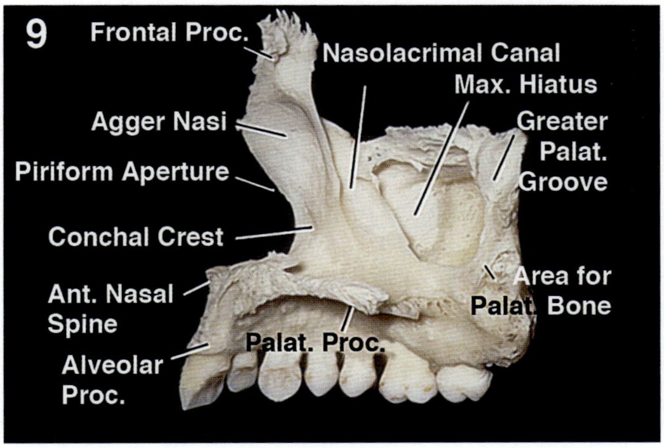

Fig. 2.9 The nasal surface of the maxillary body is responsible for most of the lateral wall of the nasal cavity. It presents the maxillary hiatus, a large opening on the posterosuperior part of the nasal surface of the maxillary body, which leads to the maxillary sinus. Inferior to the hiatus, the nasal surface contributes to the inferior meatus. Behind the hiatus, there is a rough surface for articulation with the perpendicular plate of the palatine bone. In this area, the greater palatine groove is converted into a canal by the articulation with the palatine. In front of the hiatus, a deep groove contributes to the formation of the nasolacrimal canal. The opening of the hiatus is reduced by the apposition of adjacent bones: the uncinate process of the ethmoid and descending part of the lacrimal above; the maxillary process of the inferior nasal concha below; and the perpendicular plate of palatine behind. The agger nasi, anterior to the hiatus is an elevation related to the anterior portion of the middle concha. Ant.: anterior; Max.: maxillary; Palat.: palatine; Proc.: process.

The lateral wall of the nasal cavity is formed by the nasal, maxilla, lacrimal, ethmoid, palatine, inferior nasal concha, and sphenoid bones (**Figs. 2.9, 2.10, 2.11, 2.12, 2.13, 2.14, 2.15, 2.16, 2.17, 2.18, 2.19,** and **2.20**). The nasal bone contributes with the lateral part of its inferior surface to a small anterior area of the lateral wall. The maxilla provides the inner surface of the frontal process and the nasal surface of its body, to which the inferior nasal concha attaches. The lacrimal bone, through its medial or nasal surfaces, contributes to the formation of the nasolacrimal duct and attaches to the maxilla, ethmoid, and inferior nasal concha. The medial plates of the ethmoid bone contribute to the lateral walls of the upper part of the nasal cavity. Between the medial and lateral plates, also called the laminae papyracea or orbital plate, are the ethmoid labyrinths or lateral masses, formed by ethmoidal air cells. Two or three ethmoidal conchae may project into the cavity.

The palatine bone contributes to the lateral wall with the nasal surface of its perpendicular plate. The nasal surface has two horizontal ridges—the ethmoidal and conchal crests. The ethmoidal crest is the upper ridge and articulates to the middle concha of the ethmoid bone. The conchal crest is the most inferior ridge on the nasal surface of the perpendicular plate. Together with the conchal crest of the maxilla, it gives attachment to the inferior concha. Between the ethmoidal and conchal crests, the concave area forms part of the middle meatus. Similarly, below the conchal crest, a shallow depression forms the inferior meatus of the nasal cavity. The perpendicular plate attaches between the pterygoid plate of the sphenoid and the posteromedial margin of the nasal surface of maxilla. The upper end of the perpendicular plate has two processes separated by a groove. The anteriormost process is the orbital process of the palatine bone. It attaches to the maxilla, ethmoid, and sphenoid bones and encloses an air cell that may communicate with the posterior ethmoidal air cells or the sphenoid sinus. The posteriormost process, slightly deviated medially, is the sphenoidal process. By its posterosuperior surface, the sphenoidal process articulates with the medial pterygoid plate and the undersurface of the sphenoid concha. Its medial border articulates with the ala of vomer, helping delimit the upper frame of the choana. Between these two processes is the sphenopalatine notch. With the sphenoid in place, the groove is converted into the sphenopalatine foramen and transmits the sphenopalatine vessels and posterior superior nasal nerves. It is important to note that the anterior portion of the perpendicular plate of the palatine bone projects anteriorly beyond the posterior border of the

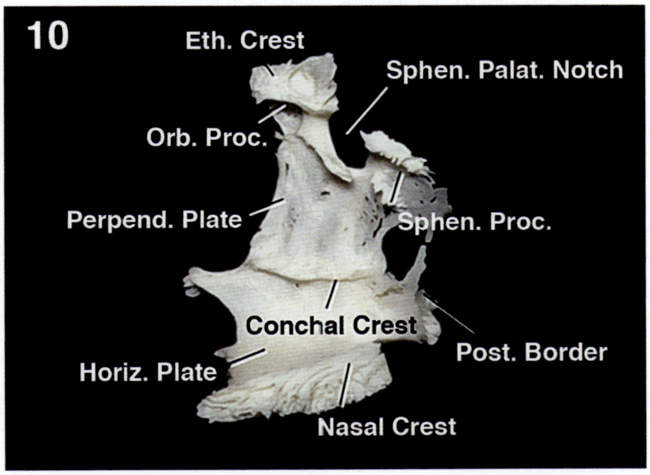

Fig. 2.10 The nasal surface of the palatine bone. The palatine bone is located at the posterior part of the nasal cavity, between the maxilla and the pterygoid process of the sphenoid. It presents horizontal and perpendicular plates. The nasal surface of the perpendicular plate presents two crests: the upper, ethmoidal crest, gives insertion to the middle nasal concha of the ethmoid, and the conchal crest gives insertion to the posterior part of the inferior nasal concha. The superior border of the perpendicular plate presents two processes, orbital and sphenoidal, separated by a deep furrow, the sphenopalatine notch. The orbital process encloses an air sinus. It has three articular and two nonarticular surfaces. It connects anteriorly with the maxilla, posteriorly with the sphenoid concha, and medially with the ethmoid. The superior non-articular surface is part of the floor of the orbit, whereas the lateral non-articular surface faces the pterygopalatine fossa. The sphenoid process is directed medially. Its superior surface connects with the sphenoid concha and the root of the medial pterygoid plate. The medial border of the sphenoid process articulates with the ala of vomer. The sphenopalatine notch is converted into a foramen by the apposition of the sphenoid bone. The foramen links the nasal cavity to the pterygopalatine fossa and transmits the sphenopalatine vessels and posterior superior nasal nerves. The posterior border of the perpendicular plate is continuous above with the sphenoid process, and articulates with the medial pterygoid plate. Eth.: ethmoid, ethmoidal; Horiz.: horizontal; Orb.: orbital; Palat.: palatine; Perpend.: perpendicular; Post.: posterior; Proc.: process; Sphen.: sphenoidal.

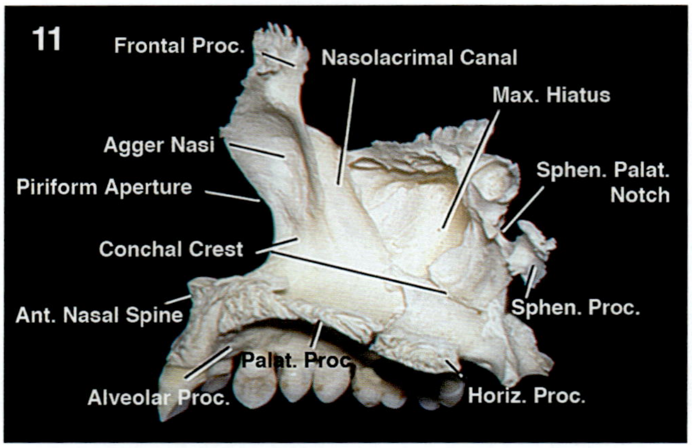

Fig. 2.11 The maxilla and palatine bone have been combined. The nasal surface of the horizontal plate of the palatine bone is concave from side to side and forms the posterior part of the floor of the nasal cavity. Its medial border forms the nasal crest for articulation with the vomer and is continuous with the nasal crest of the maxilla. The anterior border of the perpendicular plate of the palatine bone overlaps the posterior edge of the maxillary hiatus. Both conchal crests of the maxilla anteriorly and of the palatine posteriorly give attachment to the inferior nasal concha. Ant.: anterior; Horiz.: horizontal; Max.: maxillary; Palat.: palatine; Proc.: process; Sphen.: sphenoidal.

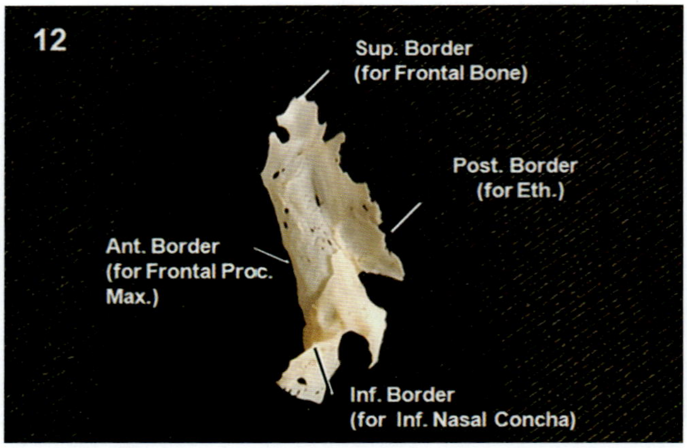

Fig. 2.12 The nasal surface of the lacrimal bone forms part of the middle meatus of the nose. Its upper and posterior part articulate with the ethmoid bone and complete some of the anterior ethmoidal cells. The anterior border articulates with the frontal process of the maxilla. Ant.: anterior; Eth.: ethmoid, ethmoidal; Inf.: inferior; Max.: maxillary; Post.: posterior; Proc.: process; Sup.: superior.

maxillary hiatus of the alveolar process of the maxilla, thus forming the posterior part of the medial wall of the maxillary sinus. The sphenoid bone contributes to the lateral wall with the most lateral part of the sphenoid concha and the medial pterygoid plate, which forms the lateral edge of the choana.

The anterior segment of the floor of the nasal cavity is formed by the maxilla and the posterior quarter by the horizontal plate of the palatine bone (**Fig. 2.11**).

The upper part of the nasal cavity is called the subfrontal space, olfactory cleft, or nasal carina,[1] and understanding its anatomy is important for approaching the anterior nasal

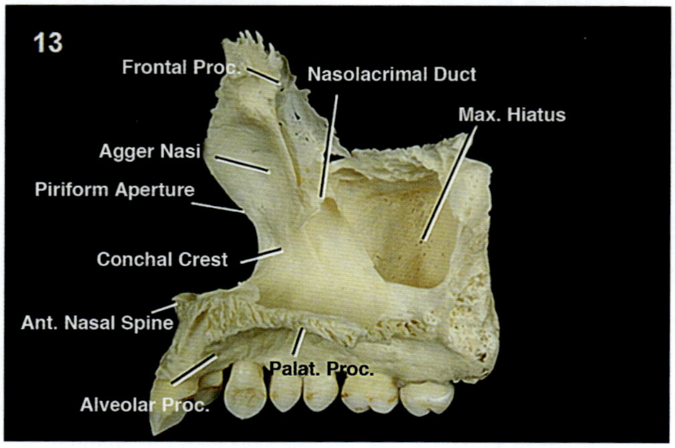

Fig. 2.13 The maxilla and lacrimal bone have been combined. The maxillary contribution to the nasolacrimal canal represents two thirds of its total circumference; the remaining one third is formed by the descending part of the lacrimal bone and lacrimal process of the inferior nasal concha. The nasolacrimal duct opens along the inferior nasal meatus. Ant.: anterior; Max.: maxillary; Palat.: palatine; Proc.: process.

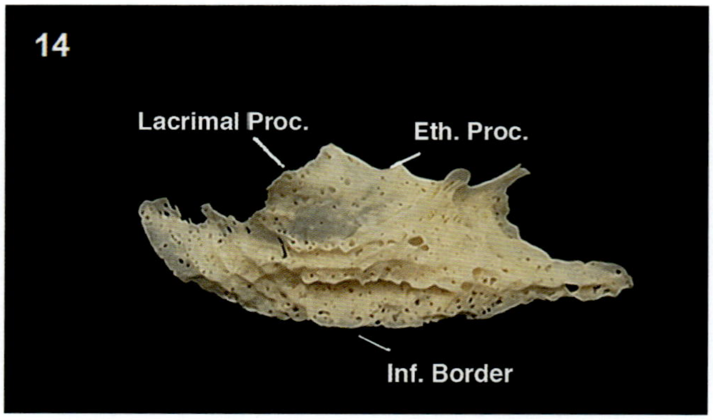

Fig. 2.14 The medial surface of the inferior nasal concha. This surface is convex and presents numerous perforations and grooves for vessels. Its superior border may be divided into three parts. The anterior part articulates with the conchal crest of the maxilla; the posterior part articulates with the conchal crest of the palatine bone; and the middle part presents three processes: lacrimal, ethmoidal, and maxillary. The lacrimal process articulates with the descending part of the lacrimal bone and edges of the nasolacrimal canal of the maxilla, helping the formation of the nasolacrimal duct. The ethmoidal process articulates with the uncinate process of the ethmoid, whereas the maxillary process forms part of the medial wall of the maxillary sinus. Eth.: ethmoid, ethmoidal; Inf.: inferior; Proc.: process.

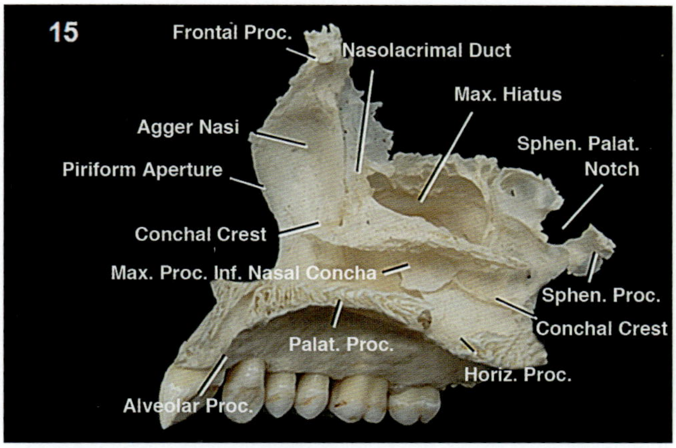

Fig. 2.15 The maxilla, palatine, lacrimal, and inferior nasal concha have been combined. The part of the body of the maxilla below the maxillary hiatus, the maxillary process of the inferior nasal concha, and the part of the perpendicular plate of palatine bone inferior to the conchal crest combine to form the inferior nasal meatus. The opening of the maxillary hiatus is reduced by the apposition of the descending part of the lacrimal concha and the maxillary process of the inferior nasal concha below and the perpendicular plate of palatine behind. Horiz.: horizontal; Inf.: inferior; Max.: maxillary; Palat.: palatine; Proc.: process; Sphen.: sphenoidal.

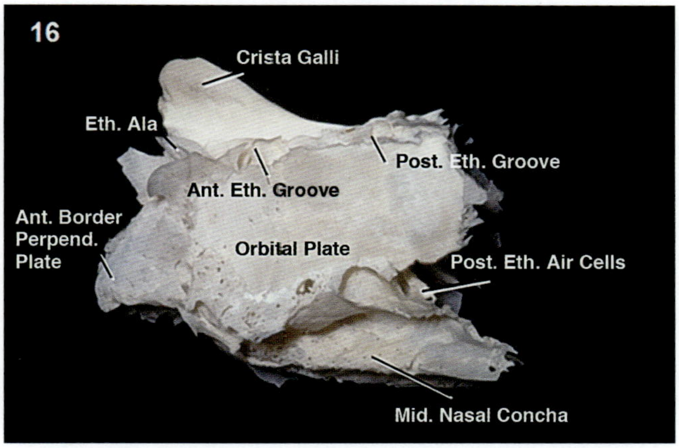

Fig. 2.16 Lateral view of the ethmoid bone. The crista galli is the thick process projecting up from the cribriform plate. Its posterior border gives attachment to the falx. Its anterior border articulates with the frontal bone by the ethmoidal alae. The anterior border of the perpendicular plate articulates with the nasal spine of the frontal bone and the crest of the nasal bones. The orbital plate of the ethmoid is the lateral vertical plate that delimits the ethmoidal air cells, forming the medial wall of orbit and covering the middle and posterior ethmoid air cells. The air cells in front of the orbital plate are completed by the lacrimal bone and the frontal process of the maxilla. The posterior surface of the ethmoidal labyrinths present large, opened air cells to be completed by the sphenoidal concha and the orbital process of the palatine bone. Ant.: anterior; Eth.: ethmoid, ethmoidal; Mid.: middle; Perpend.: perpendicular; Post.: posterior.

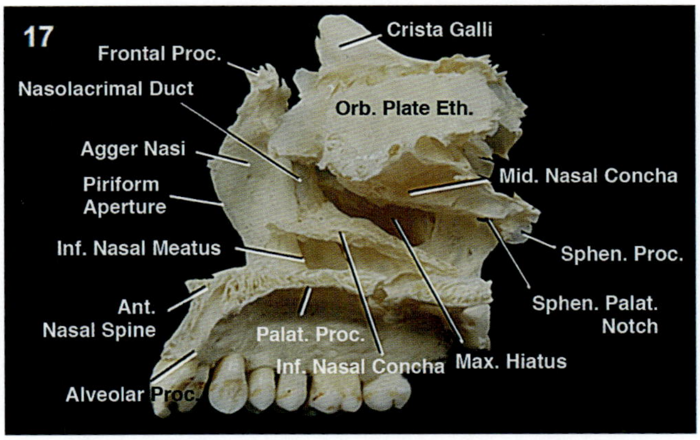

Fig. 2.17 The ethmoid has been added to the bone combination forming the lateral wall of the nasal cavity. It fits along the ethmoidal crest of the perpendicular plate of the palatine, further reducing the maxillary hiatus by the connections of the uncinate process to the maxilla, lacrimal, and inferior nasal concha. Note that the tail of the middle nasal concha is at the level of the sphenopalatine notch. This anatomical fact enables locating the sphenopalatine vessels along the lateral wall of the nasal cavity and planning for mucosal pediculated flaps. Ant.: anterior; Eth.: ethmoid, ethmoidal; Inf.: inferior; Max.: maxillary; Mid.: middle; Orb.: orbital; Palat.: palatine; Proc.: process; Sphen.: sphenoidal.

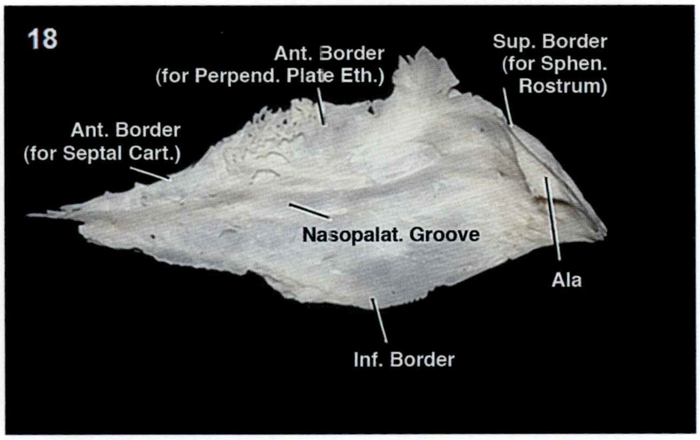

Fig. 2.18 Left lateral view of the vomer. This thin bone forms the posterior-inferior part of the nasal septum. The nasopalatine groove is the deep furrow transmitting the nasopalatine nerve and vessels. The superior border presents a deep furrow bounded by the alae, which connect to the sphenoid conchae, the sphenoidal process of the palatine, and the medial pterygoid plates, forming the superior frame of each choana. Its inferior border attaches to the nasal crest of the maxilla and palatine. The anterior border of the vomer articulates with the perpendicular plate of the ethmoid and the septal cartilage. Ant.: anterior; Cart.: cartilage; Eth.: ethmoid, ethmoidal; Inf.: inferior; Nasopalat.: nasopalatine; Perpend.: perpendicular; Sphen.: sphenoidal; Sup.: superior.

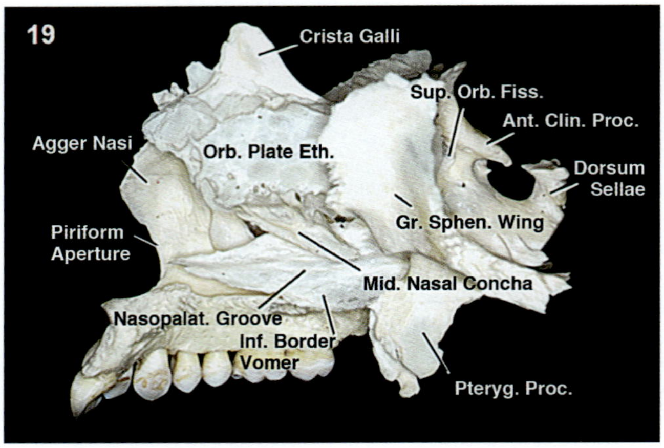

Fig. 2.19 The vomer has been added to its place inferior to the perpendicular plate of ethmoid. It attaches inferiorly to the nasal crest of the maxilla and palatine bones. Posteriorly, the vomer and ethmoid fit along the rostrum of the sphenoid. Ant.: anterior; Clin.: clinoidal; Gr.: greater; Eth.: ethmoid, ethmoidal; Inf.: inferior; Mid.: middle; Nasopalat.: nasopalatine; Orb.: orbital; Proc.: process; Pteryg.: pterygoid; Sphen.: sphenoid; Sup.: superior.

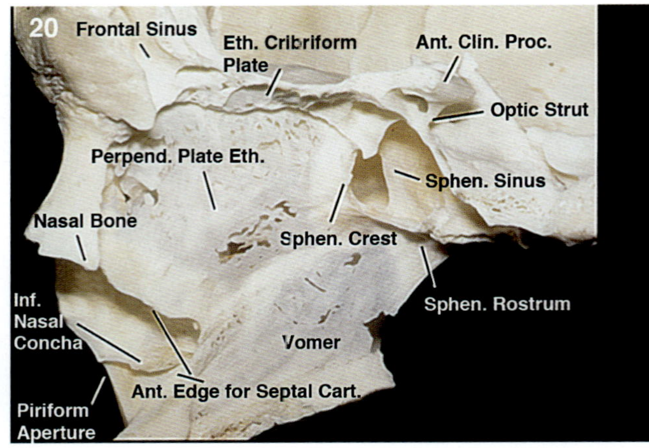

Fig. 2.20 The ethmoidal labyrinth and sphenoid concha have been removed on the left, to expose the bony nasal septum formed by the sphenoid crest, the perpendicular plate of the ethmoid, and the vomer. Ant.: anterior; Cart.: cartilage; Clin.: clinoidal; Eth.: ethmoid, ethmoidal; Inf.: inferior; Perpend.: perpendicular; Proc.: process; Sphen.: sphenoidal.

fossa, through either the transcribriform or transplanum approaches. The subfrontal space has anterior, middle, and posterior parts, named, respectively, the nasal, ethmoidal, and sphenoidal segments (**Figs. 2.21, 2.22, 2.23,** and **2.24**). The height of the nasal cavity increases from the piriform aperture to the posterior part of the nasal segment. The height is largest at the ethmoidal segment and decreases from its posterior limit to the choana. The nasal spine of the frontal bone and the nasal bones form the roof of the nasal part. The average distance between the posterior wall of the frontal sinus and the anterior edge of the cribriform plate in adults is 12.7 mm.[1] The ethmoidal segment presents the ethmoidal and cribroethmoidal foramina. The average length of the cribriform plate on the endocranial side is 20.8 mm, whereas its exocranial surface, facing the nasal cavity, averages 24.7 mm.[1] The sphenoethmoidal recess is on the posterior segment. The

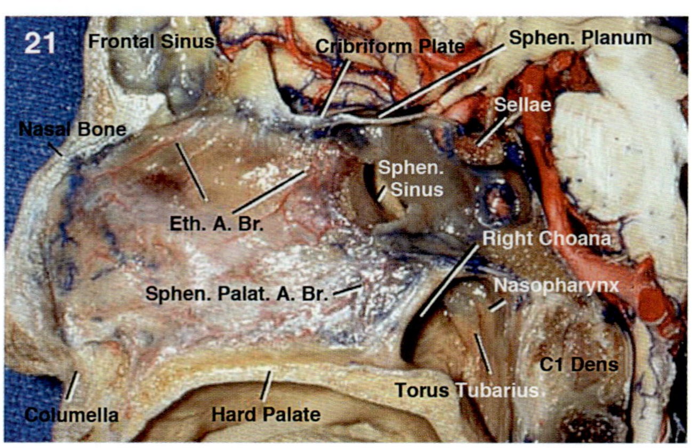

Fig. 2.21 Stepwise dissection of the nasal cavity from the midline to its lateral limit on the right side. The nasal septum has a membranous part at the columella, a cartilaginous part overlying the septal cartilage, and a bony part superoposteriorly. The bones and cartilages of the nasal septum are covered by a layer of periosteum and perichondrium, over which lie the submucosa and the mucosa of the nasal cavity and vestibule. The nasal septum and its mucosal covering vary from 5 to 13 mm in thickness. The supply for the septal mucosa derives mainly from branches of the anterior and posterior ethmoidal arteries and the septal branches of the sphenopalatine artery. A.: artery; Br.: branch, branches; C1: first cervical vertabra; Eth.: ethmoid, ethmoidal; Palat.: palatine; Sphen.: sphenoidal.

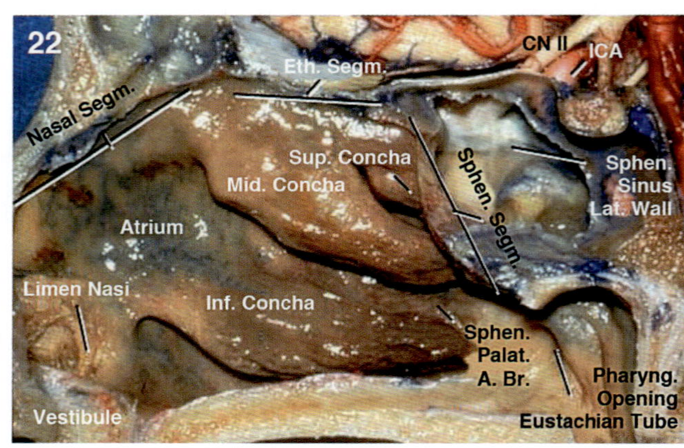

Fig. 2.22 The septum has been removed. The upper part of the nasal cavity is called the subfrontal space, which has anterior, middle, and posterior parts named, respectively, the nasal, ethmoidal, and sphenoidal segments. The height of the nasal cavity increases from the piriform aperture to the posterior part of the nasal segment. The height is largest at the ethmoidal segment and decreases from its posterior limit to the choana. The nasal spine of the frontal bone and the nasal bones form the roof of the nasal part. The limen nasi is the prominence on the lateral wall of the nasal cavity produced by the overlap between the nasal cartilages, and marks the transition between the vestibule and the nasal cavity proper. On the face, the limen nasi corresponds to the alar sulcus. The medial wall of the nasal vestibule is formed by the mobile septum, the columella. A.: artery; Br.: branch; CN: cranial nerve; Eth.: ethmoid, ethmoidal; ICA, internal carotid artery; Lat.: lateral; Mid.: middle; Palat.: palatine; Pharyng.: pharyngeal; Segm.: segment; Sphen.: sphenoidal.

average length of the planum sphenoidale up to the tuberculum sellae is 20.9 mm.[1]

The nasal septum has a membranous part at the columella, a cartilaginous part overlying the septal cartilage, and a bony part formed by the perpendicular plate of the ethmoid and vomer, attached superoposteriorly to the sphenoid crest and rostrum. The bones and cartilages of the nasal septum are covered by a layer of periosteum and perichondrium, over which lie the submucosa and the mucosa of the nasal cavity and vestibule. The nasal septum and its mucosal covering vary from 5 to 13 mm in thickness. The surface area of the septum measures 30 to 35 cm.[1] It is not uncommon that the nasal septum is deviated, frequently to the left side. When the septum is deviated, the middle concha on the concave side undergoes compensatory growth. In rare instances, the nasal septum can be pneumatized. It might happen in combination with pneumatization of the crista galli, through the frontal sinus, or by extension of the sphenoid sinus. Several pediculated flaps of nasal mucosa can be tailored to close skull base defects (**Figs. 2.25, 2.26, 2.27, 2.28, 2.29,** and **2.30**). Successfully constructing a pediculated mucosal flap relies heavily on the anatomical understanding of the vascularization of nasal cavity.

The sphenopalatine artery is the main vessel supplying the nasal mucosa. This artery arises in the pterygopalatine fossa from the maxillary artery and divides either proximal to or within the sphenopalatine foramen. It gives off the posterior lateral nasal, nasoseptal, vidian, and descending palatine arteries. The descending palatine gives off branches to the lateral wall of the nasal cavity that end up as the greater and lesser palatine arteries. On the conchae the vessels are usually embedded into deep grooves (**Fig. 2.14**), sometimes bridged by bony bars. The anterior and posterior ethmoidal arteries supply the septum, the lateral wall, and the upper part of the nasal cavity. Several arterial anastomoses are present along the nasal and septal mucosa. They include the branches of the sphenopalatine, ethmoidal, and facial arteries.

Veins draining the nasal cavity and sinuses are important pathways in the spreading of disease in this area. Arising from the dense venous network of the mucosa, the main drainage follows the arteries. The sphenopalatine vein drains toward the pterygoid venous plexus; the ethmoidal veins drain to veins of the orbit, anterior fossa, and superior sagittal sinus. The external nasal plexus drains toward the nares, to the tributaries of the facial vein, and the greater palatine veins drain toward the palatal veins.

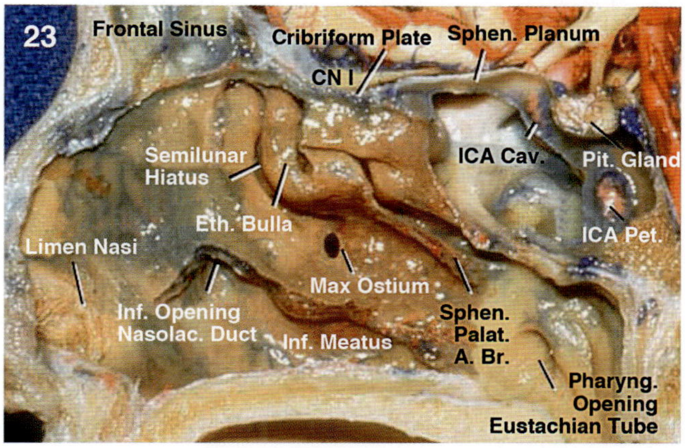

Fig. 2.23 The inferior and middle conchae have been resected, exposing the corresponding meatus. The middle meatus is limited superiorly by the attachment of the medial nasal concha, inferiorly by the attachment of the inferior nasal concha, and laterally by the lateral surface of the middle concha. The frontal, anterior, and middle ethmoidal cells and maxillary sinus open into this meatus. The middle concha is part of the ethmoid bone, attached to the skull base at the lateral limit of the cribriform plate. Posterolaterally it attaches to the lateral wall of the nasal cavity by the conchal crest. The sphenopalatine foramen is located close to the posterior attachment of the middle concha. The uncinate process of the ethmoid bone is a thin, curved bone projecting inferoposteriorly from the middle segment of the middle nasal concha. It unites with the maxilla superiorly and the inferior nasal concha inferiorly. This process is the continuation of the agger nasi, limits the semilunar hiatus inferomedially, and is inferior to the ethmoidal bullae—a rounded swelling produced by the middle ethmoidal air cells on the lateral wall of the middle meatus. Due to the variations of the connection of the uncinate process and neighboring bones, it is common to find defects on the medial wall of the maxillary sinus (fonticuli). When these defects are not covered by mucosa, they form the accessory ostia of the maxillary sinus and are more common posteroinferior to the main ostium. The ethmoidal infundibulum is the recess of the middle meatus located in front of the ethmoidal bulla. The duct of the frontal sinus, the anterosuperior ethmoidal cells, and the lacrimal, agger, frontal, and nasal cells may open through the infundibulum. The inferior meatus is deepest at the junction of its anterior and middle third, where the inferior opening of the nasolacrimal canal is located. Above the superior concha, the sphenoid sinus opens into the sphenoethmoidal recess. A.: artery; Br.: branch; Cav.: cavernous; CN: cranial nerve; Eth.: ethmoid, ethmoidal; ICA: internal carotid artery; Inf.: inferior; Max.: maxillary; Palat.: palatine; Pet.: petrous, petrosal; Pharyng.: pharyngeal; Pit.: pituitary; Sphen.: sphenoidal.

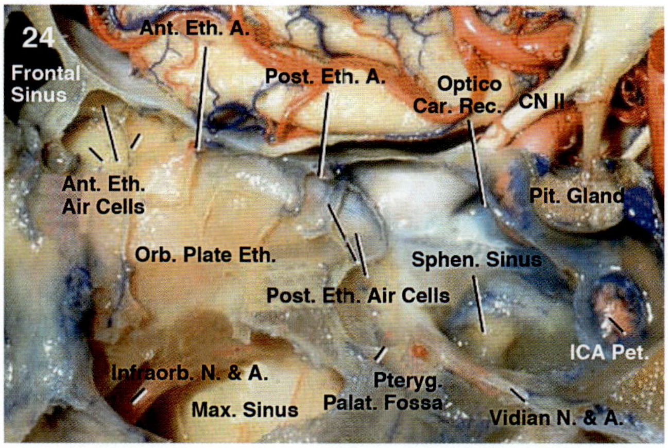

Fig. 2.24 The ethmoidal labyrinth has been resected, exposing the lateral wall of the nasal cavity, which separates from the orbit through the orbital plate. The anterior and posterior ethmoidal canals transmit the ethmoidal arteries and vessels. The anterior ethmoidal canal is located approximately at the midpoint between the nasion and the optic canal. It is located approximately 24 mm posterior to the nasion and 12 to 14 mm in front of the posterior canal. The posterior ethmoidal cells may bulge toward the anterior wall of the sphenoid sinus. The vidian canal runs along the floor of the sphenoid sinus. It transmits the vidian nerve and vessels. Following the vidian canal posteriorly leads to the location of the petrous carotid. A.: artery; Ant.: anterior; Car.: carotid; CN: cranial nerve; Eth.: ethmoid, ethmoidal; ICA: internal carotid artery; Infraorb.: infraorbital; Max.: maxillary; N.: nerve; Orb.: orbital; Palat.: palatine; Pet.: petrous, petrosal; Pit.: pituitary; Post.: posterior; Pteryg.: pterygoid; Rec.: recess; Sphen.: sphenoidal.

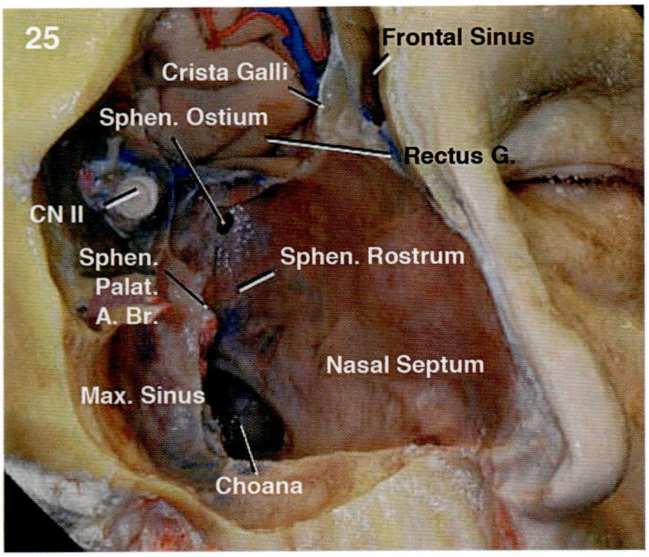

Fig. 2.25 Several pediculated flaps of mucoperiosteal and mucoperichondrium tissue can be harvested from the concha, palate, and septum, and are alternatives in closing skull base defects. A stepwise microsurgical and endoscopic dissection of the pediculated septal flap has been undertaken to clarify the steps in this procedure. During this anatomical dissection the ethmoidal labyrinth, orbital contents, and walls of the maxillary sinus have been resected to provide for extreme visualization. A.: artery; Br.: branch; CN: cranial nerve; G.: gyrus; Max.: maxillary; Palat.: palatine; Sphen.: spheno, sphenoid, sphenoidal.

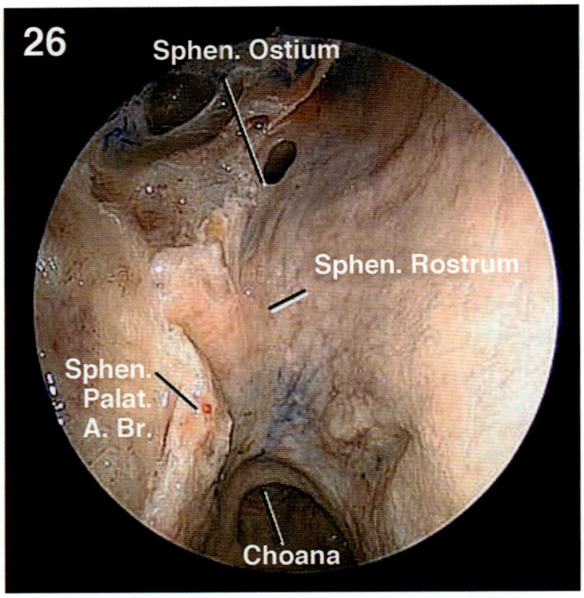

Fig. 2.26 Using the endoscope, only outfractures of the inferior and middle conchae are needed to enable visualization of the nasal septum from the cribriform plate to the nasal floor. A.: artery; Br.: branch; Palat.: palatine; Sphen.: spheno, sphenoid, sphenoidal.

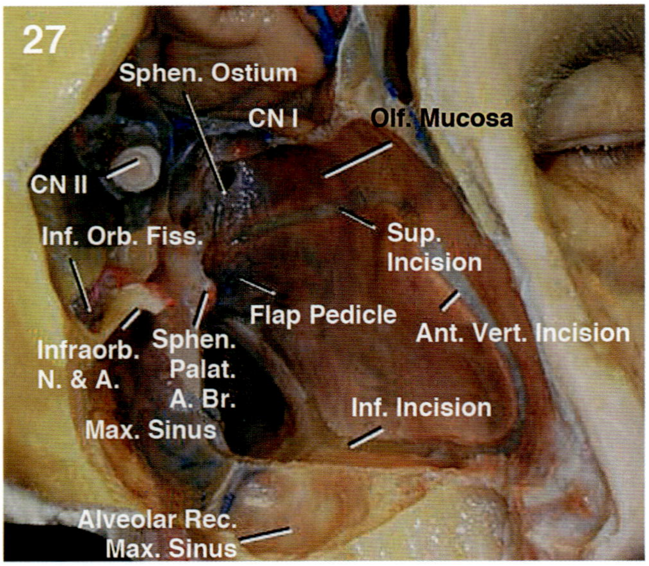

Fig. 2.27 For septal flap construction, the superior incision is parallel to the cribriform plate and located 2 cm below the superior attachment of the septum, to preserve the olfactory mucosa. The inferior incision, parallel to the nasal crest, is linked to the superior one by a vertical, anterior incision. A.: artery; Ant.: anterior; Br.: branch; CN: cranial nerve; Fiss.: fissure; Inf.: inferior; Infraorb.: infraorbital; Max.: maxillary; N.: nerve; Olf.: olfactory; Orb.: orbital; Palat.: palatine; Rec.: recess; Sphen.: sphenoidal; Sup.: superior; Vert.: vertical.

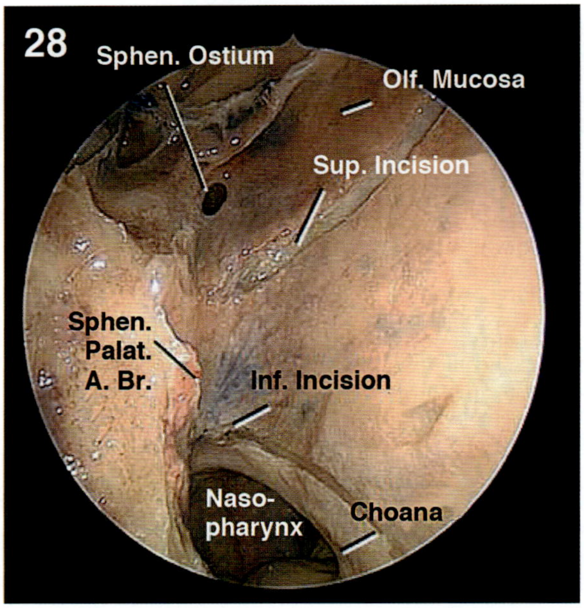

Fig. 2.28 Posteriorly, the upper incision should slant laterally along the sphenoid rostrum, close to the ostium, whereas the inferior incision follows closely the posterior edge of the septum and upper margin of the choana, below the floor of the sphenoid sinus, to preserve the posterolateral neurovascular pedicle passing through the sphenopalatine canal. All incisions should be completed before elevation of the flap. A.: artery; Br.: branch; Inf.: inferior; Olf.: olfactory; Palat.: palatine; Sphen.: spheno, sphenoid, sphenoidal; Sup.: superior.

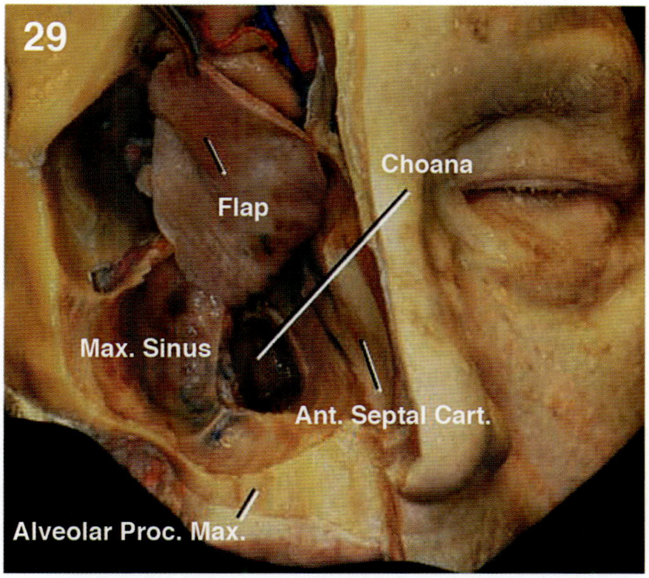

Fig. 2.29 Elevation of the septal flap starts anteriorly. Multiple modifications of the flap length and width are possible, including extension of the inferior incision to the floor of the nasal cavity and, in selected cases, bilateral harvesting. Ant.: anterior; Cart.: cartilage; Max.: maxillary; Proc.: process.

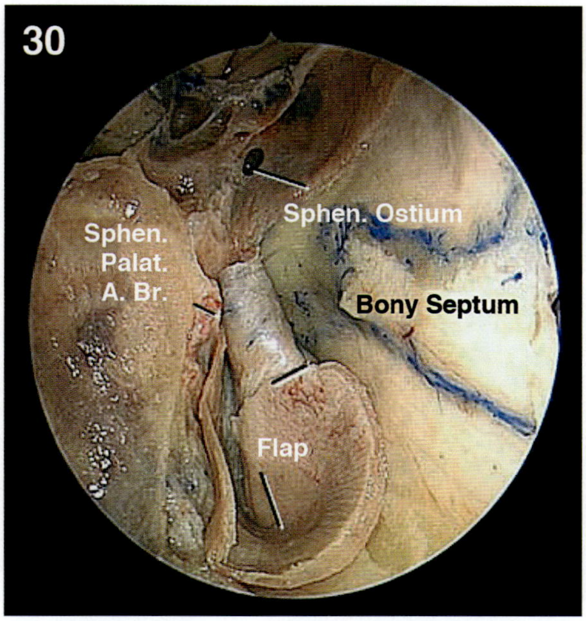

Fig. 2.30 Once harvested, the flap can be stored into the nasopharynx until the moment of closure. A.: artery; Br.: branch; Palat.: palatine; Sphen.: spheno, sphenoid, sphenoidal.

Anatomy of the Paranasal Sinuses

Ethmoidal Sinuses

The ethmoidal air cells are classically grouped into anterior, middle, and posterior cells (**Figs. 2.31, 2.32, 2.33,** and **2.34**). The anterior cells may project into the agger nasi (agger cells), toward the nasal and lacrimal bones (nasal cells and lacrimal cells, ethmolacrimal recess, or terminal cells), or the frontal cavity (frontal bulla), and open to the middle meatus through the ethmoidal infundibulum. The middle cells, in most cases, pneumatize the ethmoidal bulla. Posterosuperior ethmoidal cells can grow into the body of the sphenoid and display varying degrees of development (Onodi's cells). The posterosuperior ethmoidal cells may surround the optic canal in as many as 25% of cases[1] and reach the anterior wall of sella. The ethmoidal sinuses are supplied by branches of the ethmoidal arteries and posterior lateral branches of the sphenopalatine arteries.

Frontal Sinus

The frontal sinus arises by growth of the frontal recess or extension of its cells into the frontal bone; thus, it is considered to be derived from the ethmoidal infundibulum. The growth of this sinus starts in infancy and peaks through adolescence, being usually more prominent in males.

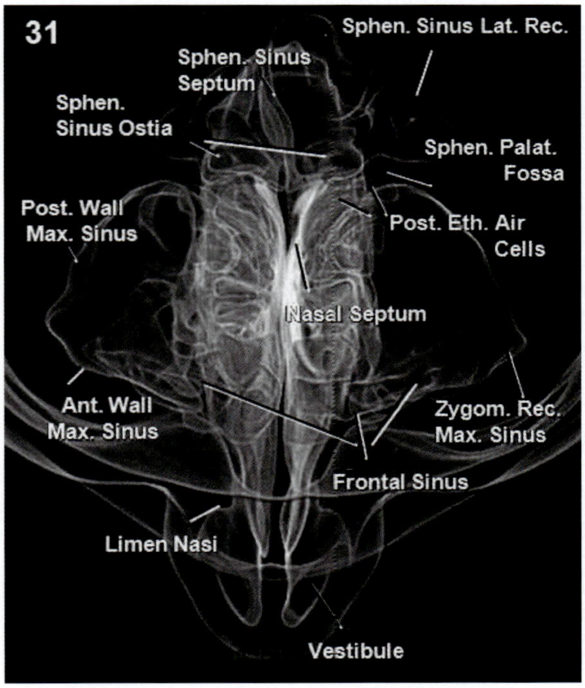

Fig. 2.31 Virtual three-dimensional (3D) radiologic reconstruction of the nasal cavity and adjacent compartments. Superior view. Ant.: anterior; Eth.: ethmoid, ethmoidal; Lat.: lateral; Max.: maxillary; Palat.: palatine; Post.: posterior; Rec.: recess; Sphen.: sphenoidal; Zygom.: Zygomatic.

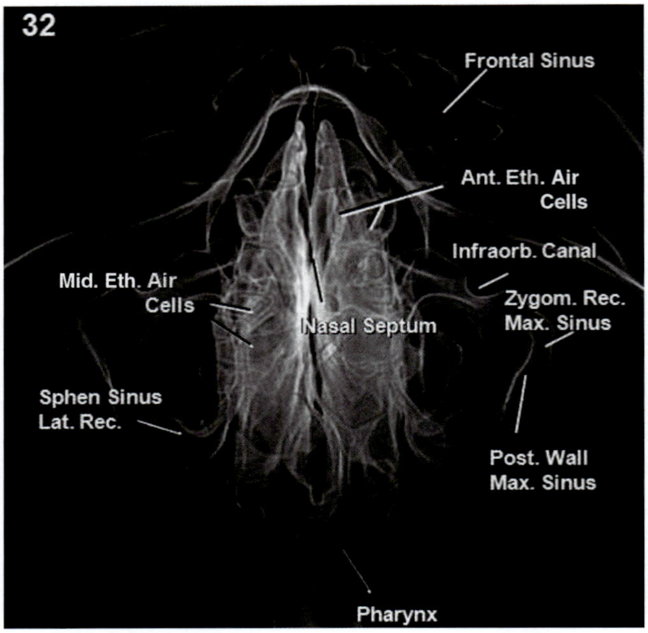

Fig. 2.32 Inferior view. Ant.: anterior; Eth.: ethmoid, ethmoidal; Infraorb.: infraorbital; Lat.: lateral; Max.: maxillary; Mid.: middle; Post.: posterior; Rec.: recess; Sphen.: sphenoidal; Zygom.: zygomatic.

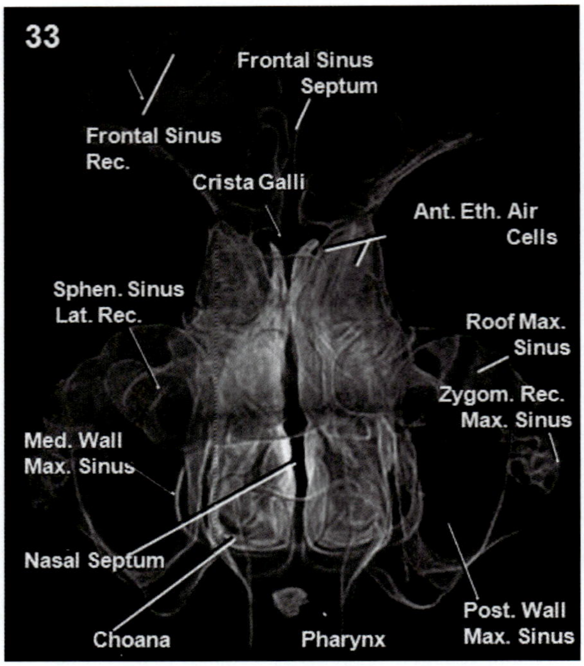

Fig. 2.33 Posterior view. Ant.: anterior; Eth.: ethmoid, ethmoidal; Lat.: lateral; Max.: maxi lary; Med.: medial; Post.: posterior; Rec.: recess; Zygom.: zygomatic.

The frontal cavity may be drained by an ostium or an infundibulum into the anterior part of semilunar hiatus in most cases. In one third of cases in which the frontal sinus drains outside the hiatus, its opening is usually anterior to the hiatus. The pneumatization of this sinus is variable. It may be aplastic, even bilaterally, or occupy almost completely the squamous and orbital parts of the frontal bone. If the orbital parts of the frontal bone are heavily pneumatized, a double floor of the orbit might be found. In some cases, the anterior edge of the olfactory fossa may protrude forward into the sinus, creating the potential for the inadvertent opening of the anterior skull base during frontal sinus procedures. The frontal sinus is supplied by the anterior falcine, supraorbital, and supratrochlear arteries.

Maxillary Sinus

The maxillary sinus is a pyramidal cavity in the body of the maxilla. Its walls correspond to the orbit (roof), alveolar (floor), and facial (anterior) and infratemporal (posterior) aspects of the maxilla (**Figs. 2.2** and **2.3**). Its apex points laterally and extends into the zygomatic process, as the zygomatic recess. The base is the lateral wall of the nasal cavity below the middle meatus and presents the maxillary hiatus (**Fig. 2.32**). The hiatus is partially closed by the inferior concha and the uncinate process of the ethmoid (**Figs. 2.2** and **2.17**), forming the ostium and a variable number of fonticuli. Through the ostium pass the posterior lateral nasal branches of the sphenopalatine artery, which provide supply for the sinus (**Figs. 2.24** and **2.25**). The medial wall may present the prelacrimal recess, which extends anterior to the nasolacrimal duct.

The alveolar canals transmit the posterior superior alveolar nerves to the molar teeth and can protrude on the posterior wall of the sinus. The posterior superior alveolar arteries take part in the supply of bone and mucosa of the maxillary sinus. Two or three branches may pierce the posterior wall of the sinus.

The roof presents the infraorbital canal for the infraorbital nerve and vessels (**Figs. 2.2, 2.24,** and **2.32**). The infraorbital vessels take part in the supply of this sinus. An infraorbital recess may project anteriorly, around the infraorbital canal.

The floor of the sinus is formed by the alveolar process and, with age, it may sink to the level of or below the nasal floor (**Fig. 2.34**). The lower the floor of the sinus, the higher the proximity of the alveoli and teeth roots, which may perforate the floor. The floor may present the alveolar or anterior recess (**Fig. 2.1**) and the palatine recess. The palatine recess may extend toward the hard palate, occasionally a few millimeters of the median sagittal plane.

The anterior wall of the sinus forms the anterior surface of the body of the maxilla and faces the oral vestibule (**Fig. 2.5**). The maxillary sinus may be incompletely divided by septa. Itis supplied by branches of the sphenopalatine, infraorbital, and posterior superior alveolar arteries.

Being on each side of the nasal cavity, the maxillary sinuses expand the concept of a natural pathway (**Figs. 2.31, 2.32,** and **2.33**) and can be used endoscopically to reach the contents of the orbit, pterygopalatine and infratemporal fossae, and cavernous sinus.

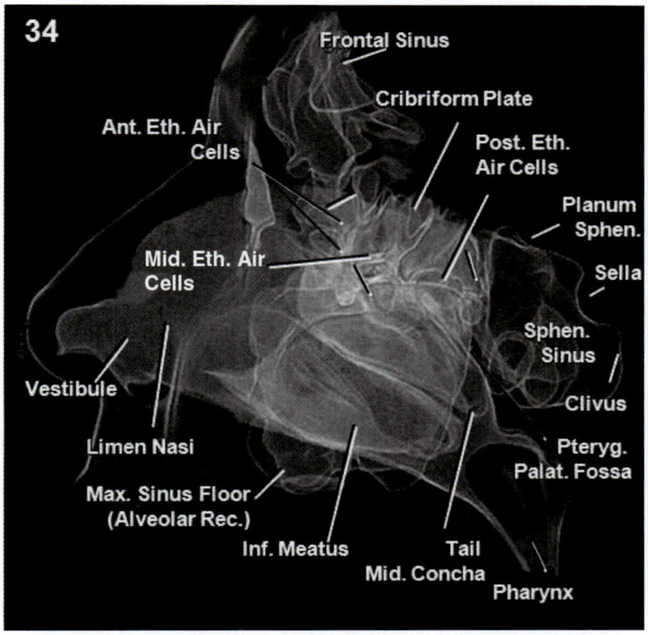

Fig. 2.34 Lateral view. The ethmoidal air cells are classically grouped into anterior, middle, and posterior cells. The frontal sinuses lie between the outer and inner layers of the frontal bone. The anterior wall of the sinus is two times thicker than the posterior wall. The floor of this cavity usually extends a little below the nasion. The frontal sinuses are frequently asymmetric, with incomplete septa producing several communicating recesses. The maxillary sinus is a pyramidal cavity in the body of the maxilla. Its walls correspond to the orbit (roof), alveolar (floor), facial (anterior), and infratemporal (posterior) aspects of the maxilla. Its apex points laterally and extends into the zygomatic process as the zygomatic recess. The anterior part of the floor can extend inferiorly as the alveolar recess. The base of this pyramidal cavity is the medial wall of the sinus, which corresponds to the lateral wall of the nasal cavity and presents the maxillary hiatus. Being on each side of the nasal cavity, the maxillary sinuses expand the concept of a natural pathway and can be used endoscopically to reach the contents of the orbit, pterygopalatine and infratemporal fossa, and ipsi- and contralateral cavernous sinus. The sphenoid sinus has an anterior wall, which faces the sphenoethmoidal recess and the posterior ethmoidal air cells; a floor, which is the roof of the nasopharynx; two lateral walls, facing the cavernous sinus, apex of orbit, and temporal fossae; a roof, formed mostly by sphenoidal planum and a posterior wall, which can be divided into an upper part, the sella, and an inferior part, the clivus. The nasopharynx is the space behind the choana, below the floor of the sphenoid sinus, and between the medial pterygoid plates. Its posterior wall is formed by the inferior clivus, the anterior rim of foramen magnum, and the C1-C2 joint. Ant.: anterior; Eth.: ethmoid, ethmoidal; Inf.: inferior; Max.: maxillary; Mid.: middle; Palat.: palatine; Post.: posterior; Pteryg.: pterygoid; Rec.: recess; Sphen.: sphenoidal.

Sphenoid Sinus

In adults, the sphenoid sinus separates the cavernous sinuses, the cavernous segments of the carotid arteries, and the optic, extraocular, and trigeminal nerves. In addition, it separates the pituitary gland from the nasal cavity (**Figs. 2.35, 2.36, 2.37, 2.38, 2.39, 2.40, 2.41, 2.42, 2.43, 2.44, 2.45, 2.46, 2.47,** and **2.48**).

At birth the sphenoid sinus presents as minute cavities within the body of the sphenoid. Its main development takes place at puberty. In early life it extends back to the presellar area and subsequently invades the area below and behind the sella turcica, reaching its full size in adolescence. Based on the degree of pneumatization, the sphenoid sinus can be classified into three types—conchal, presellar, and sellar. In the conchal type, the area below the sellae is a solid block of bone, without an air cavity, or it does not extend further from the sphenoid conchae. It is most common in children before age 12. The presellar type comprises an air cavity that goes no further posteriorly than a plane perpendicular to the sellar wall and occurs in about 11 to 24% of specimens.[2] The sellar type of sphenoid sinus is the most common, occurring in as many as 76 to 86% of cases. It comprises an air cavity that extends into the body of the sphenoid below the sella and as far posteriorly as the clivus.

Extensive pneumatization of the sphenoid sinus may produce several recesses that help delineate adjacent structures on the walls of the sinus during surgery or even provide for

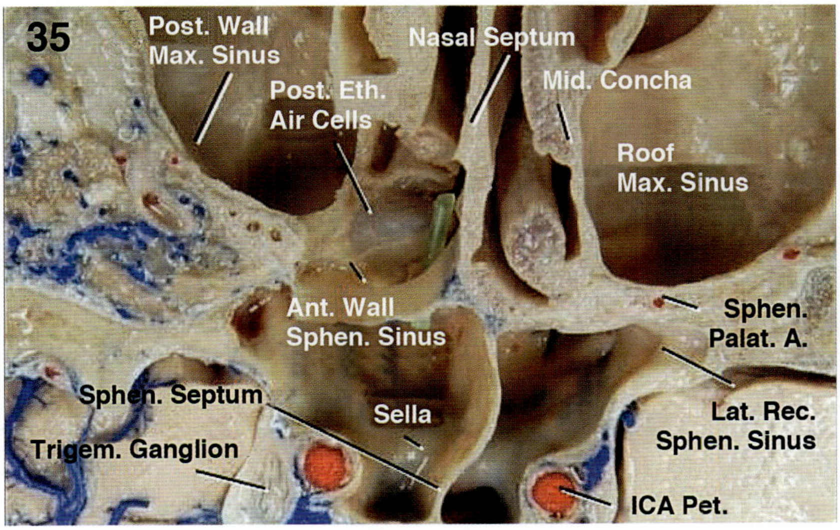

Fig. 2.35 An oblique, axial cut has been performed at the level of the nasal cavity and sphenoid sinus. The view from inferior into the upper part of the specimen exposes the roofs of the maxillary and sphenoidal sinuses and the nasal cavity above middle concha. The posterior part of the middle and superior concha on the right has been removed to expose the anterior wall of the sphenoid sinus. In this specimen, the sphenoid septum is a single, S-shaped structure, completely dividing the sinus into two cavities. A.: artery; Ant.: anterior; Eth.: ethmoid, ethmoidal; ICA: internal carotid artery; Lat.: lateral; Max.: maxillary; Mid.: middle; Palat.: palatine; Pet.: petrous, petrosal; Post.: posterior; Rec.: recess; Sphen.: sphenoidal; Trigem.: trigeminal.

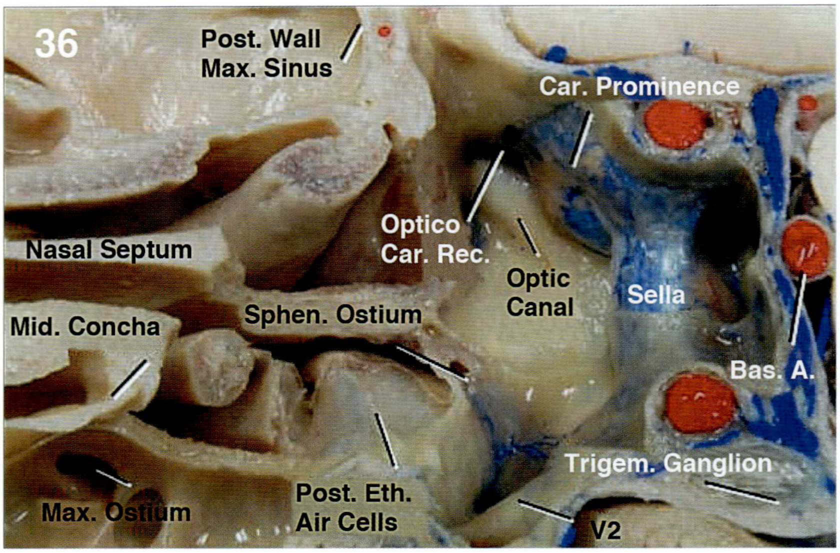

Fig. 2.36 View of the upper part of the specimen, after removal of the posterior nasal septum, sphenoid septum, and bone covering part of the sella and upper lateral wall of the sphenoid sinus. The trigeminal nerves, carotid artery, and optic canals can bulge along the lateral wall of the sphenoid sinus. A.: artery; Bas.: basilar; Car.: carotid; Eth.: ethmoid, ethmoidal; Max.: maxillary; Mid.: middle; Post.: posterior; Rec.: recess; Trigem.: trigeminal; V2: second division trigeminal nerve.

routes of access to specific areas. The sphenoidal recesses may be divided into anterior, lateral, and posterior groups.

As the sinus enlarges laterally, it may extend close to the optic canals or may even partially encircle these structures as the supra- and infraoptic recesses. The infraoptic recess located between the optic nerve and carotid artery, along the optic strut and anterior clinoid process, is the opticocarotid recess (**Fig. 2.24**). This recess is particularly helpful during surgery to locate the segments of the carotid artery inside the sphenoid sinus. The upper edge of the recess marks the position of the upper carotid ring. The lower edge marks the position of the lower carotid ring, and the carotid segment between these two areas is the clinoidal carotid (see Chapter 22, Fig. 22.6). The lateral recess extends along the greater sphenoid wing, usually below the maxillary division and lateral to the petrous carotid. As age advances, the sinus frequently undergoes further enlargement associated with absorption of its bony walls. It is not infrequent that there are gaps in the sphenoid sinus bony walls, causing the mucous membrane to lie directly against the dura mater.

When the sinus is exceptionally large inferiorly, the floor may be lower than the level of the vidian (pterygoid) canal (see Chapter 22, Fig. 22.7). In these cases the canal stands out or even may be dehiscent along the sellar floor (**Figs. 2.41, 2.42, 2.43, 2.44, 2.45, 2.46, 2.47,** and **2.48**). The sphenoid sinus may also extend into the roots of the pterygoid processes (pterygoid recess).

When the pneumatization extends posteriorly toward the clivus, it may invade the dorsum sellae (posterosuperior recess) (**Figs. 2.37** and **2.38**) or the basal part of the occipital bone (posteroinferior recess) as far as the basion.

Anterior extensions of the sphenoid sinus include septal recess (sphenovomerine bulla) and superior and inferior ethmoidal recesses. Anterior pneumatization of the sphenoid

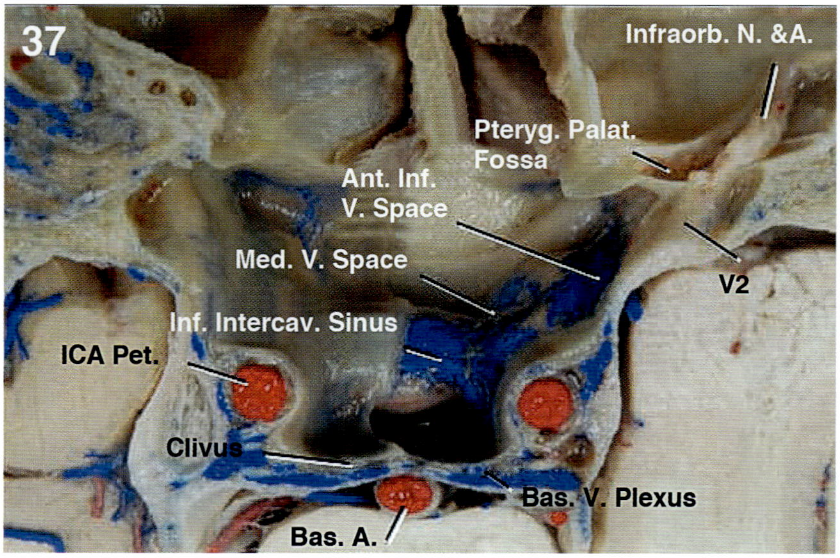

Fig. 2.37 The dura on the left half of the sella and the lateral wall of sphenoid sinus has been removed, exposing the inferior intercavernous sinus and the medial and anteroinferior venous compartments of the cavernous sinus. Transsellar connections between the cavernous sinuses may exist at any point from the anterior to the posterior mwall of the sella, including the diaphragma, or all connections may be absent. The largest and most constant intercavernous connection is the basilar venous plexus, passing posterior to the dorsum and upper clivus and connecting the posterior aspect of both cavernous sinuses. The maxillary division has been exposed along the lateral wall of the sinus. Into the pterygopalatine fossa the maxillary division sends ganglionic rami to the pterygopalatine ganglion. The largest part of the maxillary division originates the infraorbital nerve, which enters the infraorbital canal on the roof of the maxillary sinus. A.: artery; Ant.: anterior; Bas.: basilar; ICA: internal carotid artery; Inf.: inferior; Infraorb.: infraorbital; Intercav.: intercavernous; Med.: medial; N.: nerve; Palat.: palatine; Pet.: petrous, petrosal; Pteryg.: pterygoid; V.: vein; V2: second division trigeminal nerve.

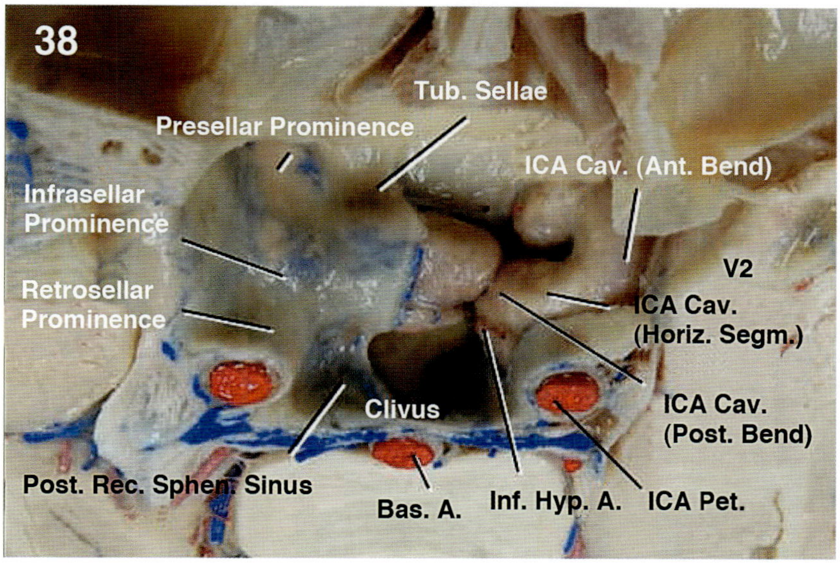

Fig. 2.38 The dura and venous structures have been removed, exposing the relationship of the carotid and pituitary gland. The infrasellar segment of the carotid prominence is located below the sellar floor and comprises the horizontal portion of the cavernous carotid. The presellar segment is located beside the anterior sinus wall and is the most frequently identified prominence related to the carotid inside the sphenoid sinus. It comprises the anterior carotid bend and the clinoidal segment of the carotid artery. The bone separating the artery and the sphenoid sinus is thinnest along the presellar part just below the tuberculum sellae. The retrosellar segment is seen on the posterolateral part of sinuses in which the pneumatization extended laterally, in the area of the dorsum. The retrosellar segment comprises the transition part between the distal petrous and the proximal cavernous carotid and is bound in place laterally by the petrolingual ligament. The posterior genu of the cavernous carotid is the origin of the inferior hypophyseal artery, which runs medially toward the posterior hypophyseal lobe and dura over the posterior part of sellar floor and anastomoses with its mate from the contralateral side. A.: artery; Ant.: anterior; Bas.: basilar; Cav.: cavernous; Horiz.: horizontal; Hyp.: hypophyseal; Inf.: inferior; Pet.: petrous, petrosal; Post.: posterior; Rec.: recess; Segm.: segment; Sphen.: sphenoid; Tub.: tuberculum; V2: second division trigeminal nerve.

sinus may put its wall in contact with the posterior part of the maxillary sinus (**Figs. 2.31, 2.35,** and **2.44**).

The cavities within the sphenoid sinus are seldom symmetrical and frequently are divided by small septa, which are usually off midline. Even when a single major septum divides the sinus (48% of cases), it is often deflected to one side.[2] It is not infrequent that paramedial sphenoid septa are linked to the carotid prominence inside the lateral walls of the sinus (**Figs. 2.43** and **2.44**).

The sphenoid sinus has an anterior wall, a floor, two lateral walls, a roof, and a posterior wall.

The anterior wall of the sphenoid sinus comprises the sphenoidal concha, ostium, and rostrum, and presents the sphenoidal crest (**Figs. 2.7** and **2.35**). The sphenoidal crest

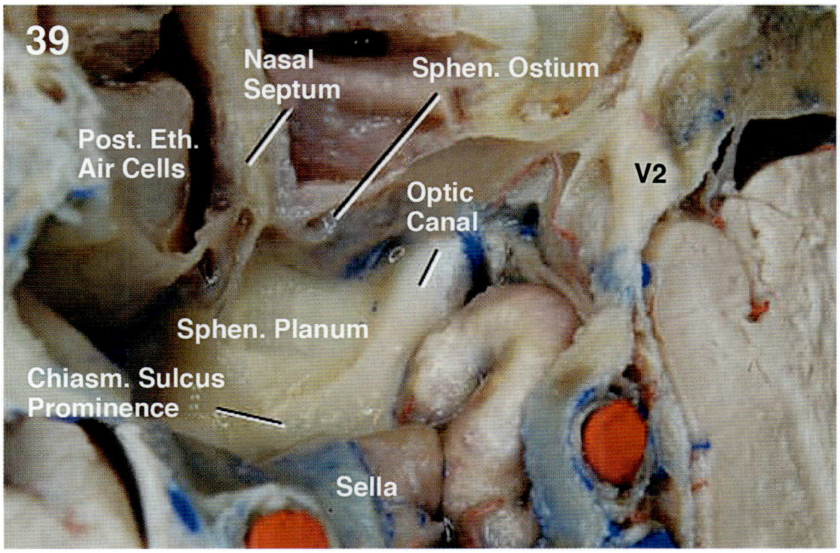

Fig. 2.39 The roof of the sphenoid sinus extends from the anterior wall to the level of the optic canals. It comprises the planum sphenoidale, the prominence of the chiasmatic sulcus, and the tuberculum sellae, below which is the sella. The sella occupies the upper part of the posterior wall of the sinus. The anterolateral parts of the roof can be occupied by the posterior ethmoidal air cells, which can surround the optic canal and reach the anterior wall of sella. Chiasm.: chiasmatic; Eth.: ethmoid, ethmoidal; Post.: posterior; Sphen.: sphenoidal; V2: second division trigeminal nerve.

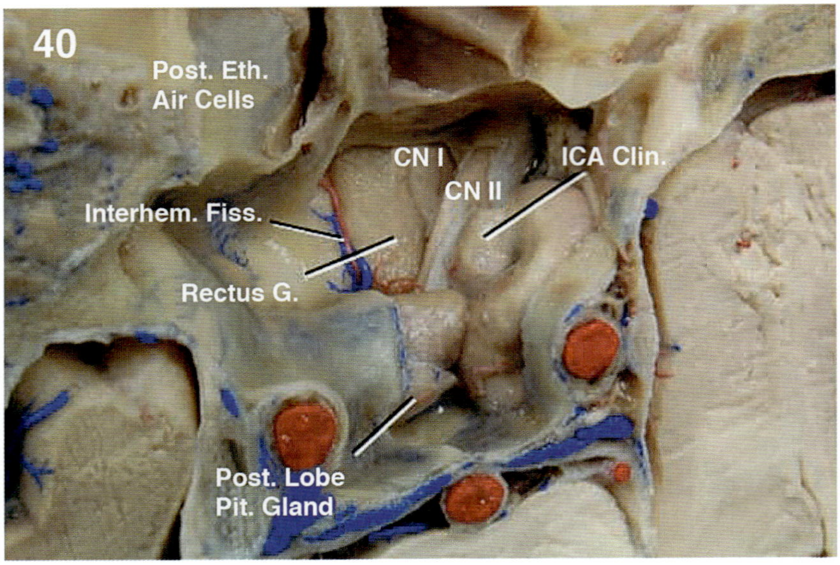

Fig. 2.40 Opening through the sphenoidal planum exposes the interhemispheric fissure, the posterior part of the rectus gyri, and the olfactory sulci and nerves, which comprise the medial part of the basal surface of cerebrum. Working through this area also enables reaching the incisural space, including the contents of the chiasmatic and lamina terminalis cisterns. Clin.: clinoid, clinoidal; CN: cranial nerve; Eth.: ethmoid, ethmoidal; Fiss.: fissure; G.: gyrus; ICA: internal carotid artery; Interhem.: interhemispheric; Pit.: pituitary; Post.: posterior.

gives attachment to the bony part of the nasal septum, formed by the vomer and the perpendicular plate of the ethmoid (**Fig. 2.20**). The anterior wall is obliquely divided into lateral and medial parts. The lateral part comprises the sphenoid conchae and posterior ethmoidal air cells. The medial part faces the sphenoethmoidal recess. The sphenoidal ostia open along the medial part of the anterior wall, closest to the sinus roof. The size, shape, and position of the sphenoid ostia are highly variable, and frequently the superior and inferior edges of both ostia are not equivalent.

The trigeminal nerves, carotid artery, and optic canals can bulge along the lateral wall, potentially causing injury to this area, such as blindness, extraocular muscle palsy, or facial numbness (**Figs. 2.36, 2.44, 2.45,** and **2.46**).

The carotid sulcus produces a prominence within the sphenoid sinus, which is maximal in the most pronounced

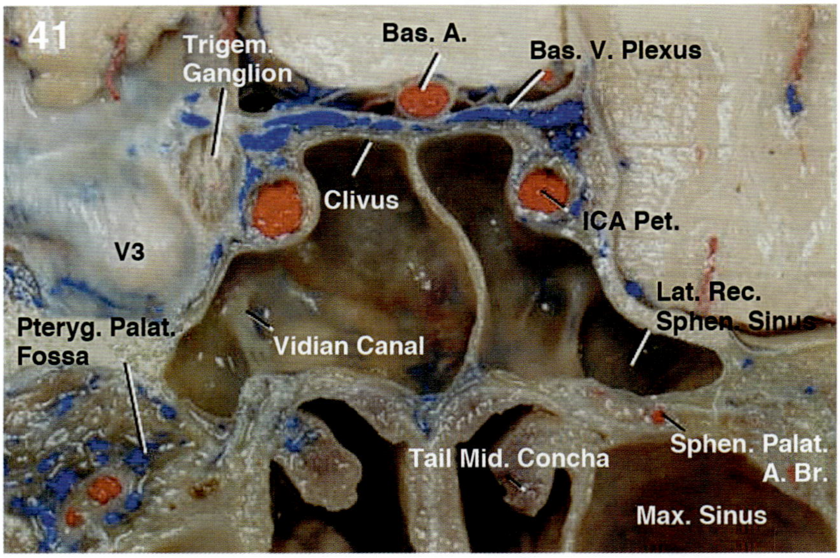

Fig. 2.41 The inferior part of the specimen is examined. The axial cut has exposed the floor of the sphenoid sinus and the nasal cavity at the level of the tail of the middle conchae. The sphenoid sinus is pneumatized to such an extent that the floor of the sinus is lower than the level of the vidian canals, making them stand out along the floor. Following the course of the vidian canal posteriorly, from the pterygopalatine fossa, takes the surgeon to the retrosellar carotid and anterior petrosal genu. On the left side, the lateral recess extends anteriorly, causing the sphenoid and maxillary sinus walls to be separated only by the contents of the pterygopalatine fossa. The inferior or clival part of the posterior wall of the sphenoid sinus can also be seen here. The clival part of the posterior wall extends from the floor of the sinus to the sella and from one petrous carotid to the other. Drilling along the clival part of the posterior wall exposes the dura of the clivus and the basilar venous plexus. Working through this area enables accessing the contents of the prepontine and the upper part of the premedullary cisterns as well as the medial parts of the cerebellopontine and cerebellomedullary cisterns. A.: artery; Bas.: basilar; Br.: branch; ICA: internal carotid artery; Lat.: lateral; Max.: maxillary; Mid.: middle; Palat.: palatine; Pteryg.: pterygoid; Rec.: recess; Sphen.: sphenoidal; Trigem.: trigeminal; V.: vein, venous; V3: third division trigeminal nerve.

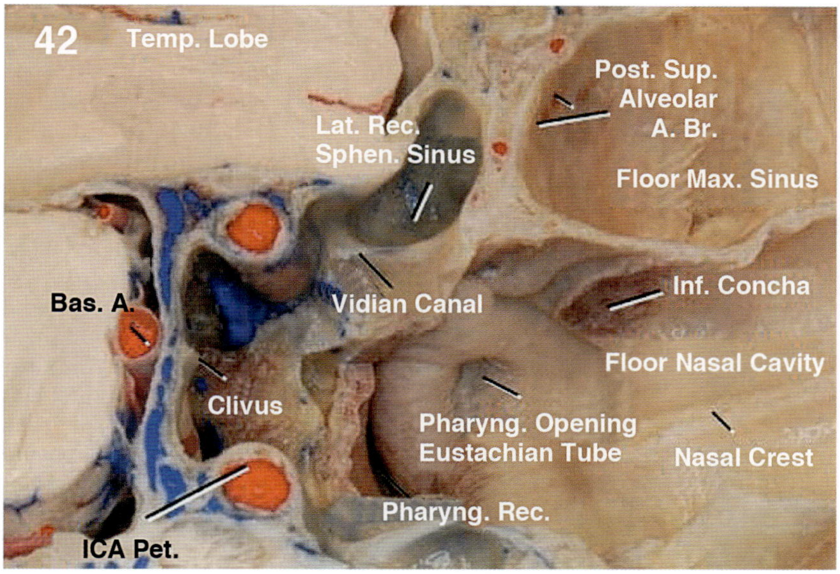

Fig. 2.42 The floor of the sphenoid sinus can be drilled down, communicating the sinus with the nasopharynx. This facilitates reaching the lower clivus and craniovertebral junction. The lateral wall of the nasopharynx presents the pharyngeal opening of the eustachian tube and pharyngeal recess. The pharyngeal recess is a landmark for the position of the cervical segment of the carotid artery. The posterior-superior alveolar arteries are branches of the pterygopalatine segment of the maxillary artery and take part in the supply of bone and mucosa of the maxillary sinus. Two or three branches may pierce the posterior wall of the sinus. A.: artery; Bas.: basilar; Br.: branch; ICA: internal carotid artery; Inf.: inferior; Lat.: lateral; Max.: maxillary; Pet.: petrous, petrosal; Pharyng.: pharyngeal; Post.: posterior; Rec.: recess; Sphen.: sphenoidal; Sup.: superior; Temp.: temporal.

pneumatized sinuses. The carotid prominence can be divided into three parts—the retrosellar, infrasellar, and presellar segments (**Figs. 2.38, 2.39,** and **2.40;** also see Chapter 22, Figs. 22.5 to 22.9). The retrosellar segment is seen on the posterolateral part of the sinuses in which the pneumatization extended laterally in the area of the dorsum. The retrosellar segment comprises the transition part between the distal petrous and the proximal cavernous carotid and is bound in place laterally by the petrolingual ligament. The distal petrous carotid encompasses the second or anterior genu and the anterior vertical petrous segments, and with or without the addition of the proximal cavernous carotid has been called the paraclival, trigeminal, or lacerum segment.[4,5] The anterior genu of the petrous carotid is located above the fibrous cartilage of the foramen lacerum, and its lateral aspect is in the extradural space between the lingual process of the sphenoid bone and the petrous apex. The anterior genu is continuous distally with the anterior vertical segment, which extends on average for 5.6 mm[4] and conceptually ends at the upper edge of the petrolingual ligament. The petrolingual ligament is an important landmark either from a lateral or a medial perspective. Looking though the middle fossa, the position of this ligament approximates a line following the upper edge of the maxillary nerve posteriorly

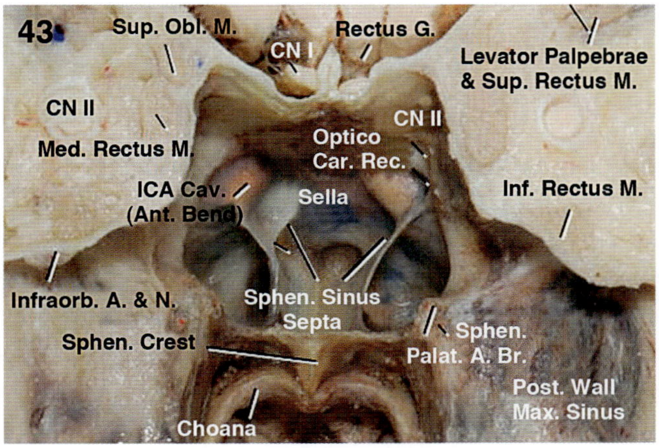

Fig. 2.43 In another specimen, a coronal cut has been performed at the level of the posterior wall of the maxillary sinus. The anterior wall of the sphenoid sinus has been removed, exposing the multiple existing septa. It is not uncommon that the sphenoid septa attach superiorly along the carotid prominences, an anatomical fact that calls for careful manipulation during its surgical removal. A.: artery; Ant.: anterior; Br.: branch; Car.: carotid; Cav.: cavernous; CN: cranial nerve; G.: gyrus; ICA: internal carotid artery; Inf.: inferior; Infraorb.: infraorbital; M.: muscle; Max.: maxillary; Med.: medial; N.: nerve; Obl.: oblique; Palat.: palatine; Post.: posterior; Sphen.: sphenoidal; Sup.: superior.

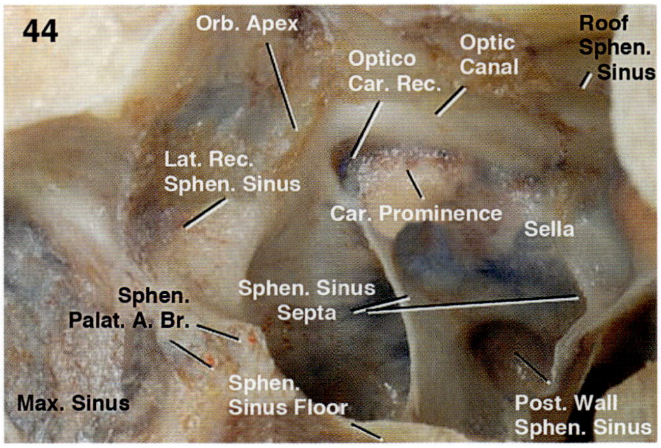

Fig. 2.44 The view along the lateral wall of the cavernous sinus. The opticocarotid recess is clearly marked. It extends along the optic strut and anterior clinoid process and has three surfaces, which face the optic canal above, the superior orbital fissure below, and the clinoid segment of the carotid posteriorly. On the inferolateral part of the anterior wall of the sphenoid sinus the sphenopalatine artery sends its nasoseptal branches, which pass along the rostrum to reach the posterior part of nasal septum. A.: artery; Br.: branch; Car.: carotid; Lat.: lateral; Max.: maxillary; Orb.: orbital; Palat.: palatine; Post.: posterior; Rec.: recess; Sphen.: spheno, sphenoid, sphenoidal.

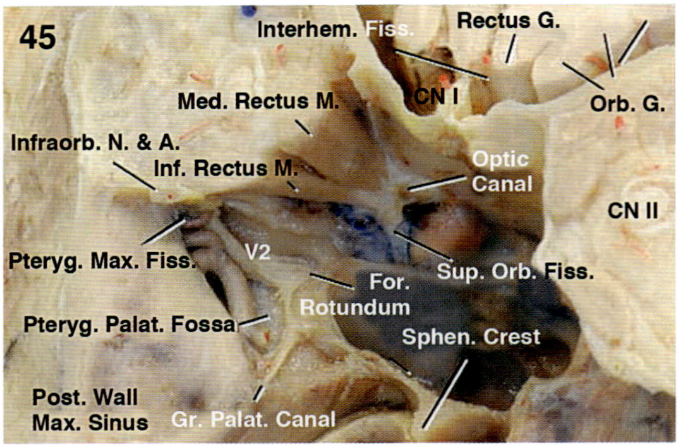

Fig. 2.45 The pterygopalatine fossa has been exposed and dissected, and the bone over the projection of the cavernous sinus along the lateral sphenoidal wall has been removed. The pterygopalatine fossa is a small, pyramidal space located below the apex of the orbit. It connects to the nasal cavity through the sphenopalatine foramen, to the orbit via the medial end of the inferior orbital fissure, and to the infratemporal fossa via the pterygomaxillary fissure. Besides the inferior orbital, pterygomaxillary, and sphenopalatine fissures, several other foramina open along its walls including the foramen rotundum, vidian canal, and greater palatine canal. A.: artery; CN: cranial nerve; Fiss.: fissure; For.: foramen; G.: gyrus; Gr.: greater; Inf.: inferior; Infraorb.: infraorbital; Interhem.: interhemispheric; M.: muscle; Max.: maxillary; Med.: medial; N.: nerve; Orb.: orbital; Palat.: palatine; Post.: posterior; Pteryg.: pterygoid; Sphen.: sphenoidal; Sup.: superior; V2: second division trigeminal nerve.

into the trigeminal ganglion (see Chapter 22, Figs. 22.11 and 22.12). When the dissection proceeds from medially, along the lateral wall of the sphenoid sinus, the petrolingual ligament is expected to be located immediately inferior to the lower edge of the abducens nerve at the point the nerve crosses the lateral surface of the carotid artery. A venous plexus, consisting of a lateral extension of the cavernous sinus, extends around the anteroinferior surface of the carotid artery within the periosteal covering of the distal part of the carotid canal.[3] It extends into the carotid canal, passing beneath the trigeminal nerve and as far as the first genu or the posterior vertical segment of the petrous carotid artery.[4] The infrasellar segment is located below the sellar floor and comprises the horizontal portion of the cavernous carotid. The presellar segment is located beside the anterior sinus wall and is the most frequently identified prominence related to the carotid inside the sphenoid sinus.

When all three parts of the carotid prominence are present and connected, they form a serpiginous bulge marking the full course of the artery (**Figs. 2.39, 2.48,** and **2.49**). According to Fujii et al,[2] the bone separating the artery and the sphenoid sinus was thinner over the retrosellar and presellar parts of the carotid prominence and thinnest along the presellar part just below the tuberculum sellae. Besides being the most vulnerable areas of covering of the carotids inside the sphenoid sinus, the presellar carotid prominences are also the areas where both carotids most approximate across the midline, reaching positions as close as 8.5 mm.[2]

The maxillary division of the trigeminal nerve can bulge along the lateral wall of the sinus, below the sella. The average length of maxillary division bulging into the sinus is 10.9 mm. (**Fig. 2.46**).[2] The maxillary division is particularly evident when the lateral recess is present. In cases of extreme pneumatization of the lateral wall, the mandibular division may be apparent. The ophthalmic division, with other contents of the superior orbital fissure, is seen as a broad prominence on the upper part of the lateral wall. Its identification is facilitated by locating the opticocarotid recess, as its upper edge corresponds to the lower edge of the recess (**Figs. 2.44, 2.45, 2.46,** and **2.47**).

The projection of the cavernous sinus along the lateral wall of the sphenoid sinus spans the area between the infrasellar carotid prominence inferiorly, which corresponds to the upper edge of the maxillary division, up to the optic canals protruding into the superolateral part of the sphenoid sinus (**Figs. 2.45** and **2.46**). The optic canal comprises the optic nerve and ophthalmic artery and has an angulation (anterior inferior decline) of 15 degrees related to the orbitomeatal line.

The roof of the sphenoid sinus extends from the anterior wall to the level of the optic canals. It comprises the planum sphenoidale, the prominence of the chiasmatic sulcus, and the tuberculum sellae, below which is the sella, on the upper

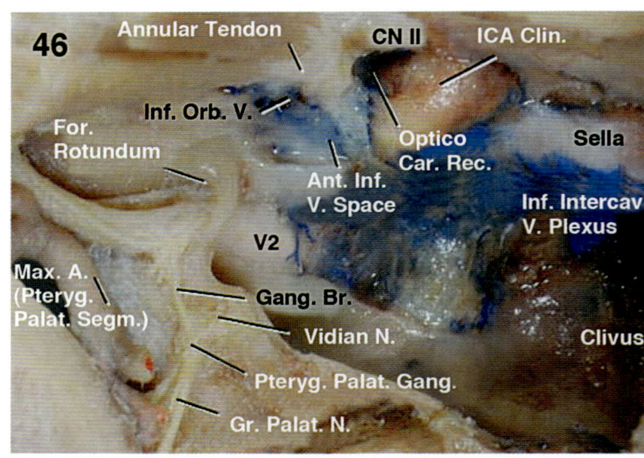

Fig. 2.46 Enlarged view. The upper border of the maxillary division marks the inferior limit of the cavernous sinus. The maxillary nerve leaves the cranium through the foramen rotundum, reaching the posterior part of the pterygopalatine fossa. Crossing the upper part of the fossa, the maxillary nerve gives off ganglionic branches toward the pterygopalatine ganglion. From this point, it deviates superolaterally to reach the upper part of the posterior surface of the maxilla. The maxillary nerve gives off the zygomatic branches and the posterior superior alveolar nerves. It eventually enters the infraorbital canal, on the roof of the maxillary sinus and orbital floor, as the infraorbital nerve. The infraorbital nerve emerges on the face, along the anterior wall of the maxillary sinus. The pterygopalatine ganglion lies behind the pterygopalatine segment of the maxillary artery, and between the maxillary nerve and the sphenopalatine canal. The sympathetic and parasympathetic roots reach this ganglion through the vidian nerve, formed by a combination of fibers of the carotid and greater petrosal nerve. The greater palatine canal is formed by the apposition of the maxilla and perpendicular plate of the palatine bone. It transmits the greater and lesser palatine vessels and nerves to the posterior nasal cavity and palate. Ant.: anterior; Br.: branch; Car.: carotid; Clin.: clinoidal; CN: cranial nerve; For.: foramen; Gang.: ganglion; Gr.: greater; ICA: internal carotid artery; Inf.: inferior; Intercav.: intercavernous; Max.: maxillary; N.: nerve; Orb.: orbital; Palat.: palatine; Pteryg.: pterygo, pterygoid; Rec.: recess; Segm.: segment; V.: vein, venous.

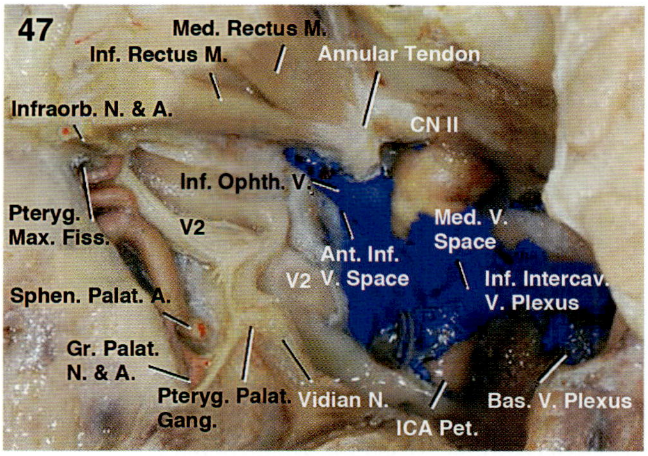

Fig. 2.47 The bone and dural covering along the lateral wall of cavernous sinus has been removed, exposing the venous compartments in and around the cavernous sinus. The venous spaces of the cavernous sinus are named according to their relationship with the cavernous carotid and include the posterosuperior, medial, and anteroinferior venous spaces. The anteroinferior venous space receives the drainage of the inferior ophthalmic vein, which may pass within or below the anular tendon. A.: artery; Ant.: anterior; Bas.: basilar; CN: cranial nerve; Gang.: ganglion; Gr.: greater; Fiss.: fissure; ICA: internal carotid artery; Inf.: inferior; Infraorb.: infraorbital; Intercav.: intercavernous; M.: muscle; Max.: maxillary; Med.: medial; N.: nerve; Ophth.: ophthalmic; Palat.: palatine; Petr.: petrous; Pteryg.: pterygoid; Sphen.: sphenoidal; V.: vein, venous; V2: second division trigeminal nerve.

part of the posterior wall of the sinus (**Figs. 2.34** and **2.39**). The anterolateral parts of the roof can be occupied by the posterior ethmoidal air cells, which can surround the optic canal and reach the anterior wall of the sella. The average distance between the carotid canals along the planum sphenoidale is 14 mm.[1] Opening through the planum sphenoidale, it is possible to approach the posteromedial portion of the anterior cranial fossa and incisura space, including the contents of the chiasmatic and lamina terminalis cistern (**Figs. 2.40, 2.49, 2.50,** and **2.51**).

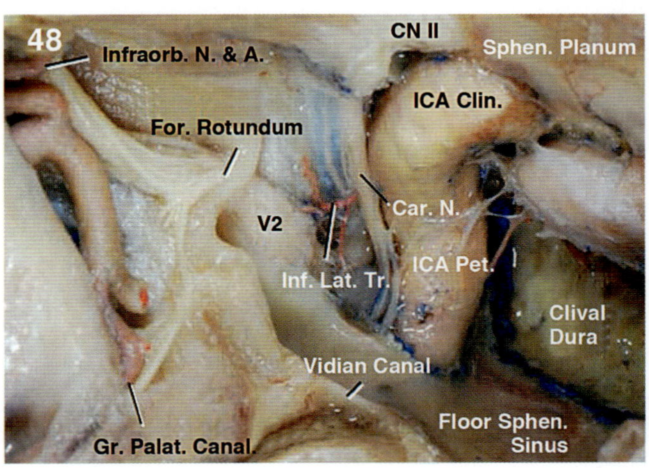

Fig. 2.48 The venous structures have been resected. The carotid nerve, a branch of the sympathetic ganglia, branches into two parts near the genu of the petrous carotid artery: a larger anterior-superior and a smaller posterior-inferior trunk. The anterior trunk gives origin to the deep petrosal nerve, which joins the greater petrosal nerve to form the vidian nerve and send twigs to the abducens and trigeminal nerves at the level of the superior orbital fissure. A.: artery; Car.: carotid; CN: cranial nerve; Clin.: clinoidal; For.: foramen; Gr.: greater; ICA: internal carotid artery; Inf.: inferior; Infraorb.: infraorbital; Lat.: lateral; N.: nerve; Palat.: palatine; Pet.: petrous, petrosal; Sphen.: spheno, sphenoid, sphenoidal; Tr.: trunk; V.: vein; V2: second division trigeminal nerve.

The floor of the sinus may be marked by the prominence of the vidian canal (**Figs. 2.41** and **2.42**). Following the course of the vidian canal posteriorly from the pterygopalatine fossa takes the surgeon to the retrosellar carotid and anterior petrosal genu. The distal portion of the petrous carotid is the most frequent site of petrous carotid branches, which occur in as many as 70% of specimens and consist of vidian and periosteal branches.[3,4] These branches usually originate from the inferior or anteroinferior surfaces of the artery. From its origin, the vidian artery courses medially an average of 11 mm along the anterior wall of the carotid canal before entering the posterior opening of the vidian canal, located at the base of the pterygoid process of the sphenoid bone, just below the floor of the sphenoid sinus and inferolateral to the anterior genu of the petrous carotid. The average diameter of the vidian branch is 0.5 mm, and all branches established an anastomosis with maxillary branches either in the pterygopalatine fossa or the vidian canal.

The posterior wall of the sphenoid sinus can be divided into a sellar part superiorly and a clival part inferiorly. Along the sellar part, the lateral limits are the pre- and infrasellar carotid prominences. On the clival part, the retrosellar carotid prominences comprise the lateral limit. The depth of the sphenoid sinus is the distance from the ostium to the

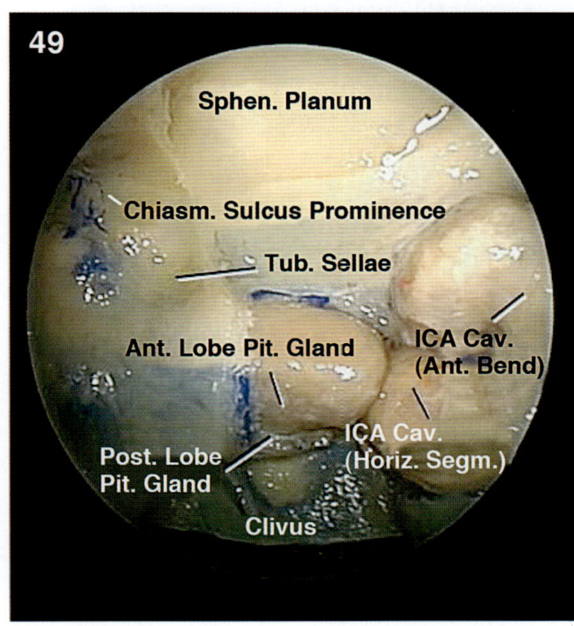

Fig. 2.49 Endoscopic dissection of the sphenoid sinus. The sphenoid sinus cavity can be considered an amplifier of the natural pathway formed by the nasal cavity. Working though this cavity can lead to several other compartments. Endoscopic exploration of the lateral wall and sellar part of the posterior wall of the sphenoid sinus is presented in Chapter 22. Ant.: anterior; Cav.: cavernous; Chiasm.: chiasmatic; Horiz.: horizontal; ICA: internal carotid artery; Pit.: pituitary; Post.: posterior; Segm.: segment; Sphen.: spheno, sphenoid, sphenoidal; Tub.: tuberculum.

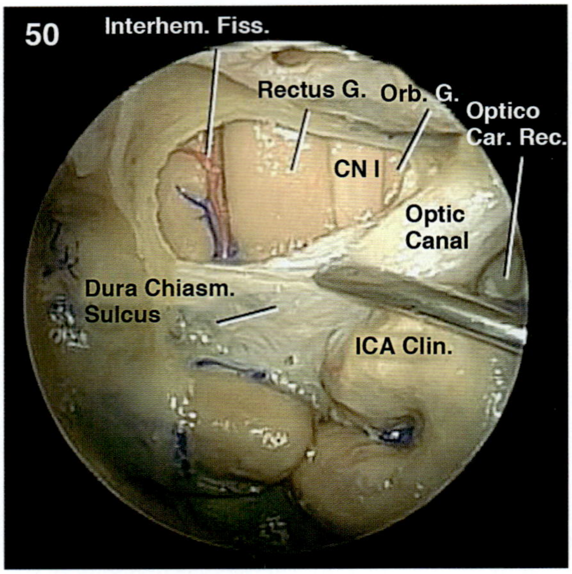

Fig. 2.50 The roof of the sphenoid sinus extends from the anterior wall to the level of the optic canals. It comprises the planum sphenoidale, the prominence of the chiasmatic sulcus, and the tuberculum sellae, beyond which is the sellar cavity on the upper part of the posterior wall of the sinus. The transition between the planum and chiasmatic sulcus is usually marked by a difference in level (tip of the dissector). This contour is followed by the dura covering the region. Car.: carotid; Chiasm.: chiasmatic; Clin.: clinoidal; CN: cranial nerve; Fiss.: fissure; G.: gyrus; ICA: internal carotid artery; Interhem.: interhemispheric; Orb.: orbital; Rec.: recess.

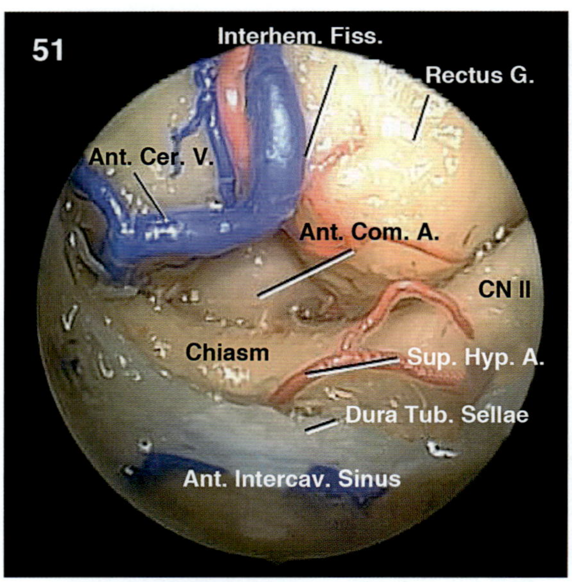

Fig. 2.51 Opening through the planum sphenoidale facilitates approaching the posteromedial portion of the anterior cranial fossa. This area is related to the posterior part of the basal surface of the cerebrum, which presents the rectus gyrus, the olfactory sulcus, and the orbital gyri. The olfactory nerve is related to the olfactory sulcus. The transplanum route may also facilitate exposing the anterior incisural space. On the center of this space the chiasm helps separate the two major cisternal compartments. Below the chiasm is the chiasmatic cistern, and above it is the center of the lamina terminalis cistern. A.: artery; Ant.: anterior; Cer.: cerebral; Com.: communicating; CN: cranial nerve; Fiss.: fissure; G.: gyrus; Hyp.: hypophyseal; Intercav.: intercavernous; Interhem.: interhemispheric; Sup.: superior; Tub.: tuberculum; V.: vein.

closest part of sella and ranges from 9 to 23 mm.[1,2] The bone of the posterior wall is thinnest along the anterior wall of sella, varying from 0.1 to 0.7 mm. Removing the bone along the sellar part of the posterior wall exposes the dura of the sella and the intercavernous sinuses (**Figs. 2.36, 2.37,** and **2.38**), and is usually accomplished during transsphenoidal approaches to sellae. Drilling along the clival part of the posterior wall exposes the dura of the clivus and the basilar venous plexus (**Fig. 2.42**). Working through this area provides access to the contents of the prepontine and the upper part of the premedullary cisterns as well as the medial parts of the cerebellopontine and cerebellomedullary cisterns (**Figs. 2.52, 2.53,** and **2.54**).

Two distances have paramount importance for surgical approaches to and through the sphenoid sinus: the distance between the nasospinale and the ostium of the sphenoid sinus, and the distance from the sphenoid ostium to the anterior wall of pituitary fossa. The average distance between the nasospinale and the ostium of the sphenoid sinus is 27.5 mm in neonates and 61.5 mm in adults, whereas the average distance between the ostium of the sphenoid sinus and the anterior pituitary wall in adults is 14.6 mm. These distances represent the path of surgical instruments and the appropriate length when working through the endonasal route.

The sphenoid sinus receives its blood supply from the sphenopalatine artery. The sellar region may also receive supply from the capsular and inferior hypophyseal arteries.

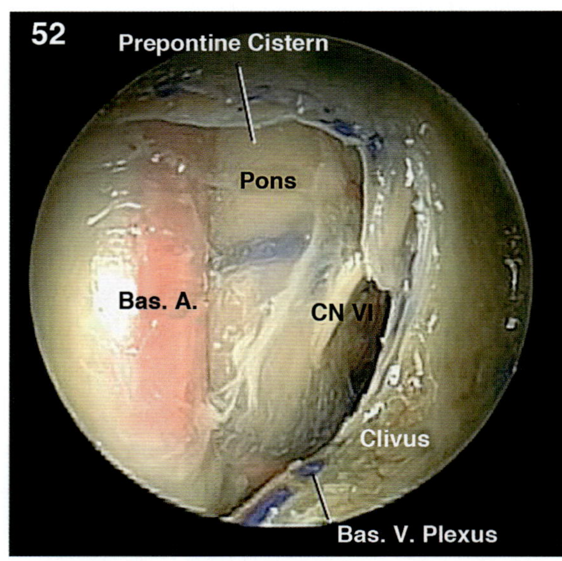

Fig. 2.52 The pituitary stalk and superior hypophyseal arteries are located into the chiasmatic cistern. The anterior cerebral arteries and branches, the anterior cerebral veins, and the anterior communicating artery complex are in the lamina terminalis cistern. The posterior wall of the sphenoid sinus is divided into an upper sellar part and an inferior clival part. The clival part extends from the floor of sella to the floor of the sinus and is on top of the nasopharynx. Opening through the clival part of the posterior wall exposes the clival dura, which contains the basilar venous plexus—the most constant connection between the cavernous sinuses. Working through this area takes the surgeon to the prepontine cistern, located between the anterior pontine arachnoidal membranes passing just medial to the abducens nerves on each side. This cistern houses the basilar trunk and origin of the anterior inferior cerebellar arteries (AICA).A.: artery; Bas.: basilar; CN: cranial nerve; V.: vein, venous.

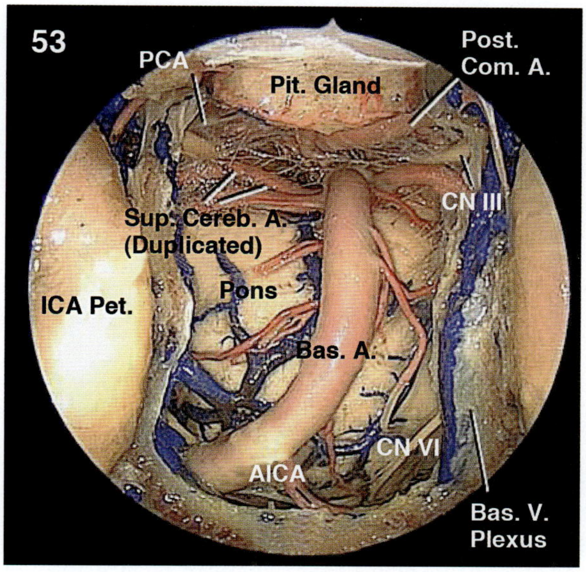

Fig. 2.53 This approach can be extended superiorly, toward the interpeduncular cistern, when removing the dorsum sellae. The interpeduncular cistern is between the oculomotor nerves on each side, and houses the basilar apex and origin of the posterior cerebral arteries. It is separated from the prepontine cistern by the inferior leaflet (mesencephalic membrane) of Liliequist's membrane. The superior cerebellar artery arises along the transition between the interpeduncular and prepontine cisterns and is duplicated on the right in this specimen. The approach can also be expanded inferiorly by removing the floor of the sphenoid sinus and working through the posterior wall of the pharynx. This provides access to the premedullary cistern and the craniovertebral junction. A.: artery; AICA: anterior inferior cerebellar artery; Bas.: basilar; Cereb.: cerebellar; CN: cranial nerve; Com.: communicating; ICA: internal carotid artery; PCA: posterior cerebral artery; Pet.: petrous, petrosal; Pit.: pituitary; Post.: posterior; Sup.: superior; V.: vein.

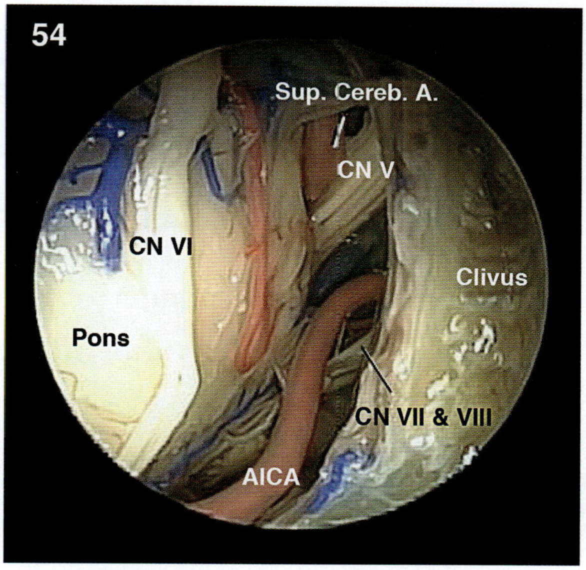

Fig. 2.54 By working laterally, beyond the abducens nerve and the anterior pontine arachnoidal membrane, it is possible to reach the medial part of the cerebellopontine cistern. This cistern houses cranial nerves V, VI, VII, and VIII and part of the trajectory of the superior cerebellar artery and the anterior cerebellar artery (AICA). It is on top of the cerebellomedullary cistern, which contains the posterior inferior cerebellar artery (PICA) and the lower cranial nerves. A.: artery; AICA: anterior inferior cerebellar artery; Cereb.: cerebellar; CN: cranial nerve; Sup.: superior; V.: vein.

References

1. Lang J. Anatomy of the Nose, Nasal Cavity and Paranasal Sinuses. New York: Thieme Medical Publishers; 1989
2. Fujii K, Chambers SM, Rhoton AL Jr. Neurovascular relationships of the sphenoid sinus. A microsurgical study. J Neurosurg 1979;50:31–39
3. Paullus WS, Pait TG, Rhoton Al Jr. Microsurgical exposure of the petrous portion of the carotid artery. J Neurosurg 1977;47:713–726
4. Osawa S, Rhoton AL Jr, Tanriover N, Shimizu S, Fujii K. Microsurgical anatomy and surgical exposure of the petrous segment of the internal carotid artery. Neurosurgery 2008;63(4 Suppl 2):210–238
5. Rhoton AL Jr. The posterior cranial fossa. Microsurgical anatomy and surgical approaches. Neurosurgery 2006;47(3 supp.):S1–S298

3 Imaging in Endoscopic Paranasal Sinus and Skull Base Surgery: Three-Dimensional Reconstruction

Rainer Guilherme Haetinger

Tips and Pearls

- Knowledge of all anatomical variations is essential to avoid surgical complications. These variations should always be described by radiologists and recognized by surgeons.
- Many lesions involving the skull base need to be investigated by both computed tomography (CT) and magnetic resonance imaging (MRI).
- Imaging of the coronal and sagittal planes is essential for lesions of the midline.
- Lesions related to the cavernous sinus are best evaluated by MRI.
- Juvenile angiofibromas are best evaluated by computed tomography angiography (CTA), including two-phase acquisition in cases of large tumors. When an invasion of the cavernous sinus is suspected, MRI is an important complementary method.
- Tumors in contiguity with the internal carotid arteries should be evaluated preoperatively with angiography and test occlusion.
- CT-cisternography is still the "gold standard" imaging method to investigate cerebrospinal fluid (CSF) fistulas.

Introduction

The role of high-quality imaging in planning surgery is paramount for a safe surgical approach and successful results. The detailed demonstration of anatomy and of the relationship between lesions and vascular and bony structures is an essential guide for the surgeon. Multislice computed tomography (MSCT) and volumetric computed tomography (VCT) provide a very reliable panorama of the anatomy because of their very thin slices (less than 1 mm) with isotropic pixels and high-speed acquisition (hundreds of images per second), allowing even greater quality in vascular studies. For the purposes of this chapter, these types of computed tomography are included in references to "CT."

A specific and very useful protocol is computed tomography angiography (CTA or CT-angiography), which is performed with a contrast media injector and later postprocessed with volume rendering (VR) (**Fig. 3.1**), maximal intensity projection (MIP), and multiplanar reconstruction (MPR) software. This method is the best choice to demonstrate the vascularity of tumors, the relation between vascular structures and the bone, as well as bony integrity.[1]

On the other hand, high-field magnetic resonance imaging (MRI), with a 1.5- and 3-tesla field, is improving the quality of imaging and the capacity to distinguish tissues and structures, mainly in the brain. Equipment with higher magnetic fields (4 to 9 tesla) is still not generally available for medical use. Magnetic resonance angiography (MRA) is also an excellent and widely used method, and may be performed with or without contrast media (preferably with contrast media) and postprocessed with the same software as used for CTA. In this method the bony structures are not visualized, and there is a very clear view of the vessels, including those inside the canals and the foramina of the skull and spine. Computed tomography cisternography (CT-cisternography) is considered the radiologic "gold standard" to investigate cerebrospinal fluid (CSF) fistulas.

This chapter presents examples, using CT and/or MRI, of lesions that may be suitable for endoscopic surgery.

Evaluation of the Paranasal Sinuses and Skull Base

The evaluation of the nose, paranasal sinuses, and skull base is done mainly by CT,[2] which provides the following essential information:

1. The degree of aeration of paranasal sinuses and integrity of the medial orbital wall and cribriform plate
2. The location of intersinus septa
3. The position of anterior skull base vessels (better demonstrated by CTA)
4. The relationship between the fovea ethmoidalis and the cribriform plate
5. The presence of anatomical variations, such as Onodi cells, basilar expansion of the sphenoid sinus, pneumatization of the anterior clinoid processes, supraorbital ethmoidal cells, dehiscence of the medial wall of the orbit (with protrusion of the orbital fat tissue toward the

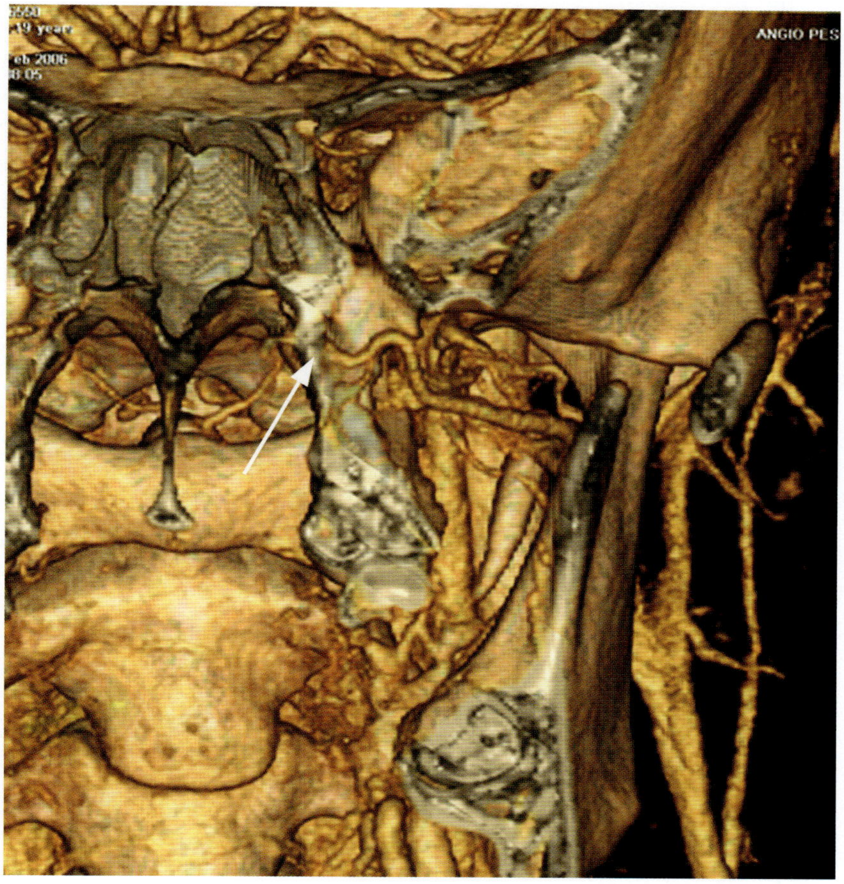

Fig. 3.1 CT-angiography with volume rendering 3D reconstruction (excluding the anterior part of the face). This postprocessed 3D reconstruction nicely shows the region of the pterygopalatine fossa and the left maxillary artery reaching the pterygopalatine foramen (*arrow*). This protocol maintains the bone, and thus it is easy to identify the pterygoid process, the inferior and superior orbital fissures, and the sphenoid sinuses.

ethmoidal labyrinth), and dehiscence of the lateral wall of the sphenoid sinus[3]

6. The presence and extent of bony dehiscences in the skull base near the internal carotid arteries, optic nerves, and cavernous sinuses

For skull base lesions, MRI is indicated to establish the following:

1. Recurrent skull base tumor
2. The intra- or extraaxial origin of tumors
3. The type of tissue located adjacent to dehiscent or destroyed bone
4. The invasion or external compression of the brain
5. The involvement of the internal carotid arteries, cavernous sinuses, vertebrobasilar system, or dural sinuses
6. The anatomical areas of potential major risk for a surgical approach, such as cavernous sinuses, Meckel's caves, optical nerves, internal carotid arteries, the vertebrobasilar system, and jugular foramina
7. The relationship between the lesion and adjacent cranial nerves
8. The presence of scar tissue and reconstructive grafts

An additional tool to evaluate the intra- and extracranial vessels is MRA, a noninvasive method that is very helpful in patients who have contraindications for iodinated contrast media, such as allergy or renal failure. It must be remembered that in cases of renal failure, the paramagnetic agent should also be avoided. The recent medical literature reports many cases of nephrogenic systemic fibrosis due to the association of renal failure with paramagnetic agents.

Digital subtraction angiography (DSA) is not used in most case, but in high-risk surgeries, mainly with involvement of arteries, it demonstrates thin but important vessels and verifies the functional integrity of the circle of Willis. In some cases it indicates the need for presurgical intravascular embolization of a vascular malformation or a vascular tumor.

Importance of Anatomy and Anatomical Variations

Arriving at a correct diagnosis requires identifying the anatomical origin of a lesion; failure to do so may lead to an incorrect differential diagnosis and a high probability of surgical complications. Therefore, radiologists and surgeons must have extensive knowledge of the complex anatomy of the skull base and face. They must be familiar with the axial, coronal, sagittal, and oblique planes. Three-dimensional (3D) reconstructions are helpful, but first the anatomy must be

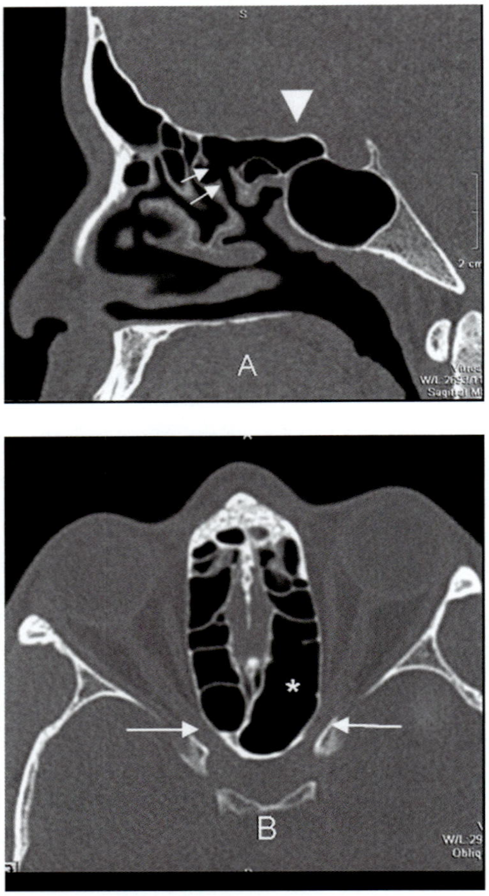

Fig. 3.2 Onodi cell. **(A)** Multislice CT image on a sagittal multiplanar reformation (MPR) exemplifying a typical Onodi cell, characterized by a posterior ethmoid cell extending backward and above the sphenoid sinus (*arrowhead*), reaching the anterior wall of the sella turcica, and also clearly demonstrating its drainage to the superior meatus (*small arrows*). **(B)** Axial plane view at the level of the optic canals (*arrows*) demonstrating the contiguity between the left canal and the ipsilateral Onodi cell (*).

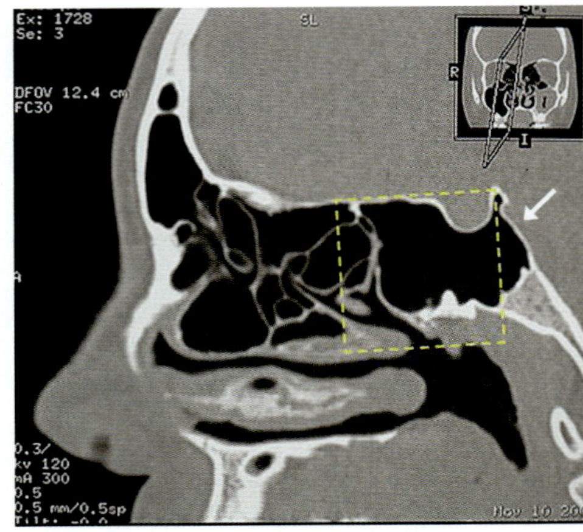

Fig. 3.3 Basilar expansion of the sphenoidal sinus. Multislice CT imaging with sagittal MFR showing the 90-degree angle with the planum sphenoidale at the dorsum sellae (*dotted square*) and the posterior extension of the sinus with a consequently thin clivus (*arrow*).

evaluated and the location of lesions determined on 2D reformations, such as MPR. It is also essential to observe the dislocation of vessels and nerves from their original topography, caused by the lesions or by anatomical variations.

There is abundant medical literature on this anatomy. So this chapter will focus on some advanced topics that are relevant to an endonasal approach to the skull base.

Anatomical variations in the posterior ethmoid or in the sphenoid sinus (e.g., Onodi cells, pneumatization of the anterior clinoid processes and pterygoid processes) may increase the risk of damage to optic nerves, internal carotid arteries,[4] maxillary and vidian nerves, as well as the anterior structures within the posterior cranial fossa, behind a very thin or dehiscent clivus (basilar expansion of the sphenoidal sinus). Variations of the *fovea ethmoidalis* may increase the risk of anterior cranial fossa damage during surgery assisted by endoscopy, as classified by Keros in 1962,[5] and referred to many times in the specialized literature. The presence of supraorbital ethmoidal cells, agger nasi cells, frontal bulla, and anterior and superior insertions of the uncinate process are also essential to determine and describe in each patient.

There are originally different types of Onodi cells, as Hungarian professor of Rhinology Adolph Onodi described in his original work.[6] The most important type that is currently used is defined as the most posterior ethmoidal cell in contiguity with the optic canal, and it typically expands backward and above or laterally to the sphenoid sinus (**Fig. 3.2**). This expansion also leads to contact between the posterior ethmoid and the internal carotid artery, which usually is related only to the sphenoid sinus. For a surgical approach into the posterior ethmoidal and sphenoidal region, knowledge of this variation is essential to avoid complications and to plan the best surgical approach. (See also the subsection Meningioma in the section Extraaxial Lesions of the Anterior Cranial Fossa, below, and a specific example in the section Meningioma of the Anterior Cranial Fossa, below.)

The basilar expansion of the sphenoidal sinus result is an extension backward to the dorsum sellae, based on a 90-degree angle with the planum sphenoidale, in association with a thin clivus (**Fig. 3.3**). This basilar expansion represents a feature of great surgical importance. Complications may occur using the endoscopic approach in endonasal surgery, in which the form of basilar expansion is critical, that is, less than 2 mm thickness of the clivus, with an incidence of 45% in a series of 750 CT examinations and 50 dry skulls reported by Haetinger in 2006.[7] There are reports in the literature of fracture, vertigo, posterior headache, vomiting, and empyema in patients with sphenoidal sinus prolongations. Recent reports of vasculitis of the basilar artery with ischemic infarction of the pons secondary to sphenoidal sinusitis, of spontaneous CSF fistula (**Fig. 3.4**), and of frequent exposure of the internal carotid arteries support the risk factors of a thin clivus due to a basilar expansion of the sphenoidal sinus.[8–12] In addition, a thin clivus is a potentially weak region in cases of a skull base fracture, and it is susceptible to traumatic CSF fistula.

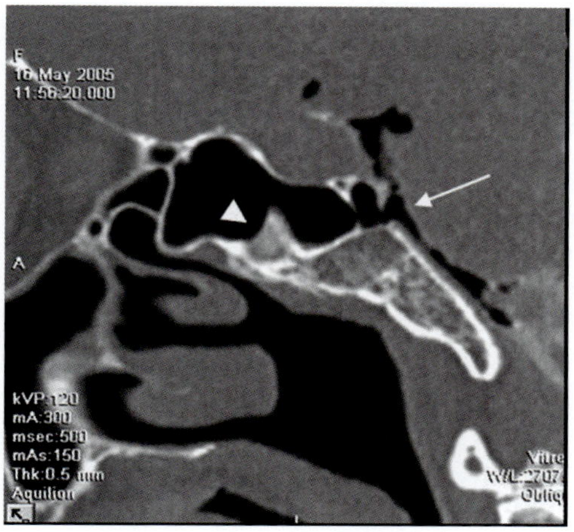

Fig. 3.4 Spontaneous CSF fistula at the clivus due to basilar expansion of the sphenoid sinus. CT-cisternography demonstrates pneumocephalus due to a CSF fistula in a patient with a dehiscent clivus (*arrow*). There is also CSF with contrast media inside the sphenoid sinus, adjacent to an intrasinusal septum (*arrowhead*).

Characteristic Findings in Imaging

The most relevant lesions related to the nose, paranasal sinuses, and skull base are listed below, with their most characteristic imaging findings.

Lesions of the Nose and Paranasal Sinuses

Solitary Polyps and Cysts

- CT: well-defined mass, low to intermediate density, rare peripheral enhancement of mucosa, no central contrast enhancement
- MRI: intermediate signal on T1-weighted imaging (T1WI), hypersignal on T2-weighted imaging (T2WI), only slight peripheral enhancement of mucosa, no central contrast enhancement on enhanced T1WI[13]

Sinonasal Polyposis

- CT: well-defined polypoid masses, low to intermediate density, with irregular peripheral contrast enhancement, without central enhancement; in advanced stages, bone remodeling is a common finding
- MRI: intermediate or mixed signal on T1WI, hypersignal or mixed signal on T2WI (with central low signal in cases of chronic secretions), with peripheral irregular enhancement on enhanced T1WI

Mucocele

- CT: filled sinus with remodeled and thinned bony wall, hyperdense content (high protein content), without contrast media enhancement
- MRI: low signal on T1WI, usually with peripheral hyperintensity of the mucosa and central hypointensity on T2WI, no enhancement on enhanced T1WI; in earlier stages, with predominant high water content, there is diffuse hypersignal on T2WI

Inverted Papilloma

- CT: soft tissue mass in the nasal cavity, usually arising from the lateral wall, extending into the maxillary sinus, or within the maxillary sinus extending into the nasal cavity, with bone remodeling and erosion; there is a variable enhancement pattern, but it is usually heterogeneous
- MRI: intermediate or slight hypersignal on T1WI, heterogeneous hypersignal on T2WI, irregular enhancing mass on enhanced T1WI; cortical bone erosion may be seen, but this aspect is better evaluated by CT

Squamous Cell Carcinoma

Squamous cell carcinoma arises in the nasopharynx from the pharyngeal mucosal space and forms a mass in the posterior and lateral wall. When clinical symptoms begin, the tumor is usually large and there is often invasion of the skull base. Extensions to the prevertebral and parapharyngeal spaces, as well as to the posterior nasal cavity and oropharynx, are also patterns of spread. Metastatic disease to the lymph nodes is very common.

- CT: soft tissue mass producing bone destruction, with irregular enhancement after contrast media injection, usually infiltrating the clivus, pterygoid process, and prevertebral space; sagittal and coronal MPR images are very important for diagnosis
- MRI: isointense on T1WI, slightly hyperintense on T2WI, and diffuse enhancement on enhanced T1WI. It is essential to obtain an enhanced series with fat suppression (fat saturation). Perineural and perivascular spread is best evaluated with these series. Eventual invasion of the cavernous sinus is best evaluated on the coronal plane.

Adenoid Cystic Carcinoma (Cylindroma, Adenocarcinoma)

This carcinoma is an aggressive malignant tumor arising from seromucous glands or surface epithelium. It may originate in a paranasal sinus, at the hard palate, or in the parotid and submandibular salivary glands. Perineural spread is common and very dangerous, mainly through the pterygopalatine fossa, the inferior and superior orbital fissure, and the cavernous sinus.

- CT: irregular and infiltrating mass, with bone remodeling and destruction, with heterogeneous enhancement after iodinated contrast media intravenous injection
- MRI: mixed signal intensity, sometimes with hyperintense hemorrhagic foci on T1WI, irregular hyperintensity on T2WI, and irregular enhancement on enhanced T1WI; it is essential to use fat suppression in the enhanced series

Esthesioneuroblastoma

The origin of this tumor is in the olfactory membrane of the upper nasal cavity, at the cribriform plate.

- CT: mass causing remodeling or destruction of the cribriform plate, usually with inhomogeneous enhancement, sometimes with areas of cystic degeneration or necrosis
- MRI: low or intermediate signal intensity on T1WI, hyperintensity or mixed intensity on T2WI, and inhomogeneous enhancement after infusion of gadolinium contrast

Non-Hodgkin's Lymphoma

- CT: lobulated soft tissue mass in nasal cavity or paranasal sinus, remodeling or destroying bone, with potential intracranial invasion; there is usually a moderate and diffuse enhancement after iodinated contrast media injection
- MRI: intermediate signal intensity on both T1WI and T2WI, with diffuse enhancement on enhanced T1WI

Extraaxial Lesions of the Anterior Cranial Fossa

Meningioma

- CT: extraaxial well-circumscribed mass, usually hyperdense (75%), sometimes isodense (25%), with homogeneous, intense, and diffuse enhancement after intravenous (IV) contrast media; about 25% have calcifications, and hyperostosis or irregular bone cortex are frequent findings
- MRI: intermediate signal on T1WI, variable signal on T2WI, sometimes with a sunburst pattern, homogeneous and intense enhancement after gadolinium in the majority of cases
- In the anterior cranial fossa, approximately 5 to 10% occur at the olfactory groove and 10 to 20% at the planum sphenoidale.[14]
- There are also atypical and malignant meningiomas that have areas of necrosis, bone destruction between the intra- and extracranial mass, and marked perifocal edema.

Craniopharyngioma

- CT: frequent tumor calcification; mixed cystic and solid mass with enhancement of the solid component and cyst wall
- MRI: variable from hypo- to hyperintense on T1WI depending on the cystic contents; mixed solid and cystic components with enhancement of the solid component and cyst wall; T2WI and fluid-attenuated inversion recovery (FLAIR) demonstrate heterogeneous signal in the solid components and cyst hyperintensity; calcification has low signal on T2WI

Frontoethmoidal Meningocephalocele (Cephalocele)

- CT: bone deformity with frontal bone displacement superiorly and nasal bones inferiorly, bifid or absent crista galli, absent or incomplete lamina cribrosa and frontal bone; there is a heterogeneous mass in continuity with the brain
- MRI: T1WI and T2WI demonstrate soft tissue mass isointense to gray matter herniated through the bony defect, without abnormal enhancement postgadolinium (but enhancement may be seen in cases of inflammation or infection)

Meningocele

- CT: similar bone deformity to meningocephalocele, but with hypodense content (CSF)
- MRI: hypointense on T1WI and hyperintense on T2WI CSF content, without brain parenchyma

Metastasis

- CT: bone destruction or permeative behavior adjacent to soft tissue, usually enhancing after IV contrast media injection
- MRI: intermediate signal in nonenhanced images, and heterogeneous enhancement postgadolinium; usually hyperintense on T2WI. It should be always considered in the differential diagnosis for solid aggressive lesions.

Aneurysm

- CT: well-delineated round or oval extraaxial lesion, which may be slightly dense in the precontrast phase, with high enhancement of its lumen after contrast media injection; there may be peripheral calcifications or not
- MRI: low ("flow void") or heterogeneous signal on T1WI and low intensity on T2WI; sometimes the signal intensity is mixed or laminated

Extraaxial Lesions of the Middle Cranial Fossa

Meningioma

- CT: extraaxial well-circumscribed mass, usually hyperdense (75%), sometimes hypodense (25%), with homogeneous, intense, and diffuse enhancement after IV contrast media; about 25% have calcifications, and hyperostosis and irregular bone cortex are frequent findings
- MRI: intermediate signal on T1WI, variable signal on T2WI, sometimes with a sunburst pattern, homogeneous and intense enhancement postgadolinium in the majority of cases; the meningioma "en plaque" is seen as a sessile thickened enhanced dura
- T2* gradient echo (GRE) is very helpful to see calcifications.
- A "dural tail" is a very common finding in this tumor (~80% of cases).

Schwannoma

When a schwannoma affects the mandibular branch from the trigeminal nerve (V3), the solid mass enlarges the foramen ovale, with components below, in the masticatory space, and above, in the middle cranial fossa. Atrophy of the masticator muscles is common.

- CT: isodense to a musculature nodule or mass before IV contrast, and diffuse but moderate enhancement after contrast media injection. Bone remodeling may be seen, especially at the foramen ovale. There may be also little cysts and hemorrhagic components.
- MRI: intermediate or low signal intensity on T1WI, variable intensity on T2WI and different modes of enhancement, from homogeneous to heterogeneous, also depending on the presence of cysts and hemorrhagic foci

Aneurysm

- CT: well-delineated round or oval extraaxial lesion, which may be slightly dense in the precontrast phase, with high enhancement of its lumen after contrast media injection; there may be peripheral calcifications or not
- MRI: patent aneurysm has "flow void" or heterogeneous signal inside; a partially thrombosed aneurysm has commonly a mixed or laminated thrombus, depending on its age, on T1WI. On T2WI the aneurysm appears as hypointense. A patent lumen may enhance on enhanced T1WI.

Metastasis

- CT: bone destruction or permeative behavior adjacent to soft tissue, usually enhancing after IV contrast media injection
- MRI: intermediate signal on nonenhanced images, and heterogeneous enhancement postgadolinium; usually hyperintense on T2WI. It should be always considered in the differential diagnosis for solid aggressive lesions.

Extraaxial Lesions of the Posterior Cranial Fossa

Chordoma

Chordomas are typically localized at the clivus (when intracranial).

- CT: bone erosion and diffuse enhancement; the tumor may also extend into the middle fossa
- MRI: intense hypersignal on T2WI, hyposignal on T1WI, diffuse enhancement on enhanced T1WI

Chondrosarcoma

Chondrosarcomas are typically localized at the petro-occipital fissure, out of the midline.

- CT: bone erosion, irregular shape, and irregular or diffuse enhancement
- MRI: intense hypersignal on T2WI, hyposignal on T1WI, irregular or diffuse enhancement on enhanced T1WI

Meningioma

- CT: extraaxial well-circumscribed mass, usually hyperdense (75%), sometimes hypodense (25%), with homogeneous, intense, and diffuse enhancement after IV contrast media; about 25% have calcifications, and hyperostosis and irregular bone cortex are frequent findings
- MRI: intermediate signal on T1WI, variable signal on T2WI, sometimes with a sunburst pattern, homogeneous and intense enhancement postgadolinium in the majority of cases; the meningioma "en plaque" is seen as a sessile thickened enhanced dura
- A "dural tail" is a very common finding in this tumor (~80% of cases).
- T2* GRE is very helpful to see calcifications.

Metastasis

- CT: bone destruction or permeative behavior adjacent to soft tissue, usually enhancing after IV contrast media injection
- MRI: intermediate signal in nonenhanced images, and heterogeneous enhancement postgadolinium; usually hyperintense on T2WI. It should be always considered in the differential diagnosis for solid aggressive lesions.

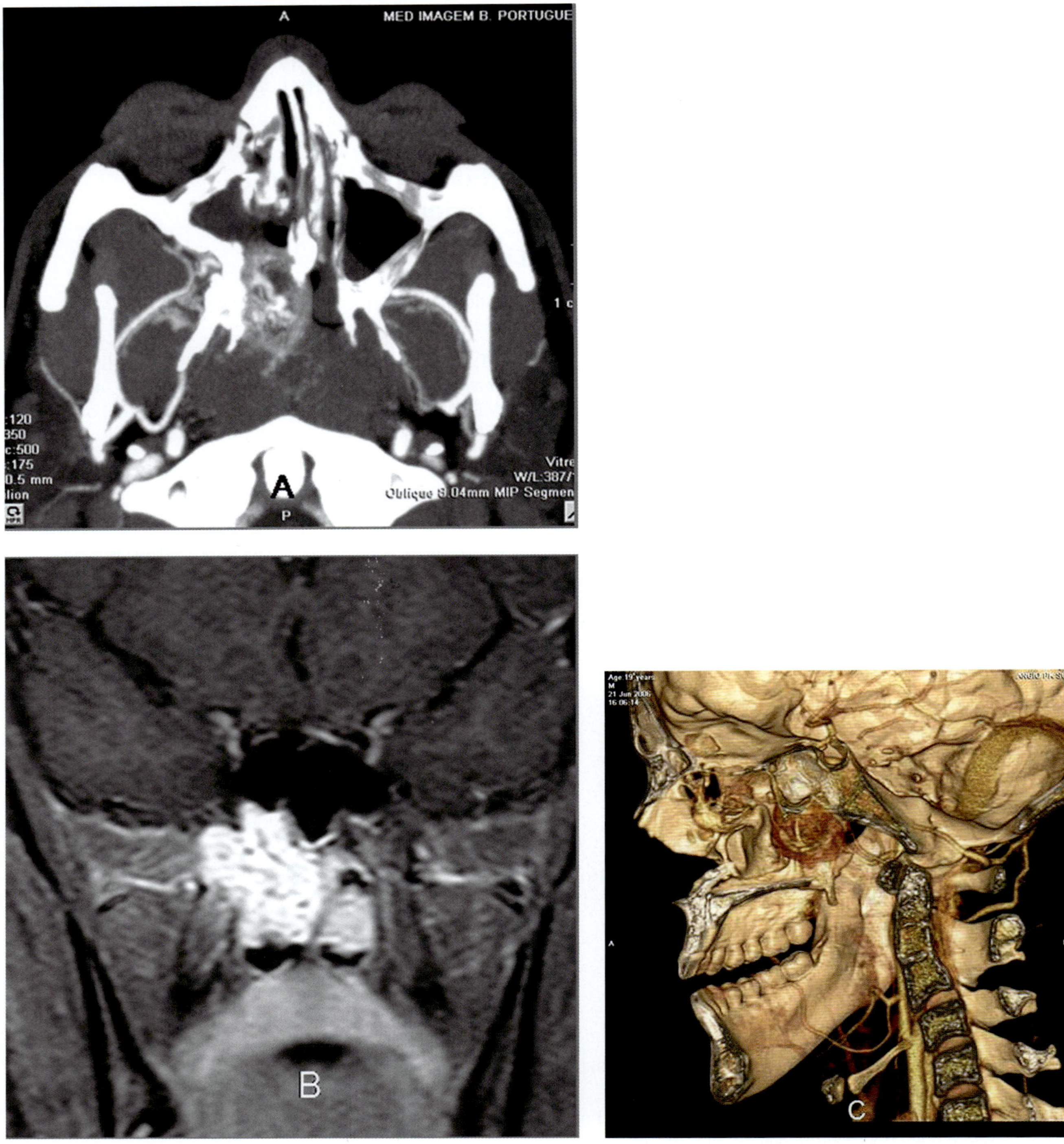

Fig. 3.5 Juvenile angiofibroma (recurrence). **(A)** CT-angiography with maximal intensity projection (MIP) technique on the axial plane, thick slice, demonstrates a high vascular tumor in the nasopharynx and choanal region, as well as the pterygopalatine fossa. The pathologic tortuous vessels are well seen in the center of the lesion, as well as their relationship with the right maxillary artery. There is also a postsurgical status on this side. **(B)** MRI T1WI postgadolinium on the coronal plane demonstrates the extension of the tumor, without intracranial involvement. **(C)** A 3D reconstruction in lateral view with volume rendering technique gives the surgeon a very helpful view of the anatomical relationships.

Aneurysm

- CT: well-delineated round or oval extraaxial lesion, which may be slightly dense in the precontrast phase, with high enhancement of its lumen after contrast media injection; there may be peripheral calcifications or not
- MRI: low ("flow void") or heterogeneous signal on T1WI and low intensity on T2WI; sometimes the signal intensity is mixed or laminated

Selected Skull Base Lesions

The following subsections provide examples of typical lesions involving the skull base, describe the different tools used for diagnosis and documentation, discuss some technical aspects, and suggest key issues to consider in the differential diagnosis.

Juvenile Angiofibroma

Juvenile angiofibroma is usually diagnosed clinically, before the radiologic examination. Teenage boys are the typical group at risk, commonly presenting with nasal obstruction and epistaxis. The objective of imaging is to establish the boundaries of the lesion; imaging is also used to evaluate recurrent or residual disease. Both CT and MRI are helpful tools to confirm the diagnosis. On MRI, considering the high grade of vascularization, T2WI demonstrates that the lesion is hyperintense in comparison with the white matter of the brain, and associated with multiple flow-void points related to larger vessels. These findings resemble a "salt-and-pepper" appearance. The enhanced T1WI depicts the entire lesion and delimits which anatomical compartments are involved. CT is important to demonstrate remodeling or destruction of the bone, usually infiltrating the pterygopalatine fossa and sometimes the skull base and the sphenoid or maxillary sinuses. The location is almost always related to the sphenopalatine foramen and the maxillary artery. CTA is a very helpful method for planning the surgical approach and for exposing all the important vascular structures related to the lesion and along the access to it. We consider CTA the method of choice for evaluating angiofibromas. From the technical point of view, larger tumors should be examined with two-phase acquisition, that is, first a true arterial phase and then a venous phase, showing the boundaries of the whole tumor (**Fig. 3.5**). It is also essential to determine if there is invasion of the cavernous sinus, which can be better diagnosed with MRI.

Meningioma of the Anterior Cranial Fossa

About 10 to 20% of meningiomas occur at the planum sphenoidale. **Figure 3.6** demonstrates an example, associated with

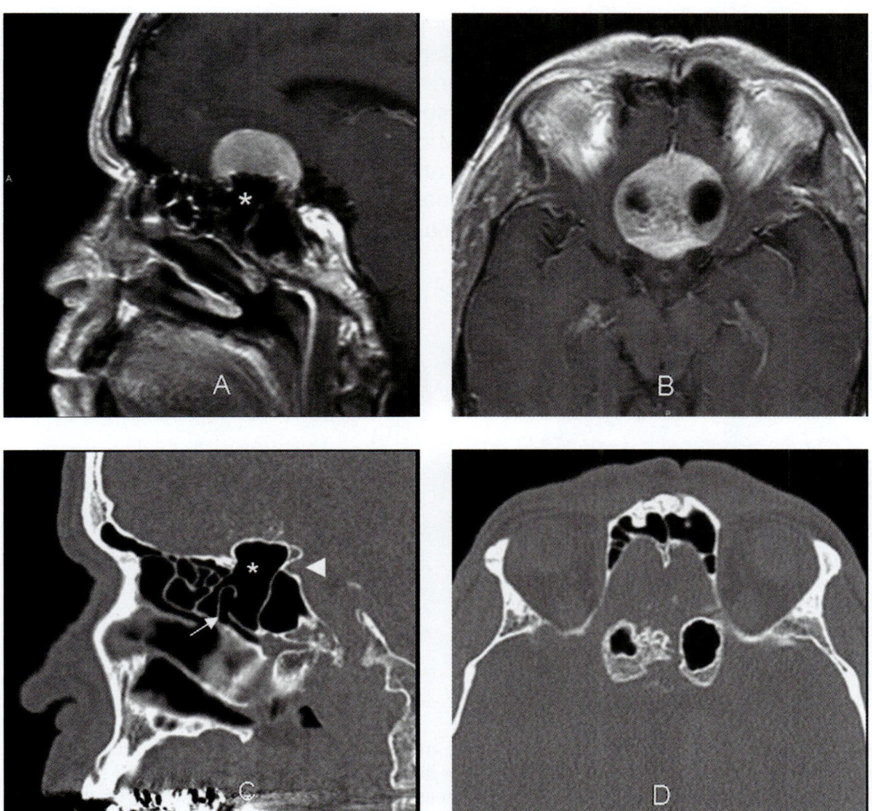

Fig. 3.6 Meningioma of the planum sphenoidale with pneumosinus dilatans. MRI T1WI postgadolinium on sagittal **(A)** and axial **(B)** planes demonstrates a solid mass above a dilated posterior ethmoid with a cranial extension (*). CT on sagittal **(C)** and axial **(D)** multiplanar reconstruction (MPR) images clearly show typical bilateral Onodi cells (*), which present as pneumosinus dilatans related to the meningioma. The sagittal plane is the best way to demonstrate the drainage of the posterior ethmoid cell (*small arrow*) and the relation between the Onodi cell and the optic canal (*arrowhead*). Calcifications inside the meningioma can also be seen on CT images. This lesion is best approached from below.

two particular findings: the presence of bilateral Onodi cells as anatomical variants and pneumosinus dilatans of these cells. The literature describes the association between pneumosinus dilatans and meningioma, as well as an arachnoid cyst or idiopathic finding. In this specific case, an endonasal surgical approach may use these Onodi cells, as they are exactly in the center of the tumor. Both CT and MRI demonstrate an extraaxial well-circumscribed mass, with homogeneous, intense, and diffuse enhancement after IV contrast media. About 25% have calcifications, and hyperostosis and irregular bone cortex are frequent findings. MRI sometimes demonstrates a sunburst pattern. This chapter discusses a meningioma only with enhanced T1WI in two planes and CT with a window for bone structures to demonstrate the combination of the lesion and the anatomical aspects for the surgical approach.

Clivus Chordoma

Chordoma is usually a well-circumscribed multilobulated mass, and it can occur anywhere along the path of the primitive notochord. About one third arise around the spheno-occipital synchondrosis in the skull base.

This tumor is typically located in the midline and is locally invasive, with bone destruction in 95% of cases. Therefore, there are many bone fragments within its matrix. CT demonstrates a mass with mixed density that may contain some low-attenuation areas that represent myxoid material.

It is important to remember that about 80% of these tumors demonstrate tumoral encasement and displacement of vessels on MRA or CTA studies. T2WI demonstrates classically high signal intensity, and T1WI demonstrates some small foci of hyperintensity, representing hemorrhage or mucoid material. Postcontrast T1WI demonstrates moderate or high enhancement, as well as some nonenhancing areas of low intensity, representing necrosis or mucinous material (**Fig. 3.7**). These tumors are often close or in direct contact with the internal carotid artery. An angiographic study with test occlusion should be performed in the preoperative evaluation.

Chondrosarcoma

Chondrosarcoma is a chondroid malignancy, and two thirds are localized in the petro-occipital fissure, followed by the anterior basisphenoid region. Chondroid calcifications are very common. On CT the enhancement may be diffuse or irregular, and bone destruction is part of its behavior. When CTA is performed, a second (venous) acquisition at the skull base might be necessary, because its total enhancement may be relatively slow. On MRI the tumor has low to intermediate signal on T1WI, characteristic hypersignal on T2WI (sometimes low-intensity foci due to calcifications may be seen), and irregular enhancement on enhanced T1WI (**Fig. 3.8**). When an MRA is performed, a venous phase is very important, for the same reason as for CTA. These tumors are also often close to or in direct contact with the internal carotid artery. An angiographic study with test occlusion should be performed in the preoperative evaluation.

Craniopharyngioma

Craniopharyngiomas are derived from remnants of the craniopharyngeal duct and can occur from the floor of the third ventricle to the pituitary gland. There are peaks of incidence at ages 10 to 14 years and 60 to 70 years. There are two main types: adamantinomatous (pediatric) and papillary (adult). Imaging findings depend on the content of the cysts. T1WI signal intensity varies depending on cyst contents, and can appear hyperintense due to protein, blood products, or cholesterol (in the classic adamantinomatous type). In the papillary variety, solid components appear isointense on T1WI.

Peripheral enhancement of the cyst wall is typical, as is diffuse heterogeneous enhancement of the solid components.

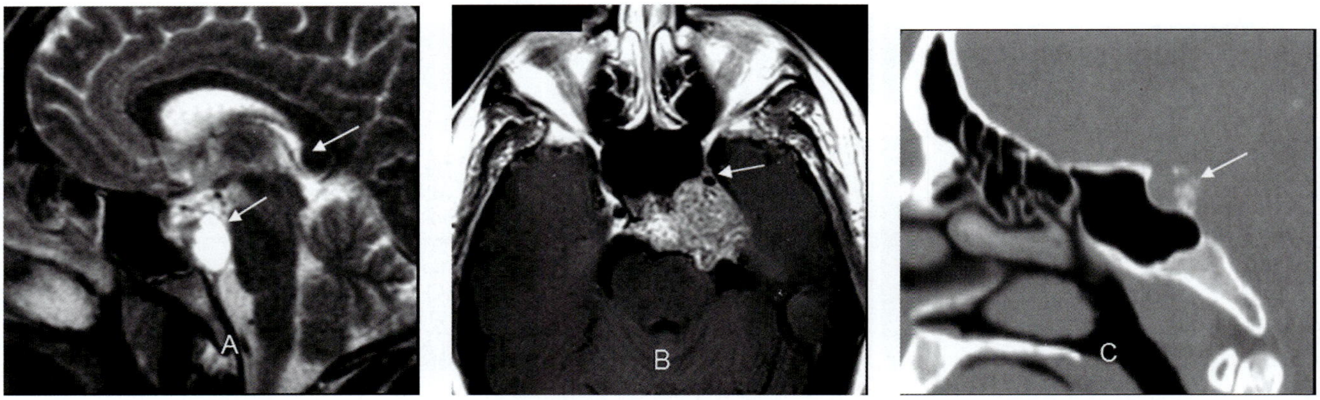

Fig. 3.7 Clivus chordoma. **(A)** MRI sagittal T2WI demonstrates a very hyperintense lesion (*arrows*) located at the dorsum sellae, projecting into the prepontine cistern. **(B)** Postgadolinium T1WI on the axial plane demonstrates an irregular enhancement and the asymmetrical growth of the tumor to the left and posteriorly, whereas the left intracavernous internal carotid artery is dislocated anteriorly (*arrow*). **(C)** CT MPR image on the sagittal plane clearly demonstrates the bony destruction at the dorsum sellae (*arrow*).

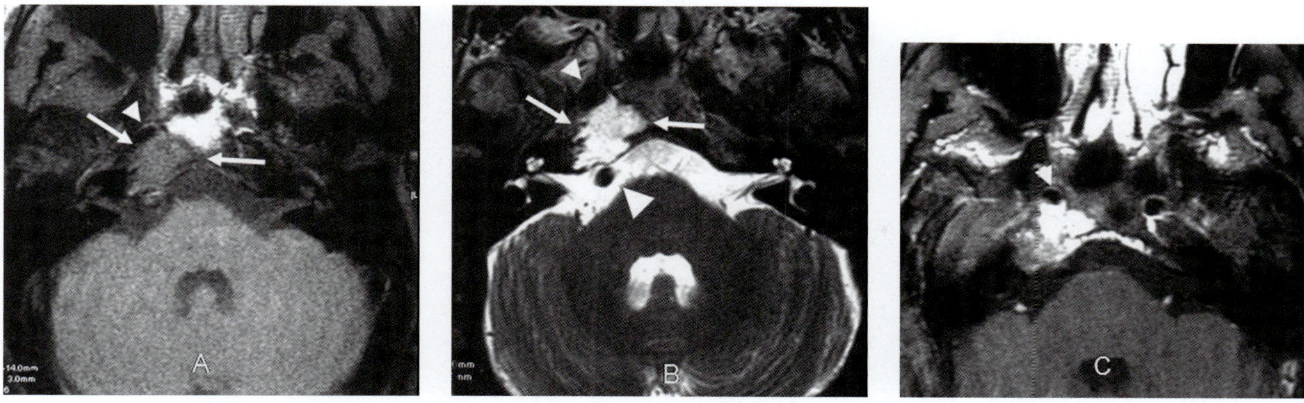

Fig. 3.8 Chondrosarcoma. Axial plane on T1WI **(A)** demonstrates an infiltrating lesion with intermediate signal intensity, on T2WI **(B)** demonstrates a characteristic hyperintensity of the lesion (*arrows*) and a close relation to the basilar artery (*large arrowhead*), and after gadolinium **(C)** demonstrates intense irregular enhancement. Note also the displacement of the right internal carotid artery caused by the tumor (*small arrowhead*).

Peripheral calcifications are very frequent, occurring in 90% of children and 70% of adults.

T2 signal is high in both solid and cystic components, but is variable depending on the content of the fluid. Calcification has a low signal on T2WI (**Fig. 3.9**).

Pituitary Macroadenoma

The pituitary macroadenoma arises from the adenohypophysis, and the most common presentation is an intra- and suprasellar solid tumor, looking like a snowman or the number 8. The size is larger than 1 cm and, when larger than 4 cm, it is called a giant adenoma. On CT the lesion is isodense to the gray matter of the brain before IV contrast media, and it enhances diffusely after the injection. Displacement of the intracavernous internal carotid arteries is common. MRI demonstrates the tumor isointense with gray matter on unenhanced T1WI, and diffuse enhancement on the enhanced T1WI. On T2WI the lesion is also isointense to the gray matter (**Fig. 3.10**).

Hemorrhagic Cystic Adenoma

Cystic adenomas of the pituitary gland may have hemorrhagic content, and it is very important to differentiate this entity from a solid pituitary macroadenoma, as shown in **Fig. 3.10** and **Fig. 3.11**. Due to hemorrhage, there is hyperintensity in the cystic tumor on unenhanced T1WI, and, due to the fluid content, hyperintensity of the cyst is also seen on T2WI. On the enhanced T1WI only a peripheral rim enhances. Compare **Fig. 3.10** and **Fig. 3.11** to see the difference.

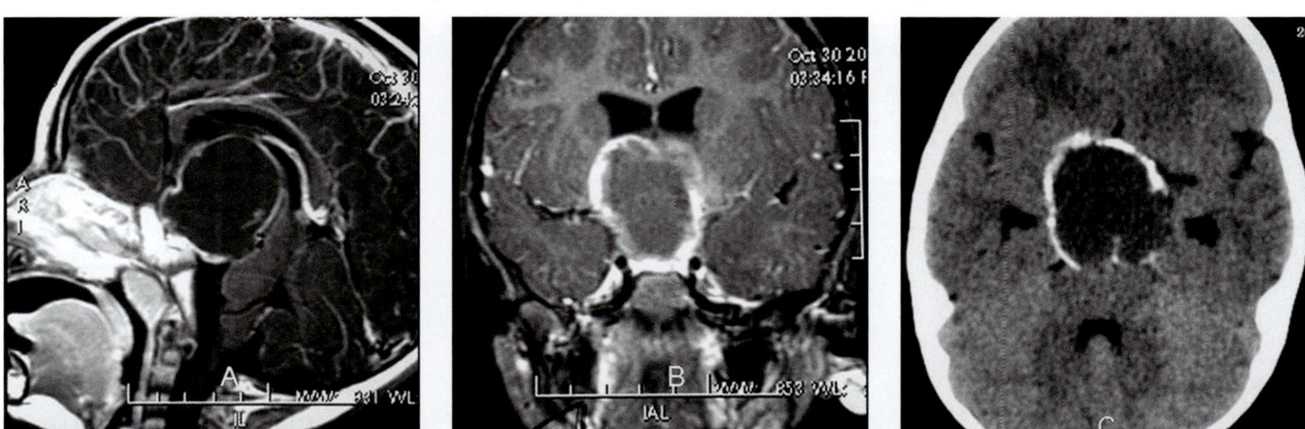

Fig. 3.9 Craniopharyngioma. MRI T1WI postgadolinium on the sagittal **(A)** and coronal **(B)** planes showing a large cystic mass at the midline above the sella turcica, hypointense inside and with peripheral enhancement. **(C)** CT axial image with soft tissue windowing demonstrates the very characteristic peripheral calcifications, as well the hypodense content of the cystic lesion. There is also a slight enlargement of the temporal horns of the lateral ventricles.

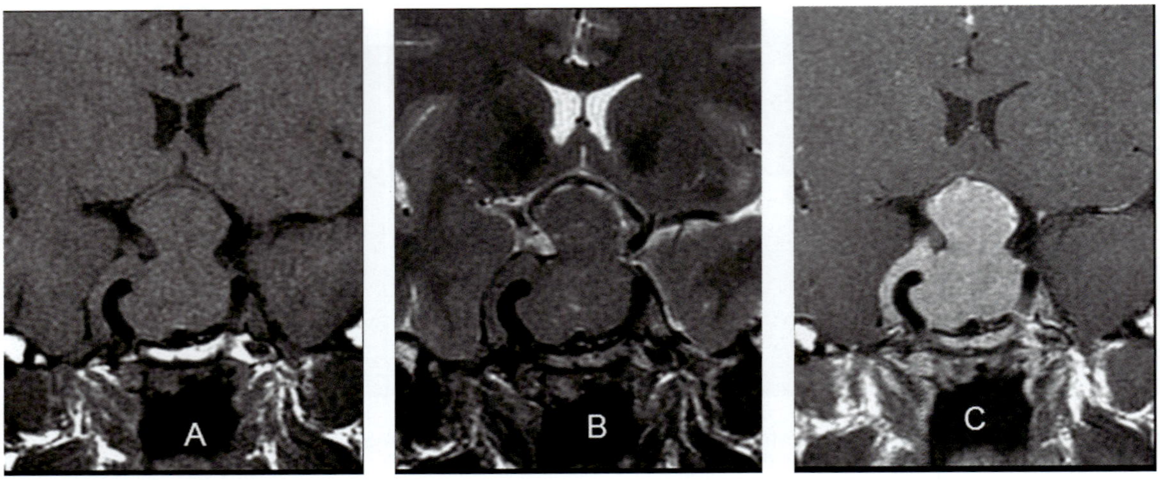

Fig. 3.10 Pituitary macroadenoma. Coronal MRI T1WI **(A)**, T2WI **(B)**, and enhanced T1WI **(C)** demonstrate a snowman-shaped homogeneous solid tumor inside and above the sella turcica, dislocating the internal carotid arteries laterally and the optic chiasma cranially. On unenhanced T1WI and on T2WI the tumor is isointense to the brain parenchyma, and its enhancement is diffuse and homogeneous.

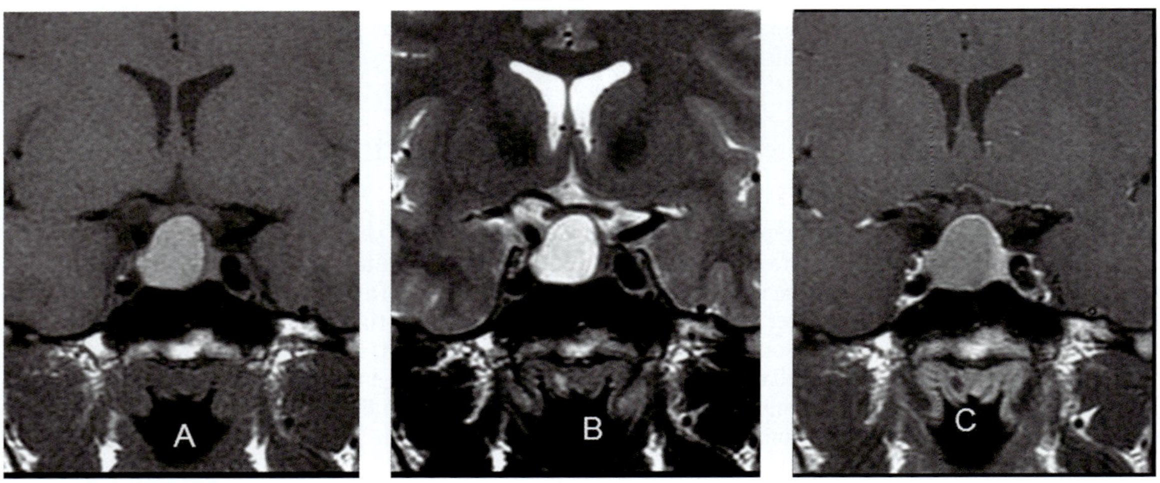

Fig. 3.11 Hemorrhagic cystic adenoma. Coronal MRI T1WI **(A)**, T2WI **(B)**, and T1WI postgadolinium **(C)** demonstrate a different behavior in comparison to a solid pituitary macroadenoma (see **Fig. 3.9**). Note the hyperintense signal inside the tumor on unenhanced T1WI **(A)** and T2WI **(B)**, which characterizes hemorrhagic content, and only a very thin peripheral enhancement after the gadolinium injection **(C)**, which demonstrates the cystic origin of the lesion. Courtesy of Leonardo L. de Macedo, M.D.

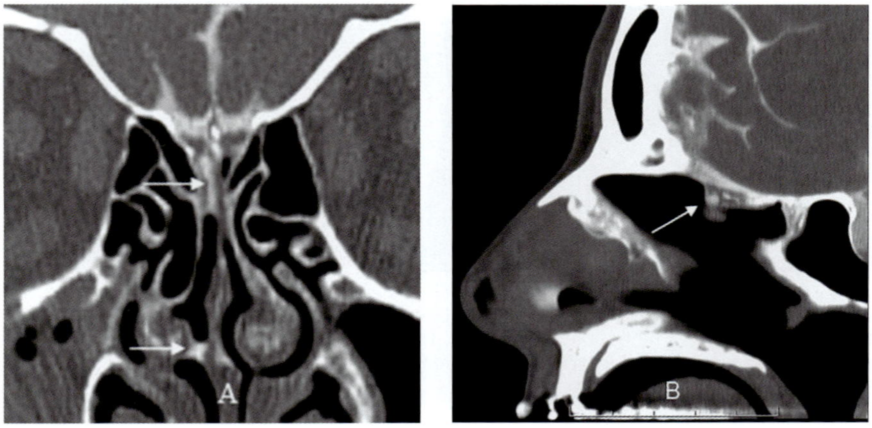

Fig. 3.12 Spontaneous CSF fistula at the lamina cribrosa. **(A)** CT cisternography on the coronal plane, ventral decubitus of the patient, demonstrates the CSF mixed with the intrathecal iodinated contrast media passing through the lamina cribrosa (*arrows*) on the right side. **(B)** The sagittal plane obtained with MPR gives a better notion of the exact location of the CSF fistula (*arrow*).

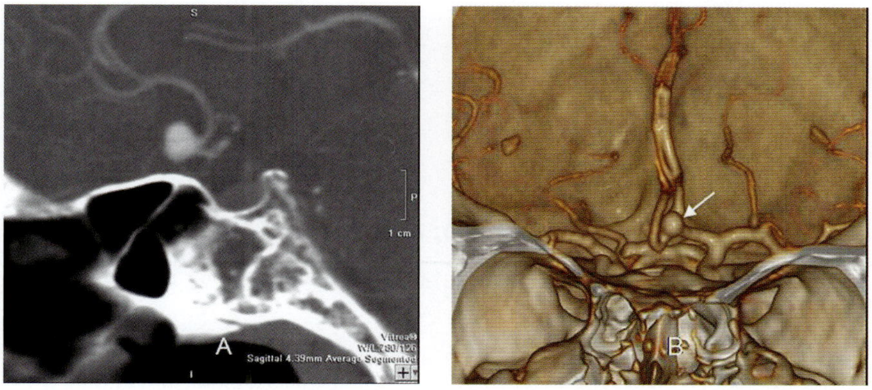

Fig. 3.13 Aneurysm of the anterior communicating artery. CTA on the sagittal plane with MIP technique **(A)** and a volume rendering 3D reconstruction in frontal view **(B)** facilitate a precise evaluation of this aneurysm.

Cerebrospinal Fluid Leak (CSF Fistula)

Cerebrospinal fluid leak may be spontaneous or secondary to trauma, tumor (especially in the pituitary gland), congenital anomalies, or surgery (complications). The most common sites are the lamina cribrosa and the fovea ethmoidalis. In some cases, fistulas have been demonstrated in the sphenoid sinus, especially in the clivus in cases of basilar expansion of this sinus and in the roof of a pneumatized pterygoid process, where it is not rare to find a point of thinning or dehiscence of the bone. The gold standard in imaging is still the CT-cisternography, using the following technique:

1. Subarachnoid injection of nonionic iodinated contrast media
2. Trendelenburg positioning of the patient for less than a minute
3. Application of cotton pledges in both nasal cavities, which will be wetted by CSF and contrast media in case of fistula
4. Prone positioning of the patient
5. Volumetric acquisition of the whole face (including the cotton plugs)
6. When necessary, performing of a second acquisition with the patient in the supine position
7. Reformation in axial, coronal, and sagittal planes (**Fig. 3.12**).

Aneurysm

The Circle of Willis is the most common location for an aneurysm (more than 90% of cases); the majority occur in the anterior communicating artery. CTA and MRA are both excellent diagnostic methods. MRA does not demonstrate the bone, and CTA can be documented with or without the bone. On CTA the lumen of the vessel and the aneurysm enhance strongly, and postprocessing is performed with MIP and VR protocols (**Fig. 3.13**). On MRI there is low ("flow void") or heterogeneous signal on T1WI and low intensity on T2WI. Sometimes the signal intensity is mixed or laminated. MRA is performed with a 3D-TOF (three-dimensional "time-of-flight") technique, a gradient-echo sequence which provides a bright vascular image based on the difference between unsaturated spins from the flowing blood and the presaturated spins of the stationary tissue (better results are obtained with intravenous contrast media).

References

1. Aygun N, Zinreich JS. Imaging of the skull base. In: Anand VK, Schwartz TH, eds. Practical Endoscopic Skull Base Surgery. San Diego: Plural Publishing; 2007:25–43
2. Stamm AC, Flávio (Nogueira) J, Harvey RJ. Revision endoscopic skull base surgery. In: Kountakis SE, ed. Revision Endoscopic Surgery. New York: Springer; 2008:289–300
3. Haetinger RG. Imaging of the nose and paranasal sinuses. In: Stamm AC, Draf W, eds. Micro-Endoscopic Surgery of the Paranasal Sinuses and the Skull Base. Berlin: Springer; 2000:53–81
4. Earwaker J. Anatomic variants in sinonasal CT. Radiographics 1993; 13:381–415
5. Keros P. Über die Praktische Bedeutung der Niveauunterschiede der Lamina Cribrosa des Ethmoids (About the practical significance of the different levels of the cribriform plate of the ethmoid). Z Laryngol Rhinol Otol Ihre Grenzgeb 1962;41:808–813.
6. Ónodi A. Der Sehnerv und die Nebennasenhöhlen der Nase (The optic nerve and the paranasal sinuses) Vienna and Leipzig: Alfred Hölder Verlag, 1907:6–34, 42–69.
7. Haetinger RG, Navarro JA, Liberti EA. Basilar expansion of the human sphenoidal sinus: an integrated anatomical and computerized tomography study. Eur Radiol 2006;16:2092–2099
8. Sorimachi T, Kamada K, Ozawa T, Takeuchi S. Basilar artery vasculitis secondary to sphenoid sinusitis—case report. Neurol Med Chir (Tokyo) 2001;41:454–457
9. Jenkins HA, Calcaterra TC. Spontaneous cerebrospinal rhinorrhea from the sphenoid sinus. Trans Sect Otolaryngol Am Acad Ophthalmol Otolaryngol 1977;84:ORL916–ORL918
10. Coiteiro D, Távora L, Antunes JL. Spontaneous cerebrospinal fluid fistula through the clivus: report of two cases. Neurosurgery 1995;37: 826–828
11. Stamm AC, Freire LAS. Cerebrospinal fluid rhinorrhea: transnasal micro-endoscopic surgery. In: Stamm AC, Draf W, eds. Micro-Endoscopic Surgery of the Paranasal Sinuses and the Skull Base. Berlin: Springer; 2000:451–463
12. Jho HD, Carrau RL, McLaughlin MR, Somaza SC. Endoscopic transsphenoidal resection of a large chordoma in the posterior fossa. Acta Neurochir (Wien) 1997;139:343–347, discussion 347–348
13. Harnsberger HR. Diagnostic Imaging: Head and Neck. Salt Lake City: Amirsys; 2005:II-2-1 to II-2-99
14. Osborn AG. Diagnostic Imaging: Brain. Salt Lake City: Amirsys; 2004: II-4-1 to II-4-83

4 Nasal Endoscopy in the Preoperative Assessment

Juan Eugenio Salas Galicia, Raúl Omar Cadena Torrero, and María Chávez Méndez

Tips and Pearls

- The preoperative evaluation of a transnasal craniotomy assisted by endoscopy must include a clinical history with complete physical examination, imaging studies, and diagnostic nasal endoscopy.
- Nasal endoscopy and computed tomography imaging are the gold standard diagnostic tools for sinonasal diseases.
- The nasal endoscopic evaluation and imaging studies should be performed preferably the day before surgery.
- A systematic preoperative nasal endoscopy is fundamental to identify the characteristics of the mucosa, mucus, secretions, and the anatomical variations of the nasal structures, including the nasal septum.
- A nasoseptal mucosa flap may be used for reconstruction of the dural or skull base defect.
- Rigid endoscopes are preferable for adult evaluation: 2.7 mm (30, 45, and 70 degrees) and whenever possible 4 mm (45 and 75 degrees). Flexible endoscopes are indicated for narrow nasal cavities or in children.
- The video equipment, the computer, and the software of high-definition imaging capture are complementary to an endoscopic evaluation of excellence.
- Systematic endoscopic nasal evaluation with digital or high definition (HD) cameras in the doctor's office provides the surgeon with training about different diseases, and provides an opportunity to acquire indispensable skills and abilities in endoscopic skull base surgery.
- The documentation of the endoscopic nasal evaluation findings in a computerized database is very important, especially in patients who have had previous surgery.
- The biopsy, the contact mucosal endoscopy, and identification of the cerebrospinal fluid (CSF) fistula with fluorescein are other applications of endoscopic nasal evaluation.
- It is mandatory, for our own benefit and that of the patient, to use the best technology we can afford.

Introduction

"A picture is worth a thousand words." The images provided by endoscopic examination are a powerful diagnostic tool in the area of otorhinolaryngology–head and neck surgery and neurosurgery, particularly for the evaluation of the nose, paranasal sinuses, and skull base region. Nasal endoscopy was first performed by Hirschmann in 1901 using a modified cystoscope, and soon after it was applied in minor surgical procedures by Reichert, Valentine, Sargnon, and Zaufal, from 1902 to 1908. The use of endoscopes for diagnostic and surgical treatment purposes presented a great development in the late 1960s with the introduction of the Hopkins cylindrical lenses, thereby improving the diagnostic and surgical capabilities of this instrument both for providing a direct vision and for photo documentation. Messerklinger introduced systematic exploration of the lateral nasal wall, confirming with his vast clinical experience that most of the diseases of the paranasal sinuses are rhinogenic. He also found that these diseases were generally related to two fundamental areas that he called the ostiomeatal complex and the sphenoethmoidal recess. His studies provided more precise knowledge of the anatomical structures and the sinonasal physiology.[1–3]

Indications

Diagnostic nasal endoscopy is indicated in the following cases:

1. Chronic obstructive rhinopathy
2. Recurrent or chronic rhinosinusitis
3. Facial neuralgia or headache, mostly associated with previous sinonasal surgery
4. Persistent rhinorrhea
5. Epistaxis
6. Epiphora
7. Chronic pharyngitis or laryngitis
8. Rhinopharynx diseases
9. Chronic or recurrent otitis media
10. Anosmia or hyposmia
11. CSF leakage (topodiagnostic)
12. Sinonasal tumors
13. Skull base tumors
14. Sinonasal and skull base tumor biopsies (when indicated)
15. Postoperative follow-up of endoscopic sinus surgery and transnasal craniectomy[2,4–6]

Contraindications

Rigid nasal endoscopy in the doctor's office under local anesthesia is usually contraindicated in uncooperative children or in apprehensive adults or psychiatric patients. For these patients, flexible endoscopy under topical anesthesia is well tolerated. General anesthesia is rarely required.

Risk Factors

In general, nasal endoscopy should be avoided in the elderly and in patients with a history of asthma and hypersensitivity, heart disease, and facial pain, and in hypervascularized tumors when their size makes it difficult to introduce the endoscope into the nasal cavity.

Complications

Complications of nasal endoscopy in the doctor's office are very uncommon and may occur due to vasoconstrictors and local anesthetics, which can occasionally cause tachycardia, hypersensitivity, and high blood pressure. Other complications are related to the procedure itself, and include injury to the mucosa, epistaxis, vagal reaction, nasofacial neuralgias, and asthmatic events. After taking into account the contraindications and risk factors listed above and these possible complications, nasal endoscopy, as a preoperative evaluation, is a safe and effective procedure of high diagnostic value.[2,3,5,6]

Equipment

Telescopes: 2.7 mm, 30, 45, and 70 degrees; 4 mm, 30 and 45 degrees; flexible nasofibrolaryngoscope, 3.5 mm/ 2.5 mm in diameter

Light source: Xenon 175 or 300 W; cold light source LED Nova 100 W (new option)

Cable of fiber optics or optic fluid (recommended for photo documentation)

Video: Analog or digital, three chips or high-definition camera (HD Image 1, Karl Storz Endoscopy, Flanders, NJ); the authors consider the high definition camera the most appropriate in terms of image

Monitor: A 19" LCD flat monitor SXGA (1280 × 1024) resolution or a 23" wide-view HD monitor (1920 × 1200) resolution[11]

Documentation: HDD and DVD video recorder or Blue-Ray HDD recorder (Sony or Panasonic); UP-D 55 digital Sony video printer

Computer Equipment

Hardware: PC: Intel dual or quad core processor; Chipset Intel motherboard; DDR2 or DDR3 memory, 4.0 Gb recommended; S-ATA-II hard disk drive, 300 MBps, 7200 Rpm, 320.0 Gb recommended; HD or full-HD capable PCI express 16× video card, 512 Mb DDR2 or DDR3 minimum; LCD monitor 20" wide screen with digital inputs (DVI or HDMI); DVD or Blu-Ray writer drive; multiple memory flash card reader; PS2 or USB keyboard; PS2 or USB laser mouse; uninterruptible power system, with at least twice the total power consumption. A mirror disk array (Raid-1) is recommended for data protection in case of hardware failure.

Macintosh HD: Intel Xeon "Nehalem" dual or quad core processor, 2.66 GHz, 3 to 8 GB memory, 640 GB hard disk; Express 18× super drive disc; Chipset motherboard, NVIDIA GeForce GT 120 with 512 MB; LED Cinema Apple Monitor, 24" display, 1920 × 1200p image

PC software: Windows XP Professional is the most stable operating system (with the Pinnacle studio 12 capture and editing software).

Mac software: XO 10.5.6 operating system with the Final Cut Pro Edition software

Data archiving system: The Karl Storz AIDA® DVD-M is the ideal system (state of the art) for data, image, and video archiving, report writing and printing, and automated storing with image or video inspection, DVD, CD-ROM, or USB stick recording. Another database solution for file control is Capturis, a powerful database developed on FileMaker Pro 10; it works on a PC or Mac platform (**Fig. 4.1**). Other options on the market are Pentax-Kay, Olympus, Ecleris, and others. Clinicians must choose a system that is appropriate for the particular needs of their daily practice.

Method

Basic Diagnostic Nasal Endoscopy

In addition to nasal endoscopy, several functional tests may also be used to evaluate the nasal cavity, including active anterior rhinomanometry and acoustic rhinometry (**Fig. 4.2**), olfactometry, and mucociliary clearance. It is important to avoid using irritating substances that can disturb the nasal mucosa. The diagnostic nasal endoscopy is performed with the patient seated or in a recumbent position, after a traditional anterior rhinoscopy (**Fig. 4.3**). The evaluation takes place without any anesthesia or vasoconstriction medication. The nasal cavity is assessed with a 2.7-mm, 30-degree endoscope, which offers a wider anterior view. The tip of the endoscope is inserted slowly and carefully into the vestibule and nasal valve region to avoid any discomfort to the patient, without touching the nasal septum or the lateral nasal wall. It is very important to visualize both nasal cavities as completely as possible. The characteristics of the mucosa, mucus, and nasal secretions are assessed, as well as the anatomical variations. This procedure is more difficult to perform with a 4-mm telescope due to its larger diameter. In this phase, cultures guided by endoscopy may be taken by using a suction-collector device (Juhn Tym-Tap®, Xomed Inc., Jacksonville, FL) or even with an ear aspirator. A cheaper alternative would be a urologic swab for culture.

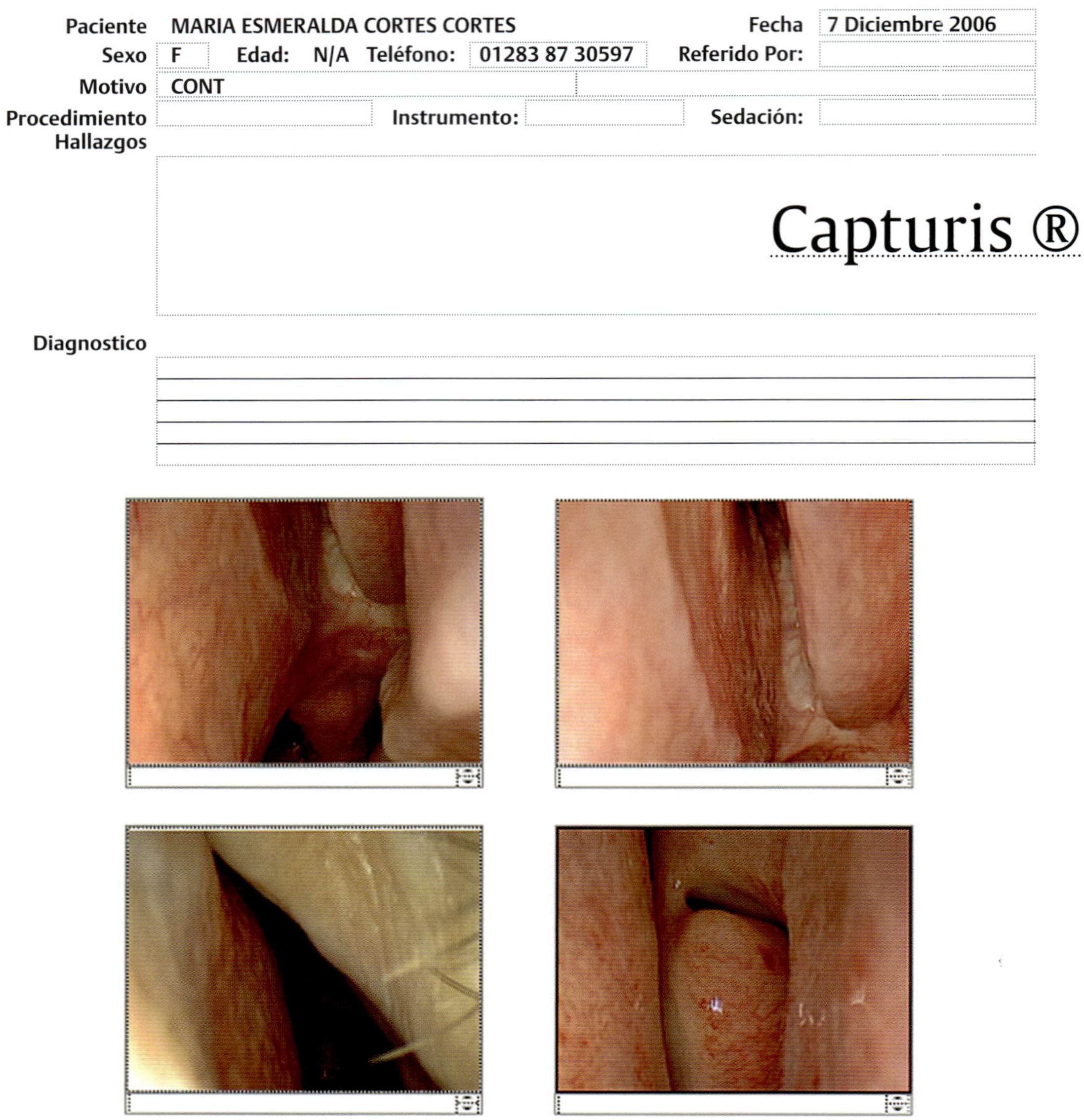

Paciente MARIA ESMERALDA CORTES CORTES Fecha 7 Diciembre 2006
Sexo F Edad: N/A Teléfono: 01283 87 30597 Referido Por:
Motivo CONT
Procedimiento Instrumento: Sedación:
Hallazgos

Capturis ®

Diagnostico

Fig. 4.1 Endoscopic Capturis report sheet.

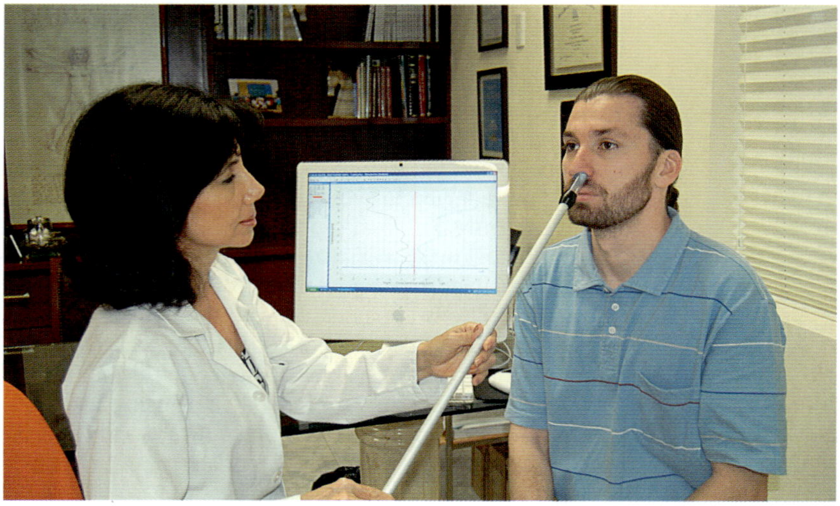

Fig. 4.2 Functional nasal test (rhinometry).

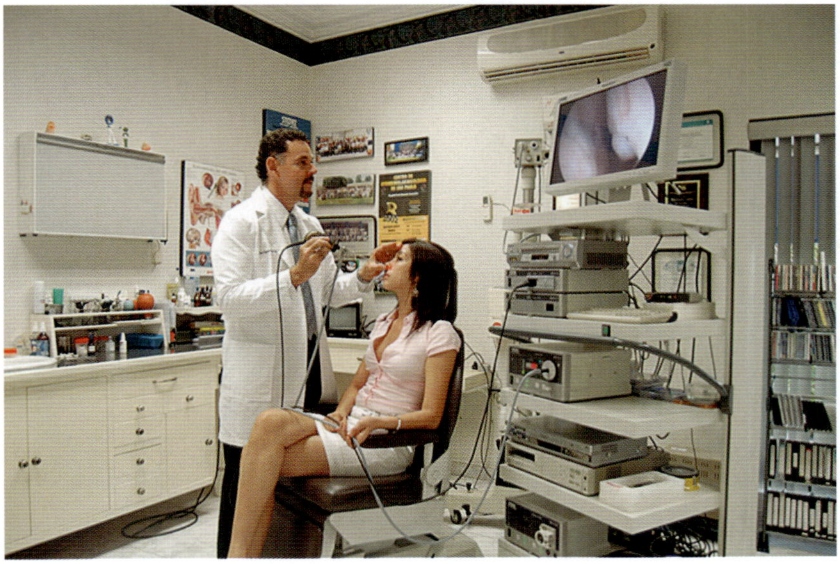

Fig. 4.3 Nasal endoscopy evaluation.

Diagnostic Nasal Endoscopy

At the completion of the basal endoscopy, the patient's nasal cavities are decongested and anesthetized with 1% oxymetazoline and 4% lidocaine atomization. After 10 minutes, nasal function tests are performed (**Fig. 4.2**). Sometimes it is necessary to reinforce the anesthesia and vasoconstriction in the middle meatus, sphenoethmoidal recess, or olfactory area, or in narrow zones where the contact endoscope may cause disturbance or pain. It is advisable to begin the endoscopy with a 4-mm, 30-degree endoscope, which gives a panoramic view of the nasal cavity. In cases of limited space, a 2.7-mm, 30- or 45-degree endoscope is recommended. Nasal endoscopy is performed in a systematic manner in the following three steps (**Figs. 4.4** and **4.5**).

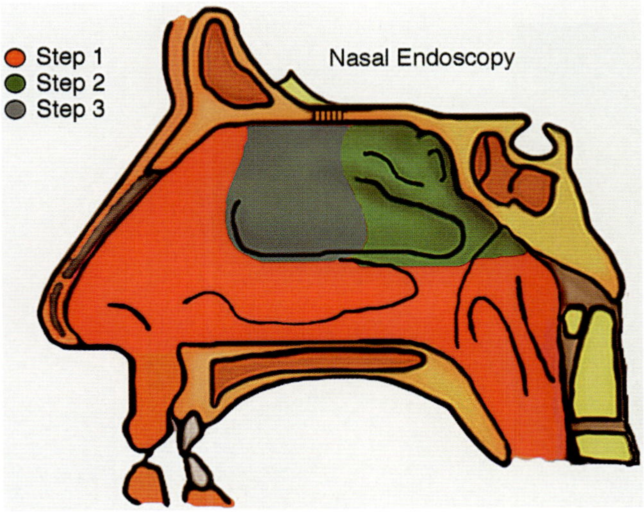

Fig. 4.4 Systematic nasal endoscopy: three steps.

1. Nasal Vestibule, Nasal Valve, Rhinopharynx, and Inferior Meatus

The examination begins by introducing the endoscope through the nostril, visualizing the vestibule and nasal valve without distortion; it is carefully slipped on the floor of the nasal cavity using the septum and inferior turbinate as anatomical parameters. These structures are inspected on the way to the rhinopharynx, paying careful attention to the end of the inferior turbinate and the eustachian tube. The endoscope is then rotated 90 degrees to visualize the ipsilateral eustachian tube. Dynamic action is assessed, requiring the patient

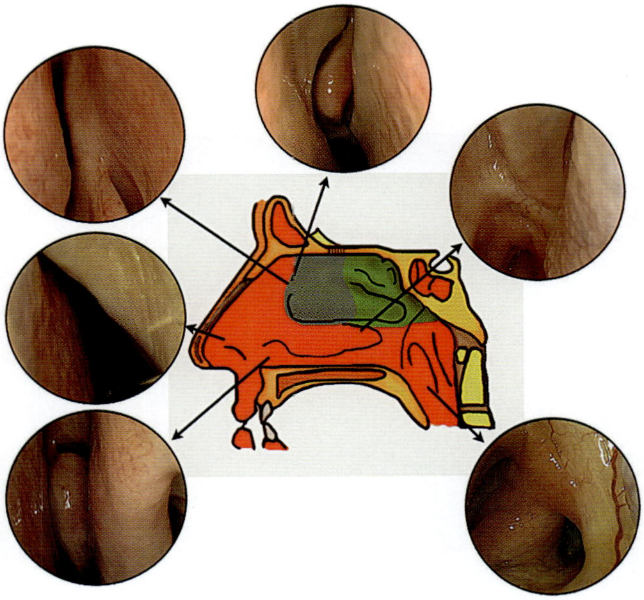

Fig. 4.5 Endoscopic images performing systematic endoscopic examination of the nasal cavity.

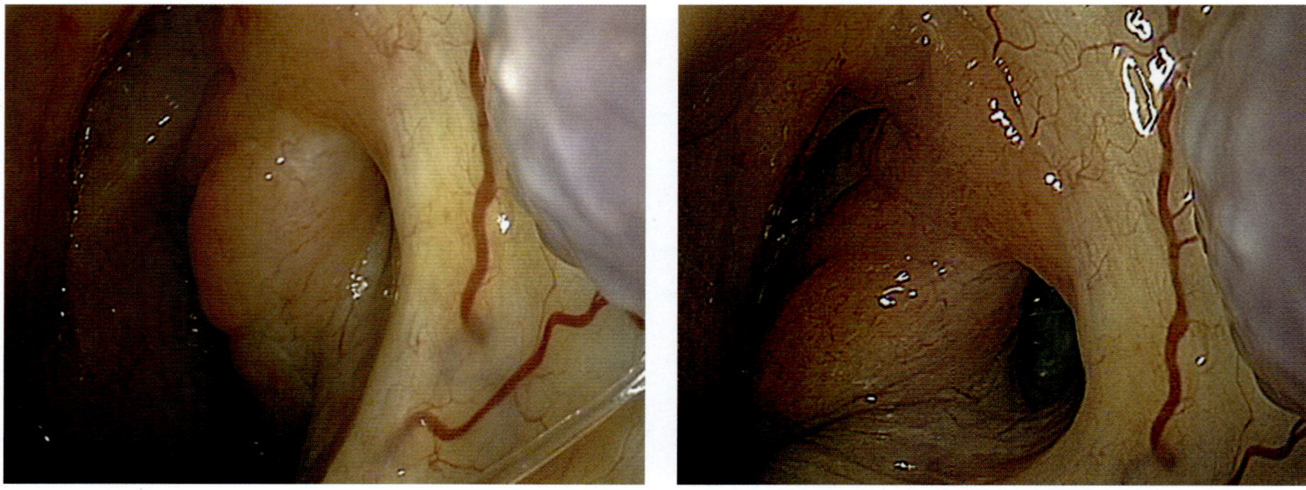

A B

Fig. 4.6 Dynamic action of the eustachian tube. **(A)** Closed. **(B)** Open.

to swallow (**Fig. 4.6**). At this point, it is possible to inspect the tubal prominence and the Rosenmüller's recess. Going back to the neutral position of the endoscope and turning it 90 degrees toward the contralateral eustachian tube (**Fig. 4.7**), the choana and the superior portion of the rhinopharynx can be visualized. The presence of adenoidal tissue or the persistence of Rathke's pouch can be observed. The endoscope is then withdrawn and turned to the inferior meatus to locate Hasner's valve, which corresponds to the final point of the nasolacrimal duct and can be expanded by gently pressing the internal cantus of the eye (tears, mucus, or purulent material will drain if there is pathology at this level).

2. Sphenoethmoidal Recess, Superior Meatus, and Posterior Olfactory Cleft

The endoscope is reintroduced between the inferior and middle turbinate, heading toward the sphenoethmoidal recess and superior meatus. With a good vasoconstriction and anesthesia, it may be possible to see the natural sphenoidal sinus ostium. This step is concluded by observing the olfactory fissure in its posterior portion, especially in patients with olfactory or taste disturbances, or when a cerebrospinal fluid (CSF) fistula and skull base tumors are suspected (**Fig. 4.5**).

3. Middle Meatus, Ostiomeatal Complex, and Anterior Olfactory Area

The endoscope surrounds the tail of the middle turbinate and goes under it. By retracting the endoscope, the middle meatus, uncinate process, hiatus semilunaris, accessory ostium, and occasionally the natural maxillary ostium, ethmoidal bulla, and frontal recess can be seen. Sometimes a Freer elevator is helpful to discretely displace the middle turbinate without fracturing it, permitting better visualization of the ostiomeatal complex. Smears and cultures can be taken

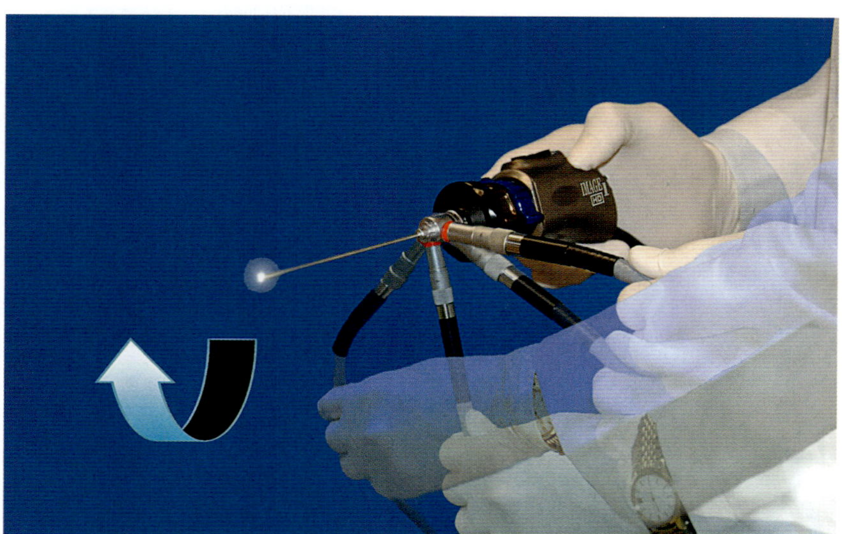

Fig. 4.7 Acquiring a lateral view with angled endoscopes by light cable rotation.

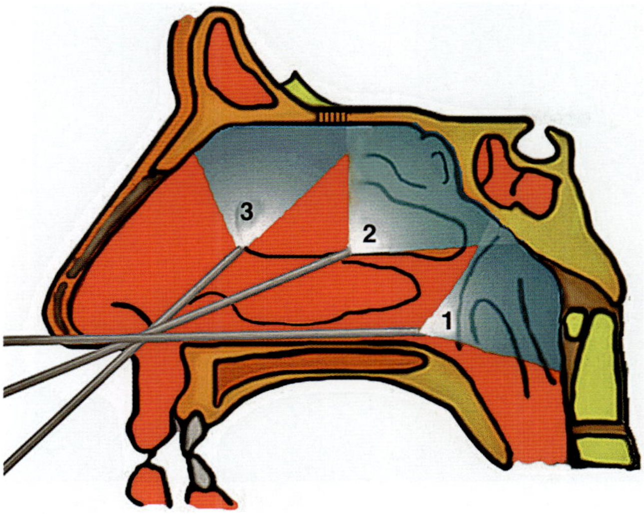

Fig. 4.8 Target nasal endoscopy: three steps in the preoperative assessment for skull base surgery.

if necessary. Finally, the endoscope is withdrawn from the middle meatus and reintroduced to assess the anterior olfactory fissure. A 2.7-mm, 30- or 45-degree endoscope is recommended (**Fig. 4.5**).[2–4,6,7,9]

Schematic Review of the Three Steps

Step 1: vestibule → nasal valve → inferior turbinate → choana → nasopharynx's posterior and superior wall → turn 90 degrees, eustachian tube orifice → Rosenmüller's recess → turn 180 degrees to the opposite side → contralateral eustachian tube and Rosenmüller's recess → retract endoscope and rotating → inferior meatus → nasolacrimal duct

Step 2: reintroduce endoscope → choana's upper edge → sphenoethmoidal recess → superior and supreme turbinates → sphenoid sinus ostium → olfactory fissure (posterior aspect)

Step 3: endoscope into the middle meatus → careful medialization of the middle turbinate (Freer); do not fracture it → sphenopalatine area → uncinate process → hiatus semilunaris → natural or accessory maxillary ostium → ethmoidal infundibulum → ethmoidal bulla → frontal recess → retracting endoscope → olfactory fissure (anterior aspect) (**Fig. 4.5**)

The areas to be visualized and documented in a nasal endoscopy as a preoperative assessment for endoscopic transnasal craniectomy (**Figs. 4.8** and **4.9**) are as follows:

- Step 1: nasopharynx → transclival/transodontoid/craniocervical junction surgical approach
- Step 2: sphenoethmoidal recess → transplanum/sellar and parasellar surgical approach
- Step 3: olfactory cleft → transcribriform approach/frontal sinusotomy (Draf III) sphenopalatine area → surgical approach: vascularized mucosal septal flap (posterior lateral nasal artery)

Complementary Endoscopic Procedures

Biopsy

A biopsy is performed, when indicated, by introducing the surgical punches always underneath and in front of the endoscope. The instruments are slowly moved ahead, ensuring their visualization on the monitor. The fiberoptic cable is lateralized if the cable hinders the movement of the surgical instrument inside the nasal cavity (**Fig. 4.7**). This procedure is an ideal opportunity for the development and improvement of the surgeon's skills and abilities in handing the endoscope and surgical instruments, which is indispensable in performing an endoscopic atraumatic surgery.

Maxillary Sinus Endoscopy

Maxillary sinus endoscopy is indicated in cases suspicious for malignancy, mycosis, cysts, polyps, or symptomatic mucocele, and for aspiration of thick secretions, cultures, and foreign bodies.[2,6,9] An approach via the canine fossa is indicated for patients older than 9 years of age; an approach

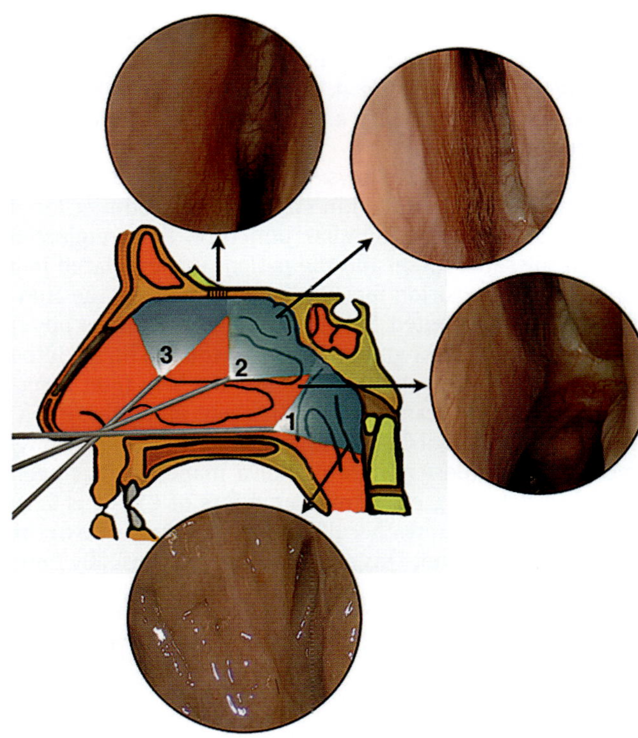

Fig. 4.9 Endoscopic images of the endonasal skull base as a preoperative evaluation.

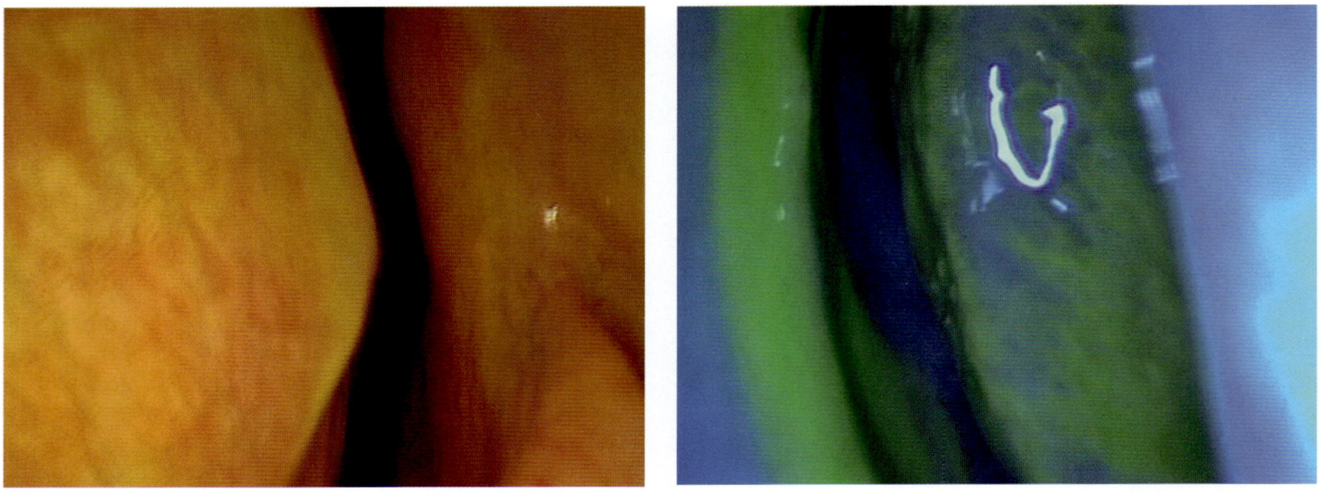

A B

Fig. 4.10 Intrathecal sodium fluorescein in the nasal cavity. (A) No filter. (B) Blue filter.

via the inferior meatus is indicated for children age 9 and younger.[2]

Localization of Cerebrospinal Fluid Fistulas Using Fluorescein and Blue Filter

After intrathecal injection of a 5% sodium fluorescein solution and performing a diagnostic nasal endoscopy, the site and exact location of a skull base defect can be determined. When the image studies do not reveal the site of the lesion, a preoperative endoscopic fluorescein test with or without a blue filter is performed (**Fig. 4.10**). Sometimes the CSF fistula is located in the middle ear, and the leak through the eustachian tube is seen.

The technique is as follows: 0.2 to 0.5 mL of 5% sodium fluorescein solution diluted in 10 cc of CSF is administered through an intrathecal lumbar puncture. It is reinjected through the same route, and the patient is then placed in a Trendelenburg position for 30 minutes, allowing the fluorescein to be distributed. Subsequently, a nasal endoscopy is performed, looking for greenish-yellow–colored liquid. If the site of the fistula is not found, the use of a blue filter is recommended, as it enhances the fluorescein; under these conditions, even minimal CSF traces appear as a glowing yellow/green. In our experience the Valsalva maneuver has been helpful in detecting even small amounts of CSF. It is very important that the intrathecal fluorescein solution be in the correct concentration. This entire procedure is usually done in the operating room as a preoperative study.[9]

Contact Endoscopy

Contact endoscopy of the nasal mucosa has great pre- and perioperative diagnostic value for the evaluation of sinonasal and skull base diseases. However, to become a standard perioperative evaluation it requires more studies, systematization, training, and experience.[10]

■ Conclusion

Routine diagnostic nasal endoscopy as a preoperative assessment for skull base surgery is paramount. It is also an opportunity for the development of the necessary skills in handling the endoscopes and surgical instruments, which is an essential requirement for adequate endoscopic surgeon training. The accurate documentation of the nasal endoscopic findings as a part of the patient file in the computer database is of the upmost importance. These data can be particularly useful and of a great value in medicolegal issues, particularly in cases of previous surgery. Moreover, the nasal endoscopy evaluates the characteristics of the mucosa, anatomical variations of the septum, and the sphenopalatine artery area. This will be important for designing and planning the confection of the pedicled vascularized nasoseptal flap, which will ultimately be used to reconstruct the great skull base and to seal occasional dural defects.

References

1. Kaluskar SK, Patil NP. Office Nasal Endoscopy in the Evaluation of Chronic Sinus Disease. Tuttlingen, Germany: Endo-Press; 2002
2. Stammberger H. Functional endoscopic sinus surgery. In: Endoscopic and Radiologic Diagnosis. Philadelphia: B.C. Decker; 1991:145–271
3. Pownell P, Minoli J, Rohrich R. Diagnostic Nasal Endoscopy. Plast Reconstr Surg; 1997:99(5):1451–1458
4. Behrbohm H, Kaschke O. In: Nasal Endoscopy. Universitätsklinikum Charité Berlin. Tuttlingen, Germany: Hals-Nasen-Ohrenklinik; 1990
5. Kennedy D. Pathogenesis of Chronic Rhinosinusitis. Penn International Rhinology Course. Advances in Management of Sino-Nasal Disease. Philadelphia: University of Pennsylvania, 2005

6. Salas JE, Chávez M, Cadena O. Evaluación endoscópica de las patologías nasosinusales. In: Stamm A, ed. Rhinology. Sao Paulo, Brazil: Komedi; 2002:28–33

7. Simmen D, Jones N. An endoscopic tour: endoscopic examination. Anatomical variations, and specific conditions. In: Manual of Endoscopic Sinus Surgery and Its Extended Applications. Stuttgart, New York: Thieme;2005:106–120

8. Castelnuovo P. Mauri S, Locatelli D, et al. Diagnostic endoscopy. In: Endoscopic Cadaver Dissection of the Nose and Paranasal Sinuses. Tuttlingen, Germany: Endo-Press; 2004:8–13

9. Stammberger H. Technique of Diagnostic Nasal Endoscopy. In: Functional Endoscopic Sinus Surgery: Endoscopic Diagnosis and Surgery of the Paranasal Sinuses and Anterior Skull Base. Tuttlingen, Germany: Braun-Druck GmbH; 2002:8–18

10. Andrea M, Dias O. Contact endoscopy of nasal mucosa. In: Storz K, ed. The World of Endoscopy. Sinuscopy/Rhinoscopy/Postrhinoscopy. Tuttlingen, Germany: 2004:210

11. Karl Storz Endoscope history since 1945. http://www.karlstorz.com

5 Transnasal Surgical Approaches for Skull Base Lesions

Eduardo Vellutini, Aldo Cassol Stamm, Shirley S.N. Pignatari, and Leonardo Balsalobre Filho

Tips and Pearls

- The nasal steps of the transnasal endoscopic surgical approaches can produce injuries that might affect the patient's quality of life.
- The best surgical approach should be chosen on an individual basis depending on the location, size, and complexity of the lesion, particularly if a subsequent reconstruction step is being considered.
- The direct transnasal surgical approach is the first choice of access for the management of most of the cases of small, well-defined cerebrospinal fluid (CSF) fistulas and also for orbital decompression.
- The bi-nostril transnasal/transseptal endonasal surgical approach is the most suitable to remove sellar tumors that are located medially in the skull base. This surgical approach allows the surgeon to use two hands, minimizing the need for or totally avoiding a septal perforation. Furthermore, it allows the creation of a vascularized nasal septal mucosal flap, which can be used for the reconstruction of the skull base.
- The extended transsphenoidal approach is ideal to remove midline intradural tumors presenting anterior extension to the planum sphenoidale or to the suprasellar region.
- Removal of malignant tumors sometimes requires extra-septal mucosal flaps for the reconstruction step, because the septal mucosa might be involved by the tumor.
- The lateral transmaxillary-transpterygoidal surgical approach is indicated to remove tumors located more laterally, especially the ones extending into the cavernous sinus region. This surgical approach permits the complete exposure of the anterior vertical segment of the internal carotid artery.

Introduction

Since the introduction of modern endoscopic surgical techniques, transnasal endoscopic skull base surgery has been indicated for the management of lesions located from the cribriform plate to the clivus and C2, showing low rates of morbidity and mortality.[1–5]

Endoscopic surgical treatment approaches for the majority of skull base lesions usually requires entering the sphenoid sinus, the most posterior of the paranasal sinuses. To enter the sphenoid sinus through the nose, knowledge and understanding of the nasal cavity and sphenoid sinus anatomy, physiology, and function are paramount. It is always important to remember that the sphenoid sinus presents close anatomical relations to important structures, such as the optic nerves, the internal carotid arteries, and the cavernous sinus.

Several surgical approaches to the sphenoid sinus have been proposed over the years, both microscopically and endoscopically. From sublabial, to transoral, to fully endoscopic transnasal approaches, much has been described.

Most of the surgical approaches developed in recent years have focused on how to avoid the most frightening complications usually related to surgeries, such as vascular and neural injuries, cerebrospinal fistula (CSF), and meningitis.

However, little attention has been given to a very important part of this surgical approach—the nasal step. Although not life threatening, some nasal complications, such as epistaxis, septal perforation, infection, and nasal obstruction, are situations that frequently lead to impairment of the patient's quality of life.

Moreover, the type of nasal approach will determine whether it is possible for the surgeon to use both hands in performing the surgery, and whether it is possible to do a cranial base reconstruction with pedicle nasal mucosal grafts. As there is a wide range of lesions in different topographies that can be treated by transnasal endoscopic surgery, the type of nasal approach as part of the procedure should be chosen individually for each patient according to the lesion's location, size, and complexity, and the need for skull base reconstruction.

If the proposed endoscopic skull base surgery is not complex, it can usually be performed by just one surgeon, and in most cases less invasive approaches are preferable. In contrast, complex lesions more often require two surgeons and a four-hand technique. In these cases, the surgical approaches are usually more invasive, with a higher chance of producing sinonasal complications and sequelae.

The introduction of the endoscope in skull base surgery facilitated the adaptation of the classic nasal surgical approaches, such as the transnasal-transseptal and direct transnasal, to a nonspeculum type of surgery. The transnasal-transeptal surgical approach allows better preservation of the nasal mucosa; however, because the approach is accomplished by using a single nostril, it does not permit the two-hand technique. In contrast, the direct transnasal approach, although creating more injury to the nasal mucosa and turbinates, allows the use of two nostrils after the resection of the posterior part of the nasal septum.

These two surgical approaches are usually sufficient to resect a wide range of tumors; however, due to the progress of endoscopic techniques in addition to the development of more complex surgeries, particularly those beyond the paranasal sinuses extending into the dura and cavernous sinus, it has been necessary to review the classic surgical approaches and to seek complementary procedures. In addition, the still significant rates of persistent CSF fistula related to the surgeries has driven surgeons to develop new approaches, combining a large exposure of the surgical field with the possibility of creating vascularized mucosal flaps, facilitating the reconstruction of the cranial base defect.[6] In complex surgeries, preoperative planning of the reconstruction step always plays an important role in determining the best surgical access.

The precise knowledge of the patient anatomy provided by imaging exams is also important when determining the best surgical approach. Computer tomography (CT) and magnetic resonance imaging (MRI) are essential for characterizing the morphologic aspects of the sphenoid sinus, for identifying its anatomical relationship with the internal carotid artery, optic nerve, cavernous sinus, and Onodi cells, and for determining the precise location of the lesion or tumor and its relationship with other important anatomical structures including the paranasal sinuses, skull base, and ethmoidal arteries. This chapter describes the transnasal surgical approaches that are most often used today.

■ Transnasal Direct (Unilateral) Approach

Indications

This surgical approach is usually indicated for lesions that do not need a wide exposure or a special skull base reconstruction. It can be used to treat patients with small unilateral CSF fistulas in the sphenoid or ethmoid sinuses and patients with unilateral medial orbital decompression.

Surgical Technique

The surgery is performed through a single nostril. If the nasal cavity is too narrow and the passage of the endoscope and operating instruments is limited because of a septal deviation, a septoplasty should be done first.

After identification of the middle and superior turbinates, the posterior region of the nasal septum, and the choanal arch, the ostium of the sphenoid sinus is probed with a seeker/palpator. The ostium lies superiorly to the choanal arch between the superior turbinate and the septum. To improve access to the posterior ethmoidal cells and to the sphenoid sinus, the superior turbinate can be removed. Exceptionally, the posterior portion of the middle turbinate can also be removed.

Following the identification of the sphenoid ostium, if the lesion is located within the sphenoid sinus, the anterior wall of the sinus is then opened, starting from the ostium region. The sphenoidotomy is carefully enlarged inferiorly, avoiding damage to the posterior septal branch of the sphenopalatine artery that crosses the anterior wall of the sphenoid sinus at this region. If both sphenoid sinuses need to be surgically exposed, the mucoperiosteum of the anterior wall and the sphenoid rostrum are displaced laterally and reserved for posterior reconstruction if necessary. The anterior wall, sphenoid rostrum, and all intersinus septa are resected, giving wide exposure to the sinus (**Fig. 5.1**).

This surgical approach is preferred mainly for the treatment of unilateral lesions. The advantages of this approach are that it provides direct access and it preserves most of the anatomical structures in the nose and the physiology of the

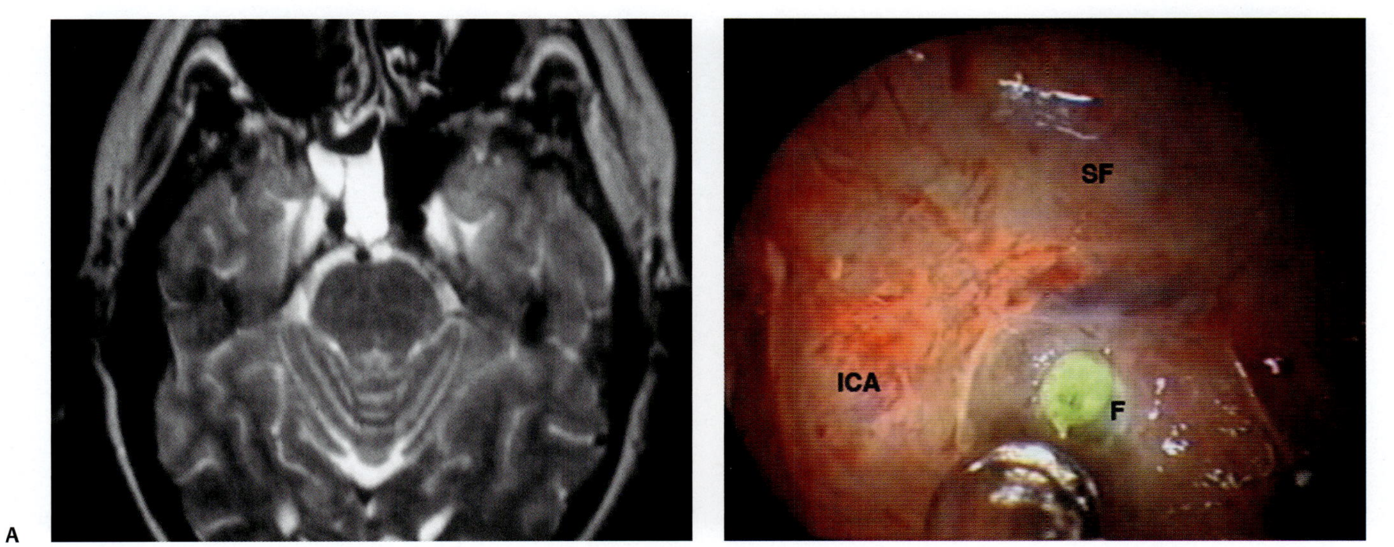

Fig. 5.1 (A) Magnetic resonance imaging of cerebrospinal fluid filling the right sphenoid sinus. **(B)** Intraoperative view through a direct nasal approach demonstrating the fistula in the right clivus, under the floor of the sella. F: clival fistula; ICA: internal carotid artery; SF: sellar floor.

nasal cavity. The disadvantage is the inability to work in both nostrils simultaneously by two surgeons.

Bi-Nostril Approach

Indications

This surgical approach is described in detail in Chapter 25. The bi-nostril approach is the one we routinely use for the treatment of all cases of midline sellar tumors, especially pituitary adenomas.

With the introduction of endoscopic techniques in sellar surgeries, new approaches have been developed, increasing the efficiency and safety of the surgical procedures. To overcome some important limitations of the method, the bi-nostril endonasal approach associated with a resection of the posterior septum has been developed.[7] It allows a four-hand technique, adding safety to the procedure and facilitating the control of bleeding and the dissection of the tumor. It improves the surgical results without compromising the nasal function. Essentially, it combines two previous surgical approaches: one side transseptal and transnasal contralaterally. As the nasal septum mucosa from one side is left intact (transseptal dissection), at the end of the procedure the posterior nasal septum mucosa remains with no perforation.

On the other side, a quadrangular-shaped flap of the posterior nasal septum mucosa is created, pediculated in its posterior edge. This mucosal window, located on the posterior region of the nasal septum, permits the surgeon also to work from that side of the nasal cavity. This mucosal flap is temporarily displaced toward the rhinopharynx or the maxillary sinus, and at the end of the surgery it can be used as a vascularized flap for cranial base reconstruction (**Fig. 5.2**).

Extended Transnasal Approach

Indications

This surgical approach is especially useful to remove midline intradural tumors that need a wider exposure, outside the boundaries of the sellar region, particularly the ones that extend to the planum sphenoidale area. The most frequent indications for this surgical access are meningiomas located on the tuberculum sellae, craniopharyngiomas, and giant pituitary adenomas.[1,2,5]

Surgical Technique

The approach comprises a bi-nostril access and a total ethmoidectomy to expose the planum sphenoidale. The nasal septal mucosa of both sides is prepared for the creation of bilateral vascularized flaps. Sometimes it is necessary to remove both middle turbinates to provide space for the surgical instruments. The sphenoid sinus is totally exposed by removing the sphenoidal floor to the lateral recess. Bone removal starts at the sellar floor, and continues to the planum sphenoidale in an arciform fashion, completely exposing the dura from these regions. Laterally, the bone removal continues to the most proximal part of the optic canal. The dura is then opened in the sellar region and, after coagulation of the intercavernous sinus, the aperture is extended to the anterior floor, laterally limited by the olfactory nerves bilaterally. In some cases, especially in patients with malignant tumors, the septal mucosa also must be removed to achieve an effective oncologic resection. In this situation other vascularized flaps can be used for the reconstruction, including the inferior turbinates, the palatal mucosa, or even pericranium, brought to the nasal cavity through the frontal sinus (**Fig. 5.3**).[8,9]

A

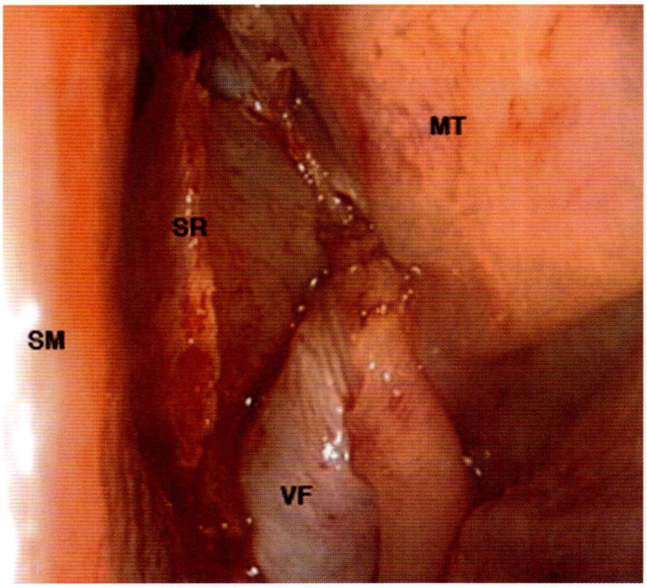

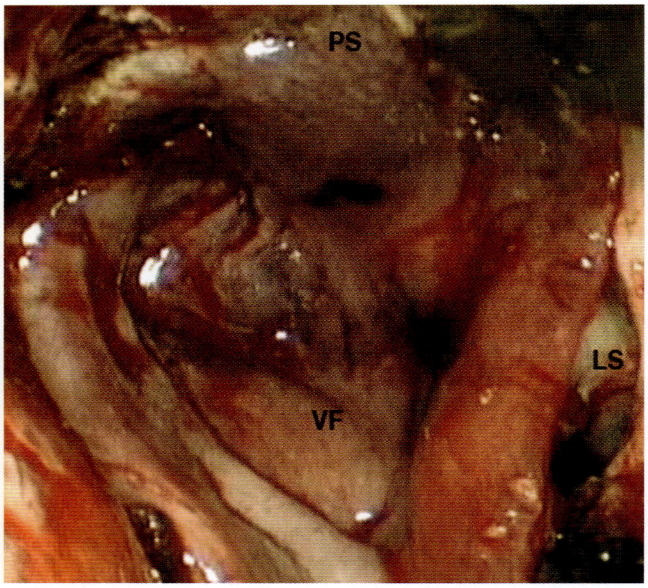

B

Fig. 5.2 **(A)** Bi-nostril approach with right transseptal and left endonasal exposure of the sphenoid rostrum. The right septal mucosa is preserved and the left one hangs on its arterial supply. MT: left middle turbinate; SM: septal mucosa of the right side; SR: sphenoidal rostrum; VF: vascularized flap of the left side. **(B)** Vascularized flap in the surgical site after tumor removal. LS: left sphenoid sinus; PS: planum sphenoidal; VF: vascularized flap.

A

B

C

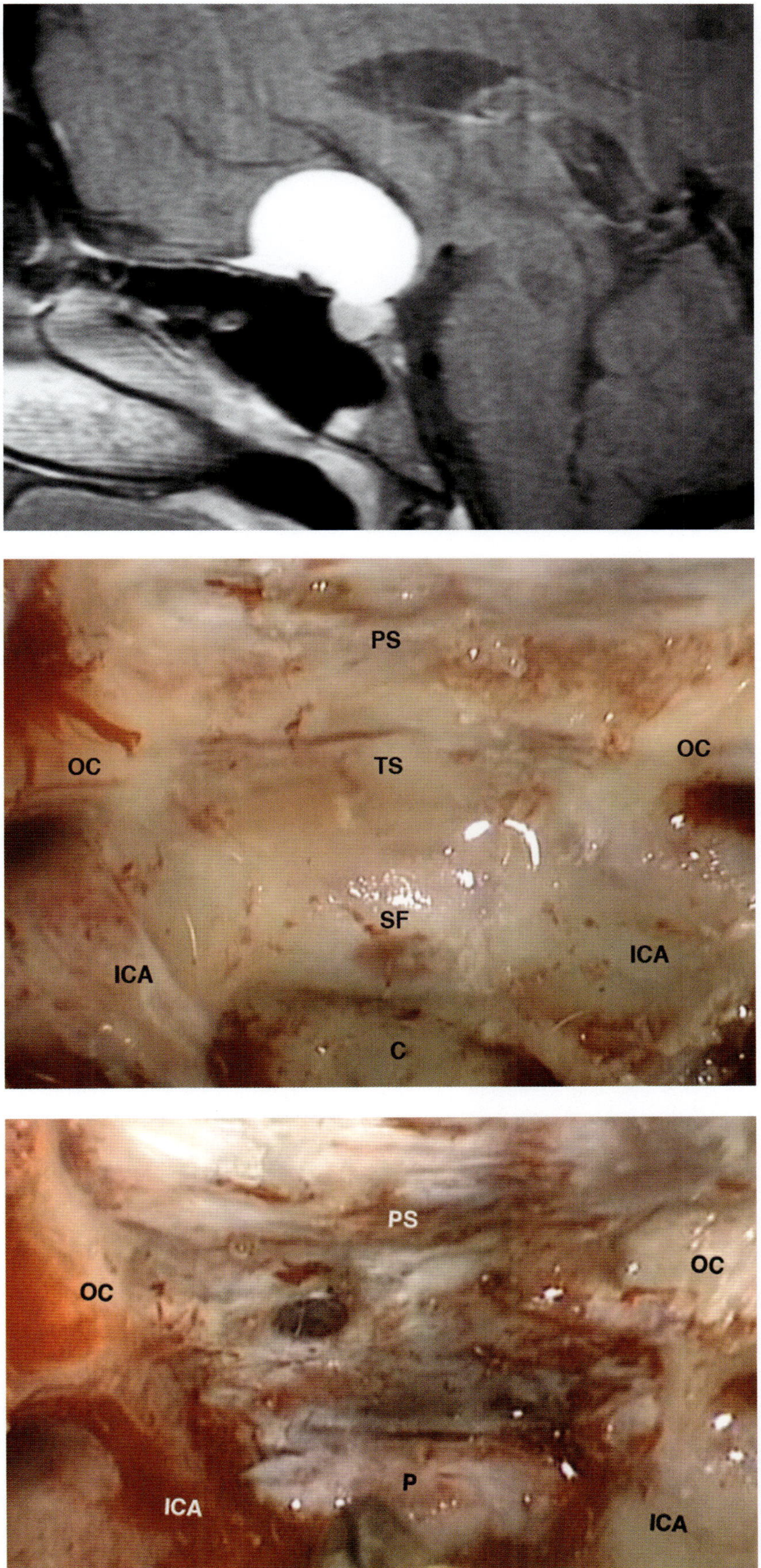

Fig. 5.3 (A) Tuberculum sellae meningioma dislocating superiorly the anterior cerebral artery complex and posteriorly the pituitary stalk and optic chiasma. **(B)** Extended transnasal approach with bone exposure through the sphenoid sinus. C: clivus; ICA: internal carotid artery; OC: optic canal; PS: planum sphenoidal; SF: sellar floor; TS: tuberculum sellae. **(C)** Surgical view after bone removal from the planum, tuberculum, and sellar floor, with exposure of the dura mater. ICA: internal carotid artery; OC: optic canal; P: pituitary gland; PS: planum sphenoidal. (*continued on next page*)

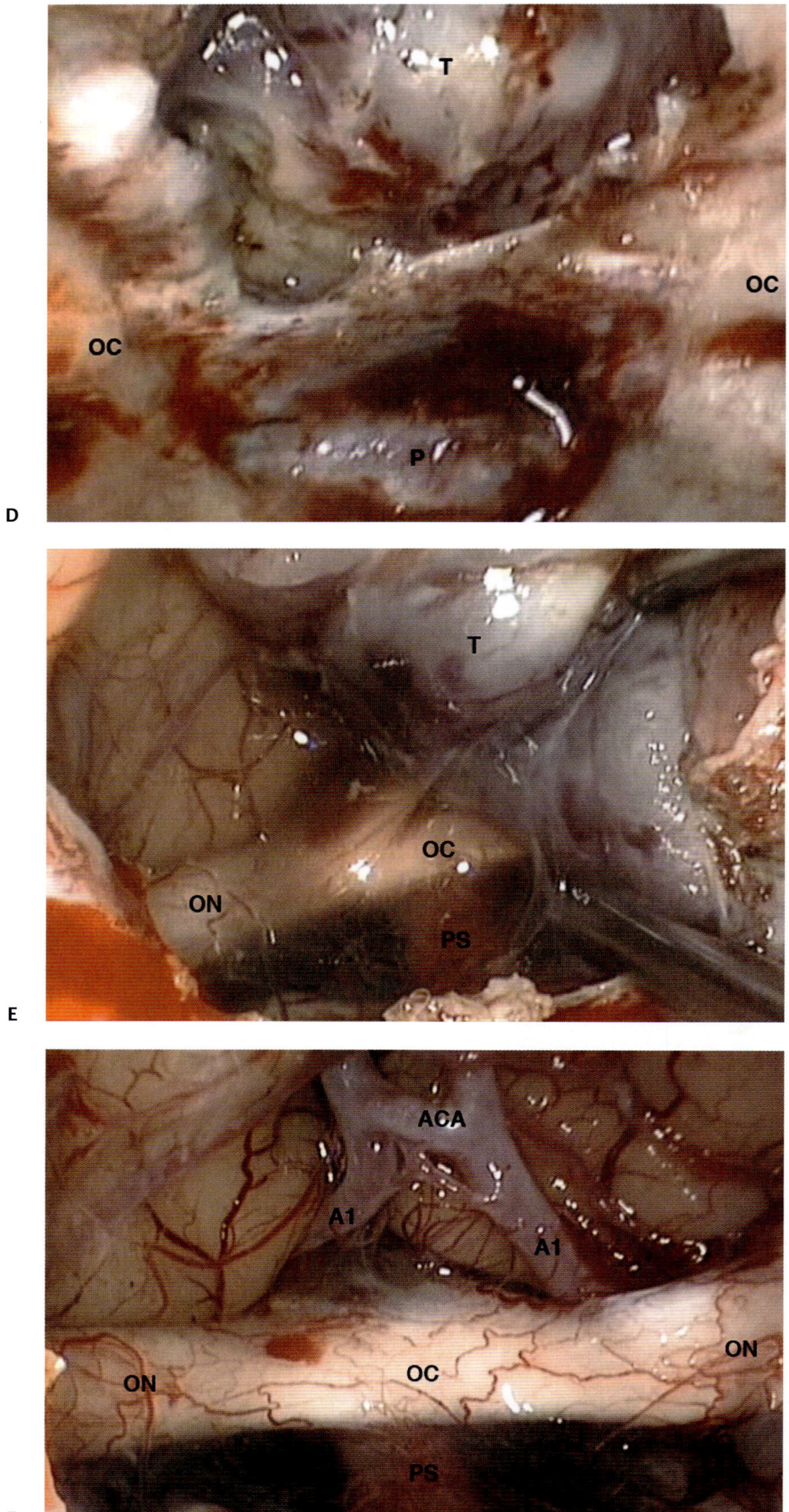

Fig. 5.3 (*Continued*) **(D)** Tumor exposure through an extended transnasal approach. OC: optic canal; P: pituitary gland, T: tumor. **(E)** Tumor dissection with preservation of the arachnoid between the tumor and the neurovascular structures. OC: optic chiasma; ON: optic nerve; PS: pituitary stalk; T: tumor. **(F)** Extended t-ansnasal approach after total tumor removal with preservation of the arachnoid and its small arteries supplying the optic chiasm. ACA: anterior communicating artery; A1: anterior cerebral artery; OC: optic chiasm; ON: optic nerve; P: pituitary stalk.

Transmaxillary-Transpterygoidal Approach (Lateral)

Indications

This surgical approach is indicated in patients with tumors that are located laterally at the skull base, or midline lesions with important lateral extension. The majority of these lesions consist of pituitary adenomas and meningiomas with cavernous sinus extension and chordomas and chondrosarcomas located more laterally.

Surgical Technique

This surgical approach comprises an endonasal bilateral access with the removal of the homolateral middle turbinate, bulla ethmoidalis, and uncinate process. The medial wall of the maxillary sinus is opened, and in some cases an endoscopic medial maxillectomy is performed.

The opening of the anterior wall of the sphenoid sinus comprises the region of the sphenopalatine foramen. Because the septal arteries and the posterior lateral nasal artery are often coagulated as part of the procedure, the nasal septal mucosal flap must be created by dissecting the contralateral mucosa. By removing a wide portion of bone, the surgeon should be able to identify the infraorbital nerve in the roof of the maxillary sinus and follow it proximally until the inferior part of the cavernous sinus. The intracavernous nerves are always located superior to the infraorbital nerve and inferior to the maxillary artery. Identification of the vidian nerve, leaving the pterygopalatine ganglion from lateral to medial on the floor of the sphenoid sinus, is important because it serves as a guide to the anterior portion of the carotid artery as it runs into the foramen lacerum.[10] This surgical approach exposes the internal carotid artery in the midline of the operative field (**Figs. 5.4 and 5.5**).

Conclusion

There are many possible transnasal endoscopic approaches for surgical management of the skull base lesions. This chapter summarized the most frequent surgical approaches currently used by our team, discussing their advantages and pitfalls, and providing tips. The development of new endoscopic surgical techniques and modern diagnostic tools has enabled skull base surgeons to perform less invasive surgery that provides maximal exposure of the surgical field and the best possibility of skull base reconstruction for each type of lesion.

A

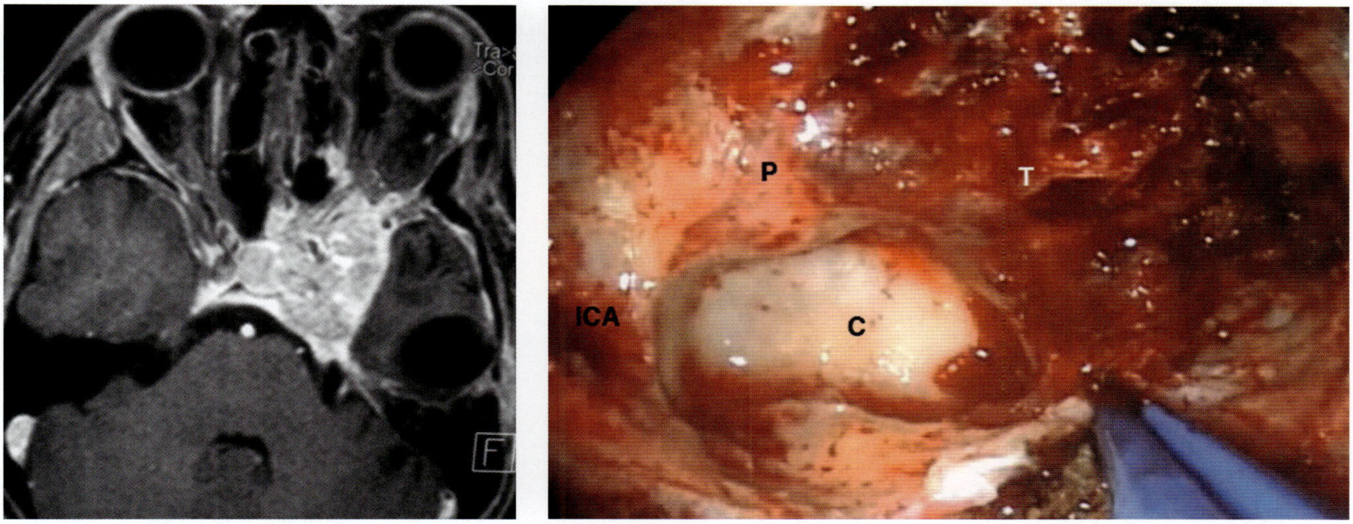

B

Fig. 5.4 **(A)** Magnetic resonance imaging demonstrating an ameloblastoma filling the left cavernous sinus. **(B)** Intraoperative view after a transmaxillary-transpterygoidal approach with exposure of the left intracavernous ameloblastoma infiltrating the pituitary gland. C: clivus; ICA: internal carotid artery; P: pituitary fossae; T: tumor.

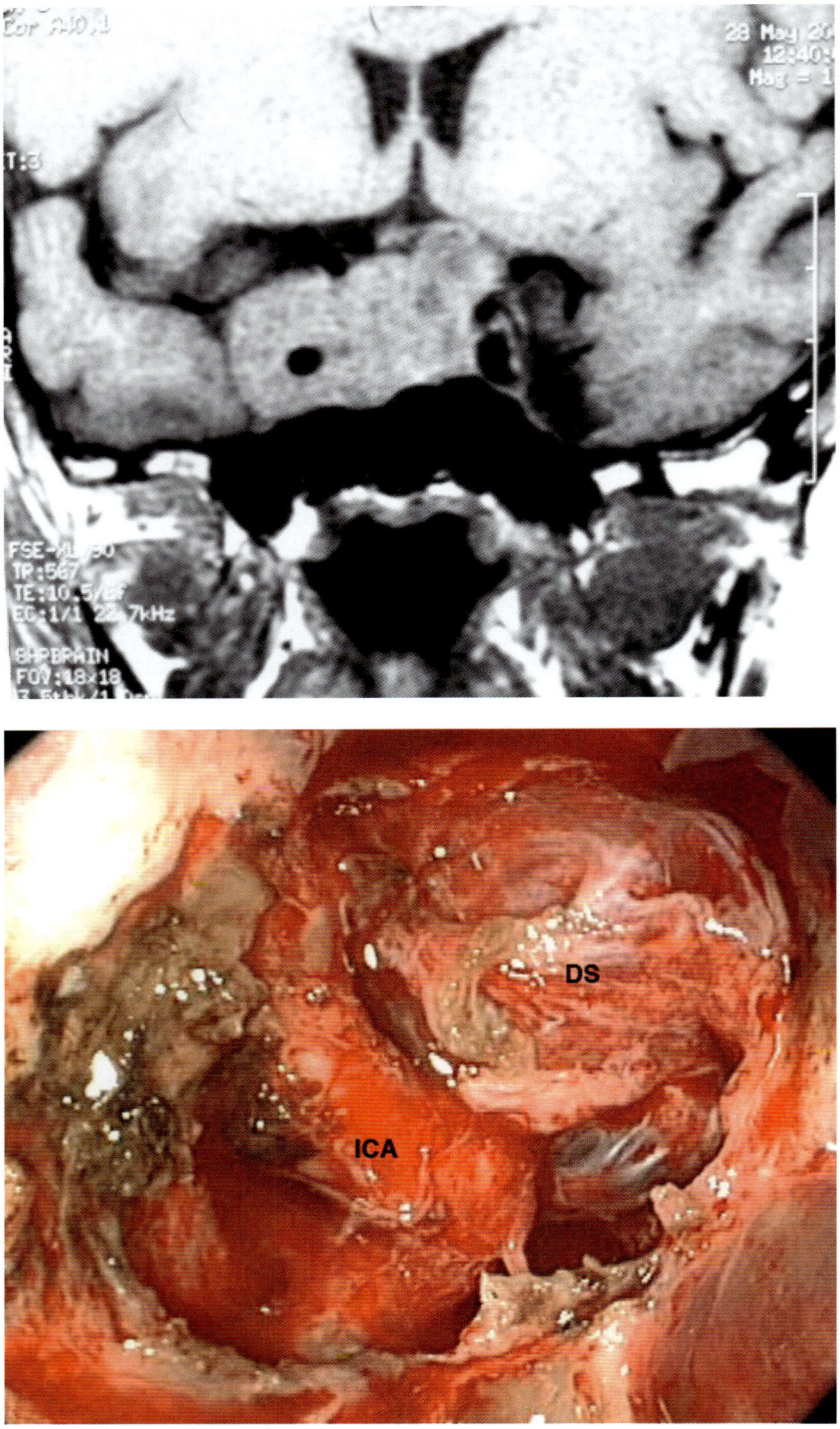

A

B

Fig. 5.5 **(A)** Magnetic resonance imaging demonstrating an adrenocorticotropic hormone (ACTH)-producing pituitary adenoma invading the right cavernous sinus. **(B)** Intraoperative view after total removal of a sellar and right cavernous sinus pituitary adenoma. DS: diaphragma sellae; ICA: right intracavernous internal carotid artery.

References

1. Cavallo LM, Prevedello DM, Solari D, et al. Extended endoscopic endonasal transsphenoidal approach for residual or recurrent craniopharyngiomas. J Neurosurg 2009;111:578–589
2. de Divitiis E, Esposito F, Cappabianca P, Cavallo LM, de Divitiis O, Esposito I. Endoscopic transnasal resection of anterior cranial fossa meningiomas. Neurosurg Focus 2008;25:E8
3. Nogueira JF Jr, Stamm AC, Vellutini E, Santos FP. Endoscopic management of congenital meningo-encephalocele with nasal flaps. Int J Pediatr Otorhinolaryngol 2009;73:133–137
4. Stamm AC, Pignatari SS, Vellutini E. Transnasal endoscopic surgical approaches to the clivus. Otolaryngol Clin North Am 2006;39:639–656, xi
5. Stamm AC, Vellutini E, Harvey RJ, Nogeira JF Jr, Herman DR. Endoscopic transnasal craniotomy and the resection of craniopharyngioma. Laryngoscope 2008;118:1142–1148
6. Hadad G, Bassagasteguy L, Carrau RL, et al. A novel reconstructive technique after endoscopic expanded endonasal approaches: vascular pedicle nasoseptal flap. Laryngoscope 2006;116:1882–1886
7. Stamm AC, Pignatari S, Vellutini E, Harvey RJ, Nogueira JF Jr. A novel approach allowing binostril work to the sphenoid sinus. Otolaryngol Head Neck Surg 2008;138:531–532
8. Harvey RJ, Nogueira JF, Schlosser RJ, Patel SJ, Vellutini E, Stamm AC. Closure of large skull base defects after endoscopic transnasal craniotomy. Clinical article. J Neurosurg 2009;111:371–379
9. Zanation AM, Snyderman CH, Carrau RL, Kassam AB, Gardner PA, Prevedello DM. Minimally invasive endoscopic pericranial flap: a new method for endonasal skull base reconstruction. Laryngoscope 2009; 119:13–18
10. Osawa S, Rhoton AL Jr, Seker A, Shimizu S, Fujii K, Kassam AB. Microsurgical and endoscopic anatomy of the vidian canal. Neurosurgery 2009;64(5, Suppl 2)385–411, discussion 411–412

6 Navigation in Endoscopic Paranasal and Skull Base Surgery

Benjamin Bleier and Rodney J. Schlosser

Tips and Pearls

- Image-guided surgery (IGS) enables enhanced preoperative planning and intraoperative surgical navigation.
- All IGS systems have common basic components and rely on optical or electromagnetic tracking systems that provide comparable surgical accuracy.
- Accuracy is based on the quality of the preoperative imaging and inherent errors in registration.
- Accuracy must be checked throughout the procedure and can only be interpreted and compensated for by sound surgical judgment and a thorough anatomical knowledge base.

Introduction

Although the basic tenets of stereotactic surgery were introduced a century ago, advances in imaging within the past 20 years have led to the widespread development and utilization of image-guided surgery (IGS) for paranasal and skull base procedures. Current IGS platforms enable detailed preoperative planning using triplanar and three-dimensional imaging as well as highly accurate intraoperative surgical navigation. Despite these advances, IGS remains subject to a variety of types of error and thus should be used only to augment sound clinical judgment and surgical expertise.

History

The recent advances in IGS have been predicated on concomitant advances in neuroradiography. The first stereotactic devices were developed in the early 1900s, although the marriage of radiography to surgical navigation did not occur until the 1940s.[1] The advent of computed tomography (CT) provided a significant improvement in image quality and led to a CT-guided frame-based system in 1976.[2] Although this development led to an increase in surgical accuracy, the stereotactic frame obstructed the surgical field, providing impetus for the development of early frameless systems in the 1980s.[3] Since that time, the use of IGS has become widely accepted and is currently endorsed by the American Academy of Otolaryngology–Head and Neck Surgery (**Table 6.1**).[4]

Table 6.1 American Academy of Otolaryngology–Head and Neck Surgery (AAO-HNS) Indications for Intraoperative Use of Computer-Aided Surgery

1. Revision sinus surgery
2. Distorted sinus anatomy of development, postoperative, or traumatic origin
3. Extensive sinonasal polyposis
4. Pathology involving the frontal, posterior ethmoid, and sphenoid sinuses
5. Disease abutting the skull base, orbit, optic nerve, or carotid artery
6. CSF rhinorrhea or conditions where there is a skull base defect
7. Benign and malignant sinonasal neoplasms

From American Academy of Otolaryngology Head and Neck Surgery: AAO-HNS Policy on Intra-Operative Use of Computer Aided Surgery. http://www.entnet.org/Practice/policyIntraOperativeSurgery.cfm.

System Components

All commercially available IGS platforms contain the same basic component features. The computer workstation functions to integrate the tracking system, computer interface, and image display into a single unit (**Fig. 6.1**).[3] The software platform is optimized to create a three-dimensional virtual data set that can be correlated to the surgical volume through a process of registration.[1]

All IGS tracking systems are designed to monitor the position of an intraoperative localization device (ILD) within the surgical volume. The ILD may be fabricated as a surgical instrument or it may attach to a preexisting instrument. Current systems employ either optical or electromagnetic technology to track the ILD (**Fig. 6.2**).[3]

Electromagnetic (EM) systems utilize a radiofrequency field to determine positional information through a receiver in the ILD. The limitations of this system include the potential for field distortion by metallic objects, the reliance on wires to communicate with the system,[3] and the need to

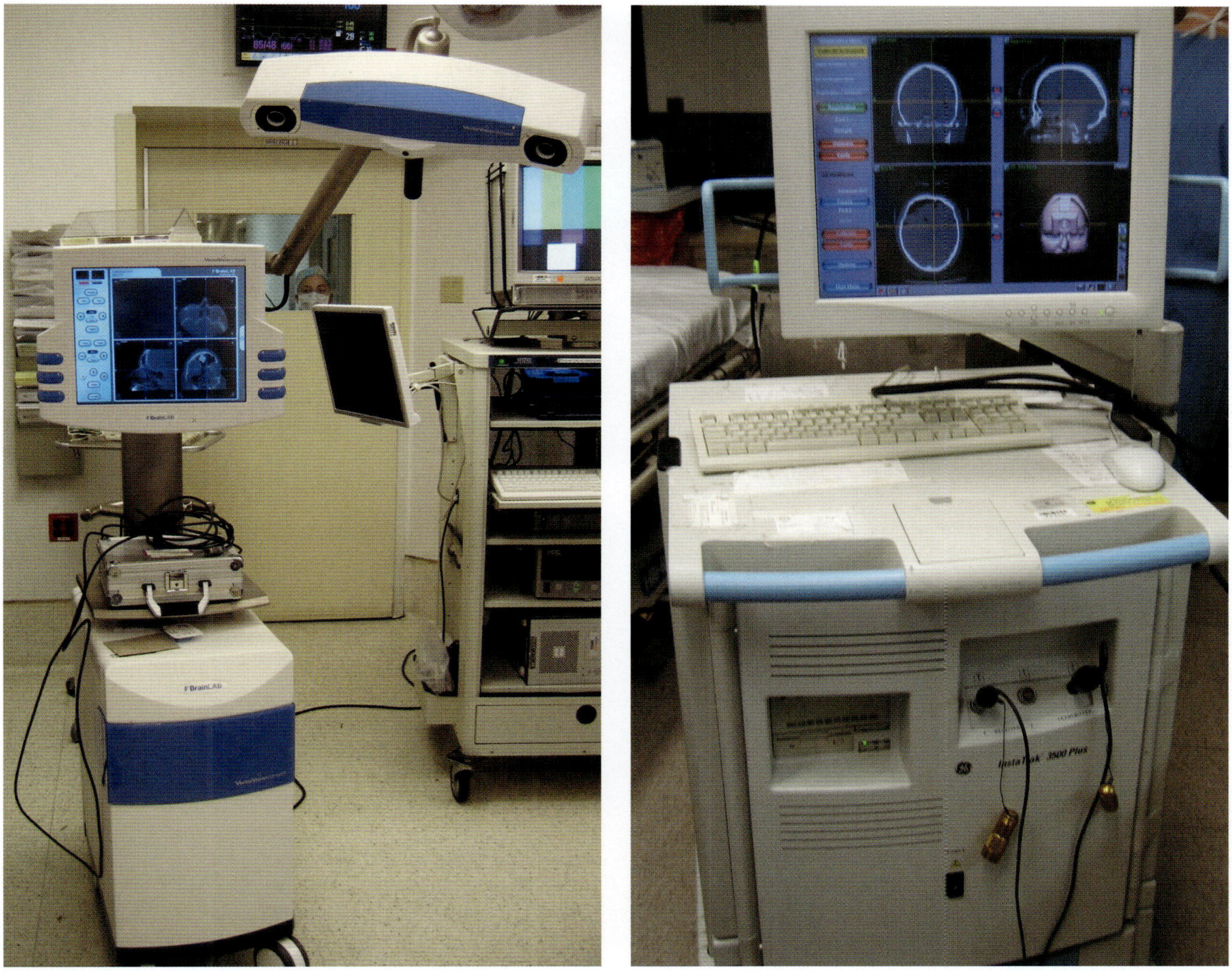

A B

Fig. 6.1 (A,B) Image-guided surgery (IGS) towers from two different manufacturers with component hardware features, including computer workstation, tracking system, computer interface, and image display.

bring the same bulky headset from the preoperative imaging to the surgery, although some studies suggest headset reuse has little effect on accuracy.[5,6]

In optical systems the ILD is composed of an array of light-emitting diodes (active tracking) or reflective spheres (passive tracking) that are captured by an overhead camera and referenced to a set of markers on a headset worn by the patient. The limitation of this system is that the operative suite must be arranged to provide an uninterrupted line of sight to the overhead camera.[3]

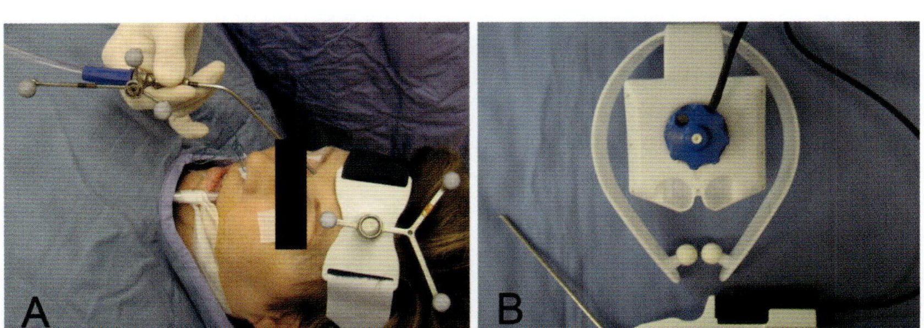

Fig. 6.2 Headsets and intraoperative localization devices (ILDs). **(A)** Optical ILD with reflective spheres on straight suction. **(B)** Electromagnetic device on prefabricated suction instrument.

Table 6.2 Common Image-Guided Surgery (IGS) Features

Hardware
Computer workstation
Tracking system
Computer interface
Image display
Intraoperative location device (ILD)
Tracking mechanism
Optical
Passive (reflective spheres or glions)
Active (light-emitting diodes)
Electromagnetic
Registration
Paired-point registration
Automatic registration
Contour registration

Registration and Calibration

Registration comprises the process of correlating the relationship between fiducial position and the corresponding point in the data-set volume. In contrast, calibration refers only to the confirmation of the relationship between the instrument tip and the ILD.[3] Registration paradigms include paired-point, contour-based, and automatic registration.

Paired-point and contour-based registration both require manual intraoperative mapping of the fiducial points that have been predefined in the virtual data set. In contour-based registration, this is followed by the acquisition of up to 500 points over fixed facial contours. The computer then calculates the registration by aligning these points with the virtual data set.

In contrast, automatic registration utilizes a headset that incorporates the fiducials in a fixed position, allowing the software platform to perform the registration automatically. In this system changes in head-frame position result in diminished accuracy (**Table 6.2**).[3]

Surgical Accuracy

Given the proximity of vital neurovascular structures in paranasal and skull base surgery, the navigational accuracy of the IGS system is of paramount concern. The degree of baseline accuracy depends on the quality of the imaging data set as well as the stability, number, and position of the fiducial points relative to the entire surgical volume. Error is then inherently introduced during the registration process, leading to subtle degradations in accuracy. Target registration error (TRE) is the best measure of navigational accuracy and can be assessed clinically by visually comparing a known anatomical landmark to its coordinate position in the virtual data set. TRE is lowest near the fiducials and may deteriorate over time due to fiducial motion, instrument deformation, and tracking errors. As such, the TRE should be assessed intraoperatively in three axes, as the two-dimensional endoscopic image may misrepresent the degree of TRE in a single axis.[3] Other sources of error include fiducial localization error (FLE) and fiducial registration error (FRE).[1]

Current systems are generally accurate to within 1.5 to 2.4mm.[3] Of note, Metson et al[7] reported an accuracy within 2 mm using the InstaTrak and Stealth Station systems with a mean degradation of 0.89 mm during the case, supporting the recommendation that the TRE should be assessed throughout the course of the procedure.

Preoperative Planning

One of the benefits of the IGS system is the ability to perform detailed preoperative planning with rapid scrolling through sequential high-resolution images in multiple axes. This allows the surgeon to map complex anatomical pathways in three dimensions and has enabled clinically relevant descriptions of the variable frontal recess anatomy.[8]

In skull base approaches, preoperative review facilitates the localization of pathology and the selection of the optimal surgical corridor.[1] The ability to perform three-dimensional reconstruction is particularly useful in characterizing morphologically complex lesions at the skull base. Rosahl et al[9] reported that in a series of 110 patients, virtual three-dimensional reconstruction enhanced surgical planning and assisted in targeting structures that would otherwise be hidden or obscured in the surgical field.

Advances in neuroimaging have also enabled the incorporation of soft tissue data into the preoperative planning stage. CT resolution is not adequate to allow for accurate delineation of soft tissue and neurovascular structures. This has been addressed by the advent of image-to-image registration (IIR) software, which allows MRI images to be coupled to CT data using anatomical landmarks to create a fusion image (**Fig. 6.3**).[10]

The intracranial vasculature may also be visualized utilizing three-dimensional CT angiography (3D-CTA), in which images are captured as the contrast bolus fills the internal carotid system, thereby enabling the simultaneous acquisition of the vascular and bony anatomy of the skull base.[10] Leong et al[11] performed 3D-CTA in 18 cases and found an accuracy of 2 mm or better, concluding that 3D-CTA provided an accurate assessment of the location of the internal carotid artery (ICA) and its relationship to the surgical field. The incorporation of diffusion-weighted MRI and positron emission tomography (PET) scanning may also prove to aid in planning approaches to metabolically active tumors.[1]

Intraoperative Image Guidance

The current literature suggests that the intraoperative use of IGS decreases surgical disorientation,[6] improves surgical

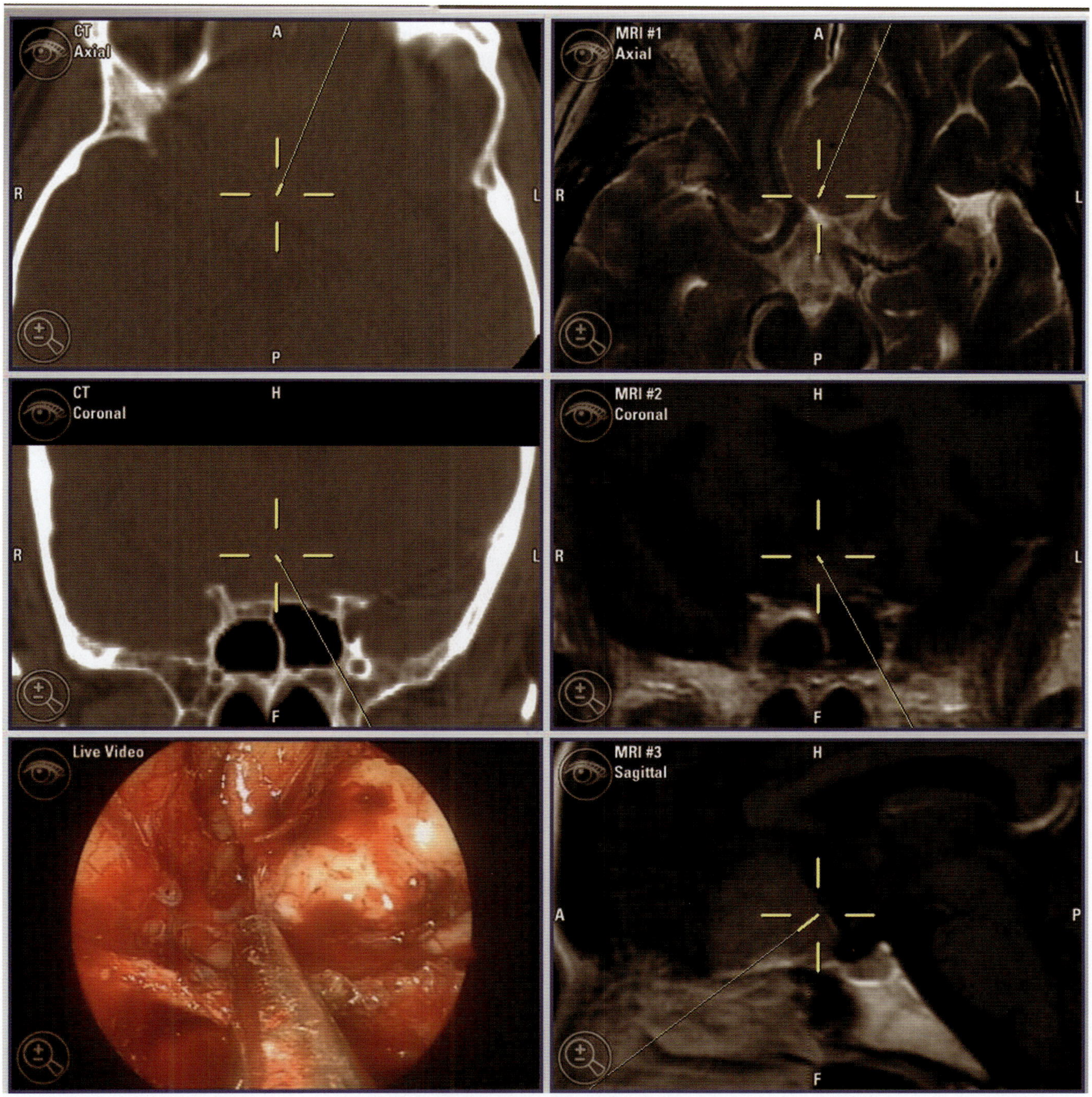

Fig. 6.3 CT/MRI fusion images demonstrate complete resection of planar meningioma.

completeness, and potentially lowers complication rates.[10] In fact, studies have demonstrated that in 50% of cases where IGS is used, the surgical strategy is adjusted based on the navigational data (**Fig. 6.4**).[12]

Image-guided surgery is particularly helpful in revision cases where the traditional anatomical landmarks may be either distorted or absent, creating a greater potential for complications. However, in a series of 110 patients undergoing sinus surgery with image guidance, Kacker et al[13] found no major complications even in revision cases.

Image-guided surgery is also valuable in both primary and revision frontal sinus surgery where complex anatomy and potential scarring may blur the border between the frontal recess and the adjacent orbit and skull base. One study noted a significant increase in successful frontal sinusotomy following the introduction of IGS in a review of 800 procedures.[14] Success rates in frontal sinus drill-out also have also been shown to trend toward improvement when using IGS.[15]

External approaches may also benefit from the use of IGS by increasing the accuracy of the osteotomy or frontal trephine sites during osteoplastic flap.[10] The use of IGS for frontal sinus obliteration was first reported by Carrau et al,[16] who suggested that IGS was more accurate than 6-foot Caldwell radiography, transillumination, and sinus trephination with probing.

Finally, the incorporation of CT/MRI fusion and 3D-CTA imaging into the virtual data set provides valuable information during tumor and skull base approaches with regard to the extent of tumor resection and clarification of boundaries between the tumor and normal adjacent soft tissue and neurovascular structures.[1]

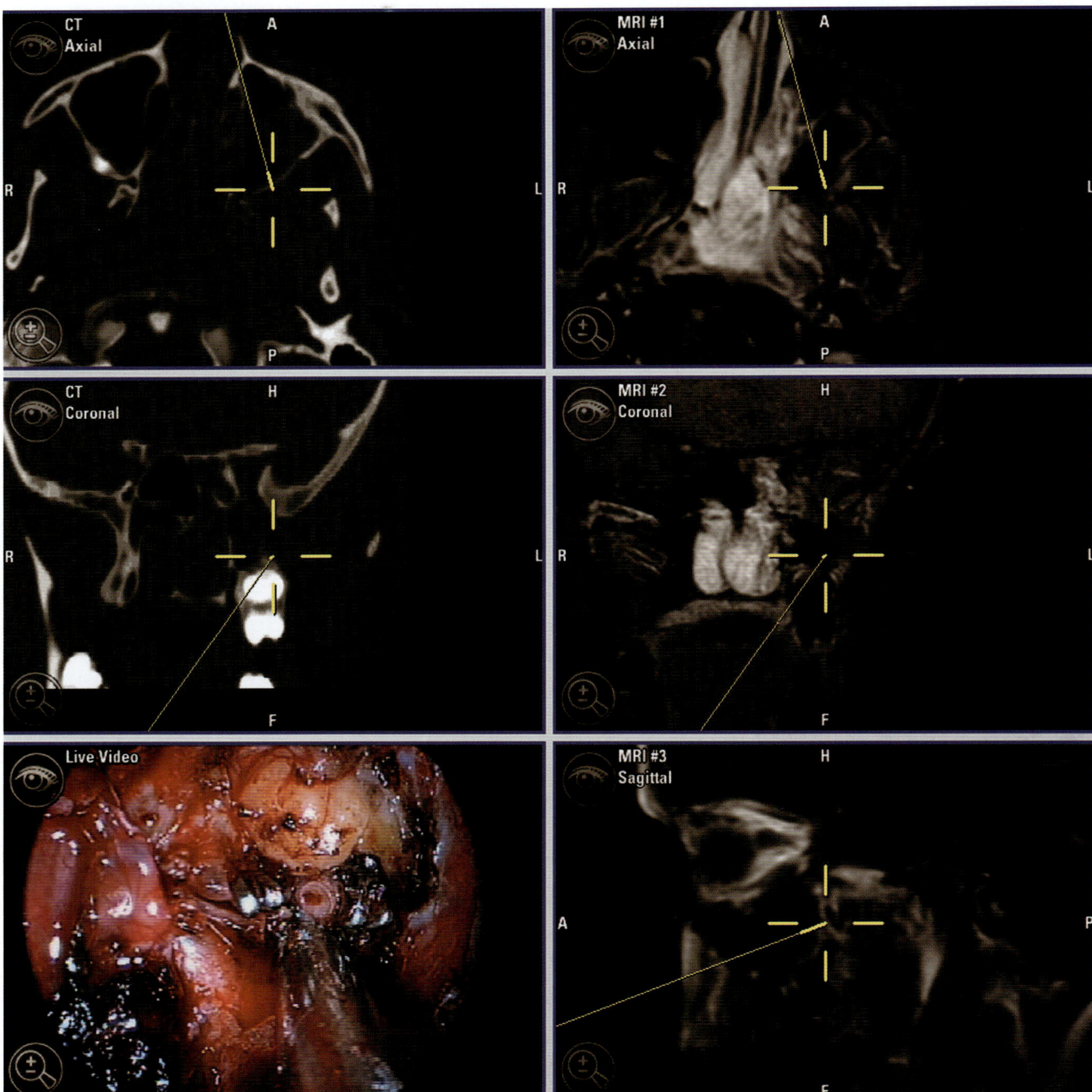

Fig. 6.4 Intraoperative triplanar CT/MRI fusion images of juvenile nasopharyngeal angiofibroma demonstrate ligation of the internal maxillary artery and the approach to the lateral extent of tumor into the infratemporal fossa.

Intraoperative Image Updating

Registration error theory is predicated on the assumption that the sinonasal anatomy remains static from the preoperative image acquisition through the duration of the procedure. However, intraoperatively bone is resected and soft tissue structures are subject to displacement secondary to gravitational, physiologic, and hydrodynamic forces. Multiple models of soft tissue shift have been described, including spring-based and finite element models that attempt to predict volumetric changes based on surface deformation, although their clinical utility has yet to be determined.[17] Although surgical judgment remains the cornerstone of anticipating discrepancies between the IGS data and the surgical field, the use of intraoperative CT and MRI have enabled real-time image acquisition and the ability to update the navigational data set as the surgery progresses.

The image quality of intraoperative CT systems is a large improvement over earlier attempts at intraoperative fluoroscopic CT,[10] although their utility is limited to evaluation of changes in the bony anatomy. Although the data are sparse, preliminary reports are favorable, and one series noted a transition to additional surgery in 30% of cases following intraoperative CT acquisition, half of which were for additional frontal recess dissection.[18]

Several reports have investigated the use of intraoperative MRI for skull base lesions and suggest that its use enables more complete tumor resection. In a retrospective study, Nimsky et al[19] reported a 27% rate of surgical modification in 200 patients based on intraoperative MRI data. However, given the cost of these systems, their practical utility has yet to be determined.

Conclusion

Although prospective studies in IGS use are impractical, a wealth of retrospective data supports the use of IGS for challenging paranasal and skull base surgery. However, IGS must be used with caution, as inherent registration and accuracy errors as well as spherical distortion by the two-dimensional endoscope can only be interpreted and compensated for by the surgeon's clinical acumen. Although IGS is not a substitute for surgical skill, it does facilitate improved preoperative planning and enhanced surgical performance.

References

1. Tabaee A, Schwartz TH, Anand VK. Image guidance in endoscopic skull base surgery. In: Anand VK, Schwartz TH, eds. Practical Endoscopic Skull Base Surgery. San Diego: Plural Publishing; 2007:57–69
2. Bergström M, Greitz T. Stereotaxic computed tomography. AJR Am J Roentgenol 1976;127:167–170
3. Citardi MJ, Batra PS. Image-guided sinus surgery. In: Kountakis SE, ed. Rhinologic and Sleep Apnea Surgical Techniques. Heidelberg, Germany: Springer; 2007:189–198
4. American Academy of Otolaryngology Head and Neck Surgery. AAO-HNS Policy on Intra-Operative Use of Computer Aided Surgery. http://www.entnet.org/ Practice/ policyIntraOperativeSurgery.cfm
5. Javer AR, Kuhn FA, Smith D. Stereotactic computer-assisted navigational sinus surgery: accuracy of an electromagnetic tracking system with the tissue debrider and when utilizing different headsets for the same patient. Am J Rhinol 2000;14:361–365
6. Metson R, Ung F. Image-guidance in frontal sinus surgery. In: Kountakis SE, ed. The Frontal Sinus. Heidelberg, Germany: Springer; 2005:201–209
7. Metson R, Gliklich RE, Cosenza M. A comparison of image guidance systems for sinus surgery. Laryngoscope 1998;108(8 Pt 1):1164–1170
8. Lee WT, Kuhn FA, Citardi MJ. 3D computed tomographic analysis of frontal recess anatomy in patients without frontal sinusitis. Otolaryngol Head Neck Surg 2004;131:164–173
9. Rosahl SK, Gharabaghi A, Hubbe U, Shahidi R, Samii M. Virtual reality augmentation in skull base surgery. Skull Base 2006;16:59–66
10. Citardi MJ, Batra PS. Revision functional endoscopic sinus surgery. In: Kountakis SE, ed. Revision Sinus Surgery. Heidelberg, Germany: Springer; 2008:251–267
11. Leong JL, Batra PS, Citardi MJ. Three-dimensional computed tomography angiography of the internal carotid artery for preoperative evaluation of sinonasal lesions and intraoperative surgical navigation. Laryngoscope 2005;115:1618–1623
12. Strauss G, Koulechov K, Röttger S, et al. Evaluation of a navigation system for ENT with surgical efficiency criteria. Laryngoscope 2006;116: 564–572
13. Kacker A, Tabaee A, Anand V. Computer-assisted surgical navigation in revision endoscopic sinus surgery. Otolaryngol Clin North Am 2005;38: 473–482, vi
14. Reardon EJ. Navigational risks associated with sinus surgery and the clinical effects of implementing a navigational system for sinus surgery. Laryngoscope 2002; **112**(7 Pt 2, Suppl 99)1–19
15. Samaha M, Cosenza MJ, Metson R. Endoscopic frontal sinus drillout in 100 patients. Arch Otolaryngol Head Neck Surg 2003;129:854–858
16. Carrau RL, Snyderman CH, Curtin HB, Weissman JL. Computer-assisted frontal sinusotomy. Otolaryngol Head Neck Surg 1994;111:727–732
17. Carter TJ, Sermesant M, Cash DM, Barratt DC, Tanner C, Hawkes DJ. Application of soft tissue modelling to image-guided surgery. Med Eng Phys 2005;27:893–909
18. Jackman AH, Palmer JN, Chiu AG, Kennedy DW. Use of intraoperative CT scanning in endoscopic sinus surgery: a preliminary report. Am J Rhinol 2008;22:170–174
19. Nimsky C, Ganslandt O, Von Keller B, Romstöck J, Fahlbusch R. Intraoperative high-field-strength MR imaging: implementation and experience in 200 patients. Radiology 2004;233:67–78

7 Anesthesia in Endoscopic Skull Base and Brain Surgery

Nelson Mizumoto

Tips and Pearls

- The choice of the anesthesia technique is determined by the tumoral pathologic characteristics, such as tumor vascularization, surrounding edema, or production of hormones by the tumor.
- The correlation between tumor localization and the adjacent structures at the skull base indicates the complications likely to occur.
- Preexisting diseases of the cardiovascular, respiratory, renal, or locomotor systems interfere with the anesthesia of the central nervous system (CNS).
- Good monitoring of hemodynamics and pulmonary ventilation is essential to both prevention and treatment of intraoperative complications.
- The anesthesiologist must be familiar with the CNS physiopathologic mechanisms and their interactions with anesthetics, to synchronize his or her actions with those of the surgical team.
- Hormone-secreting tumors or large tumors compressing the hypothalamic-pituitary neural axis may induce changes in the neuroendocrine baseline and cause a panhypopituitarism event that will affect the cardiovascular, pulmonary, osteomuscular, and hydroelectrolytic functions.
- Cardiac arrhythmias can be triggered by the surgical manipulation of structures of the CNS.[1,2]
- When the surgical field is located on a higher level than the right cardiac atrium, the presence of lesions in venous vessels at the surgical site may lead to a venous air embolism (VAE).[3]
- Whereas patient immobility is essential for surgery, the necessary dose of muscle relaxants does not always correlate with the body weight of the patient.
- The association of short- and medium-acting anesthetics provides better results than the administration of a short- or medium-duration anesthetic alone.
- If there is a risk of liquid fistula, cough must be prevented during the removal of the endotracheal tube and recovery of consciousness, because the intrathoracic pressure increases the intracranial pressure (ICP), augmenting the risk of liquor infiltration into the dura mater through the puncture sealed by the blood clot (or the grafted patch).

Introduction

Advances in neuroimage scanning techniques and the improvement of surgical equipment and of intraoperative and postoperative monitoring resources have made possible the surgical resection of tumors located at the skull base through the transnasal endoscopy approach, with lower morbidity. Nevertheless, due to the close localization of large vessels at the skull base and the intimate correlations with the hypothalamic-pituitary neural axis, the cranial nerves, the pons, and the medulla oblongata, surgical manipulation in this area can cause cardiac arrhythmias, arterial brady/tachycardia, hypo/hypertension,[4] depression of consciousness level, depression of the respiratory centers, and hydroelectrolytic alterations. Additionally, it can induce vascular lesions of difficult hemostasis and the risk of venous air embolism.

Tumor Features that Should Determine Anesthesia Selection

Pituitary tumors can cause specific alterations, which are associated with the implicated neurohormone as follows.

Cushing's Disease

Microadenoma in the anterior pituitary secretes abnormal high levels of adrenocorticotropic hormone (ACTH) and increases plasmatic cortisol, which causes several body changes. The vascular fragility makes difficult the venous and arterial access. Arterial hypertension and tachycardia interfere with the evaluation of the depth of anesthesia.[5] The use of beta-blockers to treat arterial hypertension and tachycardia is helpful, as they reduce the need for great amounts of anesthesia. In the assessment of depth of anesthesia, electrocardiogram (ECG) and invasive arterial pressure monitoring is complemented by the bispectral index (BIS),[6] which monitors the electroencephalographic activity. Cortisol-induced bone resorption leads to osteoporosis, requiring the careful handling of the patient to prevent bone fractures. The hyperaldosteronism and the hypokalemic alkalosis can cause cardiac arrhythmias, making difficult the diagnosis of cardiac arrhythmias caused by surgical procedures in areas close to the hypothalamus.[7] The conversion of muscle proteins into glucose reduces the muscular mass as well as the amount of curare necessary to ensure immobility. The hyperglycemia must be treated to prevent hyperglycemic coma, which could complicate the recovering of consciousness.

Acromegaly

Acromegaly is often associated with pituitary adenoma and is caused by the tumor's high secretion of growth hormone (GH). The resulting enlargement of the lower jaw, oral cavity, and tongue interferes with the laryngoscope during tracheal intubation. The increase of muscular mass requires a higher dose of curare for muscle relaxation, because the internal organs are also enlarged. The enlarged lungs require higher volume flow during assisted ventilation. The size of the heart also increases, but leads to interstitial fibrosis and infiltrating lymphomononuclear myocarditis, posing a risk of cardiac ischemia and making the proper procedures more difficult. A higher cardiac output is needed to perfuse the enlarged organs and muscular mass. However, despite the heart's hypertrophy, its contractility is compromised and may result in cardiac arrest.[8] The associated hyperglycemia is mediated by the excess of GH that induces resistance against insulin activity. Acromegalic patients must be fully awaken before tracheal extubation is done because the decreased ventilation caused by the partial encephalic depression, due to the residual action of anesthetics, is aggravated by the enlarged tongue that obstructs the respiratory pathways, compromising breathing.

Prolactinoma

Patients with prolactin-producing pituitary tumors who are treated with dopamine agonist drugs (e.g., bromocriptine) may present dopamine-like cardiovascular effects such as arterial hypotension and cardiac arrhythmia in a hypertensive patient.[9]

Pituitary Tumors or Tumors in the Sella Turcica Area

Whether or not these are hormone-producing tumors, they eventually compress the hypothalamic-pituitary neural axis as their volume increases, thus causing panhypopituitarism.[10] The reduction of synthesis of ACTH, GH, and thyroid-stimulating hormone (TSH) renders the patient more sensitive to anesthesia and cardiovascular depressant drugs, making it difficult to evaluate the depth of anesthesia. Again, the BIS monitor can be useful. Surgical ablation of the pituitary stalk causes sudden arterial hypotension in the immediate postsurgical period, due to adrenal insufficiency associated with decreased ACTH secretion. Lesions of the hypothalamic-pituitary neural axis can cause diabetes insipidus (DI),[11,12] leading to free water loss through the kidney and increase of sodium in the plasma, which results in hypernatremia. Diuresis may reach an output of 15 to 20 mL/kg/hour, rendering the patient hypovolemic and susceptible to arterial hypotension. Plasmatic sodium increases to 155 to 160 mEq/L and elevates plasma osmolarity to 310 to 315 mEq/L. Vasopressin must be promptly administered to prevent seizures as soon as the DI hypothesis is confirmed. Edema around the tumor indicates loss of integrity of the blood–brain barrier in that area and possible reduction of vascular-arterial reactivity, suggesting the use of anesthetics that reduce the metabolic rate and induce cerebral vasoconstriction. Intravenous anesthetics, except ketamine, reduce neuron metabolism and induce vasoconstriction.

Meningioma and Angioma

In vascularized tumors, such as meningiomas and angiomas, the discrete to moderate arterial hypotension reduces surgical bleeding, also preserving the cerebral blood flow (CBF) in the absence of intracranial hypertension (ICH). Arterial hypertension significantly increases bleeding inside the tumor and its surroundings, because there is no vasoconstrictor response to the increased arterial pressure in these areas, as a result of reduced arterial self-regulation.

■ Characteristics of Structures Adjacent to the Tumor

Invasive blood pressure (IBP) shows sudden variations in extensive arterial hemorrhage due to lesions in arteries of the skull base involved by the tumor. Immediate arterial hypotension must be induced through higher doses of anesthetics or the use of arterial vasodilators. However, the reduction of blood flow may cause brain ischemia. Some drugs that induce arterial hypotension through systemic vasodilation (e.g., sodium nitroprusside and halogenated anesthetics) also lead to cerebral vasodilation, thus increasing both intracranial blood and intracranial pressure. If necessary, the carotids must be compressed. Blood components must be available for transfusion because the hemorrhage can be difficult to control.

Venous Air Embolism

The proximity of the field of tumor access to the venous sinus may cause venous injury and a venous air embolism (VAE). Air bubbles in the superior cava vein increase the central venous pressure (CVP), and once they reach the cardiac chambers they augment the pressure in the right atrium and hinder blood output through the right ventricle. Air bubbles passing through capillary vessels in lung alveoli also hinder the blood flux. Therefore, hypotension and tachycardia ensue. Pulmonary perfusion reduces and compromises gaseous exchanges in the alveoli, with the consequent fall of exhaled CO_2 [end-tidal carbon dioxide concentration (E_T-CO_2)] and O_2 saturation in arterial blood. Cardiac Doppler detects air bubbles inside the cardiac chambers. The prophylaxis against VAE consists of volume adjustment to prevent the negative balance in the volume replacement and the use of 6 to 8 cm of peak end-expiratory pressure (PEEP) H_2O. Treatment consists of warning the surgeon, reducing the proclivity and aspiration of air bubbles through the inserted catheter, with the orifices positioned in the superior cava vein and in the right atrium, and, if needed, administering a rapid infusion of volume and compression of jugular veins (if possible). In cases of hypotension, administer vasopressor medication.

Arrhythmias and Blood Pressure Changes Associated with Surgical Procedures

Arrhythmias and changes in arterial pressure, emerging from surgical manipulation of the hypothalamus or of the brainstem, require the immediate warning of the surgeon to reduce harmful stimulation of the CNS, because the stronger the stimulus, the worse the cardiovascular alterations will be. The increase of the depth of anesthesia reduces both arrhythmias and blood pressure changes. Nevertheless, the stimulus continues, and a more serious lesion of the CNS may occur despite the reduced impact on the cardiovascular tract. Intense changes in arterial pressure, as a consequence of surgical manipulation of the brainstem and of the bulb, may signal changes in the patient's respiratory pattern during awakening because of the vicinity of the respiratory centers to the bulbar cardiovascular centers. The intensive manipulation of the bulb may compromise the recovery of consciousness because the ascending reticular activating system (ARAS), responsible for wakefulness, is situated in this area.

When a tumor is compressing cranial nerves, tracheal intubation must be maintained to avoid pulmonary infection, because the glossopharyngeal (IX) and the hypoglossal (II) nerves are responsible for the sensitivity of the larynx, pharynx, and trachea as well as for bronchial motility. Dysfunction of these nerves reduces sensitivity to any substance in the oropharyngeal tract and causes difficulty in swallowing, thus facilitating the aspiration of substances into the trachea and bronchi.

The excessive manipulation of the oculomotor nerve (III) induces pupillary dilation that interferes with the neurologic assessment. In such cases, early awakening is necessary to allow the assessment of consciousness degree and motor activity as well.

Patient's Monitoring

Electrocardiography identifies the source of cardiac arrhythmias, whereas the invasive arterial pressure promptly shows either hypo- or hypertension states. Central venous pressure helps in volume replacement and in the diagnosis and treatment of venous air embolism. Capnography and oxygen saturation indicate changes in pulmonary ventilation and variations in the ventilation/perfusion ratio. Intrathoracic pressure guides adjustments in ventilation and curare dosing. Doppler, BIS, and curare-action monitoring are supporting tools during anesthesia.

Patient's Positioning for Transnasal Approach

The positions that favor venous drainage from the brain and reduce intracranial pressure are as follows:

1. The head must be above the cardiac atrium to favor venous drainage by gravity, because the encephalic segment of the venous system does not have valves.
2. The optimum positioning for the transnasal approach is dorsal decubitus with an approximately 20-degree inclination of the bench, and an extended neck.
3. Flexion or rotation of the neck must be avoided to prevent compression of the internal jugular vein.
4. It is important to carefully check and remove any form of external compression of the neck.
5. Excessive volume of intravascular infusion and the rise of intrathoracic pressure must be avoided to prevent increasing the central venous pressure.
6. The surgical field is better exposed with the head-above-the-heart position that also reduces local hemorrhage. However, because the surgical field is higher than the heart, the opening of any venous system may lead to VAE. Note that for each 13 cm of head elevation above the heart, there is a correspondent 10 mm Hg reduction in the cerebral perfusion pressure. Therefore, the distance between the surgical field and the heart must be considered when arterial hypotension is induced to diminish arterial hemorrhage. Moreover, the invasive arterial pressure transducer must be positioned at the median point of the head.
7. When a graft is needed to seal a liquoric fistula, the positioning of flexed legs and internal rotation of the right thigh must be carefully done, especially with patients suffering from Cushing disease and osteoporosis, to prevent pathologic fractures.

Action of Anesthetics

The selected anesthetics must not contribute to the increase of intracranial pressure if it is already high. Anesthetics reduce the neuronal metabolic rate, but the necessary concentrations to provide encephalic protection may be too high, causing cardiovascular depression and systemic arterial hypotension, which reduces cerebral perfusion. In such cases, arterial hypotension is curbed with volume infusion and, if necessary, the association of a vasopressor drug. The depth of anesthesia should not be decreased because the metabolic rate would increase and elevate ICP.

Intravenous Anesthetics (Droperidol, Barbiturates, Propofol, Remifentanil)

These drugs depress the cardiovascular system without causing vasodilation. Some undesirable effects in the CNS, however, may occur. High doses of fentanyl (200 mg/kg) may increase the metabolic rate and activate the limbic system, inducing electroencephalogram (EEG) hyperactivity similar to a convulsive seizure.[12] Etomidate in subclinical doses may stimulate EEG activity in patients with a history of convulsive crises.[13,14] Ketamine increases cerebral blood flow and therefore strongly elevates neuronal metabolic rates, which may lead to convulsive crises.[15]

Inhalation Anesthetics

Besides reducing the metabolic rate, halogenated anesthetics cause a certain degree of cerebral vasodilation by interfering with the intrinsic mechanism of cerebral arteries that regulates neuronal metabolic reduction and vasoconstriction. Therefore, although halogenated anesthetics reduce neuron metabolism, they also induce cerebral vasodilation due to their action upon the arterial muscular fibers. As the cerebral vasodilation increases the volume of encephalic blood, the intracranial pressure is also increased. In the presence of deep hypocapnia, enflurane may evoke EEG activity similar to convulsive crises.[16]

Anesthetics that depress functional neuron activity also reduce their metabolic rate and therefore do not damage nerve cells, because they also decrease cellular oxygen intake. However, the neuronal metabolic rate may already be reduced by an existing low oxygen delivery associated with hypoxia or deep hypocapnia or due to an accentuated state of poor encephalic perfusion or deep anemia.

When PaO_2 is lower than 60 mm Hg, cerebral arterial dilation takes place in response to hypoxia, as an attempt to maintain oxygen delivery through the increased blood flow to the brain. In the process, as PaO_2 reduces to 30 mm Hg, this cerebral reflex action is unable to sustain the delivery of oxygen to the neurons.

The induction of hypocapnia to reduce cerebral blood volume and intracranial pressure may lead to ischemia when $PaCO_2$ reaches values below 25 mm Hg, as a consequence of intensive vasoconstriction in areas of the brain in which the vascular reactivity is preserved. Cerebral perfusion pressure (CPP) results from the difference between the mean arterial pressure (MAP) and the intracranial pressure (ICP). The increase of ICP or the reduction of MAP that results in CPP levels lower than 40 mm Hg is extremely damaging to the brain. Sharp and acute lowering of the hematocrit count may compromise cerebral vascular reactivity.

Perioperative Management of Endoscopic Transnasal Sellar Surgery

Before anesthesia induction, it is important to check for possible preexisting oculomotor lesions. The eyes must be protected with cream or gel that does not contain atropine in the formulation, to avoid mydriasis, which would later interfere with the neurologic assessment.

- The tracheal intubation probe should be properly positioned and well fixed to prevent accidental extubation during the surgical manipulation of the transnasal access or during intraoperative procedures such as single-lung intubation through the endotracheal passage. Ventilation must be checked through auscultation, and the oral cavity must be filled with a small tampon to prevent blood or serum access to the oropharyngeal area and consequent aspiration into the trachea and bronchi.
- Soft tissues at the site of the surgical access are infiltrated with adrenaline to reduce intraoperative bleeding, but excess adrenaline leads to hypertension, tachycardia, and extrasystole. To counter these cardiovascular alterations, the infusion of short-acting anesthetics should be increased and, if needed, beta-blockers and arterial hypotensors should be added.
- For skull base surgeries, the immobility of the patient is of utmost importance, due to the complexity of the brain structures that may either be involved in the surgical field or be next to it. Therefore, the depth of anesthesia and the dosage of muscle relaxant must be properly considered according to the patient's physical and clinical characteristics.

Postoperative Care

- To help the graft's sealing a cerebrospinal fluid (CSF) leak, the introduction of a drainage catheter in the lumbar subarachnoid space may be required for continuous liquid drainage in the postoperative phase. The anesthesiologist is the best-prepared professional to perform the lumbar puncture and to insert the catheter, due to his familiarity with these procedures. Furthermore, the drainage of liquor through the fistula during the intraoperative phase may have caused liquoric hypotension, thus making it more difficult to localize the subarachnoid space during the lumbar puncture.
- The prevention of coughing during extubation is essential and must be done as soon as the patient recovers consciousness, because the intrathoracic pressure increases the risk of CSF leak if the dura mater has been injured.

References

1. Schaller B. Trigemino-cardiac reflex during transsphenoidal surgery for pituitary adenomas. Clin Neurol Neurosurg 2005;107:468–474
2. Stober T, Sen S, Anstätt T, Bette L. Correlation of cardiac arrhythmias with brainstem compression in patients with intracerebral hemorrhage. Stroke 1988;19:688–692
3. Duke DA, Lynch JJ, Harner SG, Faust RJ, Ebersold MJ. Venous air embolism in sitting and supine patients undergoing vestibular schwannoma resection. Neurosurgery 1998;42:1282–1286, discussion 1286–1287
4. Bauer DF, Youkilis A, Schenck C, Turner CR, Thompson BG. The falcine trigeminocardiac reflex: case report and review of the literature. Surg Neurol 2005;63:143–148

5. Torpy DJ, Mullen N, Ilias I, Nieman LK. Association of hypertension and hypokalemia with Cushing's syndrome caused by ectopic ACTH secretion: a series of 58 cases. Ann N Y Acad Sci 2002;970:134–144

6. Ali Z, Prabhakar H, Bithal PK, Dash HH. Bispectral index-guided administration of anesthesia for transsphenoidal resection of pituitary tumors: a comparison of 3 anesthetic techniques. J Neurosurg Anesthesiol 2009; 21:10–15

7. Rath GP, Chaturvedi A, Chouhan RS, Prabhakar H. Transient cardiac asystole in transsphenoidal pituitary surgery: a case report. J Neurosurg Anesthesiol 2004;16:299–301

8. Colao A, Marzullo P, Di Somma C, Lombardi G. Growth hormone and the heart. Clin Endocrinol (Oxf) 2001;54:137–154

9. Luchsinger A, Velasco M, Urbina A, et al. Comparative effects of dopaminergic agonists on cardiovascular, renal, and renin-angiotensin systems in hypertensive patients. J Clin Pharmacol 1992;32:55–60

10. Arafah BM, Prunty D, Ybarra J, Hlavin ML, Selman WR. The dominant role of increased intrasellar pressure in the pathogenesis of hypopituitarism, hyperprolactinemia, and headaches in patients with pituitary adenomas. J Clin Endocrinol Metab 2000;85:1789–1793

11. Shah S, Har-El G. Diabetes insipidus after pituitary surgery: incidence after traditional versus endoscopic transsphenoidal approaches. Am J Rhinol 2001;15:377–379

12. Tempelhoff R, Modica PA, Bernardo KL, Edwards I. Fentanyl-induced electrocorticographic seizures in patients with complex partial epilepsy. J Neurosurg 1992;77:201–208

13. Krieger W, Copperman J, Laxer KD. Seizures with etomidate anesthesia. Anesth Analg 1985;64:1226–1227

14. Ebrahim ZY, DeBoer GE, Luders H, Hahn JF, Lesser RP. Effect of etomidate on the electroencephalogram of patients with epilepsy. Anesth Analg 1986;65:1004–1006

15. Ferrer-Allado T, Brechner VL, Dymond A, Cozen H, Crandall P. Ketamine-induced electroconvulsive phenomena in the human limbic and thalamic regions. Anesthesiology 1973;38:333–344

16. Neigh JL, Garman JK, Harp JR. The electroencephalographic pattern during anesthesia with Ethrane: effects of depth of anesthesia, PaCo2, and nitrous oxide. Anesthesiology 1971;35:482–487

8 Postoperative Care in Skull Base Surgery

Parul Goyal, Devyani Lal, and Peter H. Hwang

Tips and Pearls

- Immediate postoperative care after endoscopic skull base procedures should focus on monitoring for neurologic complications, cerebrospinal fluid leaks, and endocrine disturbances.
- Patients should be monitored in an intensive care unit after surgery.
- The most common endocrine disturbances after endoscopic skull base surgery involve disruption of fluid homeostasis. Therefore, it is important to measure fluid intake and output very closely after surgery.
- Adequate postoperative care in the office after discharge should be aimed toward optimizing wound healing and ensuring patent paranasal sinus outflow tracts.

Introduction

Postoperative care after endoscopic skull base surgical procedures is important in ensuring optimal outcomes. Initially, postoperative care focuses on diagnosis and treatment of neurologic, rhinologic, and systemic problems that may arise in the immediate postoperative period. Long term, adequate postoperative care is necessary to ensure patent and functional sinus ostia.

General Care

Certain aspects of postoperative care start even before the patient leaves the operating room. At the completion of the procedure, it is important to communicate with the anesthesia team to ensure as smooth an emergence and extubation as possible. Avoidance of excessive coughing or "bucking" on the endotracheal tube helps to minimize bleeding and risk for disruption of grafts at the reconstruction site. If a lumbar drain is placed for the purpose of cerebrospinal fluid (CSF) diversion after skull base reconstruction, it is left unclamped at the time of extubation to minimize large changes in intracranial pressure.

In the recovery room, patients should be monitored closely with particular attention to neurologic status. For patients who have undergone more extensive skull base resections, postoperative observation in the intensive care unit may be indicated to facilitate close monitoring of neurologic status and fluid balance.

Packing

Various packing materials and protocols have been described for patients after endoscopic skull base surgery, both to support graft materials at the site of reconstruction as well as to promote hemostasis. In cases where a small skull base defect has been repaired, or where no CSF leak has occurred, a minimal amount of absorbable packing may be sufficient; absorbable gelatin sponges, fibrin glue, and polymerized hydrogel are among the many options for bioabsorbable packing material. However, in cases where a large defect has been repaired using composite grafting materials, it may be desirable to support the graft with additional nonabsorbable packing. For example, an inflatable balloon in the form of a Foley catheter or a posterior epistaxis pack may be placed against the graft to support the skull base repair for several days postoperatively. Nonabsorbable sponges or gauze may also be used. Packing removal should be done with extreme care so as not to disrupt the surgical repair, and endoscopic debridement of the repair site should be deferred for several weeks until definitive closure of the repair site has been ascertained. Because patients often find packing removal to be among the most uncomfortable parts of the postoperative process, our practice is to avoid large amounts of packing after endoscopic procedures whenever possible, balancing functional necessity for packing against patient comfort.

Antibiotics

There are no standardized recommendations for postoperative antibiotic use after endoscopic skull base surgical procedures. The procedures can best be classified as clean-contaminated procedures given the fact that instruments and graft materials must be passed through the nose to the operative site, allowing for contamination by nasal flora. Standardized regimens of antibiotics have been described in patients undergoing open skull base surgical procedures.

Kraus and colleagues[1] investigated the use of a standardized regimen of antibiotics in patients undergoing traditional (open) skull base surgical procedures. Their study included 211 patients, 90 of whom were treated with a standard regimen of ceftazidime, metronidazole, and vancomycin for a mean of 7.7 days. Patients who were treated with this standard regimen had significantly fewer infectious complications when compared with patients treated with various other antibiotic regimens.

With regard to endoscopic skull base procedures, the existing data suggest that endoscopic procedures may be associated with a lower likelihood of severe postoperative infections compared with open skull base procedures, perhaps due to qualitative differences between endoscopic and nonendoscopic techniques. Thus, endoscopic skull base surgery may have different perioperative antibiotic requirements. Brown and colleagues[2] investigated the role of prophylactic postoperative antibiotics after endoscopic skull base surgery. Their study included 90 patients treated for pituitary tumors, encephaloceles, meningiomas, and craniopharyngiomas. Intravenous antibiotics were given at the time of induction and were continued for 24 to 48 hours postoperatively until the patients' nasal packing was removed. The authors had no cases of intracranial infections or meningitis. However, 21% of the patients did need outpatient antibiotics within the first 3 months for nasal or sinus cavity infections.

In our practice, patients undergoing endoscopic skull base surgery receive a single preoperative dose of an intravenous antibiotic. Postoperatively, the use of antibiotics varies according to the extent of skull base resection and the amount of packing used. Smaller cases such as pituitary tumor resection are not treated with postoperative antibiotics, whereas larger skull base resections are treated prophylactically with a 2-week course of amoxicillin-clavulanate or quinolone. This may help to decrease the relatively high rate of postoperative sinus infections described by Brown et al.[2] Patients who develop sinusitis are treated in a culture-directed fashion.

Cerebrospinal Fluid Leak

Reconstruction of the skull base is a critical part of endoscopic skull base surgery. The goal of reconstruction is to create a watertight seal so that complications associated with a persistent CSF leak can be avoided. Many different algorithms have been described for reconstruction after endoscopic skull base procedures.[3–5] Although there is inadequate evidence to support one algorithm over another, vascularized flap reconstruction in general provides more favorable closure for large skull base defects. At the conclusion of endoscopic skull base surgery, careful inspection of the operative site facilitates visualization of most CSF leaks that may be present. Occasionally it can be difficult to identify a CSF leak at the time of surgery when the CSF may be obscured by blood, clots, and nasal secretions. Intrathecal fluorescein can be used to help identify and localize occult CSF leaks. However, its role as a routine intraoperative diagnostic tool is limited by the fact that it must be injected before the start of the procedure.

It is important to assess patients postoperatively for a CSF leak. In most instances, patients who have a postoperative CSF leak manifest the leak in the first 24 to 48 hours after surgery. However, it is important to search for a delayed leak when the patient is seen in outpatient follow-up. Some patients with a postoperative CSF leak may have obvious clear rhinorrhea, making the diagnosis straightforward. Other patients may have subtle signs, in which case imaging studies (computed tomography cisternogram) or surgical reexploration may be indicated. Nasal drainage that can be collected can be sent for β-2-transferrin assay to differentiate CSF from nasal secretions. In most institutions, this assay is not performed in the hospital's own laboratory and must be sent to a different facility. It is often not practical to wait several days for the results of the testing; thus the diagnosis of a CSF leak is often made based on history and clinical suspicion, before the results of such tests are available.

After a CSF leak is diagnosed, treatment options include lumbar drainage for CSF diversion versus surgical reexploration. Cases in which a meticulous, layered reconstruction was performed at the time of surgery may initially be managed with lumbar drainage to allow for any small leak sites to seal. Patients who continue to have a persistent leak after a 48- to 72-hour trial of lumbar drainage should be taken back to the operating room for reexploration and revision of the reconstruction.

Bleeding

Although some degree of postoperative oozing is unavoidable after endoscopic skull base surgery, bleeding can typically be controlled at the conclusion of surgery with relatively limited amounts of nasal packing (or no packing). Thus our practice is to avoid large amounts of packing at the conclusion of endoscopic procedures. Patients are told before surgery to expect some minor oozing and expression of clots from the nose.

Heavy bleeding that occurs postoperatively is most commonly related to arterial injury. During the course of transsphenoidal surgery, the posterior septal branch of the sphenopalatine artery can be injured. Similarly, the anterior and posterior ethmoid arteries may be subject to injury during anterior cranial base surgery. Arterial nasal bleeding can be managed with nasal packing, surgical exploration and control, or, for posterior bleeding, angiography and embolization. We prefer the option of surgical exploration and control in most patients with suspected bleeding from branches of the sphenopalatine artery. If the bleeding site can be localized, the area can be controlled directly with bipolar cauterization. Alternatively, endoscopic techniques can be used to ligate the sphenopalatine artery as the vessel exits the sphenopalatine foramen. At our institutions, this method is preferred over embolization because of its effectiveness and low morbidity.

Injury to the carotid artery is rare, but can have serious immediate and long-term consequences. Patients typically present with profuse bleeding. Direct surgical repair is generally not feasible, and the best chance for control is by way of angiography and endovascular treatment.[6,7] When patients present with profuse bleeding, it is important to control the bleeding and stabilize the patient by applying direct pressure at the bleeding site. A large Foley catheter or other form of nasal packing can help stabilize the bleeding enough to allow for angiography.

Postoperative Debridement

It is important to ensure patent sinus ostia after endoscopic skull base surgical procedures to avoid postoperative sinus obstruction and sinusitis. Our routine care includes postoperative endoscopy approximately 2 weeks after surgery. Debris and crusting can be removed from areas that are not adjacent to areas of skull base reconstruction. It is important to avoid aggressive debridement because manipulation can disrupt grafts at the site of skull base reconstruction. At subsequent follow-up visits, endoscopy is used to ensure patent sinus ostia and satisfactory healing at the surgical site. Saline nasal irrigations can be used after the first few weeks to help clear residual debris and crusting.

Endocrine Dysfunction

Patients undergoing parasellar skull base surgery are commonly vulnerable to transient or permanent derangements in the hypothalamic-pituitary-adrenal axis.[8] Changes in the water-sodium balance result from abnormalities of antidiuretic hormone (ADH). Also, patients with functioning pituitary tumors may have unique hemodynamic and endocrine changes associated with conditions such as acromegaly, Cushing's disease, or thyrotoxicosis.

Diabetes Insipidus

Diabetes insipidus (DI) is a common complication of transsphenoidal pituitary surgery, occurring in 0.5 to 25% of cases.[9] DI typically manifests 1 to 2 days after pituitary surgery and is characterized by polyuria with dilute urine. Urine output can range from 4 to 18 L/day, with a urine specific gravity less than 1.005.[10] After endoscopic pituitary surgery, most patients are awake and oriented, with increased thirst and polydipsia. Therefore, critical hypernatremia (over 150 mmol/mL), severe volume contraction, and hyperosmolality are rare.[9] DI is transient in most patients and usually resolves by the third postoperative day.[10] Hensen and colleagues[11] found DI in 31% of patients in the early postoperative period, but in only 6% one week after surgery. Permanent DI requires the degeneration of 90% of the magnocellular neurons bilaterally and is very uncommon.[10]

Table 8.1 Differential Diagnoses of Polyuria Following Pituitary Surgery

Cause	Features
Diabetes insipidus (DI)	Line specific gravity <1.005 Hypernatremia
Diuresis of perioperatively administered intravenous fluids	Urine specific gravity >1.005 Low to normal sodium levels Increased body weight
Glycosuria (diabetes mellitus)	Falsely elevated serum, urine osmolarity Increased serum and urine glucose Falsely decreased sodium levels

A triphasic DI may occur in some patients with complete stalk resection.[10] The first phase of transient DI over 1 to 3 days is followed by a period of antidiuresis 1 week later due to the release of ADH from degenerating neurons. In this second phase, patients may have hyponatremia and hypoosmolarity. Permanent DI follows these first two phases.

Screening for DI is performed by measuring intake and output, serial plasma osmolarity, serum chemistry, and urine specific gravity. Urine output >250 mL/hour over two consecutive hours supports the diagnosis of DI. Other causes of increased postoperative urine output must be considered (**Table 8.1**). Increased body weight with normal or low sodium and urine specific gravity >1.005 suggests postoperative fluid diuresis. This is a self-limited homeostatic response and should not be treated. Hypernatremia with urine specific gravity less than 1.005 is seen in DI. Elevated serum glucose with hyperglycemia is suggestive of glycosuria.

Treatment of DI is directed to restoring electrolyte homeostasis. Patients with intact thirst mechanisms, stable sodium levels, and stable osmolarity should be monitored closely with accurate measurements of intake-output and serum electrolytes. Water deficit should be accurately calculated, and fluid can be replaced orally or intravenously over a period of 24 to 48 hours. Treatment with desmopressin [deamino-8-D-arginine vasopressin (DDAVP)], a synthetic ADH analogue, is considered if there is significant discrepancy between fluid intake and output, serum sodium above 145 mEq/L, or when polyuria interferes with sleep.[9] DDAVP administered intranasally, orally, subcutaneously and intravenously is quick and effective. An initial 1 µg of DDAVP subcutaneously and an oral dose of 0.1 mg are equally effective.[10] Urine output and serum electrolyte monitoring is mandatory as hyponatremia can occur.

Syndrome of Inappropriate Antidiuretic Hormone and Other Causes of Postoperative Hyponatremia

Delayed hyponatremia is common following pituitary surgery, being present in 9 to 25% of patients.[10] In such patients, ADH is secreted in spite of hyponatremia. Free water intake exceeds free water excretion, and increased urinary sodium excretion in the context of inappropriately concentrated urine is observed. The syndrome of inappropriate antidiuretic hormone (SIADH) is diagnosed by the presence of low serum sodium (usually <135 mEq/L), serum hypo-osmolarity, hyperosmolar urine with excess sodium excretion (>40 mEq/L), and euvolemia. Patients usually exhibit symptoms about 1 week after surgery. Symptoms include confusion, delirium, agitation, headache, appetite loss, nausea, vomiting, and lethargy. Seizures may occur if sodium levels drop below 115 mmol/L.

Cerebral salt wasting (CSW), adrenal insufficiency, hypothyroidism, and hyperglycemia are other factors that can contribute to postoperative hyponatremia. SIADH has a delayed onset, and this helps distinguishing SIADH from other causes of hyponatremia (**Table 8.2**). CSW is the renal loss of sodium after intracranial surgery, causing hyponatremia and hypovolemia. SIADH is characterized by euvolemia or mild hypervolemia, with decreased uric acid level with normal blood urea nitrogen (BUN) and creatinine. In contrast, CSW patients have volume contraction, elevated BUN and creatinine, and may have increased uric acid level. Patients with CSW lose weight, whereas patients with SIADH gain weight.

Adrenal insufficiency is important to rule out in early postoperative hyponatremia. Cortisol inhibits ADH secretion, and deficient or absent cortisol levels cause increased ADH secretion, leading to impairment in excreting free water.[12] Treatment with cortisone replacement corrects hyponatremia. Hypothyroidism may cause hyponatremia by poorly understood mechanisms.[10] Hyperglycemia may cause "pseudo"-hyponatremia by drawing intracellular water into the extracellular space due to increased intravascular osmotic load.

Therapy for hyponatremia is based on its severity, acuteness of onset, and associated symptoms. In SIADH, fluid restriction is the key. Fluid intake is restricted to less than 1000 mL/day, and serum electrolytes are measured at least daily.[10] If sodium levels do not improve over the next several days, then fluid restriction to less than 600 mL is initiated. Although mild cases of SIADH may be managed on an outpatient basis, severely hyponatremic patients must be treated as inpatients. Refractory SIADH or patients with severe symptomatic hyponatremia (<120 mEq/L, with headache, nausea, vomiting, altered mentation, or seizures) may need treatment with intravenous hypertonic saline. Over-rapid correction must be avoided to prevent central pontine myelinolysis. The correction rate should not exceed 1 mmol/L/hour in the acute setting, and 0.5 mmol/L/ hour in the chronic setting.[9,10] Hypertonic therapy should not be used for more than 12 to 24 hours; it should be discontinued once there is partial correction and resolution of symptoms. Serum electrolytes should be measured frequently (every 6 hours). Intravenous urea may also be used as an adjunct in severe hyponatremia.

Diabetes insipidus and SIADH are the most common causes of disruption in fluid homeostasis postoperatively, and the clinical features of these disorders are summarized in **Table 8.3**.

Table 8.2 Causes of Hyponatremia Following Pituitary Surgery

Cause	Features
Syndrome of inappropriate antidiuretic hormone (SIADH)	Delayed onset at 1 week Euvolemia
Cerebral salt wasting	Early postoperative onset Hypovolemia
Adrenal insufficiency	Early postoperative onset Low serum cortisol Hyponatremia responsive to cortisol therapy
"Pseudo"-hyponatremia	Early postoperative onset Falsely decreased sodium due increased glucose levels (diabetes mellitus, Cushing's disease, acromegaly)

Other Endocrine Considerations and Perioperative Management

Perioperative stress dosing with glucocorticosteroids is controversial. The rationale for administering steroids is based on the assumption that surgery may disturb the hypothalamic-pituitary-adrenal axis (HPA). If patients have preoperative cortisol deficiency, perioperative steroids are indicated. A dose of 50 to 100 mg of intravenous hydrocortisone every 6 hours, then tapered to the oral preoperative dose, is usually used. Patients with Cushing's disease require postoperative cortisol level assessment to determine results form surgery, and in these patients perioperative steroids may be avoided.

Acromegaly is associated with major cardiac-related morbidity and mortality. Hypertension and left ventricular failure may be seen in about half these patients.[9] Diastolic dysfunction and cardiomyopathy, conduction abnormalities, and coronary artery disease may be present. Airway obstruction

Table 8.3 Characteristics of Diabetes Insipidus (DI) Versus Syndrome of Inappropriate Antidiuretic Hormone (SIADH)

	DI	SIADH
Onset	1–2 days after surgery	1 week after surgery
Symptom/sign	Polyuria, polydipsia	Chemistry: hyponatremia Symptoms rare
Serum osmolarity	Hypertonic (>310 mOsm/L)	Hypotonic (<275 mOsm/L)
Serum sodium	Increased (>145 mEq/L)	Decreased (<135 mEq/L)
Urine volume	High (4–18 L)	Low
Urine osmolarity	Low (<200 mOsm/L)	High (>100 mOsm/L)
Treatment	Supportive Hydration Hypertonic saline	Fluid restriction Hypertonic saline

Source: Modified from Nemergut EC, Dumont AS, Barry UT, Laws ER. Perioperative management of patients undergoing transsphenoidal pituitary surgery. Anesth Analg 2005;101(4):1170–1181.

may occur secondary to hypertrophic facial bones and soft tissue or laryngeal stenosis, leading to difficulties in intubation. Obstructive sleep apnea (OSA) is also common in these patients. Postoperatively, close monitoring of patients' airway and cardiac status is important. Patients with acromegaly have brisk diuresis following tumor resection, and early DDAVP should be avoided.[13]

Cushing's disease patients commonly have systemic hypertension, electrocardiogram (ECG) abnormalities, and left ventricular hypertrophy.[9] OSA is common. Impaired glucose tolerance (60%) and frank diabetes mellitus (in one third) are common. Tight glycemic control must be achieved in these patients to correct polyuria and unmask any underlying DI.

Thyrotoxicosis and hyperthyroidism due to thyroid-stimulating hormone (TSH)-producing adenoma are rare. However, these tumors are larger and more invasive at the time of diagnosis due to initial treatment for other causes of hyperthyroidism. Therefore, these tumors may be associated with higher blood loss. Hyperthyroidism should be controlled preoperatively.

Conclusion

Endoscopic skull base surgery is a rapidly advancing field, and regimens for postoperative care continue to evolve. There is little consensus on the specifics of postoperative care for these patients. The most commonly encountered postoperative problems include neurologic sequelae, endocrine disturbances, bleeding, and cerebrospinal fluid leaks. Postoperative care should be directed toward carefully monitoring and treating patients for these types of problems.

References

1. Kraus DH, Gonen M, Mener D, Brown AE, Bilsky MH, Shah JP. A standardized regimen of antibiotics prevents infectious complications in skull base surgery. Laryngoscope 2005;115:1347–1357
2. Brown SM, Anand VK, Tabaee A, Schwartz TH. Role of perioperative antibiotics in endoscopic skull base surgery. Laryngoscope 2007;117: 1528–1532
3. Kassam A, Carrau RL, Snyderman CH, Gardner P, Mintz A. Evolution of reconstructive techniques following endoscopic expanded endonasal approaches. Neurosurg Focus 2005;19:E8
4. Tabaee A, Anand VK, Brown SM, Lin JW, Schwartz TH. Algorithm for reconstruction after endoscopic pituitary and skull base surgery. Laryngoscope 2007;117:1133–1137
5. Sonnenburg RE, White D, Ewend MG, Senior B. Sellar reconstruction: is it necessary? Am J Rhinol 2003;17:343–346
6. Pepper JP, Wadhwa AK, Tsai F, Shibuya T, Wong BJ. Cavernous carotid injury during functional endoscopic sinus surgery: case presentations and guidelines for optimal management. Am J Rhinol 2007;21:105–109
7. Lippert BM, Ringel K, Stoeter P, Hey O, Mann WJ. Stentgraft-implantation for treatment of internal carotid artery injury during endonasal sinus surgery. Am J Rhinol 2007;21:520–524
8. Ciric I, Ragin A, Baumgartner C, Pierce D. Complications of transsphenoidal surgery: results of a national survey, review of the literature, and personal experience. Neurosurgery 1997;40:225–236, discussion 236–237
9. Nemergut EC, Dumont AS, Barry UT, Laws ER. Perioperative management of patients undergoing transsphenoidal pituitary surgery. Anesth Analg 2005;101:1170–1181
10. Dumont AS, Nemergut EC II, Jane JA Jr, Laws ER Jr. Postoperative care following pituitary surgery. J Intensive Care Med 2005;20:127–140
11. Hensen J, Henig A, Fahlbusch R, Meyer M, Boehnert M, Buchfelder M. Prevalence, predictors and patterns of postoperative polyuria and hyponatraemia in the immediate course after transsphenoidal surgery for pituitary adenomas. Clin Endocrinol (Oxf) 1999;50:431–439
12. Raff H. Glucocorticoid inhibition of neurohypophysial vasopressin secretion. Am J Physiol 1987;252(4 Pt 2):R635–R644
13. Jane JA Jr, Thapar K, Kaptain GJ, Maartens N, Laws ER Jr. Pituitary surgery: transsphenoidal approach. Neurosurgery 2002;51:435–442, discussion 442–444

II Evolving Concepts in Endoscopic Skull Base and Brain Surgery

9 Classification of Endonasal Approaches to the Ventral Skull Base

Carl H. Snyderman, Harshita Pant, Ricardo L. Carrau, Daniel M. Prevedello, Paul A. Gardner, and Amin B. Kassam

Tips and Pearls

- Otolaryngologists and neurosurgeons have collaborated to apply endoscopic principles to the treatment of cranial base tumors.
- The ventral skull base can be divided into modular units that can be approached individually or in combination to provide access to various pathologic processes.
- A transfrontal approach accesses the most anterior portion of the anterior cranial fossa.
- A transcribriform approach extends from the posterior table of the frontal sinus to the planum sphenoidale and along the coronal plane, to the medial wall of the orbit on either side.
- A transplanum approach is limited laterally by the optic canals and anteriorly by the posterior ethmoidal arteries.
- A transsellar approach is the standard approach to the sella but may be used to access other areas of the skull base.
- A transclival approach is divided into upper, middle, and inferior thirds. The upper third is related to the dorsum sellae. The middle third is related to the sphenoidal clival recess between the clival internal carotid arteries (ICAs). The inferior third is determined from the level of foramen lacerum to the foramen magnum.
- The body of C2 is usually the inferior limit of exposure in a transodontoid approach, which can be estimated by a line that touches the inferior border of the nasal bone and the posterior aspect of the hard palate projected to the cervical spine.
- The midpoint of the orbital roof may be reached by resection of the medial orbital wall and displacing the orbital contents.
- Intraconal dissection of orbital tumors is performed between the medial and inferior rectus muscles with preservation of extraocular motor function.
- A transpterygoid approach is a preliminary step to accessing the other modules in the coronal plane at the middle and posterior fossa.
- The cavernous sinus may be approached medial or lateral to cavernous ICA.
- Meckel's cave can be accessed above the petrous ICA.
- The approaches below the petrous ICA are infrapetrous, supracondylar, and transcondylar. The jugular foramen can be accessed lateral to the occipital condyle.

Introduction

We live in an era of minimally invasive surgery where many traditional open surgical approaches are being replaced by endoscopic approaches. In otolaryngology, endoscopic sinus surgery has become the standard of care for the treatment of inflammatory diseases and many benign and malignant sinonasal tumors. In neurosurgery, endoscopes have had a limited role and have been primarily used as an adjunct to open microscopic procedures, including surgery for pituitary tumors,[1,2] posterior fossa nerve decompression, and intracranial aneurysms. In recent years, otolaryngologists and neurosurgeons have collaborated to apply endoscopic principles to the treatment of cranial base tumors.[3] Development of endonasal cranial base surgery required an understanding of the skull base anatomy from an endoscopic perspective, the development of technologies adapted for intranasal use, and the concept of team surgery with an otolaryngologist and a neurosurgeon operating simultaneously and synergistically.

Introducing a new surgical concept often has three main phases of development: technical feasibility, safety and complications, and treatment outcomes. A critical examination of the outcomes begets new innovations or modifications of techniques, and this cycle repeats itself. We previously reported on the technical aspects of endonasal surgery of the cranial base and described new endoscopic surgical approaches to the ventral skull base.[4–6] Our experience over the last decade with more than 1000 entirely endoscopic surgeries demonstrated that endonasal cranial base surgery can be performed with acceptable morbidity. Reporting of treatment outcomes requires verification and comparison of experiences at multiple medical centers. A comparison of surgical series is made difficult by the variety of surgical approaches to the ventral skull base, diverse pathology and biology, and lack of standard measures of outcome.

Endonasal surgery of the cranial base began with pituitary surgery[1,2] and gradually progressed to encompass neighboring regions of the cranial base. It became apparent that the sphenoid sinus was the starting point for access to most of the cranial base and it contained the most critical anatomical structures, including the optic nerves and internal carotid arteries (ICAs). A surgical extension from the sphenoid sinus to adjacent areas of the ventral skull base can proceed in all directions with basic orientation along the sagittal and coronal planes. Thus, the ventral skull base can be divided into modular units that can be approached individually or in combination to provide access to various pathologic processes.[4–6]

As endonasal techniques evolve and become more widespread, a classification scheme is necessary to facilitate effective teaching of these techniques, preoperative planning, comparison of reported surgical series, and to refine surgical techniques. Here, we report our classification system based on our surgical experience with endonasal skull base surgery.

Methods

A retrospective analysis of all patients undergoing endonasal skull base surgery for all types of pathology at the University of Pittsburgh Medical Center from 1998 to 2006 was performed. A tumor registry was maintained on all patients with approval of the medical center's institutional review board. The ventral skull base was divided into anatomical subunits based on the relationship of these to key anatomical structures such as the internal carotid artery, cavernous sinus, optic nerve, and bony landmarks.

The classification scheme is shown in **Table 9.1**. In the sagittal plane, these endoscopic approaches extend anteriorly to the frontal sinus, inferiorly to the second cervical vertebra, and laterally to the jugular foramen and parapharyngeal carotid artery. It is useful to subcategorize the approaches in the coronal plane that correspond to the anterior, middle, and posterior cranial fossae. The anterior coronal plane extends from the midline across the roof of the orbits. The middle coronal plane includes the cavernous sinus, petrous apex, Meckel's cave, and the infratemporal skull base that is above the level of the petrous ICA. The posterior coronal plane includes the occipital condyle, extends along the inferior surface of the petrous bone below the level of the petrous ICA to the jugular foramen, and includes adjacent extracranial structures (parapharyngeal space).

Table 9.1 Classification of Endonasal Approaches to the Ventral Skull Base

- Sagittal plane
  - Transfrontal
  - Transcribriform
  - Transplanum (suprasellar)
  - Transsellar
  - Transclival
    - Superior: dorsum sellae
    - Middle: midclivus
    - Inferior: foramen magnum
  - Transodontoid
- Coronal plane
  - Anterior (anterior cranial fossa)
    - Supraorbital
    - Transorbital
  - Middle (middle cranial fossa)
    - Transpterygoid
    - Transcavernous
      - Medial
      - Lateral
    - Medial petrous apex
    - Suprapetrous (middle fossa) Meckel's cave
  - Infratemporal skull base
  - Posterior (posterior cranial fossa)
    - Transcondylar
    - Infrapetrous
    - Parapharyngeal space
    - Medial (jugular foramen)
    - Lateral

Surgical Approaches

More than 1000 endonasal skull base procedures were performed for a variety of pathologic processes including intracranial and extracranial neoplasms. For the purpose of this study, the first 700 patients were included. Although the largest number of patients had pituitary adenomas (39%), the majority of these were macroadenomas with extrasellar extension. There were more than 50 pediatric patients (<18 years). Approximately 23% were younger than 35 years and 25% were older than 62 years.

Using the classification scheme shown in **Table 9.1**, surgical approaches were categorized according to the predominant approach (**Fig. 9.1**). The sphenoid sinus was selected as a starting point for most endonasal procedures because of the key anatomical structures surrounding the sinus: ICA, optic nerves and chiasm, cavernous sinus, pituitary gland, and basilar artery. Many patients required surgical access via multiple anatomical modules, depending on the extent of the pathology and the need to expose key anatomical structures for tumor resection.

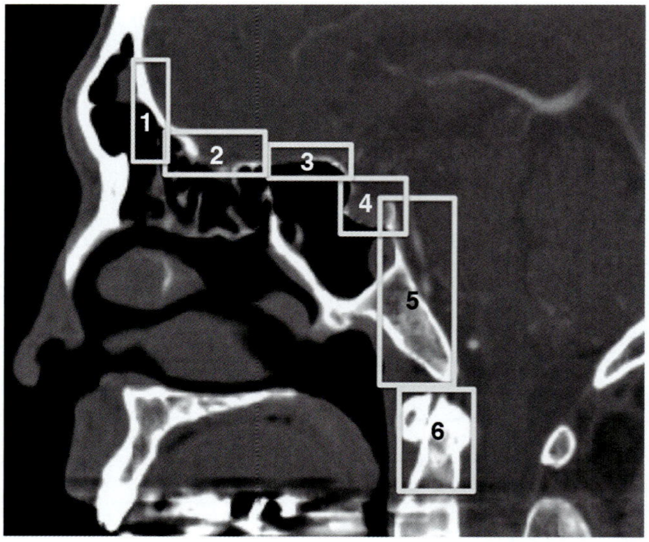

Fig. 9.1 Distribution of EEA surgical approaches. Some of the surgical approaches are grouped. 1: transfrontal; 2: transcribriform; 3: transplanum; 4: transsellar; 5: transclival; 6: transodontoid.

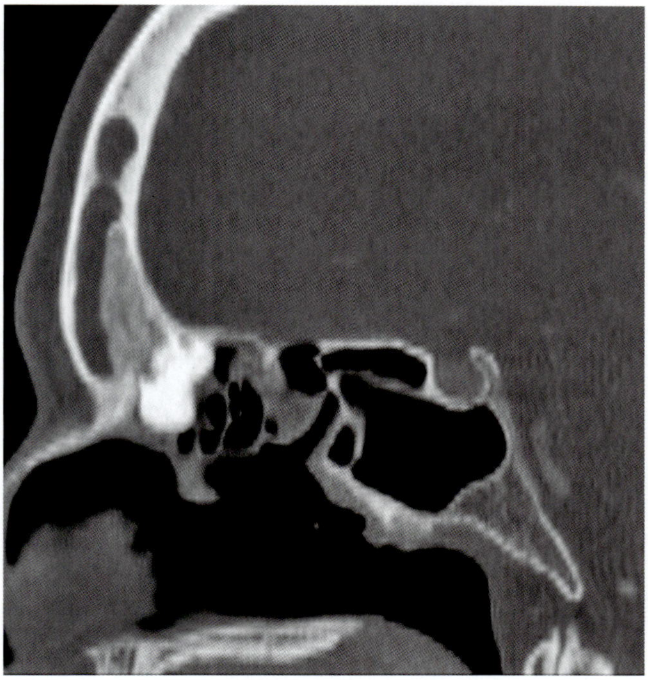

Fig. 9.2 Computed tomography (CT) scan at the sagittal plane of a nasal dermoid cyst with a tract extending through the skull base at the foramen cecum. This is an example of a disease treated with a transfrontal approach.

Sagittal Plane

Transfrontal Approach (Fig. 9.2)

A transfrontal approach accesses the anterior cranial fossa. It starts by bilateral frontal recess clearance, an access via the superior septal window to facilitate a modified endoscopic Lothrop (MEL) or a Draf 3 procedure in which a single maximum-sized frontal sinus ostium is created. Dissection posterior to the attachment of the middle turbinate to the skull base preserves olfaction and avoids violation of the cribriform plate and cerebrospinal fluid (CSF) leak. Common pathologies requiring a transfrontal approach include chronic frontal sinusitis, frontal sinus mucocele, fibro-osseous tumors, and nasal dermoid cysts. In pediatric patients with dermoid cysts, the cyst is opened intranasally and the septum is resected up to the skull base. Bone surrounding the sinus tract is drilled to the level of the dura with complete removal of epithelium lining the cyst.

Transcribriform Approach (Fig. 9.3)

The final surgical resection with this approach is analogous to the classic craniofacial resection. The cribriform plates are commonly resected for sinonasal malignancies (including esthesioneuroblastoma) and olfactory groove meningioma. First, the intranasal portion of the tumor is debulked to the plane of the skull base to define the attachment to the cribriform plate, and this attachment is cauterized with bipolar electrocautery. A complete sphenoethmoidectomy is performed bilaterally and a Draf 3 procedure performed to define the anterior resection margin. The nasal septum is transected along the sagittal plane from the crista galli anteriorly to the sphenoid rostrum approximately 1 cm inferior to the tumor attachment to the septum. This defines the inferior resection margin. The tumor is devascularized by cauterizing and transecting the anterior and posterior ethmoidal arteries, along the fovea ethmoidalis, midway along its course from the orbital margin and lateral lamella. The bone of the anterior cranial base in the periphery of the tumor is thinned with a coarse diamond drill to the resection margins, anteriorly to the posterior table of frontal sinus, posteriorly to the planum sphenoidale, and laterally to the medial orbital walls. The thinned bone is gently fractured and elevated inferiorly off the overlying dura.

The dura is cauterized and incised longitudinally along the lateral orbital margins, taking care to avoid injury to cortical vessels. The crista galli is removed with a drill, and the attached falx cauterized and transected. This facilitates rotating the dural specimen posteriorly. Dural incision along its posterior margin allows removal of the entire dural specimen en bloc. When indicated, the olfactory bulbs and nerves are elevated inferiorly off the overlying brain and transected at the level of the posterior dural margin. In the sagittal plane, the surgical defect extends from the posterior table of the frontal sinus to the planum sphenoidale and along the coronal plane, to the medial wall of the orbit on either side. For selected cases with small ipsilateral tumors, an ipsilateral resection of the anterior cranial base with preservation of olfaction on the contralateral side can be performed.

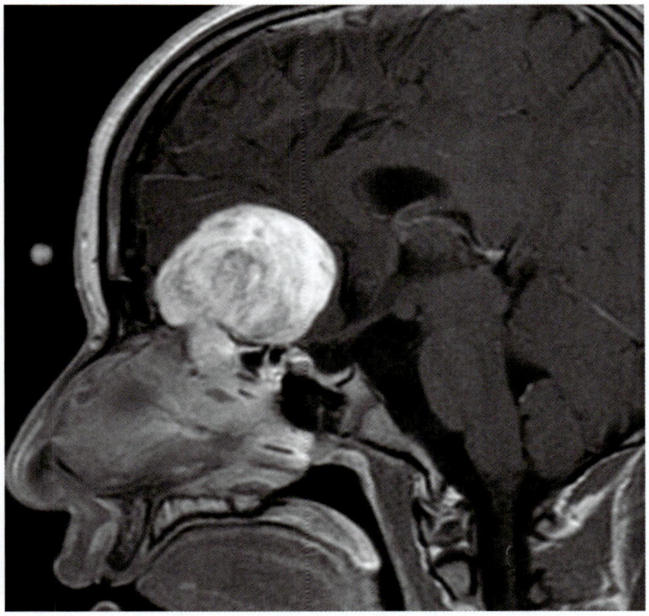

Fig. 9.3 Magnetic resonance imaging (MRI) scans of a large olfactory groove schwannoma that was completely resected using an endonasal transcribriform approach.

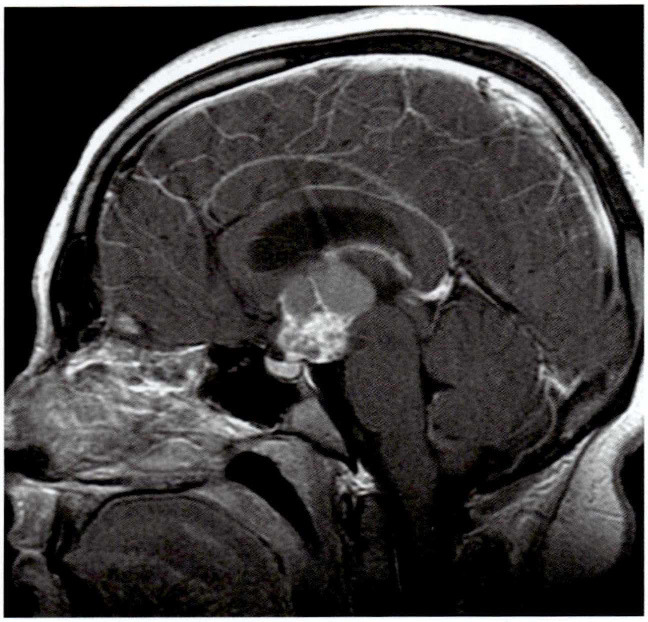

Fig. 9.4 Preoperative MRI scan of a suprasellar tumor (craniopharyngioma) removed using a combined transsellar and transplanum approach. If the pituitary gland is not involved, it can be preserved by transposition of the gland.

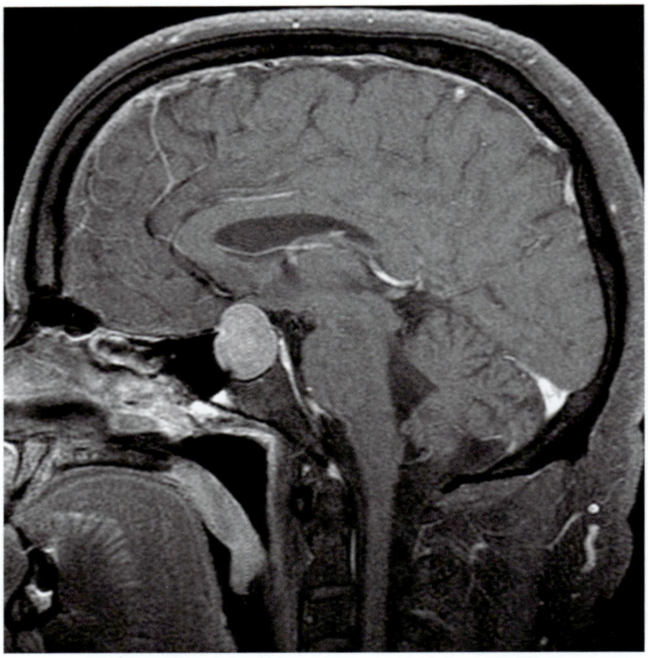

Fig. 9.5 Preoperative MRI scans of a pituitary macroadenoma. A predominantly transsellar approach is used. The tuberculum sellae may be removed for additional suprasellar exposure in selected cases.

Transplanum Approach (Fig. 9.4)

A transplanum approach is often combined with the transcribriform and transsellar approaches for tumors involving the cribriform plate or suprasellar tumors (craniopharyngiomas, pituitary macroadenomas). The course of the optic nerves and the medial optic-carotid recesses are visualized and the central planum is carefully thinned with a drill with copious irrigation to avoid thermal injury to the optic nerves, and the underlying dura is exposed. The anterior limit of resection is the fovea overlying the posterior ethmoid sinuses and cribriform plates. Removal of the tubercular strut overlying the superior sagittal sinus is frequently necessary. The superior intercavernous sinus is transected to open the suprasellar area and visualize the pituitary stalk and optic chiasm when necessary.

Transsellar Approach (Fig. 9.5)

A transsellar approach is the standard approach to the sella but may be used to access other areas of the skull base. The anterior face of the sella is removed to the margins of the cavernous sinus in all four directions. Bone overlying the ICA and cavernous sinus may be removed to allow lateral displacement of the ICA. Pituitary tumors may be followed into the medial cavernous sinus posterior to the anterior genu of the cavernous ICA.

Transclival Approach (Fig. 9.6)

The clivus extends from the dorsum sellae to the foramen magnum. Transclival approaches may be divided into superior, middle, and inferior approaches. A transclival approach provides direct access to the brainstem and vertebrobasilar arterial system. Common tumors in this area include meningiomas and chordomas. Rarely, an aneurysm that cannot be treated by endovascular means or with significant mass effect may be accessed via this approach and clipped.[7] The pituitary gland can also be transposed to access the upper clivus and posterior clinoids with preservation of pituitary function (superior transclival or posterior clinoid approach). This may be necessary with craniopharyngiomas and meningiomas that arise posterior to the infundibulum or gland. The pituitary ligaments (lateral fibrous connective tissue) are detached with preservation of some vascular supply from the superior hypophyseal arteries. The gland is displaced superiorly, pedicled on the pituitary stalk. It is necessary to remove the posterior planum to provide room for displacement of the gland.

Removal of the middle and lower thirds of the clivus requires identification of the course of the ICA laterally in its paraclival segment. The vidian artery is a useful landmark for identifying the second genu of the ICA (petrous/horizontal ICA transitioning to vertical/paraclival/cavernous ICA).[8] The bone between the paraclival carotids and below the sella (clival recess) is drilled. The pharyngeal fascia and bone inferior to the sphenoid sinus is removed to provide additional

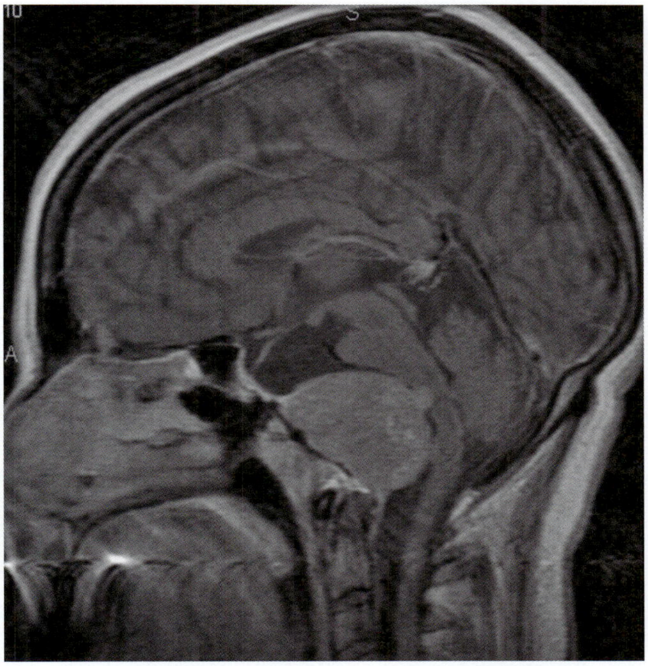

Fig. 9.6 Preoperative MRI scans of a clival chordoma with intracranial extension. The tumor abuts the basilar artery and deforms the brainstem posteriorly.

exposure. The abducens nerve in Dorello's canal is at risk of injury laterally at the level of the paraclival carotids from direct or thermal damage. Neurophysiology is key to preventing these types of injury.

Transodontoid Approach (Fig. 9.7)

A transodontoid approach is commonly utilized to decompress the brainstem in rheumatoid arthritis patients with degeneration of the upper cervical spine due to compressive pannus.[9] The body of C2 is usually the inferior limit of exposure. The posterior nasal septum is resected to the floor of the nasal cavity to provide room for bilateral instrumentation. The sphenoid sinus is opened for orientation and visualization of the course of the ICA. The nasopharyngeal mucosa, medial to the eustachian tubes, is cauterized and resected along with the underlying musculature. Caution should be observed laterally because the parapharyngeal carotid arteries may course medially deep to the eustachian tubes. Dense pharyngeal fascia is elevated from the underlying cortical bone and resected. The clival bone is drilled to the inferior margin at the foramen magnum. The ring of C1 vertebra is identified and removed with the drill. The opening is enlarged laterally with Kerrison bone rongeurs, and the foramen magnum is enlarged by removing the lower third of the clivus. At this point, the odontoid is exposed and the central bone is excavated with the drill until a thin shell remains. It is then detached at its junction with the body of C2 and dissected free from surrounding ligaments. Alternatively, the tip of the dens may be more easily dissected free prior to detachment from the body. Removal of pannus by blunt and sharp dissection or with an ultrasonic aspirator is performed until pulsations are observed (denoting adequate decompression) or the tectorial membrane is resected.

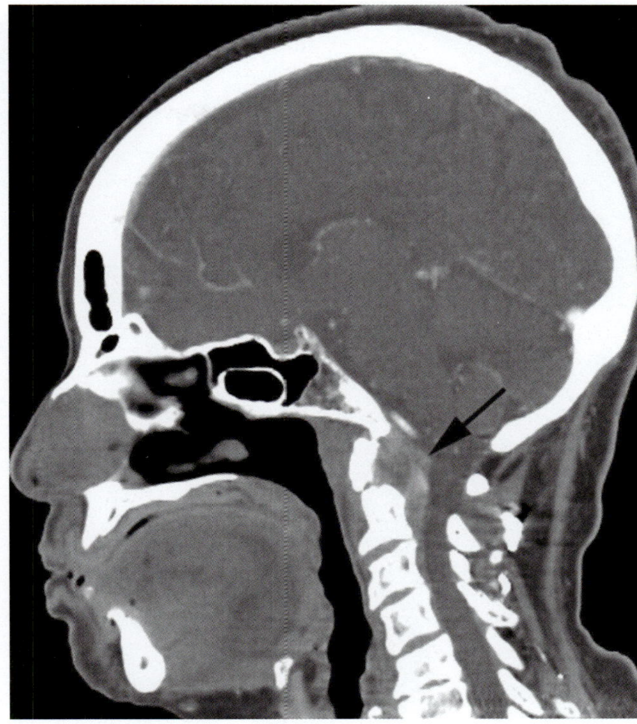

Fig. 9.7 Preoperative CT scan of a patient with brainstem compression secondary to rheumatoid degeneration (*arrow*). Decompression is achieved with removal of the odontoid process to the body of C2 and pannus resection.

Anterior Coronal Plane

Supraorbital Approach (Fig. 9.8)

A supraorbital approach provides access to tumors of the anterior cranial base that extend laterally across the orbital roof. The most common tumors in this area are meningiomas and fibro-osseous tumors. The midpoint of the orbital roof may be reached by resection of the medial orbital wall and displacing the orbital contents. The lamina papyracea is fractured and elevated from the underlying periorbita to the level of the cranial base. The anterior and posterior ethmoidal arteries are identified on the orbital side of the cranial base, cauterized, and transected. Elevation of periorbita continues across the orbital roof. Lateral access is facilitated by a binostril approach with resection of the superior nasal septum.

Transorbital Approach (Fig. 9.9)

A transorbital approach may be used for access to tumors located within the orbit. The dissection can be extraconal or

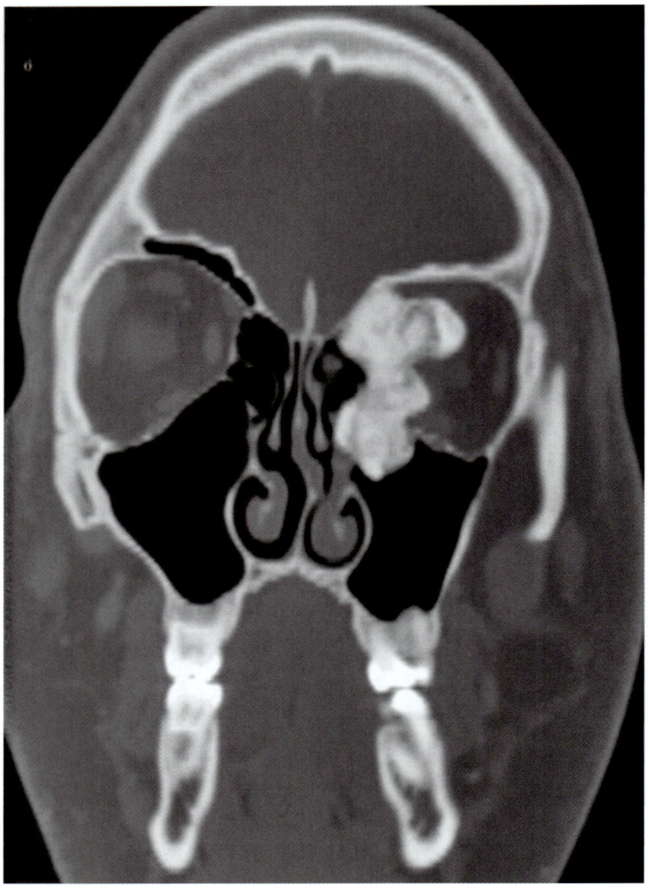

Fig. 9.8 A CT scan at the coronal plane demonstrating benign fibro-osseous tumor of the left orbit.

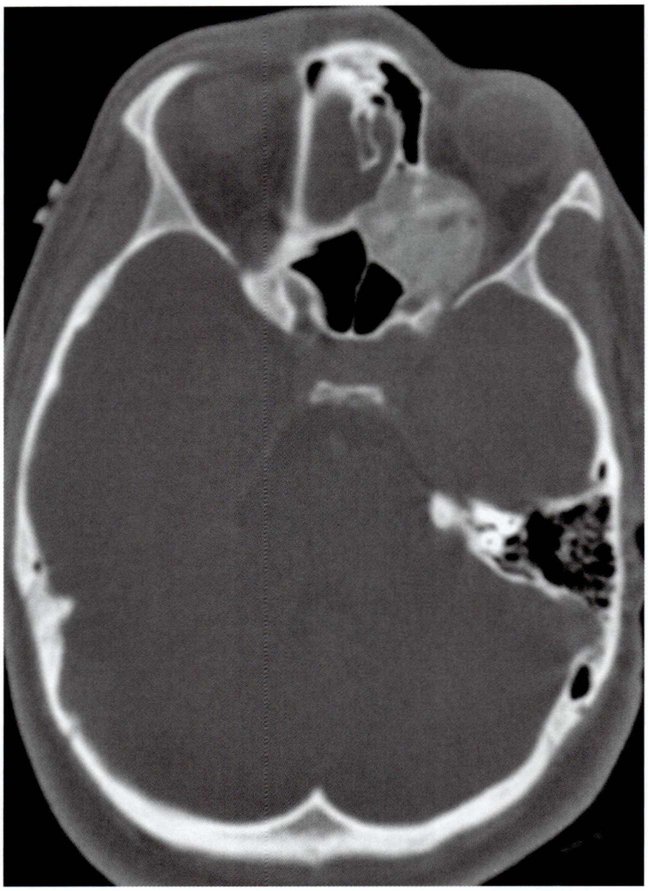

Fig. 9.9 A CT scan at the axial plane demonstrating a benign fibro-osseous tumor of the left superior orbit causing optic nerve compression.

intraconal. Intraconal dissection of orbital tumors is performed between the medial and inferior rectus muscles with preservation of extraocular motor function. This is often facilitated by external retraction of these muscles with the assistance of a neuro-ophthalmologist.

Middle Coronal Plane

Transpterygoid Approach (Fig. 9.10)

A transpterygoid approach is a preliminary step to accessing the other modules in the middle coronal plane. In isolation, it provides exposure of the lateral recess of the sphenoid sinus, especially when there is extensive pneumatization of the sinus. This is necessary for the treatment of meningoceles of the lateral recess.[10,11] The transpterygoid approach is the first step in localizing the petrous ICA, and provides access to the ventral skull base superior and inferior to the petrous ICA. A large middle meatal antrostomy is performed and the sphenoidotomy is completed. The sphenopalatine arteries are identified at the foramen and ligated and transected. The thin bone of the posterior maxillary wall is then removed with Kerrison rongeurs, and the contents of the pterygopalatine space are elevated from the underlying base of the pterygoid bone and displaced laterally. The pterygoid (vidian) canal and its contents are identified inferolateral to the lateral recess of the sphenoid sinus. The infraorbital nerve (second division of the trigeminal nerve) is identified along the orbital floor and followed to the foramen rotundum superolateral to the lateral recess of the sphenoid sinus. The intervening bone is removed with rongeurs to fully expose the lateral recess and provide visualization of the lateral wall overlying the middle fossa.

Transcavernous Approach

The cavernous sinus may be approached medial or lateral to cavernous ICA. Pituitary macroadenomas extending posterior to cavernous ICA can be approached directly via a transsellar approach. Removing the overlying bone decompresses the cavernous sinus and ICA, allows lateral displacement of the ICA, and increases access to the area behind the ICA. There are limited indications for operating in the lateral cavernous sinus. Most tumors in this area are inseparable from the cranial nerves, and tumor dissection results in loss of cranial nerve function. When indicated, access to lateral cavernous

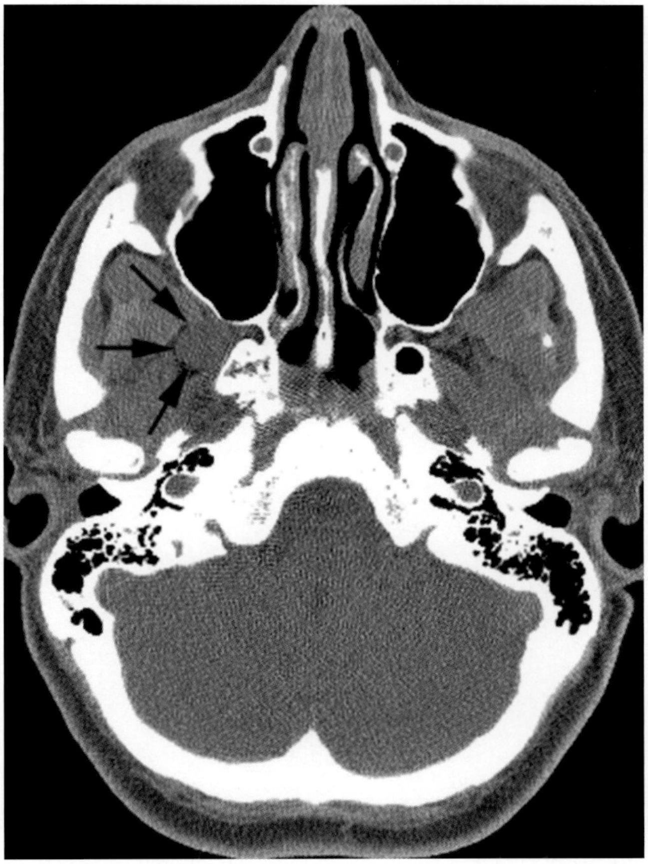

Fig. 9.10 A CT scan in the axial plane demonstrating a round lesion in the medial aspect of the infratemporal fossa (*arrows*). A transmaxillary associated with a transpterygoid approach is necessary to provide direct endoscopic visualization of the lesion that is immediately lateral to the pterygopalatine fossa.

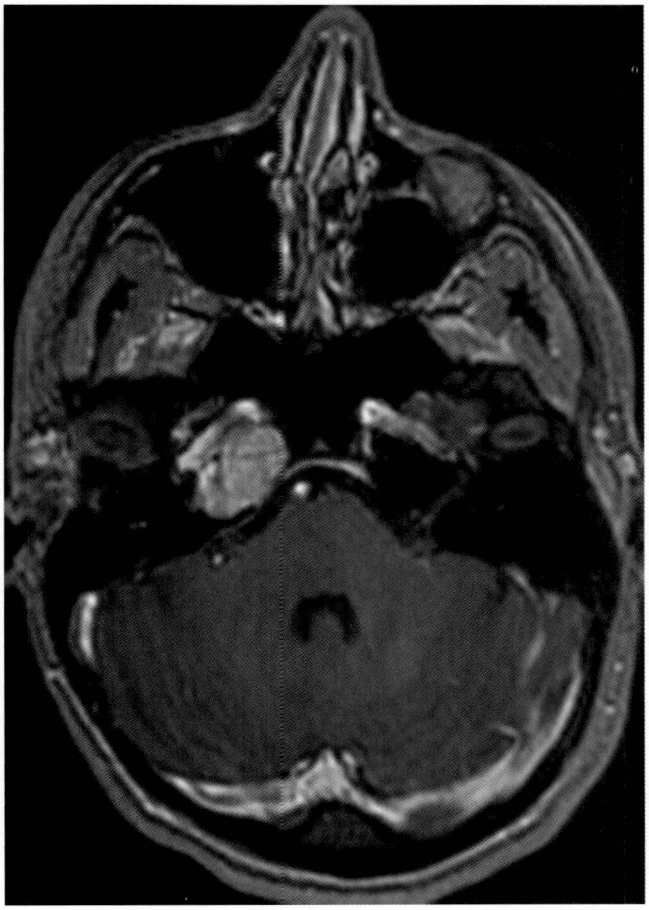

Fig. 9.11 An MRI scan with contrast of a right petrous apex lesion. This lesion that was already bright in T1 proved to be a cholesterol granuloma. It was resected by an endonasal approach to the petrous apex.

sinus is achieved using a suprapetrous approach to the middle cranial fossa (see below).

Petrous Apex Approach (Fig. 9.11)

Expansile lesions of the petrous apex may be approached medially through the sphenoid sinus, posterior to the paraclival ICA.[12] Indications for this approach include cholesterol granuloma of the petrous apex with medial expansion into the sphenoid sinus (most common), and selected benign and malignant tumors, such as chondrosarcomas. A wide sphenoidotomy is performed, and the anatomical landmarks are identified. Expansion of the lesion into the sinus is usually apparent. After removal of the sphenoid floor and intrasinus septations, bone overlying the petrous apex is thinned with a drill by vertical stroke motions parallel to the paraclival ICA. If necessary, clival bone over the brainstem can be thinned to enlarge the opening into the petrous apex. A remaining thin shell of bone is then removed with Kerrison rongeurs up to the edge of the ICA. The contents of the lesion are removed with suction and irrigation. Occasionally, lateralization of the ICA is necessary to increase exposure when there is minimal medial expansion of the lesion. In such cases, a transpterygoid approach is used to identify the paraclival course of the ICA.

Suprapetrous Approach (Middle Fossa) (Fig. 9.12)

Tumors with intracranial extension along the trigeminal nerve or involving Meckel's cave can be approached using a suprapetrous approach, superior to the petrous ICA. A transpterygoid approach is first performed to identify the course of the ICA and fully expose the lateral recess of the sphenoid sinus. The second division of the trigeminal nerve (V2, maxillary nerve) can be visualized on the roof of the maxillary sinus and followed posteriorly to the foramen rotundum, superolateral to the pterygoid canal. The bone surrounding the pterygoid canal is carefully drilled away toward the second genu of the ICA. Once the second genu of ICA is identified, bone can be thinned further in the angle between the vidian nerve and V2. The surface of the middle fossa over Meckel's cave is approached as the angle between vidian nerve and V2 narrows.

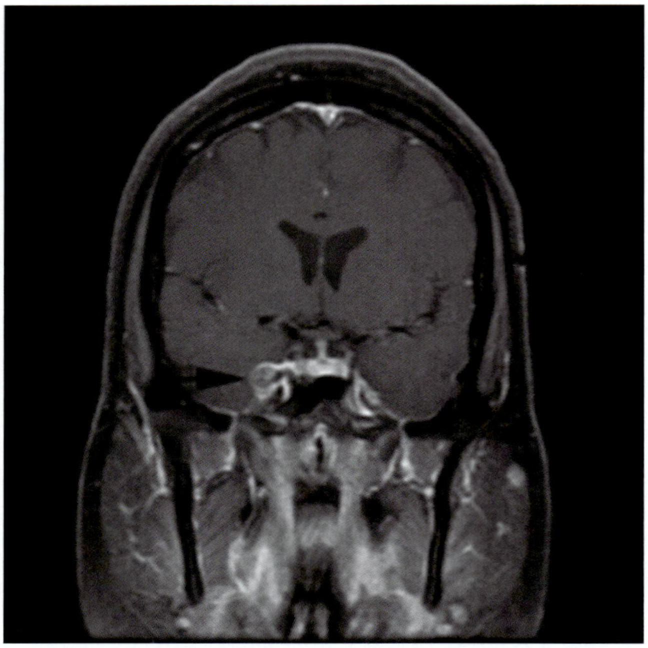

Fig. 9.12 Preoperative MRI of a lesion in the Meckel's cave superior and lateral to the right internal carotid artery (*single arrow*). This lesion can be accessed by an endoscopic endonasal suprapetrous approach.

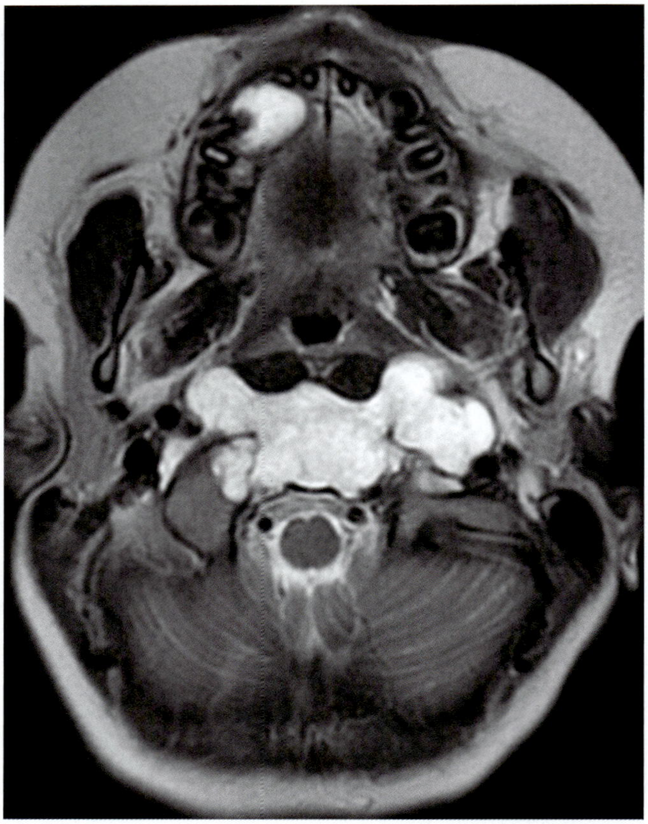

Fig. 9.13 Preoperative MRI in the axial plane showing an extensive chordoma of the skull base involving the lower clivus, the occipital condyles with extension to the parapharyngeal space. This tumor was resected using an endoscopic endonasal approach combining the modules for the posterior fossa (transclivus, transodontoid) and the inferior coronal plane (transcondylar).

Posterior Coronal Plane (Fig. 9.13)

Infrapetrous Approach

Tumors involving the petrous apex and infratemporal skull base are approached inferior to the petrous ICA. This may be the preferred approach for petrous apex lesions that do not expand medially, where there is a narrow space between the brainstem and paraclival ICA and poor sphenoid sinus pneumatization.[12] Following a transpterygoid approach, the curve of the lateral pterygoid plate can be followed laterally to the foramen ovale, where the third division of the trigeminal nerve (V3, mandibular nerve) is situated superficial to the petrous ICA and is a valuable landmark for the extracranial ICA. Bone inferior to the petrous ICA can then be removed extensively to access the petrous apex from below.

Transcondylar Approach

Dissection in the coronal plane at the level of the foramen magnum is most commonly performed for chondrosarcomas, chordomas, and meningiomas. A transodontoid approach[9] is first performed with removal of the clivus from the floor of the sphenoid sinus to the foramen magnum and identification of the ring of C1 vertebra. A transpterygoid approach[11] may also be necessary for more lateral exposure with resection of the medial aspect of the eustachian tube. Medial condyle resection, lateral to the foramen magnum, must be performed carefully with intraoperative monitoring of cranial nerve XII (hypoglossal nerve). Up to 50% of the condyle can be resected without creating craniocervical instability. Chondrosarcomas and chordomas can extend laterally across the skull base to involve the hypoglossal canal, and further lateral extension can involve the jugular foramen.

Parapharyngeal Space Approach

The endonasal parapharyngeal space approach provides access to extracranial structures lateral to the pterygopalatine space and below the infratemporal skull base. An endoscopic medial maxillectomy is necessary for adequate lateral and inferior exposure. Lateral exposure can be augmented by endonasal resection of the pyriform aperture (Denker's approach). The entire posterior and lateral walls of the maxillary sinus may then be removed accordingly. Attachments of the pterygoid muscles to the lateral pterygoid plate are transected and the posterior edge of the lateral pterygoid plate is followed to foramen ovale. If isolation of the parapharyngeal ICA is necessary, the medial portion of the eustachian tube is transected and the cartilaginous canal followed laterally to the ICA. Dissection may then proceed medial or lateral to the parapharyngeal ICA. A medial approach leads to the jugular foramen.[13,14]

Discussion

The ventral skull base is anatomically complex and encompasses multiple distinct regions including the floor of the anterior cranial fossa (from the frontal sinus to the sella and laterally over the orbits), the medial and inferior walls of the middle cranial fossa, the midline skull base of the posterior fossa (from the posterior clinoids to the foramen magnum), the anterior craniovertebral junction, and the infratemporal skull base (from the pterygoid plates to the jugular foramen along the inferior surface of the petrous bone). The ventral skull base can be divided into several endoscopic surgical modular units that can be identified by definite bony landmarks and critical vascular and neural structures. The sphenoid sinus is the starting point for these approaches due to its central location in the sagittal and coronal planes and important anatomical landmarks.

Classifying endonasal approaches to the ventral skull base helps organize our thinking and facilitates modification of current approaches and the development of new approaches. This schema is based on the endoscopic anatomy and is intuitive because we routinely view the skull base anatomy in sagittal and coronal planes on radiologic images and intraoperative navigational systems. Also, the starting point for most cranial base procedures is the sphenoid sinus, practically situated at crossroads of the sagittal and coronal planes. Furthermore, the surgical regions are modular and can be combined to encompass the extent of the pathology. The most important "real estate" in the ventral skull base is the ICA, a limiting factor in accessing various structures and regions, and this classification emphasizes the important anatomical relationships of the ICA. Notably, this classification system has few limitations. Several surgical modules can be combined to access a specific tumor, further modules can be added, and these modules are applicable to all age groups, including pediatric patients.[15,16]

Conclusion

This classification system divides the ventral skull base into two major anatomical modules based on their orientation in the sagittal and coronal planes, and the sphenoid sinus as the epicenter. Modules in the sagittal plane extend from the frontal sinus to the upper cervical spine and the coronal plane, from the midline to the jugular foramen. An anatomically based classification for endonasal skull base approaches allows uniform reporting and comparison of results and facilitates learning. Emphasis of anatomical relationships encourages preservation of function and avoidance of complications. The modular nature of the classification system provides flexibility and allows specific tailoring of surgical approaches to the disease process.

References

1. Jho HD, Carrau RL, Ko Y. Endoscopic pituitary surgery. In: Rengachary SS, Wilkins RH, eds. Neurosurgical Operative Atlas, vol. 4. New York: Thieme Medical Publishers, 1995
2. Carrau RL, Kassam AB, Snyderman CH. Pituitary surgery. Otolaryngol Clin North Am 2001;34:1143–1155, ix
3. Mehta RP, Cueva RA, Brown JD, et al. What's new in skull base medicine and surgery? Skull Base Committee Report. Otolaryngol Head Neck Surg 2006;135:620–630
4. Kassam A, Snyderman CH, Mintz A, Gardner P, Carrau RL. Expanded endonasal approach: the rostrocaudal axis. Part I. Crista galli to the sella turcica. Neurosurg Focus 2005;19:E3 http://www.aans.org/education/journal/neurosurgical/July05/19-1-3.pdf
5. Kassam A, Snyderman CH, Mintz A, Gardner P, Carrau RL. Expanded endonasal approach: the rostrocaudal axis. Part II. Posterior clinoids to the foramen magnum. Neurosurg Focus 2005;19:E4 http://www.aans.org/education/journal/neurosurgical/July05/19-1-4.pdf
6. Kassam AB, Gardner P, Snyderman C, Mintz A, Carrau R. Expanded endonasal approach: fully endoscopic, completely transnasal approach to the middle third of the clivus, petrous bone, middle cranial fossa, and infratemporal fossa. Neurosurg Focus 2005;19:E6 http://www.aans.org/education/journal/neurosurgical/July05/19-1-6.pdf
7. Kassam AB, Mintz AH, Gardner PA, Horowitz MB, Carrau RL, Snyderman CH. The expanded endonasal approach for an endoscopic transnasal clipping and aneurysmorrhaphy of a large vertebral artery aneurysm: technical case report. Neurosurgery 2006;59(1, Suppl 1):E162–E165, discussion E162–E165
8. Vescan AD, Snyderman CH, Carrau RL, et al. Vidian canal: analysis and relationship to the internal carotid artery. Laryngoscope 2007;117:1338–1342
9. Kassam AB, Snyderman C, Gardner P, Carrau R, Spiro R. The expanded endonasal approach: a fully endoscopic transnasal approach and resection of the odontoid process: technical case report. Neurosurgery 2005;57(1, Suppl):E213, discussion E213
10. Tosun F, Carrau RL, Snyderman CH, Kassam A, Celin S, Schaitkin B. Endonasal endoscopic repair of cerebrospinal fluid leaks of the sphenoid sinus. Arch Otolaryngol Head Neck Surg 2003;129:576–580
11. Al-Nashar IS, Carrau RL, Herrera A, Snyderman CH. Endoscopic transnasal transpterygopalatine fossa approach to the lateral recess of the sphenoid sinus. Laryngoscope 2004;114:528–532
12. Snyderman CH, Kassam AB, Carrau R, Mintz A. Endoscopic approaches to the petrous apex. Operative Techniques in Otolaryngology 2006;17:168–173
13. Zimmer LA, Hirsch BE, Kassam A, Horowitz M, Snyderman CH. Resection of a recurrent paraganglioma via an endoscopic transnasal approach to the jugular fossa. Otol Neurotol 2006;27:398–402
14. Kassam AB, Gardner P, Snyderman C, Carrau R, Zimmer L, Hirsch B. Mintz: Endoscopic, expanded endonasal approach to the jugular foramen. Operative Techniques in Neurosurgery: Management of Jugular Foramen Tumors 2005;8:35–41
15. Kassam A, Thomas AJ, Snyderman C, et al. Fully endoscopic expanded endonasal approach treating skull base lesions in pediatric patients. J Neurosurg 2007;106(2, Suppl)75–86
16. Pirris SM, Pollack IF, Snyderman CH, et al. Corridor surgery: the current paradigm for skull base surgery. Childs Nerv Syst 2007;23:377–384

10 Endoscopically Assisted Bimanual Operating Technique

Daniel B. Simmen, Hans Rudolf Briner, and Nick Jones

Tips and Pearls

- The bimanual technique has expanded the range of benign and malignant tumors that can be removed.
- The bimanual technique enables the surgeon to obtain optimal visualization of the operative field.
- The surgeon can keep the suction tip in the operative field and keep it free from blood at all times while having the other hand free for precise instrumentation.
- The second surgeon is responsible for directing the endoscope and keeping a steady image of the operative field displayed on the video monitor.
- This technique combines the advantages of the endoscopic technique with the key advantages of being able to operate with both hands.
- This team approach has the potential to improve the quality of the operation.
- Teaching and learning is enhanced as the two surgeons can interact and help one another at all times.
- Interdisciplinary operations can be performed with neurosurgeons or maxillofacial surgeons, and integrate the experience of each specialist.

Introduction

Today, endoscopic surgery of the paranasal sinuses is among the most frequently performed rhinosurgical procedures. It can be an effective solution in patients with chronic rhinosinusitis who have responded poorly to medical therapy.[1] The indications for endoscopic surgery of the paranasal sinuses have been constantly expanding, so much that even complex procedures of the frontal sinuses and anterior skull base can now be performed endoscopically. Besides inflammatory diseases, the range of indications has expanded to include the removal of benign and malignant tumors.

Basic Principles of Endoscopic Sinus Surgery

Diseases of the paranasal sinuses are common and may seriously affect the patients' quality of life. With an incidence of 3 to 5%, chronic rhinosinusitis is the most prevalent disease.[2] Many patients with chronic rhinosinusitis often show an inadequate response to pharmacologic therapy. Endoscopic surgery of the paranasal sinuses offers an effective therapeutic option in these cases. As a result, endoscopic sinus surgery is now among the most widely practiced rhinosurgical procedures. Since endoscopic sinus surgery was first described over 30 years ago, we have witnessed impressive advances in operating techniques. Better endoscopes, better video cameras, and improved operating instruments have made it possible to view all of the paranasal sinuses and perform surgical procedures through the natural nasal orifice.[3,4] The indications for endoscopic sinus procedures are constantly being expanded. Today even complex procedures of the lateral nasal wall and frontal sinus are performed endoscopically as well as specific operations of the anterior skull base, clivus, through the sphenoid sinus, and intracranially can be performed endoscopically. Besides inflammatory conditions, the range of indications has expanded to include the removal of benign and malignant tumors.

In the classic technique, the surgeon holds the endoscope in one hand and uses the other hand to perform the operation.[5–7] This one-hand technique has its limitations. It is particularly difficult to remove bone and tumor tissue and control bleeding with just one hand.[8,9] These difficulties have engendered a need for endoscopic surgeons to use both hands while operating. In this bimanual technique an assistant holds the video endoscope, thus freeing both of the surgeon's hands so that he or she can deal more effectively with the challenging situations that arise in endoscopic operations (**Fig. 10.1**). The assistant is responsible for directing the endoscope and keeping a steady image of the operative field displayed on the video monitor. This technique differs from procedures done under a microscope. Although the microscope enables surgeons to operate with both hands, the endoscopic technique is advantageous in that it provides a close-up, dynamic view of all the paranasal sinuses. It also eliminates the problem of a loss of light caused by instruments in the path of the microscope light beam, because the endoscopic light source is always "on site." The endoscopically assisted bimanual technique thus combines the advantages of the endoscopic technique with the key advantages of the operating microscope the ability, namely to operate with both hands (**Fig. 10.2**). The endoscopically assisted bimanual technique was first described by May et al in 1990. Despite the advantages of the bimanual technique, the classic one-hand technique is still more widely practiced. A major

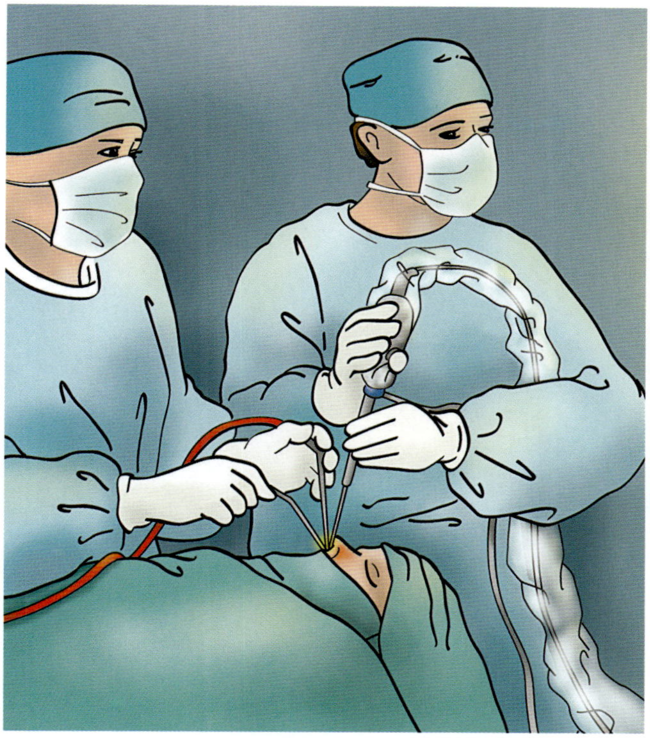

Fig. 10.1 In the bimanual technique an assistant holds the video endoscope, thus freeing both of the surgeon's hands.

reason for this is the fact that the bimanual technique requires an extra assistant. Technical advances such as shaver technology and instruments with built-in suction channels have also made it easier to operate with one hand. However, the advantages of the bimanual technique, especially the improved visualization of the operative field owing to the constant presence of a suction tip, make it possible to perform more complex procedures on the paranasal sinuses with greater safety and precision. This particularly applies to the more severe forms of chronic rhinosinusitis with polyposis.

The bimanual technique is also advantageous for revision procedures, tumor resection, and skull base and brain surgery. Moreover, a recent study has documented a reduction in operating time when the bimanual technique is used.[10] The shorter operating time lead to lower costs, and this saving more than offsets the added costs for the extra assistant. Complex endoscopic skull base surgery and surgery of the brain would not be possible without this bimanual assisted technique.

Advantages of the Endoscopically Assisted Bimanual Operating Technique

Operating with Both Hands

In the endoscopically assisted bimanual technique, the assistant holds and directs the endoscope with the attached video camera. The image is transmitted to a video monitor. The surgeon watches the monitor and has both hands free for manipulating the surgical instruments (**Fig. 10.3**). This re-creates the feel of two-hand open surgery that is already familiar to most surgeons, meaning that established operating skills can be transferred to endoscopic skull base procedures.

Suction Tip Stays in the Operative Field; Fewer Instrument Changes

Surgical procedures on the paranasal sinuses can cause relatively heavy bleeding, which may obscure the surgeon's view of the operative site. Clear visualization of the operative site is essential for anatomical orientation, and therefore the extravasated blood should be removed as rapidly as possible. In the classic one-hand technique, the surgeon must pull out frequently and exchange the operating instrument for a suction

A

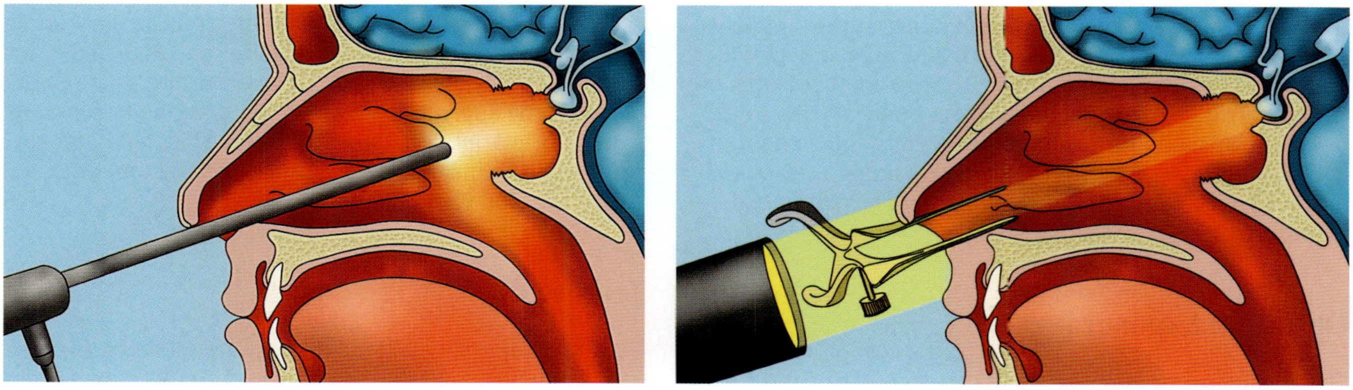

B

Fig. 10.2 The endoscopically assisted bimanual technique combines the advantages of the endoscopic technique with the key advantage of the operating microscope, namely the ability to operate with both hands. The endoscope facilitates bringing the optical device very close to the operating field with optimal image and light quality **(A)**, whereas the microscope has only a straight channel for the optical visualization and loses some light at the entrance into the nostril **(B)**.

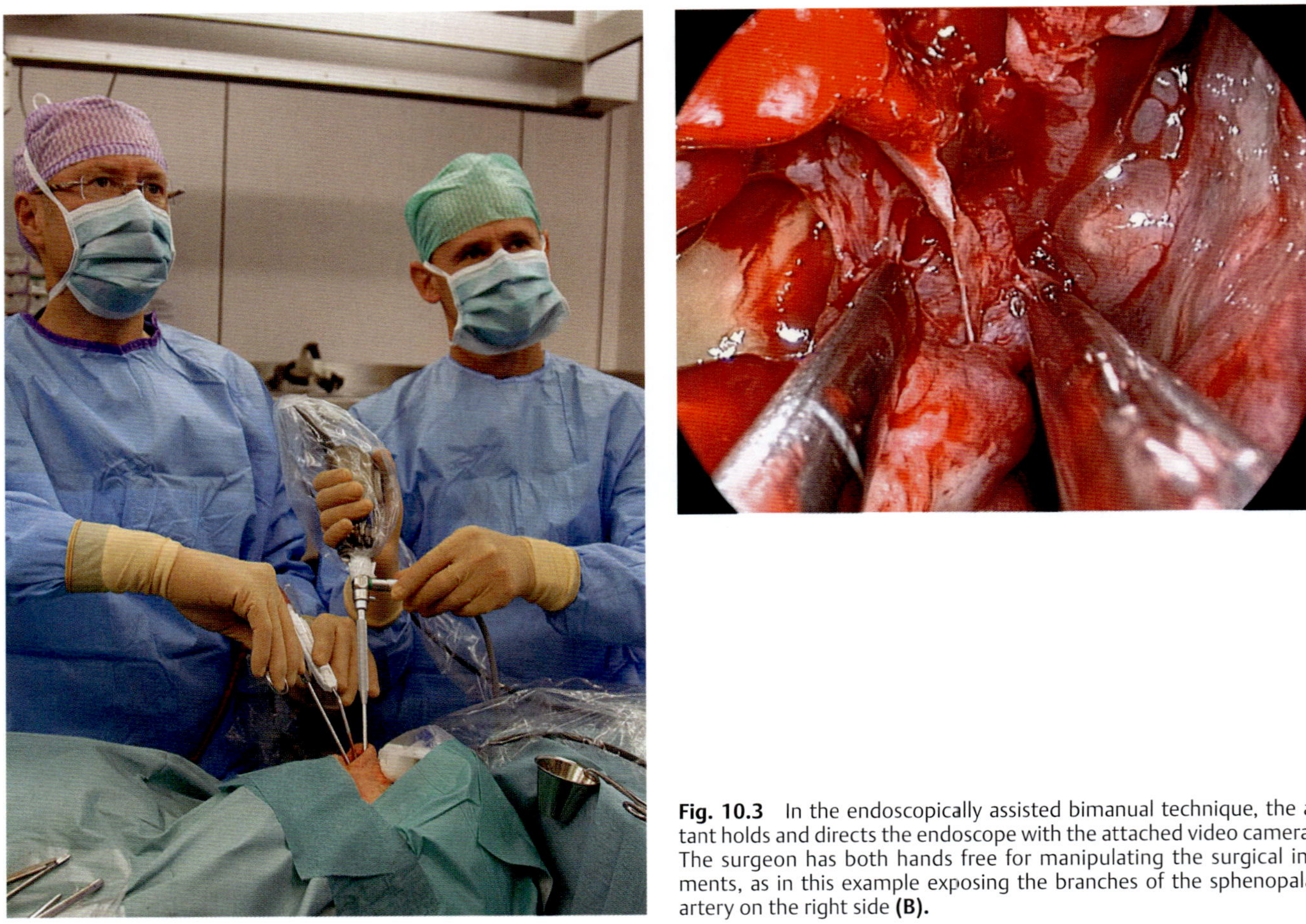

A

B

Fig. 10.3 In the endoscopically assisted bimanual technique, the assistant holds and directs the endoscope with the attached video camera **(A)**. The surgeon has both hands free for manipulating the surgical instruments, as in this example exposing the branches of the sphenopalatine artery on the right side **(B)**.

tip. These frequent instrument changes not only prolong the operation but also increase the likelihood that the distal lens of the endoscope will become soiled or smeared. With the bimanual technique, the surgeon can keep the suction tip in the operative field at all times while having the other hand free for cutting tissue. In this way the operative field remains largely free of blood, resulting in better visualization and anatomical orientation and less frequent instrument changes. This is the major reason why the operating time is approximately 20% shorter with the bimanual technique than with the one-hand technique. The ability to keep the suction tip in the operative field also facilitates bone removal with a drill or burr. The suction tip can provide a constant removal of irrigating fluid during drilling, thus maintaining a clear view of the operative site and causing less compromise of endoscopic vision by the irrigating fluid.

Optimum Exposure

The bimanual technique facilitates better operative exposure because the second instrument can be used to retract tissues. For example, the suction tip can be used to push the middle turbinate gently medially toward the nasal septum, making it easier to see into the ethmoid and simplifying the operation. In tumor resections it may be necessary to retract tumor tissue that is obscuring other structures (**Fig. 10.4**).

Holding and Cutting

The bimanual technique allows for greater precision in the manipulation and cutting of tissues. For example, the surgeon can use the suction tip to hold the tissue in place while simultaneously resecting it with a scissors (**Fig. 10.5**). This precise cut results in a smaller wound surface than removing tissue by applying traction with a grasping forceps, and results in less intraoperative bleeding. The "hold-and-cut" technique eliminates the danger of removing too much tissue by avulsion with a grasper.

Teamwork

The endoscopically assisted bimanual technique requires an assistant who actively participates in the procedure by controlling the camera position. This may be an advantage as it offers a constant opportunity to discuss intraoperative situations as a team. For example, the second surgeon may direct attention to critical anatomical structures that the surgeon

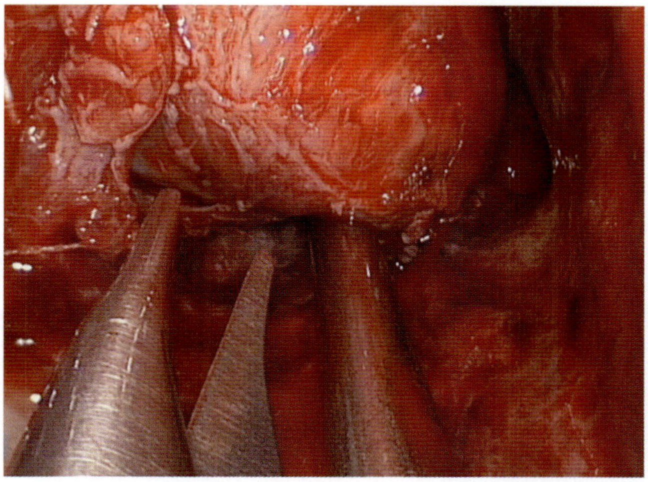

Fig. 10.4 In tumor resections it may be necessary to retract tumor tissue that is obscuring other structures, as in this example of a neurinoma of the infratemporal fossa in the pterygopalatine space on the right side.

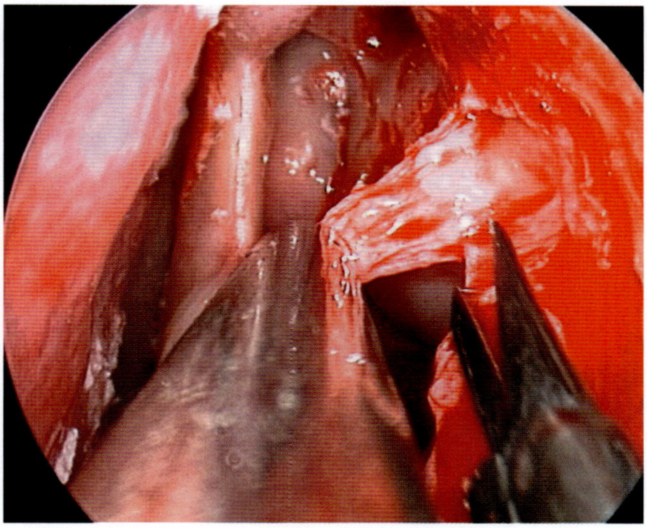

Fig. 10.5 The surgeon can use the suction tip to hold the tissue in place while simultaneously resecting it with a scissors.

might otherwise be too busy to notice right away. By promoting an ongoing, mutual exchange of information on anatomical and conceptual issues, this team approach has the potential to improve the quality of the operation. Furthermore, an interdisciplinary team can carry out a procedure together as team, combining the approach with tumor removal and closure of the defect in one operation. Each step of the operation is performed by the individual whose expertise is best suited to that aspect of the operation.

Training

The bimanual technique is ideal for training purposes. The experienced surgeon can assist an inexperienced colleague and can take over the procedure at any time. This enhances the specific advantage of having two surgeons involved in the case at all times during the whole operation.

Theater Setup and Technical Aspects

The essential part of the equipment for the endoscopically assisted bimanual operating technique is a video camera attached to the endoscope. The camera image is transmitted to the video monitor, which provides the surgeon with the necessary orientation. The assistant holds the endoscope and is responsible for maintaining an optimum visual display of the operative field. Separating the two tasks—keeping the operative field on the camera screen and performing the operation—requires good communication between the two surgeons. The surgeon gives the assistant instructions on what part of the operative field to focus on. This requires some degree of training during initial team formation, but we know from experience that smooth and effective teamwork can be established within a short time, often in a matter of minutes.

Several years of experience with this technique have shown that coordination between surgeon and assistant runs like clockwork almost automatically after just a few sessions, and that communication during the operation focuses almost entirely on the details of the operation itself, rather than on issues of coordination.

In the operating theater, the surgeon and assistant sit or stand next to each other. The video monitor is placed on the opposite side so that the operators can watch it without having to turn their heads. This is best from an ergonomic standpoint and makes it easier to operate for an extended period of time without experiencing neck strain (**Fig. 10.6**). A nurse keeps the surgical instruments ready near the foot of the table next to the video monitor so that they can be passed during the procedure. Whenever possible, an extra video monitor should be set up so that the nurse can follow the procedure more closely and anticipate the need for particular instruments.

It is advantageous to place the anesthesia equipment at the foot of the operating table, because space at the head of the table is limited due to the operating team, scrub nurse, operating instruments, and additional technical equipment (video cart, navigation unit).

Practical Hints

Ergonomic Handling of the Endoscope

The endoscope may be held with one or both hands, depending on which is more comfortable for the second surgeon.

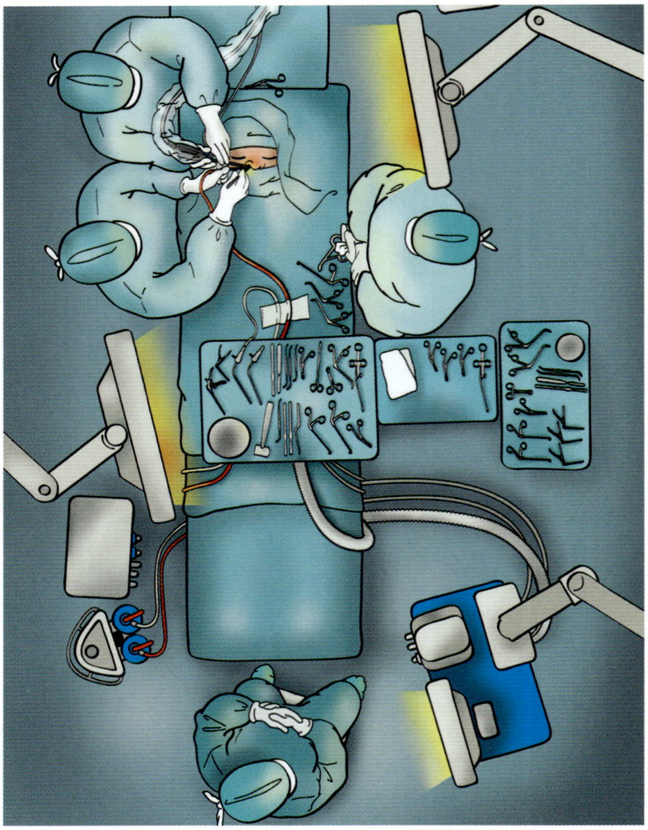

Fig. 10.6 The two surgeons sit or stand next to each other. The video monitor is placed on the opposite side so that the operators can watch it without having to turn their heads. This is best from an ergonomic standpoint and makes it easier to operate for an extended period of time without experiencing neck strain.

The flexible cold light cable should be brought out of the top or side of the operative area so that it will not interfere with the first surgeon. This also applies to the connecting cable for the video camera. Placing the patient's head in a slightly hyperextended position will make it easier to control the endoscope and will also create some additional room for the surgeon.

Stabilizing the Endoscope in the Nasal Vestibule

A stable position of the endoscope is essential for maintaining a good video image. This is achieved by gently bracing the endoscope against the roof of the nasal vestibule (hypomochlion) (**Fig. 10.7**). In this way the assistant can direct the scope more precisely and eliminate a shaky image. The surgeon can facilitate insertion of the endoscope by using both instruments to gently spread open the tissue at the narrowest point in the nasal vestibule, the nasal valve. This will also prevent smearing of the lens during endoscope insertion. This "one-nostril approach" is the workhorse for most endonasal rhinosurgical and rhinoneurosurgical procedures.

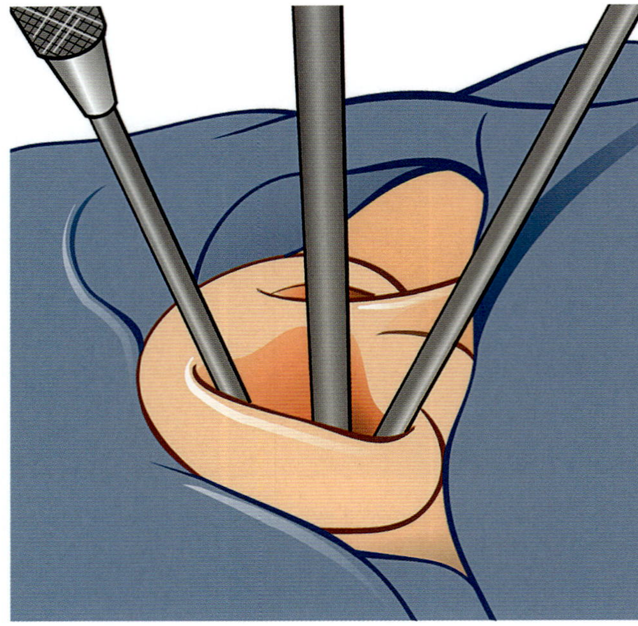

Fig. 10.7 A stable position of the endoscope is essential for maintaining a good video image. This is achieved by gently bracing the endoscope against the roof of the nasal vestibule (hypomochlion).

Cleaning the Endoscope

If the endoscope lens is slightly soiled, it can often be cleaned by rinsing it with water. This is most easily done by directing the irrigating fluid along the shaft of the endoscope and removing the fluid with the suction tip, which is always present in the field. In this way the lens can be cleaned and the operation can be continued without delay. If the lens is more heavily soiled, however, it should be withdrawn and cleaned mechanically.

Holding and Cutting

By working with both hands, the surgeon is able to fix the targeted tissue with one instrument (a suction tip or grasper) and cut it with a second instrument. This allows high surgical precision. It results in a smaller wound surface than is produced by traction with a grasping instrument, and there is less bleeding. This technique also reduces the danger of removing too much tissue (**Fig. 10.5**).

Retraction of Structures and Tissue

One difficulty in operating on the paranasal sinuses is the tight confines of the anatomical passages. Inflammatory mucosal changes or tumor tissue will often further restrict the space that is available to the surgeon. With the bimanual technique, one instrument (e.g., the suction tip) can be used for tissue retraction. This improves visualization and increases

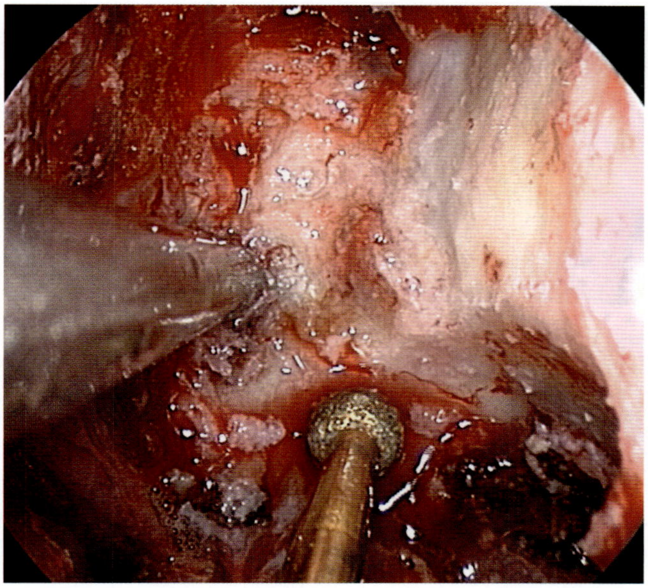

Fig. 10.8 Especially in extended skull base surgery, a significant amount of bone often has to be removed to access deeper spaces, as in this example of a fibrous dysplasia of the posterior skull base demonstrating orbit and optic nerve decompression on the left side.

surgical precision (**Fig. 10.4**). In our experience, careful retraction of the middle turbinate toward the nasal septum also makes it easier to work in the ethmoid.

Drilling and Suction

An endoscopic drill or burr is frequently used for bone removal. With the bimanual technique, the suction tip can remain in the operative field and is always on standby for clearing the field of irrigating fluid and drilling debris. This improves visualization and reduces soiling of the lens. Even prolonged drilling in the frontal sinus or sphenoid sinus can be done without difficulty. It is important, however, for the assistant to position the endoscope carefully so that the lens is not damaged by the drill. Especially in extended skull base surgery a significant amount of bone often has to be removed to be able to access deeper spaces (**Fig. 10.8**).

Coagulation and Suction

Heavy bleeding is not uncommon in sinus operations, particularly when operating near the branches of the sphenopalatine artery. This arterial bleeding must be controlled by electrocoagulation. With the bimanual technique, the suction tip is constantly available to keep extravasated blood from pooling in the operative field. The bleeding vessel can be precisely cauterized with a conventional monopolar or bipolar instrument. The bimanual technique also eliminates the danger that a cautery instrument with a built-in suction channel may become clogged by coagulated blood (**Fig. 10.9**).

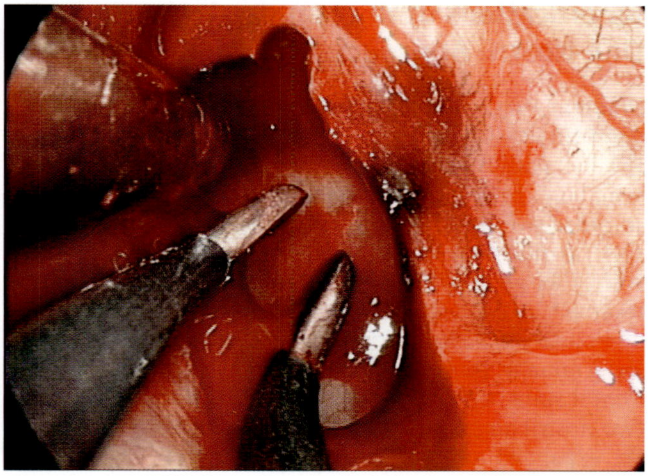

Fig. 10.9 The bimanual technique also has the advantage of suctioning and coagulating at the same time. This example shows significant venous bleeding from an intersinus septum in the sphenoid sinus that is cauterized under optimal vision with a bipolar device.

Navigation and Drilling

The endoscopically assisted bimanual operating technique is also advantageous when used in conjunction with a navigation system. The suction tip, for example, may function as the tracking instrument for surgical navigation. We know from experience that the suction tip spends the most time in the operative field, making it an excellent navigation sensor for all phases of the operation (e.g., drilling at anatomically challenging sites such as the frontal sinus and sphenoid sinus) (**Fig. 10.10**).

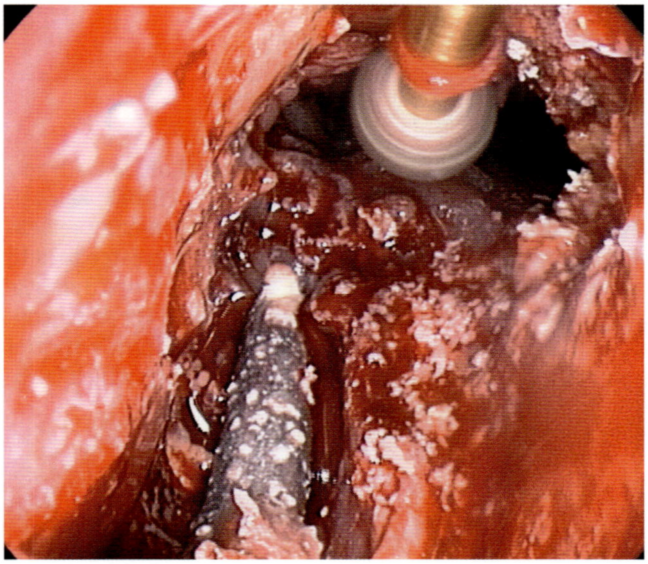

Fig. 10.10 The bimanual technique is also advantageous when used in conjunction with a navigation system. The suction tip, for example, may function as the tracking instrument for surgical navigation. In this example the suction is placed on the posterior wall of the frontal sinus while the drill work completes the access to the anterior skull base.

Modifications of the Standard One-Nostril Approach

Different surgical teams involved in skull base and rhinoneurosurgery have developed modifications tailored to their specific skills and experiences over time. In the posterior skull base, by resecting the posterior part of the septum, a so-called two-nostril approach has developed over time. This specific modification allows one channel to be used transnasally for guiding the endoscope and the other pathway is reserved for the surgeon. This specific setup is ideal for interdisciplinary work and more extended procedures, especially intracranially. For anterior skull base operations and for the frontal sinus, a septal window is mandatory to carry out a two-nostril approach. The advantage of this modification is the expanded angle and crossover of the midline to reach areas that would not be possible to reach with the ipsilateral approach.

Depending on the surgical team involved, there as been another modification in some institutions where the two surgeons sit opposite one another so that they both have full freedom for moving and handling, and each surgeon has his or her own monitor to work off. The goal for all modified setups should always be that the ergonomic posture is ideal for both surgeons and that each surgeon has the best position for his or her bimanual work or for guiding the endoscope. There is not just the one and only setup for the bimanual assisted technique; each institution has to build a team and setup that is tailored to its specific demands and possibilities that apply to each operating room (**Fig. 10.11**). This is a dynamic process that will always be adapted to new inventions and technical developments that require an open and flexible team that is able to adapt its operating room to microsurgical principles and therefore improve the surgical safety and outcome.

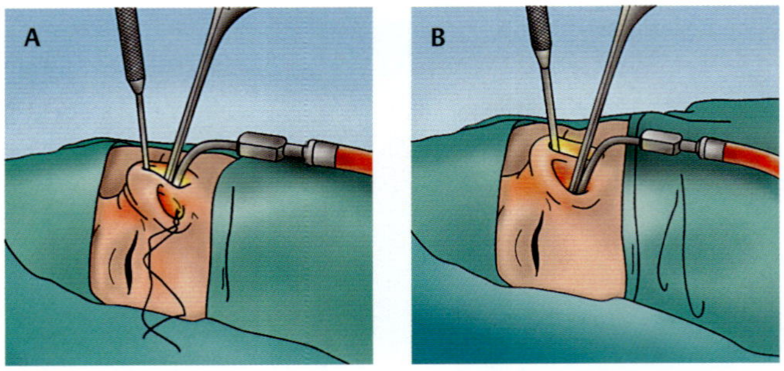

Fig. 10.11 The bimanual technique can be modified in many ways from the classic approach through one nostril **(A).** In the posterior skull base, by resecting the posterior part of the septum, a so-called two-nostril approach has developed over time **(B).** This specific modification allows one channel to be used transnasally for guiding the endoscope, and the other pathway is reserved for the surgeon. This specific setup is ideal for interdisciplinary work and more extended procedures, especially intracranially.

Conclusion

The bimanual endoscopic sinus surgery technique leads to a significant reduction in operation time for chronic rhinosinusitis. The bimanual technique appears to confer more benefit in more complex cases and be of even greater benefit in more complex procedures such as the endoscopic removal of paranasal sinus tumors, although this has yet to be confirmed objectively. The patient may benefit from a shorter operation time, the surgeon has better visibility, which facilitates more precise microsurgical work, and this may in turn reduce the incidence of complications. There may be potential economic advantages because of the increased efficiency in the use of operating room facilities.

References

1. Damm M, Quante G, Jungehuelsing M, Stennert E. Impact of functional endoscopic sinus surgery on symptoms and quality of life in chronic rhinosinusitis. Laryngoscope 2002;112:310–315
2. Hedman J, Kaprio J, Poussa T, Nieminen MM. Prevalence of asthma, aspirin intolerance, nasal polyposis and chronic obstructive pulmonary disease in a population-based study. Int J Epidemiol 1999;28:717–722
3. Krouse JH, Christmas DA Jr. Powered instrumentation in functional endoscopic sinus surgery. II: A comparative study. Ear Nose Throat J 1996;75:42–44
4. Simmen D, Jones N. Endoscopic Sinus Surgery and Extended Applications. New York: Thieme Medical Publishers; 2005
5. Kennedy DW. Functional endoscopic sinus surgery. Technique. Arch Otolaryngol 1985;111:643–649
6. Rice DH. Basic surgical techniques and variations of endoscopic sinus surgery. Otolaryngol Clin North Am 1989;22:713–726
7. Stammberger H. Endoscopic endonasal surgery—concepts in treatment of recurring rhinosinusitis. Part II. Surgical technique. Otolaryngol Head Neck Surg 1986;94:147–156
8. Arnholt JL, Mair EA. A 'third hand' for endoscopic skull base surgery. Laryngoscope 2002;112:2244–2249
9. May M, Hoffmann DF, Sobol SM. Video endoscopic sinus surgery: a two-handed technique. Laryngoscope 1990;100:430–432
10. Briner HR, Simmen D, Jones N. Endoscopic sinus surgery: advantages of the bimanual technique. Am J Rhinol 2005;19:269–273

11 Technical Innovations and Robotic Skull Base Surgery

David W. Kennedy and John M. Lee

Tips and Pearls

- Although some endoscopic surgery was performed early in the 20th century, it was really the development of rod optics by Professor Harold H. Hopkins that made this a truly viable possibility.
- Walter Messerklinger used the improved endoscopes to examine nasal mucociliary clearance in fresh cadavers and to perform detailed nasal endoscopies in the late 1960s and early 1970s.
- Several surgeons began performing some endoscopic surgeries in the late 1970s and early 1980s in Europe. Kennedy researched and modified the techniques and introduced what he termed functional endoscopic sinus surgery (FESS) in the United States.
- Skull base surgery began being performed in the late 1980s, but has continued to expand with improved technologies and improved skull base defect closure.
- Through-cutting instruments and microdebriders now permit removal of tissue and bone without inadvertent stripping of nasal cavity mucosa, markedly improving healing. Curved microdebriders have significantly helped with frontal recess mucosal preservation.
- High-definition camera technology now enables endoscopic surgery to be performed from a monitor with exceptional detail.
- The endoscope tip can be kept clean with pedal-operated flushing systems and endoscope sheaths, markedly improving the consistency of visualization.
- Stereotactic computer-aided navigation with fused preoperative CT and MRI scans are useful for endoscopic skull base surgery, and intraoperative CT scanning with low-dose scanners is now a viable option for real-time updates of computer aided navigation.
- Endonasal monopolar and bipolar electrical cautery devices provide multiple options for hemostasis control, but the ideal suction bipolar forceps for intracranial use is not yet available.
- High-speed drills facilitate rapid bone removal, and suction irrigation drills facilitate the safe removal of bone in critical areas, with excellent visualization and the availability of different curvature shafts.
- Robotic skull base surgery holds significant promise for expanding skull base surgery, as the arms and instruments become finer, providing the ability to perform fine manipulations in confined areas that are currently impossible.

Introduction

Intranasal surgery has undergone tremendous change and evolution throughout the last century. Along with an improved understanding of anatomy and physiology, technical advances in visualization, imaging, and instrumentation have provided surgeons with better access to treat a variety of paranasal sinus diseases. As more experience and skill was gained, the boundaries of endoscopic sinus surgery expanded to the skull base and intracranial cavity. This chapter highlights the key technical innovations that have provided the stimulus and tools for this exciting and growing field.

History

The origins of nasal endoscopy can be traced back to 1901 when Hirschmann used modified cystoscopes to examine the sinonasal cavity.[1,2] These cystoscopes consisted of a series of glass lenses interspersed by air. In 1902, Reichert was then credited with performing the first endoscopic sinus surgery using a 7-mm endoscope through oroantral fistulas to perform maxillary sinus manipulations.[3] It was not until 1925 that Maltz promoted diagnostic endoscopy of the sinonasal cavity and coined the term "sinoscopy."[1] However, issues with illumination and depth of field prevented its widespread acceptance and use. Perhaps the most significant technical innovation in the history of endonasal surgery was the development of the rod optic endoscopic system by Harold H. Hopkins in the 1960s. By using glass spacers in between a series of glass lenses, optical image quality improved dramatically with better resolution, wider depth of field, and a sixfold increase in light intensity. This rod-optic system was then introduced to Karl Storz, whose medical instruments company refined what would be become the modern endoscope.[4,5]

Using the improved endoscope, Messerklinger studied nasal mucociliary clearance in fresh cadavers and wrote a book on clinical endoscopic diagnosis.[6] It was not long before Messerklinger, Draf, Wigand, and others began performing endoscopic nasal procedures.[7] After visiting these surgeons Kennedy introduced endoscopy to North America, validated the principles in a rabbit model, further developing the techniques and introducing the term *functional endoscopic sinus surgery* (FESS). In conjunction with Heinz Stammberger, the first-ever course in functional endoscopic sinus surgery was taught at Johns Hopkins University in 1985.[8] Over the last 20-plus years, endoscopic sinus surgery has become the standard of care for chronic sinus disease refractory to medical therapy. As further experience and skill was gained, both otolaryngologists and selected neurosurgeons recognized the potential for the endoscope in skull base and intracranial surgery. Although the first hesitant steps in skull base surgery were made in the 1980s, one decade later multiple institutions had begun popularizing the use of endoscopy in pituitary surgery, evolving from a combined microscopic and endoscopic technique to an exclusively endoscopic transsphenoidal approach.[9–13] As techniques and technologies have evolved, the boundaries of endoscopic transnasal surgery have expanded to the anterior skull base and parasellar and paraclival regions. Described below are some of the most important innovations to have occurred that enabled this dramatic evolution.

Visualization

Since the invention of the rod-optic system, there has been more refinement rather than evolution of the endoscope itself. The large variety of zero-degree and angled endoscopes in both 4- and 2.7-mm diameters provide the endoscopic surgeon with numerous options to navigate the paranasal sinus cavity. However, perhaps the most dramatic evolution has occurred in the development of the wide-angle, 45-degree endoscope, which enables both direct forward vision and a deflected angle of view close to that achieved by a 70-degree endoscope, while at the same time providing improved illumination. Such endoscopes make it easier for surgeons, particularly those such as neurosurgeons who are less familiar with passing endoscopes intranasally, to operate under endoscopic control. One drawback of the endoscope is the two-dimensional mono-ocular image that is created. This has engendered some reservation among neurosurgeons who are familiar with the three-dimensional (3D) binocular view of the microscope. Multiple successful and innovative attempts have been made to produce 3D images with either dual-channel endoscopes or dual cameras, and even computer-generated endoscopic 3D views. Excellent pictures can be generated as a result of the dual-channel endoscope, and this technology has now been incorporated as the standard visualization arm in robotic surgery.[14] However, technical issues such as the larger endoscope size, the necessity for special goggles or headsets, and especially an inability to appropriately rotate a 3D image while turning an angled endoscope have prevented its adoption in standard transnasal endoscopic surgery.[15] Although the latter is not an issue with single-channel 3D endoscope technology, the 3D quality is inferior, and, as a result, it has not proven significantly advantageous at this point in time.

One area that has evolved dramatically in visualization is the camera technology used to project images from the endoscope onto a monitor. The original tube cameras had poor light sensitivity, especially in a field with any blood and generated poor color rendition. This often meant that the surgeon would be dependent on looking through the endoscope to operate safely. However, these concerns were subsequently addressed with light-sensitive charge-coupled device (CCD) cameras that produce improved images, and more recently with high-definition cameras and monitors, providing an excellent image so that endoscopic surgery can now routinely be performed from a monitor with exceptional detail. In addition to an improved ability to teach endoscopic techniques, operating from a screen also facilitates two-surgeon and potentially four-hand techniques, which are useful in skull base surgery (**Fig. 11.1**).

Through-Cutting Instruments and Microdebriders

Although early endoscopic sinus surgery decreased the extent of surgery compared with traditional external approaches or

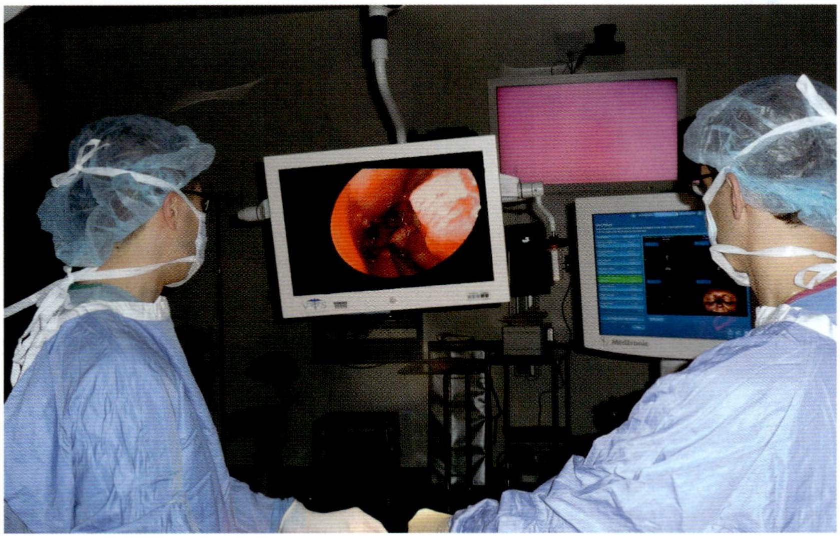

Fig. 11.1 Two-person, four-hand technique for endoscopic skull base surgery.

headlight transnasal techniques, early instruments largely consisted of Blakesley forceps, which tended to strip mucosa and create significant postoperative scarring and persistent inflammation.[7,16] Drawing from orthopedic surgery, fine through-cutting instruments were developed for intranasal use. Both straight and 45-degree through-biting instruments enabled surgeons to cut through both bone and mucosa while preventing inadvertent stripping of nasal cavity epithelium. These instruments have also proved to be especially important when removing bony partitions along the skull base and also within the frontal recess and sphenoid sinus.[17] Blunt manipulation of bony septations adjacent to the skull base or internal carotid artery can lead to disastrous outcomes if unpredictable bony breaks are created. More recently, hand instrumentation has begun to be developed for transnasal skull base and intracranial surgery. This surgery requires very fine and somewhat longer instrumentation and atraumatic suction devices. In addition, the tip of the instrument should ideally not move when the instrument is activated, as may happen with some of the typical forceps and scissors designed for sinus surgery. Continued improvement of the range of instrumentation designed for transnasal craniectomy is anticipated.

The concept of through-cutting instruments has also evolved via powered instrumentation. Microdebriders were originally developed for small-joint arthroscopy and joint removal. In 1996, Setliff[18] and Parsons[19] introduced this device for nasal use, thus facilitating sinus tissue and bone removal. Subsequent improvements in blade and power technology, as well as the addition of angled blades have significantly revolutionized our surgical techniques (**Fig. 11.2**). The combination of sharp tissue removal and concurrent suction allow for excellent visualization while reducing the risk of mucosal stripping. In addition to removal of benign inflammatory disease, this technology has also been a useful adjunct in the initial debulking of certain tumors such as inverted papillomas and other benign and malignant lesions, thus enabling the sites of attachment to be carefully identified. However, beyond the bony confines of the sinonasal cavity, the potential for orbital, intracranial, and vascular injury limits the safety and utility of the microdebrider.

Electrical Devices

Early in endoscopic sinus surgery, it was believed that lasers would be an excellent tool for the removal of sinonasal tissue and for providing hemostasis control. Although a wide variety of lasers were tried, including KTP (potassium titanyl phosphate) and YAG (yttrium-aluminum-garnet), it soon became apparent that collateral damage from lasers was a significant problem, with increased scarring and long healing times.[20,21] However, there were a couple of key innovations that have since evolved from the use of lasers. Schuman and Pineyro[22] modified the YAG laser technique by using constant warm isotonic irrigation. Their observation of warm water irrigation causing nasal vasoconstriction is a concept that is still often employed today, especially in a very vascular surgical field.[23] Second, the pulsed holmium:YAG laser suggested by Shapshay et al[24] often resulted in blood splashing back onto the lens each time the laser was fired. Consequently, Shapshay et al. developed the precursor device that would later be modified into the Endo-Scrub pump and sheath, which irrigates and cleans the tip of the endoscope (**Fig. 11.3**).[24] This has become an important addition to endoscopic equipment, as it facilitates good visualization despite a bloody operative field.

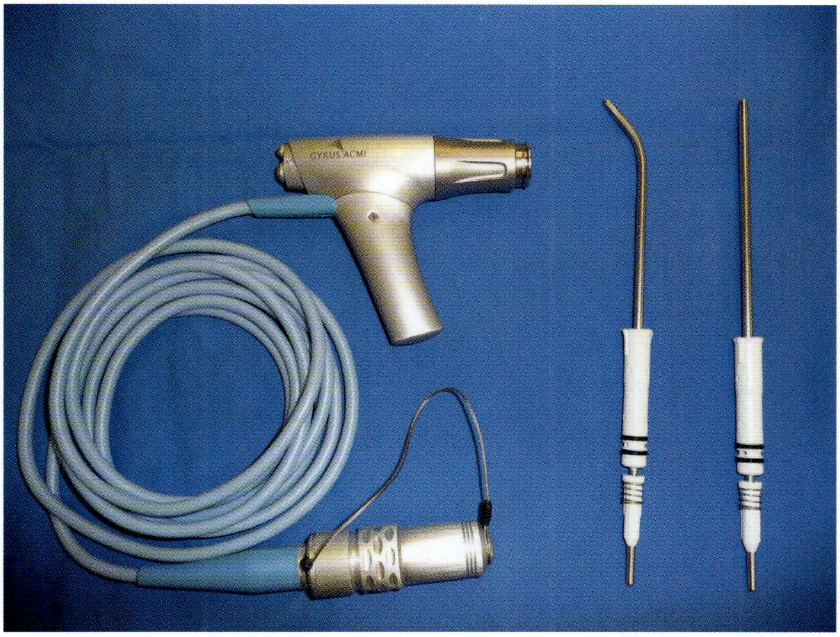

Fig. 11.2 Powered instruments: Gyrus ACMI (Southborough, MA) microdebriders.

A

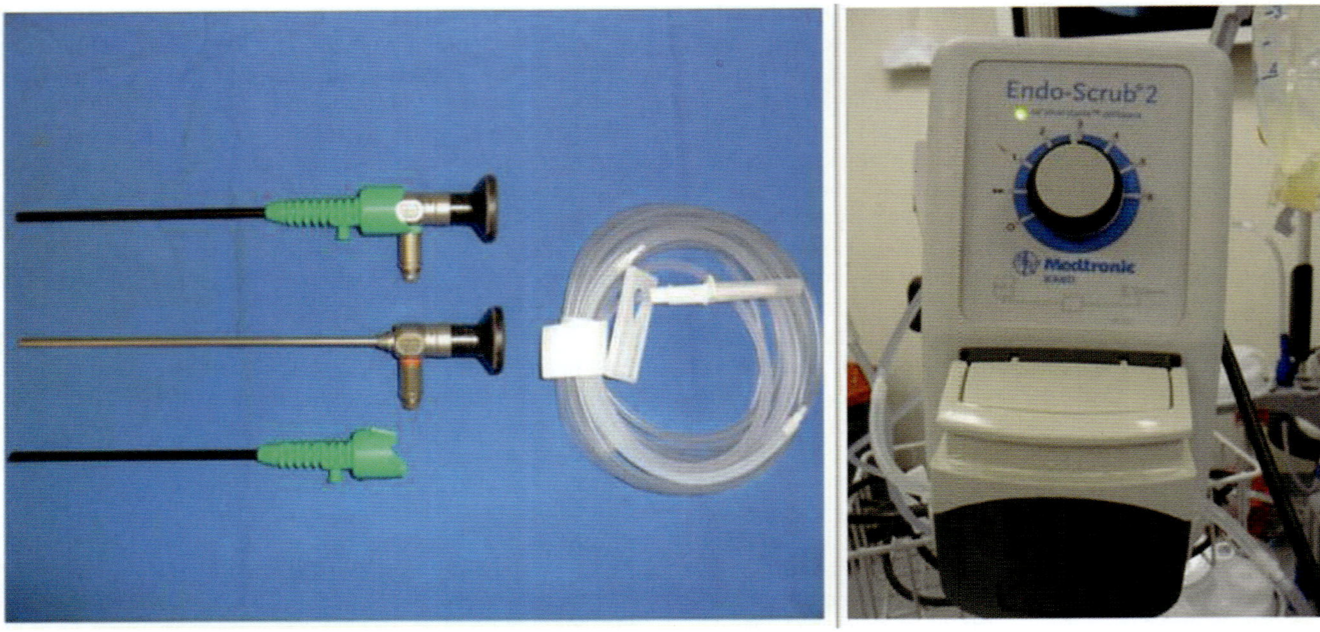

B

Fig. 11.3 **(A,B)** Medtronic (Jacksonville, FL) Endo-Scrub.

In the realm of hemostasis control, cautery devices have also been adapted to endonasal use. Suction monopolar cautery is useful for bleeding primarily located in the lower nasal cavity. Concerns over thermal transmission causing collateral damage limit its use near the skull base, orbit, and internal carotid artery. To address these areas, various endonasal bipolar cautery devices have been developed (**Fig. 11.4**). When combined with suction, these electrical devices have proven to be especially useful for both control of bleeding and skull base tumor dissection and resection. However, the ideal bipolar cautery for transnasal intracranial use has yet to be developed.

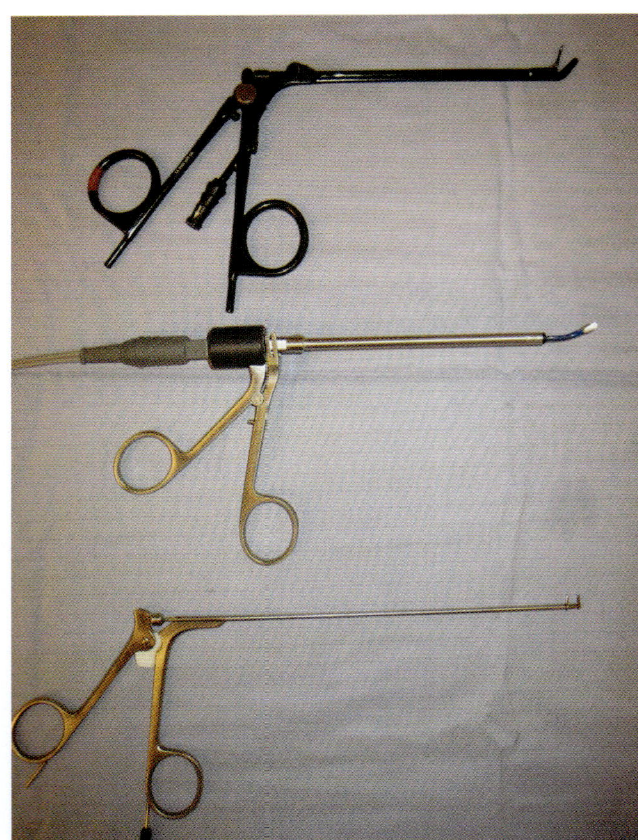

Fig. 11.4 Endonasal bipolar cautery devices.

Suction Irrigation Drills

As more knowledge was gained with endoscopic sinus surgery, it soon became apparent that there were clinical entities such as thick osteitic bone and osseous neoplasms that could not be removed with hand instruments alone. The introduction of suction irrigation drills provided the surgeon with a single instrument that could drill bone, irrigate saline, and suction the surgical field. This innovation facilitated safe drilling in critical areas while the other hand operated the endoscope. Over the years, these drills have been modified and improved with stronger torque, different degrees of angulation, and a large variety of drill bits that enable surgeons to access areas such as the frontal sinus and the skull base.[25]

Imaging (Image-Guidance and Intraoperative)

Computer-aided interactive imaging has become a significant technical innovation for procedures within the sinonasal cavity. The complicated and variable anatomy, combined with the fact that bony walls of the paranasal sinuses provide reliable boundaries of surgery as long as dissection is maintained within the rigid bony framework, made this an ideal early application for this technology. The foundation of all image guidance systems involves registration, whereby preoperative computerized images are correlated to fixed anatomical landmarks. Subsequent calibration of instruments determines the accuracy of the interactive intraoperative guidance. Two main technologies exist in today's image guidance systems, with either optically based or electromagnetic tracking devices. Although neither system is infallible, computer-aided image guidance can be particularly useful in preoperative planning with triplanar views (**Fig. 11.5**).[26,27] In the realm of skull base surgery, image guidance with fused preoperative magnetic resonance imaging (MRI) and computed tomography (CT) scans can offer tremendous information for surgery within the intracranial vault.

All current computer-assisted imaging is based on the preoperative scans. Recently, low-dose intraoperative CT has become a viable option and demonstrated its utility in endoscopic surgical procedures (**Fig. 11.6**).[28] Although the use of intraoperative scanning extends the operative time, it demonstrates residual bony partitions that may be left even by skilled sinus surgeons, and, in more complicated cases, enables real-time intraoperative updates of the computer-assisted image guidance. In the near future, single units that combine intraoperative CT and image guidance will be available on the market. In addition to speeding up the intraoperative update of the image guidance system, such units, by providing a low-dose CT scan prior to the initiation of surgery, will obviate the need for image guidance registration.

The next frontier of imaging in endonasal surgery involves surgical suites that can incorporate both intraoperative CT and MRI scanning with image guidance technologies. Although there are valid concerns about the extremely expensive nonferromagnetic instrumentation for MRI, real-time MRI updates enable surgeons to confirm the adequacy of skull base and intracranial soft tissue tumor resection. However, because of the expense of these systems, they have been adopted on only a very limited scale to date.

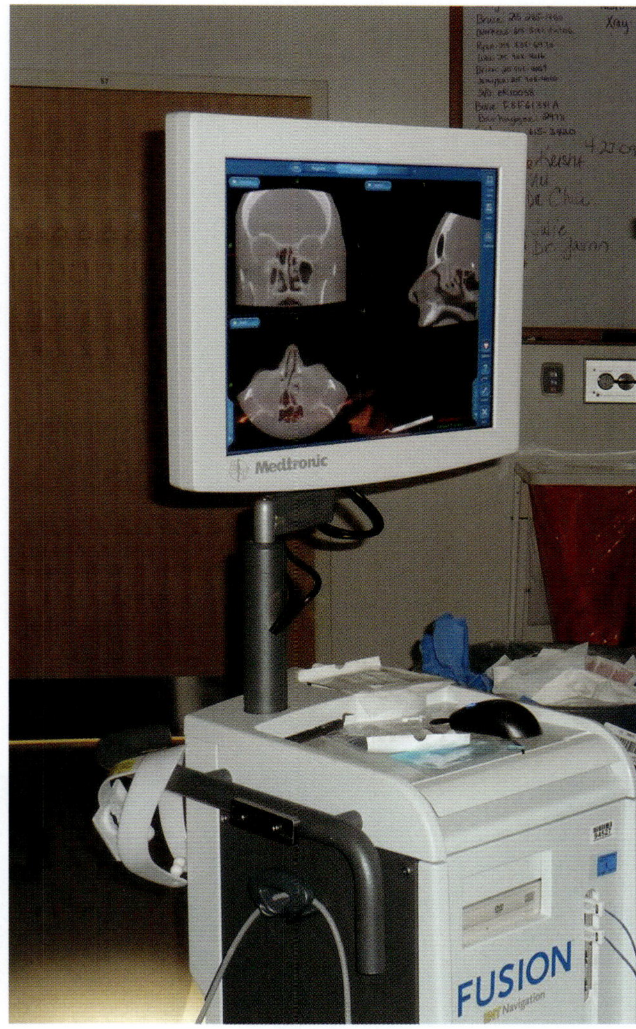

Fig. 11.5 Medtronic (Jacksonville, FL) Fusion image guidance system.

Robotic Skull Base Surgery

Originally introduced for cardiac surgery, the surgical robot has been most widely utilized for prostatic surgery. However, it holds significant promise in the future for skull base surgery.[14] This technology places the surgeon at a remote station with a three-dimensional (3D) view of the operative field and controls that can manipulate the robotic arms that perform the surgery (**Fig. 11.7**). In the field of head and neck surgery, transoral robotic surgery (TORS) has provided excellent access to many areas of the upper aerodigestive tract.[29–32] However, the limitation of TORS for skull base surgery is that the endoscope and robotic arms are placed transorally, thus limiting access rostral to the soft palate. The telescope and, in particular, the size of the robotic arms are currently still too large for transnasal skull base surgery. Although a preclinical investigation has shown that access to the skull base can be improved with an incision of the soft palate and concurrent hard palate resection, as well as placing robotic arms transcervically, there are clearly some significant current limitations for robotic skull base surgery.[33] An approach using bilateral sublabial approaches for transantral robotic access to the skull base has also been described and demonstrated to be feasible with current instrumentation size in a cadaveric model.[34]

A 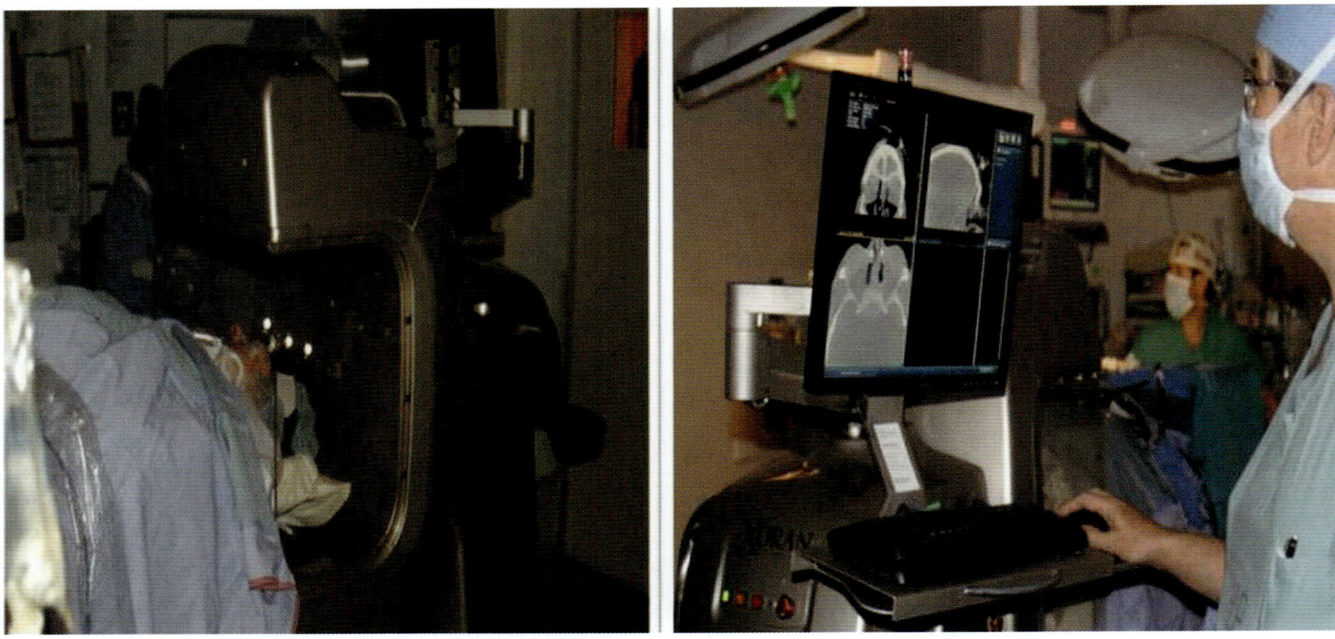 B

Fig. 11.6 (A,B) Xoran (Ann Arbor, MI) xCAT intraoperative computed tomography.

A 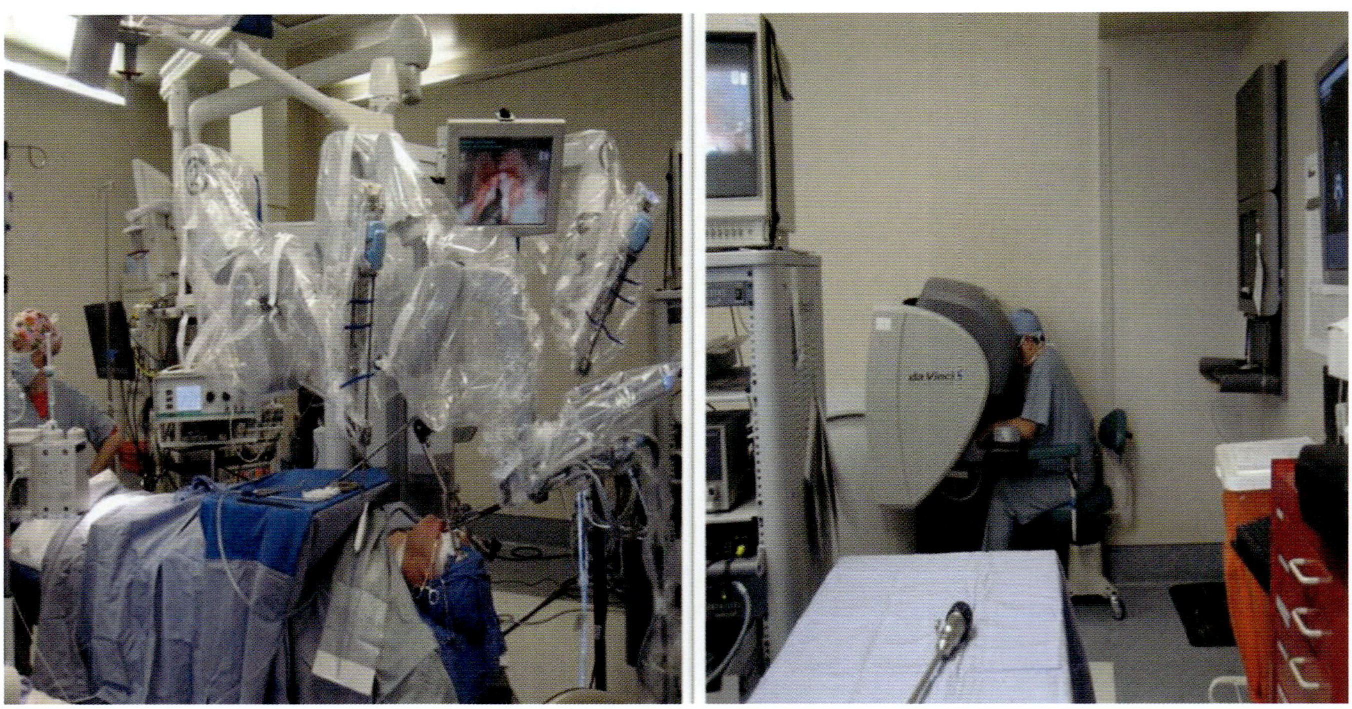 B

Fig. 11.7 (A,B) Surgical robot: the Intuitive Surgical Inc. (Sunnyvale, CA) da Vinci surgical system.

The potential for robotic skull base surgery and robotic neurosurgery is enormous. The robot facilitates fine manipulations that are simply impossible with free-hand surgery. For instance, the articulated arms can be maneuvered to apply vascular clips, remove tumor, or cauterize bleeding around corners in a manner not possible with current instrumentation. In addition, any tremor is eliminated, a critical asset when operating in areas of vital anatomy with lengthy instrumentation. Finally, the potential to sew dura robotically has been demonstrated. Further evolution of instrumentation, additional reduction of the size of the robotic arms, and the availability of 5-mm stereoscopic endoscopes should facilitate transnasal access. Such innovation will significantly expand the potential for transnasal intracranial surgery, as well as for other forms of neurosurgery with significantly reduced necessity for brain retraction and its associated morbidity.

Conclusion

Since its introduction in the mid-1980s, the spectrum of intranasal endoscopic surgery has evolved and grown from treatment of benign inflammatory disease to resection of skull base and intracranial tumors. Much of this advancement can be traced to the technical innovations that have occurred in visualization, instrumentation, and imaging. However, equally as important has been the concurrent refinement and improvement in surgical technique, including our ability to close skull base defects. As the boundaries of endonasal surgery continue to be expanded, limitations of access and instrumentation will continue to provide further impetus for technical innovation and growth, with the goal of continuing to reduce patient morbidity.

References

1. Jacobs JB. 100 years of frontal sinus surgery. Laryngoscope 1997;107(11 Pt 2):1–36
2. Woodham J. History of the development of surgery for sinuses. In: The Sinuses. New York: Raven; 1995:3–14.
3. Pownell PH, Minoli JJ, Rohrich RJ. Diagnostic nasal endoscopy. Plast Reconstr Surg 1997;99:1451–1458
4. Jennings CR. Harold Hopkins. Arch Otolaryngol Head Neck Surg 1998; 124:1042
5. Morgenstern L. Harold Hopkins (1918-1995): "let there be light . . .". Surg Innov 2004;11:291–292
6. Messerklinger W. Endoscopy of the Nose. Baltimore: Urban & Schwarzenberg; 1978
7. Hosemann W. Surgical treatment of nasal polyposis in patients with aspirin intolerance. Thorax 2000;55(Suppl 2):S87–S90
8. Vining EM, Kennedy DW. The transmigration of endoscopic sinus surgery from Europe to the United States. Ear Nose Throat J 1994;73:456–458, 460
9. Yaniv E, Rappaport ZH. Endoscopic transseptal transsphenoidal surgery for pituitary tumors. Neurosurgery 1997;40:944–946
10. White DR, Sonnenburg RE, Ewend MG, Senior BA. Safety of minimally invasive pituitary surgery (MIPS) compared with a traditional approach. Laryngoscope 2004;114:1945–1948
11. Nasseri SS, Kasperbauer JL, Strome SE, McCaffrey TV, Atkinson JL, Meyer FB. Endoscopic transnasal pituitary surgery: report on 180 cases. Am J Rhinol 2001;15:281–287
12. Cappabianca P, Cavallo LM, Colao A, et al. Endoscopic endonasal transsphenoidal approach: outcome analysis of 100 consecutive procedures. Minim Invasive Neurosurg 2002;45:193–200
13. Jho HD, Carrau RL, Ko Y, Daly MA. Endoscopic pituitary surgery: an early experience. Surg Neurol 1997;47:213–222, discussion 222–223
14. Ballantyne GH, Moll F. The da Vinci telerobotic surgical system: the virtual operative field and telepresence surgery. Surg Clin North Am 2003;83:1293–1304, vii
15. Kennedy DW. Technical innovations and the evolution of endoscopic sinus surgery. Ann Otol Rhinol Laryngol Suppl 2006;196:3–12
16. Moriyama H. Healing process of sinus mucosa after endoscopic sinus surgery. Am J Rhinol 1996;10:61–66
17. Kennedy DW, Bolger WE, Zinreich SJ. Diseases of the Sinuses: Diagnosis and Management. Hamilton, Canada: BC Decker; 2001:197–210
18. Setliff RC III. The hummer: a remedy for apprehension in functional endoscopic sinus surgery. Otolaryngol Clin North Am 1996;29:95–104
19. Parsons DS. Rhinologic uses of powered instrumentation in children beyond sinus surgery. Otolaryngol Clin North Am 1996;29:105–114
20. Berci G, Cuschieri A. Karl Storz, 1911–1996. A remembrance. Surg Endosc 1996;10:1123
21. Knappe V, Frank F, Rohde E. Principles of lasers and biophotonic effects. Photomed Laser Surg 2004;22:411–417
22. Schuman DM, Pineyro R. Functional Aqualaser sinuscopy: a safe technique for the treatment of severe nasal polyposis. J Clin Laser Med Surg 1994;12:333–337
23. Kassam A, Snyderman CH, Carrau RL, Gardner P, Mintz A. Endoneurosurgical hemostasis techniques: lessons learned from 400 cases. Neurosurg Focus 2005;19:E7
24. Shapshay SM, Rebeiz EE, Bohigian RK, Hybels RL, Aretz HT, Pankratov MM. Holmium: yttrium aluminum garnet laser-assisted endoscopic sinus surgery: laboratory experience. Laryngoscope 1991;101: 142–149
25. Chandra RK, Schlosser R, Kennedy DW. Use of the 70-degree diamond burr in the management of complicated frontal sinus disease. Laryngoscope 2004;114:188–192
26. Anon JB, Klimek L, Mosges R, Zinreich SJ. Computer-assisted endoscopic sinus surgery. An international review. Otolaryngol Clin North Am 1997;30:389–401
27. Palmer JN, Kennedy DW. Historical perspective on image-guided sinus surgery. Otolaryngol Clin North Am 2005;38:419–428
28. Jackman AH, Palmer JN, Chiu AG, Kennedy DW. Use of intraoperative CT scanning in endoscopic sinus surgery: a preliminary report. Am J Rhinol 2008;22:170–174
29. Weinstein GS, O'Malley BW Jr, Snyder W, Hockstein NG. Transoral robotic surgery: supraglottic partial laryngectomy. Ann Otol Rhinol Laryngol 2007;116:19–23
30. Weinstein GS, O'Malley BW Jr, Snyder W, Sherman E, Quon H. Transoral robotic surgery: radical tonsillectomy. Arch Otolaryngol Head Neck Surg 2007;133:1220–1226
31. O'Malley BW Jr, Weinstein GS, Snyder W, Hockstein NG. Transoral robotic surgery (TORS) for base of tongue neoplasms. Laryngoscope 2006;116:1465–1472
32. Genden EM, Desai S, Sung CK. Transoral robotic surgery for the management of head and neck cancer: a preliminary experience. Head Neck 2009;31:283–289
33. O'Malley BW Jr, Weinstein GS. Robotic anterior and midline skull base surgery: preclinical investigations. Int J Radiat Oncol Biol Phys 2007; 69(2, Suppl)S125–S128
34. Hanna EY, Holsinger C, DeMonte F, Kupferman M. Robotic endoscopic surgery of the skull base: a novel surgical approach. Arch Otolaryngol Head Neck Surg 2007;133:1209–1214

III Tips and Pearls in Paranasal Sinus Approaches

12 Maxillary and Ethmoid Sinuses in Skull Base Surgery

Nobuyoshi Otori, Kiyoshi Yanagi, and Hiroshi Moriyama

Tips and Pearls

- Appropriate ethmoidal and maxillary surgery makes it easy to perform subsequent skull base surgery.
- The maxillary sinus is a large unique cavity, but the ethmoid sinus is divided into small air cells.
- The lamina papyracea is perpendicular in the front, but inclines inward in the rear.
- Through-cutting forceps are primarily used for effective preservation of sinus mucosa, prevention of injury, and improved mucosal healing process.
- Understanding of the location of the uncinate process (basal lamellae I), bulla ethmoidalis (basal lamellae II), ground lamellae (basal lamellae III), and superior turbinate (basal lamellae IV) is important because they serve as an anatomical landmark during the operation.
- The bone septa in the ethmoid air cells are sufficiently excised to make them as smooth as possible, and a unique cavity is created.
- If the maxillary sinus is opened prior to the posterior ethmoidal surgery, the lower half of the ethmoid sinus becomes widened, bleeding is less problematic, and the opening of the most posterior ethmoid sinus is easier.
- The maxillary sinus is inspected with a 70-degree oblique scope, and then a curved forceps is inserted through fontanelle and a small hole is made through the inferior nasal meatus.

Introduction

Endoscopic ethmoidal surgery and maxillary surgery are the first step in endoscopic skull base surgery. Ethmoid air cells are removed to make the ethmoid sinus unique cavity. The ostium of the maxillary sinus is opened to make a large communication to nasal cavity. These operations make it easy to perform subsequent skull base surgery.

This chapter describes the anatomy and basic techniques of endoscopic sinus surgery for the ethmoid sinus and the maxillary sinus.

Anatomy of Ethmoid Sinus and Maxillary Sinus

The maxillary sinus is large unique cavity, but the ethmoid sinus is divided into 10 to 20 small air cells. Therefore, when the surgeon approaches the skull base via the ethmoid sinus, it is necessary to make the ethmoid sinus a unique cavity by removing a partition of these small air cells.[1–3]

The airflow tract of the frontal sinus, anterior ethmoid sinus, and maxillary sinus are called the ostiomeatal complex (OMC) or the ostiomeatal unit (OMU) (**Fig. 12.1**). It includes the ostium of the frontal sinus, the nasofrontal duct, the ostium of the maxillary sinus, the ethmoidal infundibulum, the semilunar hiatus, and the middle meatus.[4]

The lamina papyracea is perpendicular in the front, but inclines inward in the rear.[4] In addition, the front of the lamina cribrosa is more remarkable than the rear.

The anterior ethmoid sinus is composed of the uncinate process (basal lamella I) and the bulla ethmoidalis (basal lamella II). There is a ground lamella (basal lamella III, basal lamellae of middle turbinate) behind the anterior ethmoid sinus.[3] The rear of the ground lamella is a posterior ethmoid

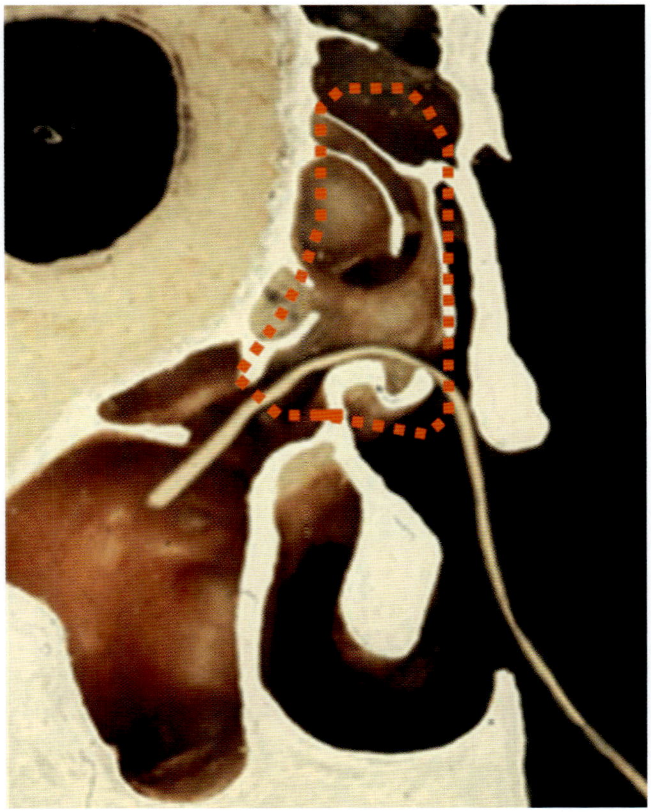

Fig. 12.1 The ostiomeatal complex.

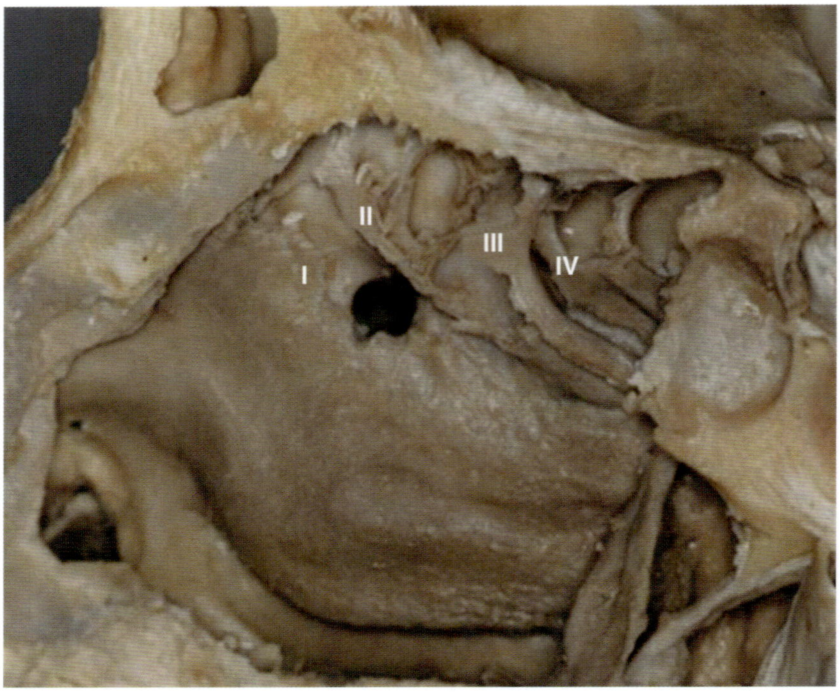

Fig. 12.2 Basal lamellae I to IV on the lateral wall of the nasal cavity.

sinus. When the surgery advances into the posterior ethmoid sinus, a skull base appears above. The next lamella is a superior turbinate (basal lamellae IV). The rear of the lamella is an anterior wall of the sphenoid sinus (**Fig. 12.2**).

There is sphenopalatine foramen at the end of the ground lamella, and the sphenopalatine artery flows into a nasal cavity from there. In addition, the anterior ethmoidal artery is at the front edge of the ground lamella.

When the posterior ethmoid sinus grows toward the upper part of the sphenoid sinus, an Onodi cell is formed. In this case the optic canal contacts a rear wall of the posterior ethmoid sinus[3,4] (**Fig. 12.3**).

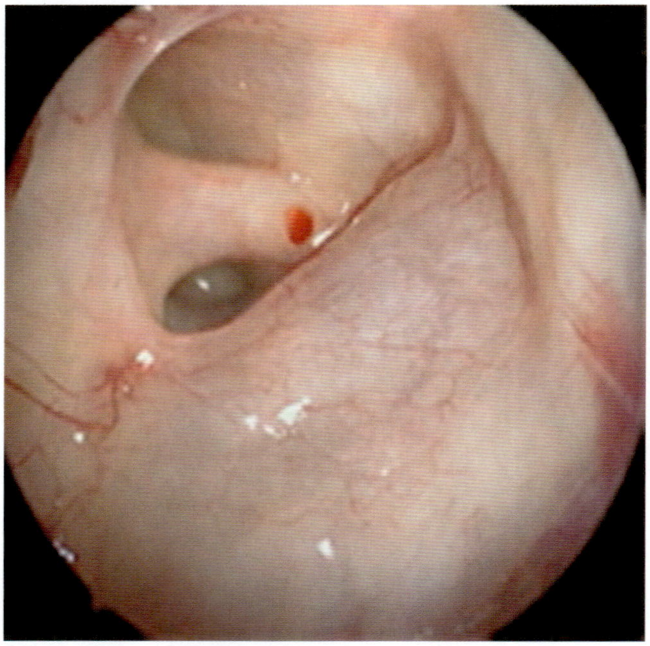

A

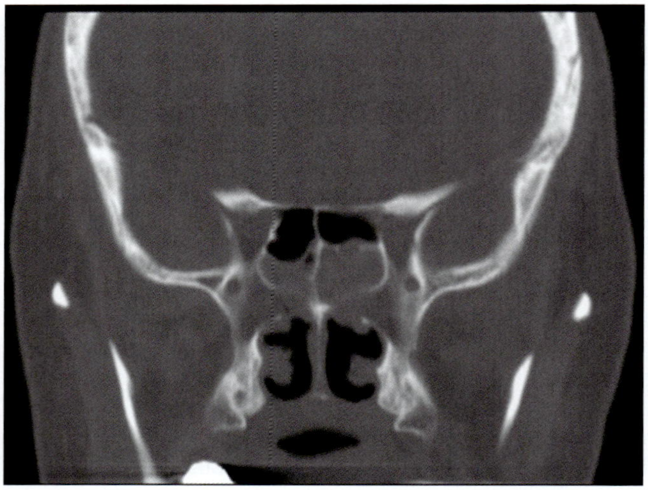

B

Fig. 12.3 Endoscopic view **(A)** and computed tomography (CT) scan **(B)** of the optic canal in the Onodi cell.

Equipment and Forceps Used for Ethmoid and Maxillary Surgery

Ethmoidal and maxillary surgery cannot be performed properly using only conventional forceps.[5–7] In addition to Grunwald forceps, a thin forceps, curved forceps, and a microdebrider are also prepared. These instruments facilitate the treatment of lesions of various sites and enable safe and accurate surgery. Curved and flexible aspiration tubes are prepared in addition to the conventional ones. Rigid endoscopes, 0 and 70 degrees with a diameter of 4 mm, are chiefly used, and endoscopes of 30 and 45 degrees are occasionally used.

The selection of forceps is important not only for a safe and accurate operation but also for obtaining good results postoperatively. The through-cutting forceps are used primarily (**Fig. 12.4**). They are preferred for effective preservation of mucosa and for prevention of injury. Morphologically, the orbit and brain are separated from the paranasal sinuses with a paper-thin bone wall, and periodically part of these bony separations will have dehiscence (**Fig. 12.5**). Accordingly, pulling the mucosa, lamella, and the bone plate with cup-type forceps is extremely dangerous. Through-cutting forceps are used for safe manipulation in opening the maxillary sinus orifice and for removal of the mucosa and lamella of the ethmoid sinus.

Surgical Techniques[5,6]

Understanding the location and variations of the middle turbinate is important, because it serves as an anatomic landmark during the operation. Once the middle turbinate is confirmed, it is pressed medially to widen the middle nasal meatus, and the anterior/posterior ethmoid sinuses are opened by approaching from the middle nasal meatus. In patients with an aerated middle turbinate concha bullosa, the outer wall of the middle turbinate is removed, and then the air cells of the middle turbinate are opened.

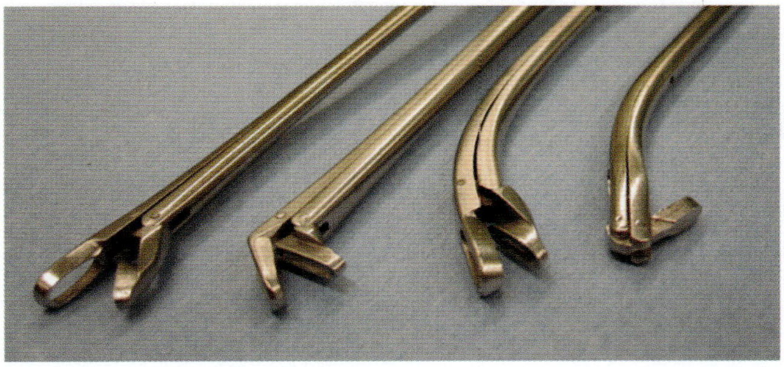

Fig. 12.4 Through-cutting forceps.

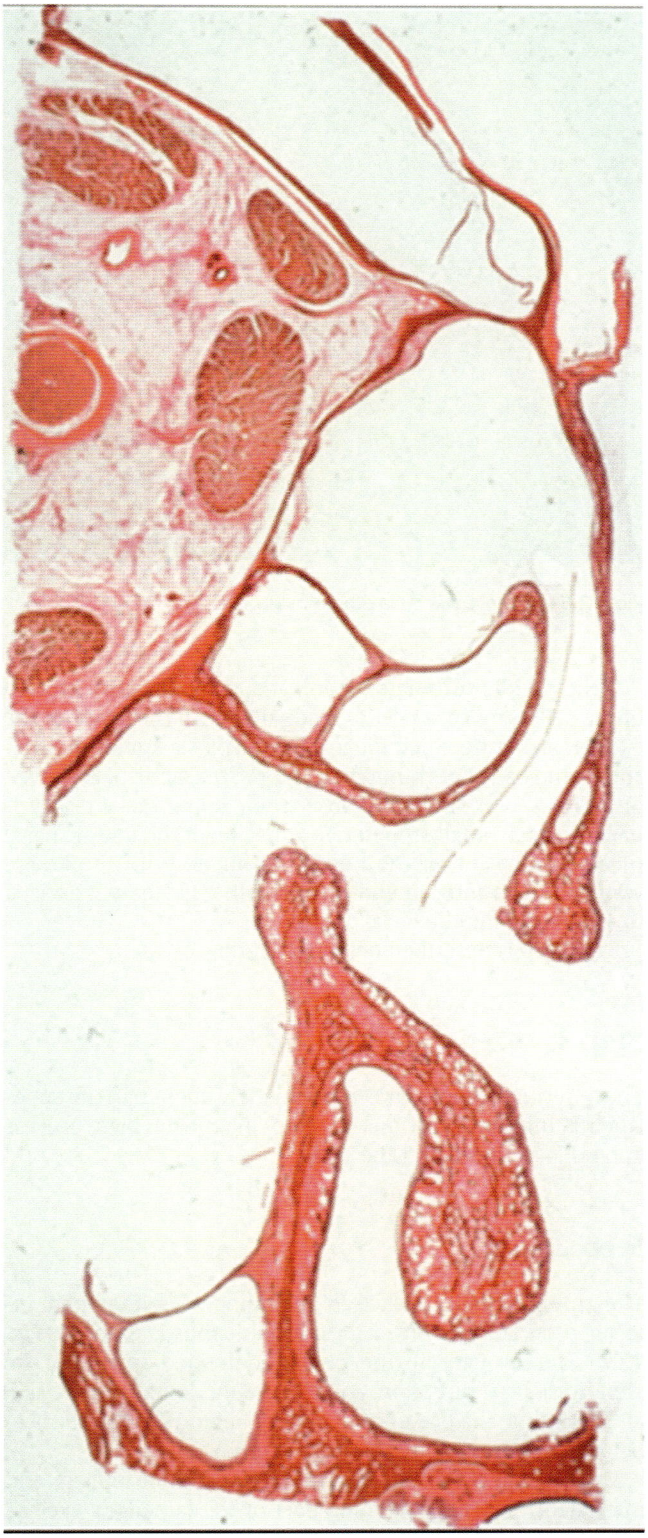

Fig. 12.5 Microscopic view of the coronal section.

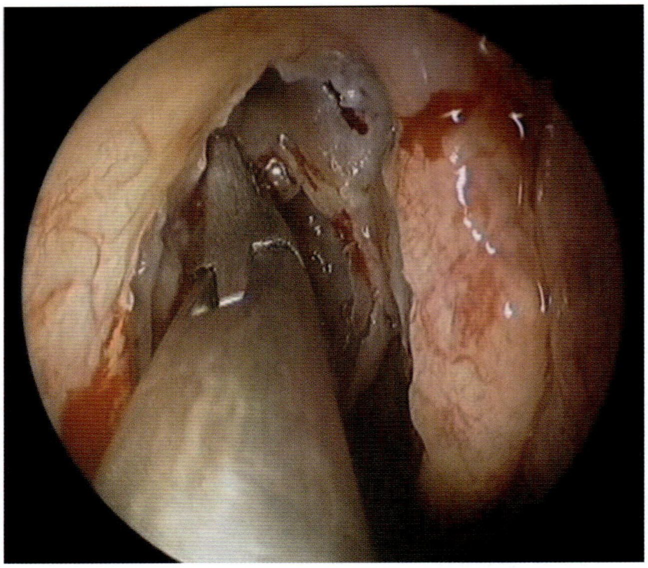

Fig. 12.6 Remove the bulla ethmoidalis.

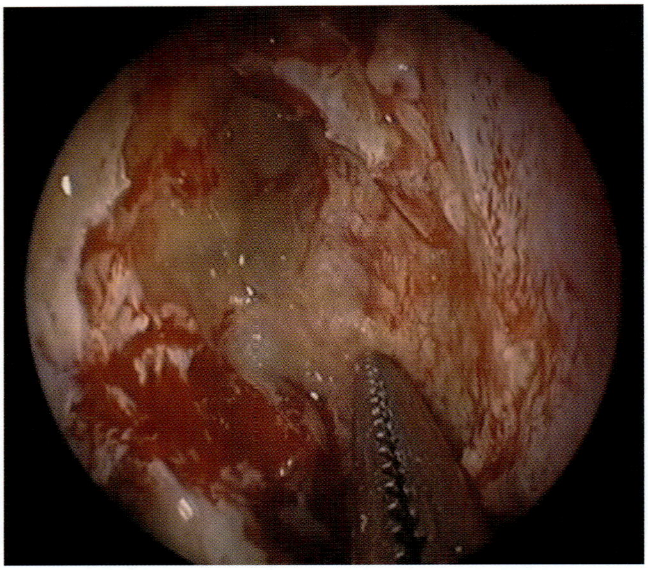

Fig. 12.7 Excise the ground lamella.

If the middle turbinate is removed, compensatory growth of the septal mucosa occurs gradually to fill the space of the excised structure. Such mucosal hyperplasia sometimes becomes the cause of rhinorrhea and postnasal drip. However, in patients with a narrow nose (their upper nasal cavity is narrow), to avoid postoperative adhesion of the middle nasal meatus (adhesion of the middle turbinate with the lateral wall), only the anterior end of the middle turbinate is excised to secure the middle nasal meatus.

Each step is described below in detail.

Step 1

The anterior ethmoid air cells are widely opened in the superior and inferior directions by removing the uncinate process and bulla ethmoidalis (**Fig. 12.6**).

Step 2

The ground lamella is excised beginning from its medial inferior part, and the posterior ethmoid sinus is entered (**Fig. 12.7**). The through-cutting forceps is directed upward in the superior lateral direction, and the ground lamella is excised, at which time the presence of a space behind the lamella is to be confirmed, and only that part is removed.

Then, using a through-cutting forceps, bone punch, and microdebrider, the remaining part of the lamella is excised (**Fig. 12.8**). To avoid postoperative scar formation, the bone septa in the ethmoid sinus are sufficiently excised to make them as smooth as possible, and a unique cavity is created. The mucosa of the limiting wall in the ethmoid sinus is to be left intact to the greatest extent possible, and the bone surface is not to be exposed. Such precaution is effective in achieving early postoperative epithelialization. When operating within the ethmoid sinus, attention must be paid to the thin bone wall (lamina papyracea or medial orbital wall) that separates the orbit. In paranasal sinus surgery, injuries to the medial orbital wall are the most frequent. When a through-cutting forceps is used, the lamina papyracea is not injured even if the forceps is manipulated while orienting it at the right angle to the lamina papyracea. If the use of a cup-type forceps is required, it is to be held parallel to the lamina papyracea; in patients with good pneumatization and a high ethmoid roof, it is held anteriorly where the ethmoid roof is especially high and the lateral wall of the cribriform plate is thin and shows a sharp elevation. Caution is required because

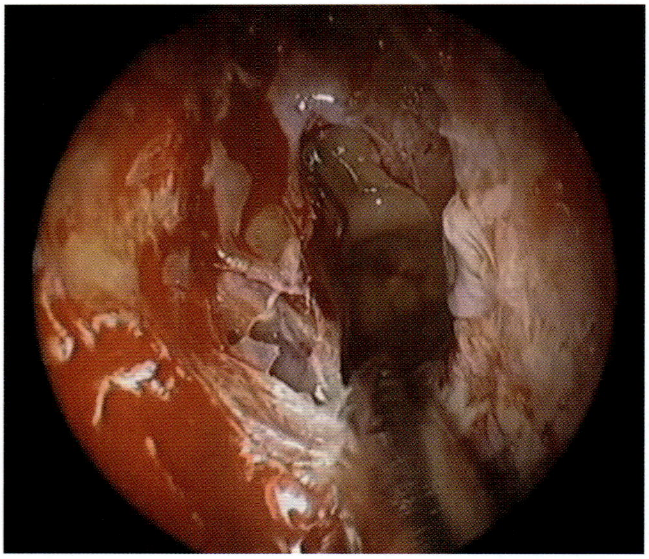

Fig. 12.8 Remove the ground lamella and enter the posterior ethmoid sinus.

the ethmoidal artery and nerve exist along this region. Also, constant attention is to be paid to the presence of the optic canal superolaterally.

Step 3

The basal lamella IV is opened in this step. Then the most posterior ethmoid sinus is entered. But if the maxillary sinus is opened first, the lower half of the ethmoid sinus becomes widened, bleeding is less problematic, and the opening of the most posterior ethmoid sinus is easier. In addition, because the position of the posterior wall of the maxillary sinus is confirmed, localization of the depth of the most posterior ethmoid sinus cell and sphenoid sinus is made easier. Therefore, opening the fontanelle of the maxillary sinus prior to the opening of basal lamellae IV is an alternative approach.

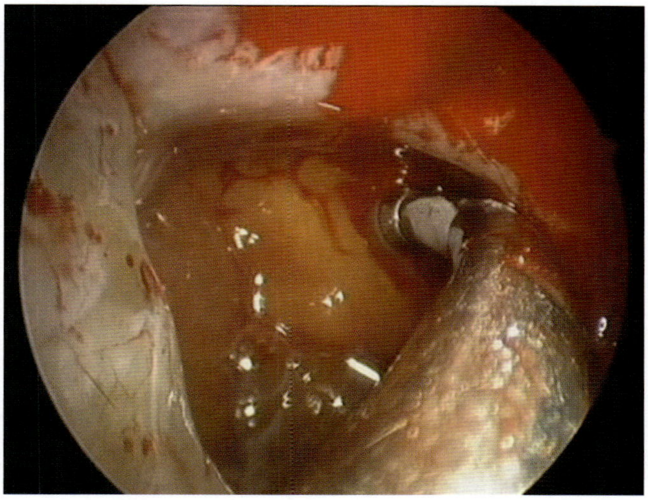

Fig. 12.9 Maxillary surgery under the view of 70-degree endoscope.

Step 4

Using a curved sharp detachment knife, the fontanelle of the maxillary sinus is incised to establish a communication route with the maxillary sinus. The posterior half of the fontanelle is removed using a curved through-cutting forceps; the anterior half is removed using a backbiting forceps, and the transitory region between the maxillary and the ethmoid sinuses is smoothed by removing the septa using a lateral forceps. In patients in whom the fontanelle is positioned laterally, the fontanelle is opened as wide as possible using a curved backbiting forceps. The cavity of the maxillary sinus is inspected with a 70-degree oblique scope. Depending on the situation, a small hole is made through the inferior nasal meatus. A forceps is inserted through this hole as well as fontanelle, and diseased mucosa (at the anterior and inferior walls) is excised (**Fig. 12.9**).

As another approach to the maxillary sinus, implanting a catheter from the gingiva is sometimes performed. The endoscope and forceps are inserted from there. In addition, medial maxillectomy, that is, removing the medial wall of the maxillary sinus together with the inferior turbinate, is another approach. In comparison with the ordinary endonasal approach, the endoscopic field of view and manipulation improve.

Treatment of the Sinus Mucosa

Excision of the mucosa is to be avoided as much as possible. For reversible pathologic changes, diseased mucosa is preserved and its normalization through improvement in aeration and drainage is awaited. For irreversible lesions showing severe edema and hypertrophy, subepithelial lesions are excised with a cutting instrument, and the mucoperiosteum is left intact (exposure of the bone surface is to be avoided) (**Fig. 12.10**). With this method, the inflammation of the

A

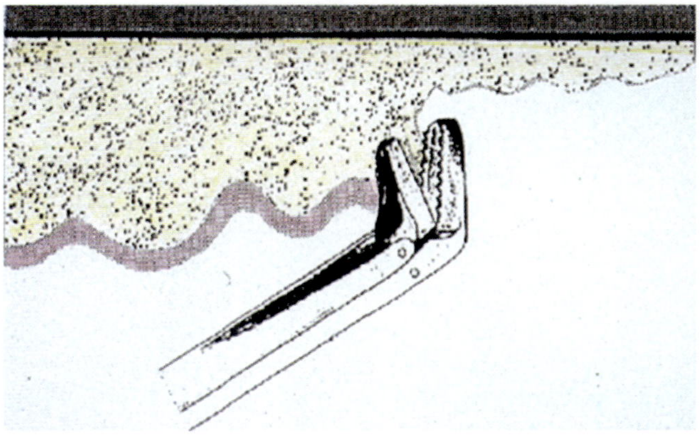

B

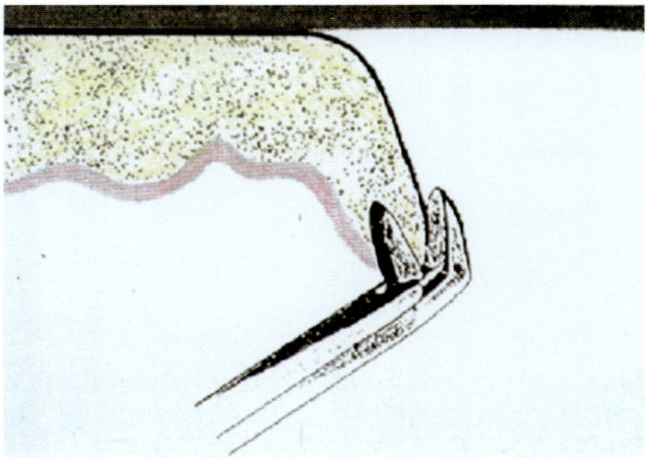

Fig. 12.10 **(A)** Mucosal preservation with through-cutting forceps. **(B)** Mucosa is not preserved with cup-type forceps.

preserved subepithelial tissue disappears, and healthy mucosal epithelium is regenerated.[8] The original paranasal cavity is to be maintained.

When the bone surface is exposed as a result of the elimination of the mucosa and periosteum, edematous tissue first covers the exposed bone surface and soon undergoes scarring. In such tissue, regeneration of mucosal epithelium is delayed, and a long period of time is required for the tissue to be covered with mucosal epithelium that extends from that surrounding it. Mucosal epithelium that regenerates after elimination of all mucosa has only a small number of ciliated cells, and thus its excretory function is poor.[8] Accordingly, the peripheral outlines of the ethmoid sinus and maxillary sinus, such as the mucosa of the ethmoid roof, medial orbital wall, orbital floor, and lateral wall of the maxillary sinus, are to be left intact as much as possible. A thin connective tissue should be left on the bone surface; the peripheral bony boundary surface should not be exposed by any means. Such treatment facilitates ciliated epithelialization of the mucosa, and recovery of the ciliary function should occur.[9]

References

1. Takahashi K. Vorlaufige Mitteilung uber die Erforsdiung des Luftstromweges in dcr Nase des Menschcn in vivo. Z Laryngol Rhinol Otol 1992; 11:203–208
2. Takahashi R. Intranasal operation of chronic ethmoiditis. (in Japanese) Shujutsu 1950;4:134–145
3. Takahashi R. Intranasal operation of chronic ethmoiditis. In: Takahashi R, ed. A Collection of ENT Studies. Tokyo: Department of ORL, Jikei University School of Medicine; 1971:372–389
4. Ashikawa R, Ohkushi H, Ohmae T. Clinical effects of endonasal sinusectomy with reconstruction of the nasal cavity (Takahashi's method). Rhinology 1981;19:93–100
5. Moriyama H, Ozawa M, Honda Y. Endoscopic endonasal sinus surgery. Approaches and post-operative evaluation. Rhinology 1991;29:93–98
6. Moriyama H, Ozawa M, Honda Y. Technique for endoscopic endonasai sinus surgery. Am J Rhinol 1991;5:137–141
7. Ohnishi T, Esaki S, Iwasaki M, et al. Endoscopic microsurgery of the ethmoid sinus. Am J Rhinol 1990;4:119–127
8. Moriyama H, Yanagi K, Ohtori N, et al. Healing process of sinus mucosa after endoscopic sinus surgery. Am J Rhinol 1996;10:61–66
9. Asai K, Haruna S, Otori N, Yanagi K, Fukami M, Moriyama H. Saccharin test of maxillary sinus mucociliary function after endoscopic sinus surgery. Laryngoscope 2000;110:117–122

13 Frontal Sinus Management in Skull Base Surgery

Kristin Seiberling and Peter-John Wormald

Tips and Pearls

- Exposure of the entire skull base is necessary for removal of skull base tumors approaching the frontal sinus. A complete sphenoethmoidectomy is typically first performed with clearance of the skull base.
- A modified Lothrop procedure (Draf 3 or frontal drillout) is performed when lesions are anterior to the anterior ethmoidal artery. Those lesions posterior to the anterior ethmoidal artery may be removed with exposure of the frontal sinus ostium without a modified Lothrop procedure.
- Lesions located in the region of the planum sphenoidale may be removed without exposure of the frontal sinus ostium.
- The modified Lothrop procedure involves the removal of the superior portion of the septum, the floor of the frontal sinus, and the intersinus septum.
- Frontal sinus trephines may be placed to help guide the dissection during the modified Lothrop procedure.
- On average the combined frontal sinus ostium stenoses by approximately 30% over time; therefore, the largest possible opening should be made during the modified Lothrop procedure.

Introduction

The endonasal approach to skull base tumors requires a complete understanding of the endoscopic anatomy of the ventral skull base and surrounding structures. The anterior skull base consists of the frontal bone, fovea ethmoidalis, and intervening cribriform plates. Posteriorly the fovea ethmoidalis attaches to the planum sphenoidale. The first step in the removal of skull base tumors endonasally is complete clearance of the entire skull base. This is accomplished by performing a bilateral sphenoethmoidectomy followed by exposure of the frontal sinus. The surgical approach to the frontal sinus during the removal of skull base tumors depends on the extent and location of the lesion.

Prior to planning the surgery, the surgeon must review the preoperative images and evaluate the extent of the tumor along the parasagittal plane. Lesions located anteriorly along the skull base require maximum visualization of the frontal sinus and skull base, which necessitates a modified endoscopic Lothrop (MEL) procedure (**Fig. 13.1A**).

A

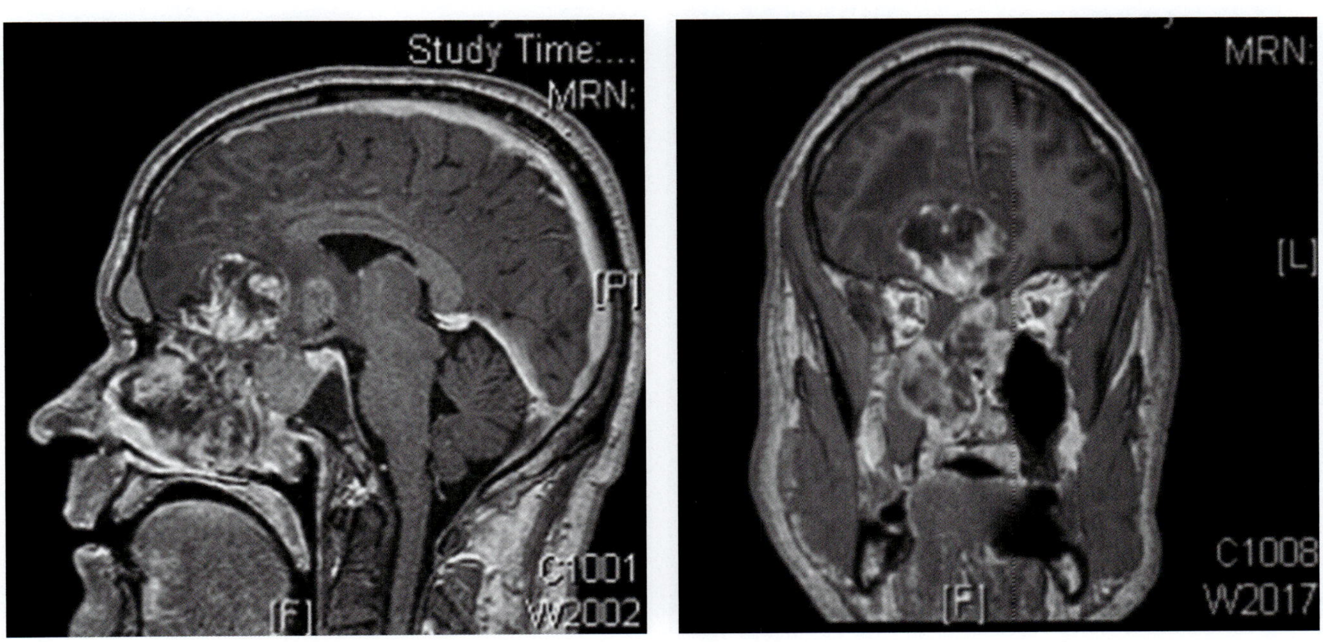

B

Fig. 13.1 Parasagittal **(A)** and coronal **(B)** magnetic resonance imaging (MRI) scans demonstrate a large T4 adenocarcinoma approaching the posterior table of the frontal sinus.

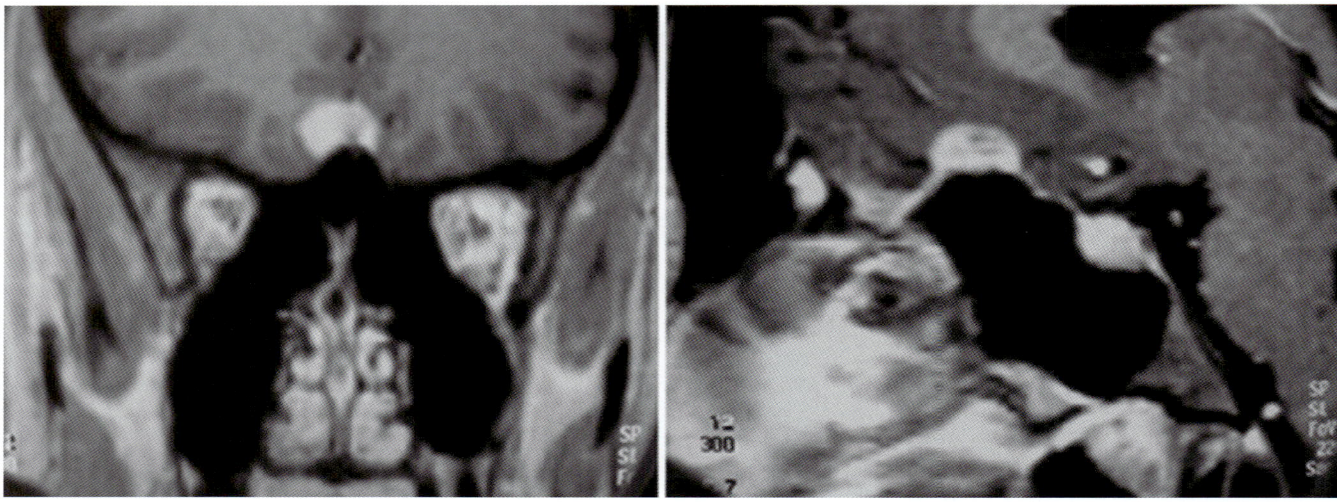

A B

Fig. 13.2 Parasagittal **(A)** and coronal **(B)** MRI scans of a small posterior based meningioma.

Although each case must be individualized, it is thought that if the tumor approaches the region of the anterior ethmoidal artery, a MEL should be performed. The anterior ethmoidal artery is located between the frontal sinus ostium and upward continuation of the anterior face of the bulla ethmoidalis (**Fig. 13.1B**). The MEL facilitates accurate delineation of the skull base anteriorly at the level of the olfactory fossa. Lesions located in the posterior region of the anterior skull base may be removed with the identification of both frontal sinus ostia without a MEL (**Fig. 13.2**). If the tumor does not extend past the planum sphenoidale, identification of the frontal sinus ostia may not be necessary (**Fig. 13.3**).

■ Surgical Anatomy

The frontal recess/sinus is a challenging area to approach surgically, given its proximity to the thin cribriform plate medially, the orbit laterally, and the anterior ethmoidal ar-

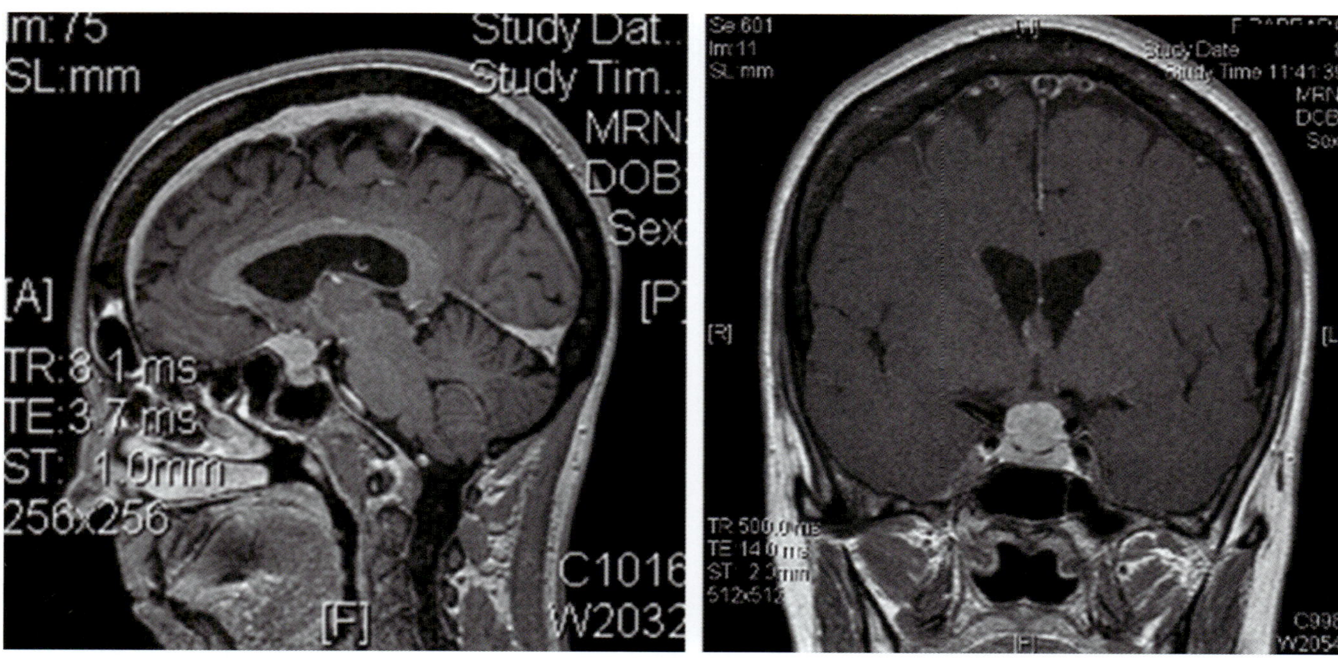

A B

Fig. 13.3 Parasagittal **(A)** and coronal **(B)** MRI scans of a suprasellar meningioma. This tumor did not extend past the planum sphenoidale, which allowed for removal without dissection of the frontal recess.

tery posteriorly. To access the frontal sinus, one must first understand the relationship of the drainage pathway of the frontal sinus to the surrounding structures.

In addition, to perform a MEL procedure, one must also grasp the relation of the frontal recess and frontal sinus to the frontal process of the maxilla, the nasal septum, the middle turbinate, the lacrimal sac, and the olfactory fossa. The thick bone of the frontal process of the maxilla, otherwise known as the frontal beak, forms the anterior wall of the frontal recess.

Anterior to the middle turbinate this bone continues to cover the lacrimal sac. The orbit is found posterior to the axilla of the middle turbinate. As long as the dissection is carried anterior or superior to the axilla, the orbit is not at risk. Another area of concern when drilling during a MEL procedure is the skull base in the region of the olfactory fossa.

To safely perform a MEL procedure one must have a strong grasp of the anatomy of the forward projection of the skull base, which forms the frontal T. The frontal T is located at a point where the middle turbinate attaches to the skull base at the anterior end of the olfactory fossa and marks the point of entry where the olfactory neurons are found. The olfactory neurons are a reliable marker for the level of the skull base used during the MEL procedure.

Modified Endoscopic Lothrop (Draf 3 or Frontal Drillout)

The MEL procedure (also known as the Draf 3 or frontal sinus drillout) was originally described by Lothrop[1] in 1914 and revised by Draf[2] in 1991 and Gross et al[3] in 1995. It involves the removal of the superior portion of the septum, the floor of the frontal sinus, and the intersinus septum, thus creating the largest possible opening between the frontal sinus and the nasal cavity (**Fig. 13.4**). This technique effectively exposes the posterior table of the frontal sinus and identifies the level of the skull base at its anteriormost extent.

In patients who have tumors that occupy the anterior skull base, a MEL is performed to delineate the level of the skull base anterior to the tumor. This enables the entire skull base to be skeletonized, facilitating tumor removal.

Surgical Technique

Prior to starting the procedure, relevant CT scans are reviewed for the anatomy of the frontal recess and dimensions of the frontal sinus. A review of the axial, coronal, and parasagittal scans is necessary to determine the anatomy and outflow tract of the frontal sinus. Image guidance is setup and used during the procedure. We routinely use image guidance in all our MEL and skull base procedures. Image guidance enables confirmation of the position of the first olfactory neurons, which mark the level of the skull base in the region of the olfactory fossa.

The surgery is begun with a zero-degree endoscope that is used for the majority of the procedure. This is switched to a 30-degree scope only at the end of the procedure when the frontal beak is taken down. The nasal septum, the region of the axilla of the middle turbinate and nasal vault, is injected with local anesthetic.

Using a powered microdebrider the mucosa over the frontal process of the maxilla superior and lateral to the axilla of the middle turbinate is removed up to the roof of the nose. Subsequently a 2 × 3 cm septal window is created, enabling instruments to be used from both sides of the nose, facilitating the dissection.

The posterior landmark for the septal window is the anterior edge of the middle turbinate (**Fig. 13.5**). The septal window is widened superiorly to the roof of the nose and inferior to the point where instruments may be passed easily from one side of the nose to the other. The surgeon must be

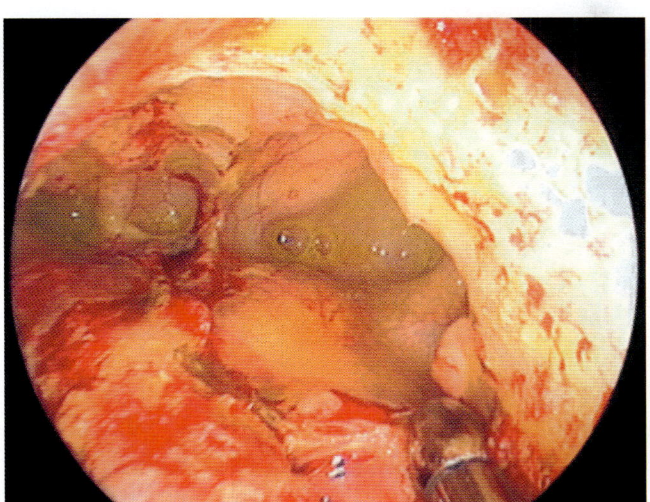

Fig. 13.4 Endoscopic view of the frontal sinus after a modified Lothrop.

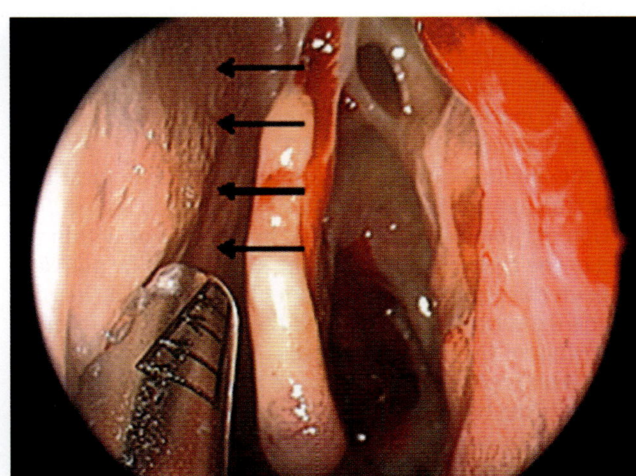

Fig. 13.5 The posterior edge of the septal window begins at the anterior edge of the middle turbinate (*black arrows*).

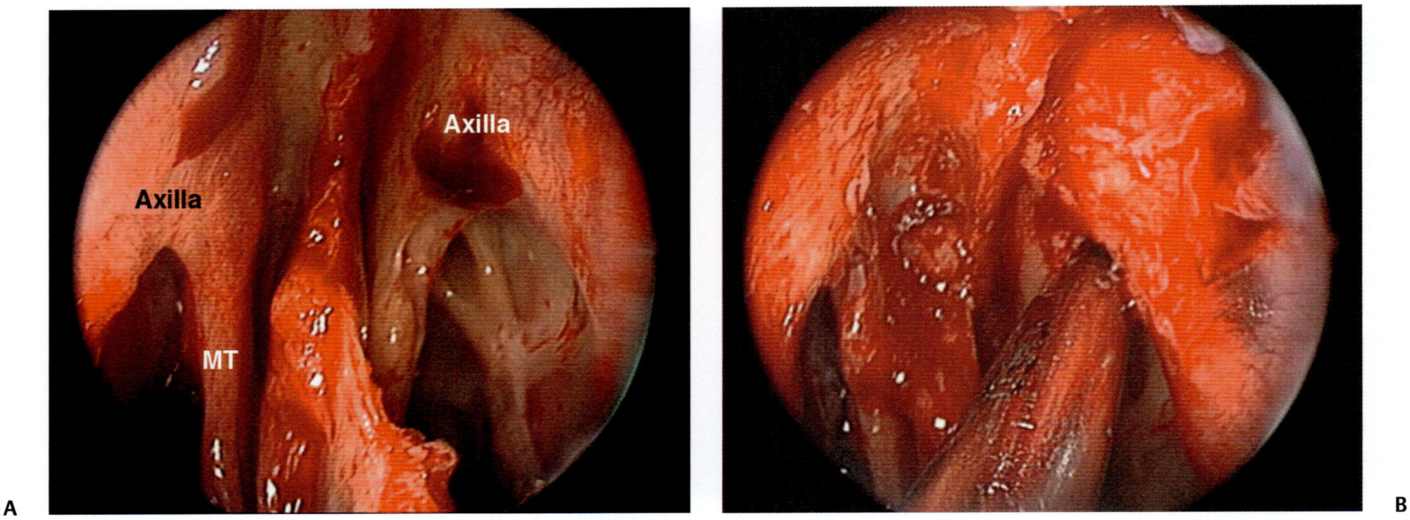

Fig. 13.6 **(A)** View through the septal window shows the axilla of both middle turbinates (MT). **(B)** Through the septal window, the microdebrider is easily placed under the axilla of the contralateral middle turbinate.

able to place instruments through the septal window and under the axilla of the contralateral middle turbinate. Anteriorly, the septum is removed until both middle turbinates, the axilla, and the frontal process of the maxilla are clearly visualized (**Fig. 13.6**).

Once the septal window has been created, the frontal sinus is approached. A frontal sinus mini-trephine may be placed to help identify the drainage pathway and guide the dissection. This step is routine for endoscopic sinus surgery cases but often omitted for skull base cases. Prior to the placement of the mini-trephine, the coronal computed tomography (CT) scan is reviewed to determine the superior and lateral extent of pneumatization of the frontal sinus.

Intracranial penetration can occur if the trephine is placed higher than the extent of aeration of the frontal sinus. In most patients a mini-trephine may be safely placed at the level of the superior orbital rim or medial aspect of the eyebrow. The skin landmarks for trephine placement can be visualized by drawing an imaginary horizontal line from the medial aspect of one eyebrow to the other. The midpoint of this line is marked, and a point 1 cm lateral to the midline is estimated along this line (**Fig. 13.7**).

At this point the skin is infiltrated with local anesthetic and a stab incision is made with a No. 15 blade scalpel. The incision may be placed in existing frown lines or within the hairs of the eyebrow; however, the skin should be pulled to the point corresponding to the above landmarks. The incision is widened with iris scissors and the drill guide is inserted and anchored firmly onto the bone. While gently irrigating, the drill bit is placed into the guide and pulled in and out as it contacts the bone.

This motion avoids overheating of the drill and skin and bone burns. Penetration of the anterior wall of the frontal sinus may be felt as the drill bit falls into the sinus. A guidewire is introduced into the sinus, and the frontal cannula is rotated over the guidewire and anchored firmly into the bone. Fluorescein-stained saline in a syringe is placed onto the cannula, and correct placement of the trephine is verified by aspirating air, blood, mucus, or pus.

Once the correct position of the trephine has been confirmed, fluorescein-stained saline is flushed into the nasal cavity. The fluorescein saline creates a pathway that may be followed directly to the frontal sinus. In addition, while drilling in the region of the frontal sinus, fluorescein saline is frequently flushed to mark the posterior extent of the dissection (skull base).

Once the drainage pathway of the frontal recess is determined, a 3.2 cutting burr (Medtronic ENT, Jacksonville, FL, USA) is used to remove the bone of the frontal process of the maxilla directly above and lateral to the axilla. To facilitate

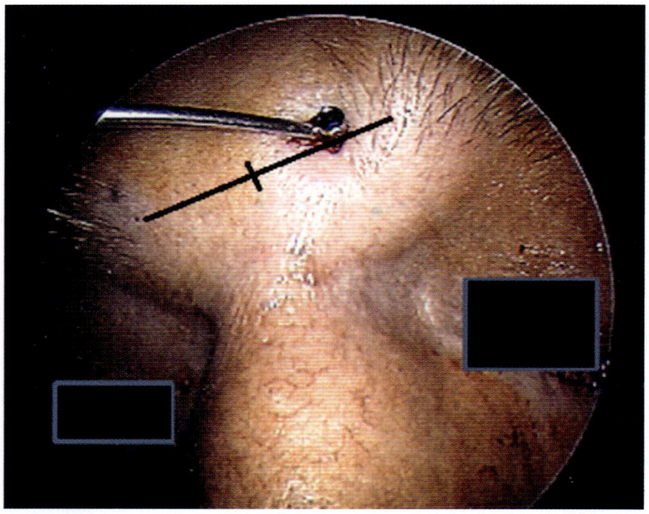

Fig. 13.7 Landmark for the mini-trephine is demonstrated by a line drawn from the medial aspect of the left and right eyebrow and a point 1 cm lateral to the midpoint of that line.

the dissection of the lateral nasal wall, the instrument is placed through the septal perforation from the contralateral nostril.

The bone is removed laterally until a small portion of skin or lacrimal sac is exposed. The exposed skin will mark the lateral extent of the dissection. The dissection is performed superiorly and laterally following the fluorescein-stained pathway up toward and into the frontal sinus. The floor of the frontal sinus is removed with the cutting burr.

The bone anterior to the frontal ostium, the frontal beak, is removed, taking care not to dissect medially at this point, which would put the skull base at risk. The majority of this dissection is done with the straight 3.2 cutting burr; however, occasionally a curved burr will facilitate the removal of the floor and anterior wall (frontal beak).

Once the floor of the frontal sinus has been entered on one side, the same steps are repeated on the other side. Up to this point no medial dissection has been performed. It is only after the skin has been exposed laterally on both sides and the floor of the frontal sinus opened that the dissection is brought medially.

Before this dissection is begun, the anterior extent of the skull base olfactory fossa needs to be delineated. The suction curette (Medtronic ENT) is used to push the mucosa in the olfactory fossa posteriorly exposing the first olfactory neuron. This marks the anterior extent of the skull base and the region of the frontal T. This is confirmed with image guidance.

The dissection can now be brought anterior to the forward projection of the skull base without placing the skull base at risk. This is accomplished with a 30-degree endoscope and curved 40-degree Finesse cutting burr (Medtronic ENT). The frontal sinuses are connected and the intersinus septum is taken down completely. The anterior frontal bone is removed until there is a smooth transition between the frontal sinus and nasal cavity without any ridges. The final step of the dissection is to remove the bone over the forward projection of the skull base at the frontal T. To do this, the exact position of the skull base is again identified using image guidance (axial scans), and the position is confirmed by identifying the first olfactory neuron.

Normally the first structure visualized is the anterior ethmoidal nerve followed closely by the first olfactory neuron. Using either a diamond 5-mm skull base burr or 3.2 round cutting burr (both available from Medtronic ENT), the bone over the olfactory fossa is removed within 1 mm of the nerve. At the end of the MEL an oval-shaped ostium is created. Although the ultimate size is dictated by the individual patient anatomy, the largest possible ostium should be created to avoid circumferential scarring and postoperative stenosis. As a rough guide, the ostium stenoses by 30% over time.[4]

Approach to Anterior Skull Base Tumors

In anterior skull base tumors, the skull base must be cleared in its entirety from the planum sphenoidale to the frontal

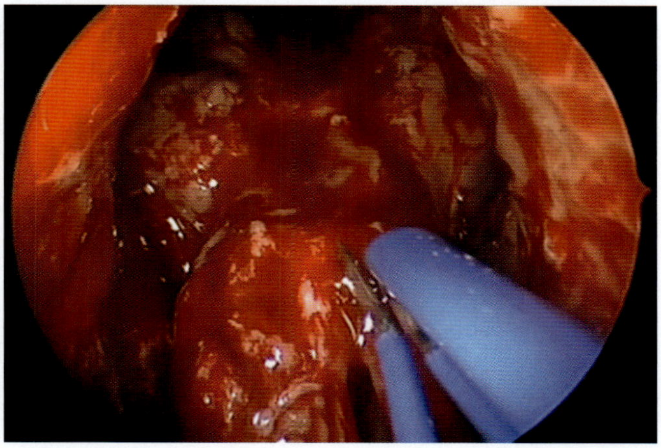

Fig. 13.8 The frontal sinus ostium has been opened with a modified Lothrop procedure exposing the skull base. The suction bipolar is seen on the frontal T.

sinus. This is accomplished with a complete sphenoethmoidectomy and modified Lothrop procedure as described above. The septum is taken down to completely expose the skull base (**Fig. 13.8**).

The anterior and posterior ethmoidal arteries are identified and cauterized. Osteotomies are performed around the tumor, and the attachment of the falx cerebri to the crista galli is cut. The skull base is dropped into the nasal cavity and the tumor is removed. Once the tumor has been removed there remains a defect from the posterior table of the frontal sinus to the planum sphenoidale. The defect is measured and a fascia lata graft is harvested.

A multilayered closure is achieved using two layers of fascia lata placed in an underlay and onlay fashion followed by the Hadad pedicled nasal septal flap.[5] The first layer of fascial lata is tucked between the dura and skull base defect. To anchor the graft anteriorly, two small rivets are made with a drill and the graft is tightly pulled through (**Fig. 13.9**).

To facilitate placement of the graft through the hole, a stitch is placed at the edge of the graft and the needle is used to thread the graft through the hole. The stitches are then tied to secure the graft in place. The second layer of fascia is placed in an overlay fashion followed by the pedicled septal mucosal flap, fibrin glue, Gelfoam, and BIPP (bismuth iodoform paraffin paste) nasal gauze packing. The nasal pack is removed after 7 to 10 days. This closure facilitates patency of the frontal ostium as the skull base heals postoperatively.

Approach to Posteriorly Based Anterior Skull Base Tumors

The approach to the frontal sinus in posteriorly based skull base tumors depends on the tumor location in relation to the planum sphenoidale. As discussed above, tumors located posteriorly along the skull base do not require a MEL for exposure of the frontal sinus (**Fig. 13.2**).

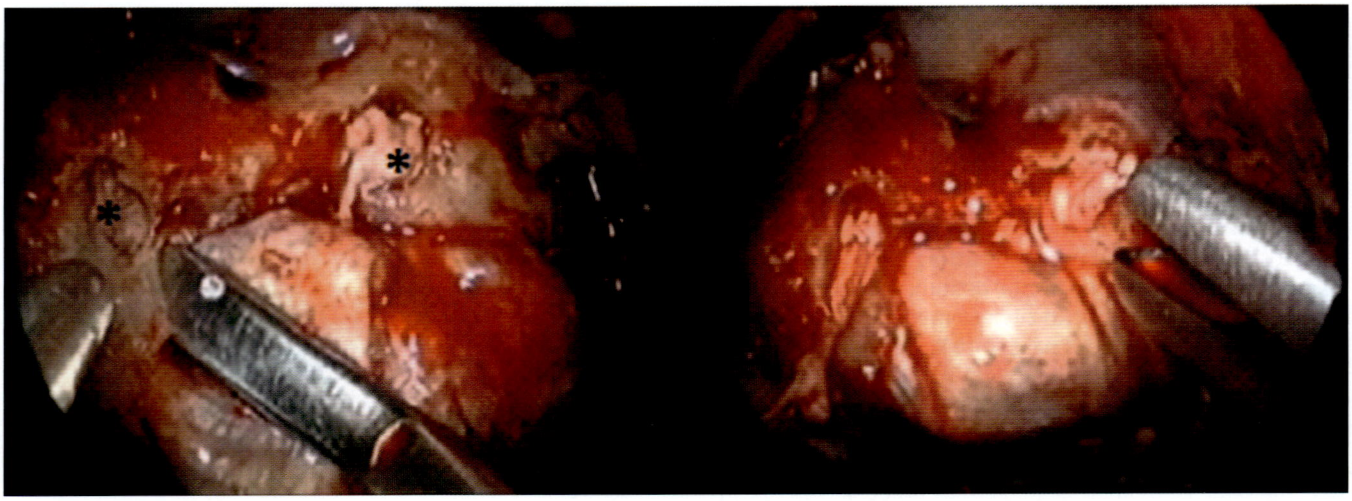

Fig. 13.9 **(A,B)** Riveting technique for anterior skull base closure. The rivets are indicated by asterisks.

However, the majority of these tumors require the frontal sinus ostium to be opened and the surrounding region of the skull base cleared. This is accomplished with a frontal sinusotomy. Prior to opening the frontal sinus, bilateral complete sphenoethmoidectomy with clearance of the skull base is performed.

This is followed by an uncinectomy and axillary flap to expose the agger nasi cell. The anterior wall of the agger nasi cell is removed with a Hajek Koffler punch (Karl Storz Endoscopy, Flanders, NJ). The drainage pathway of the frontal sinus is reviewed on the axial, coronal, and parasagittal CT scans. Intervening cells are removed, and the frontal sinus ostium is identified and exposed bilaterally without performing a MEL procedure (**Fig. 13.10**).

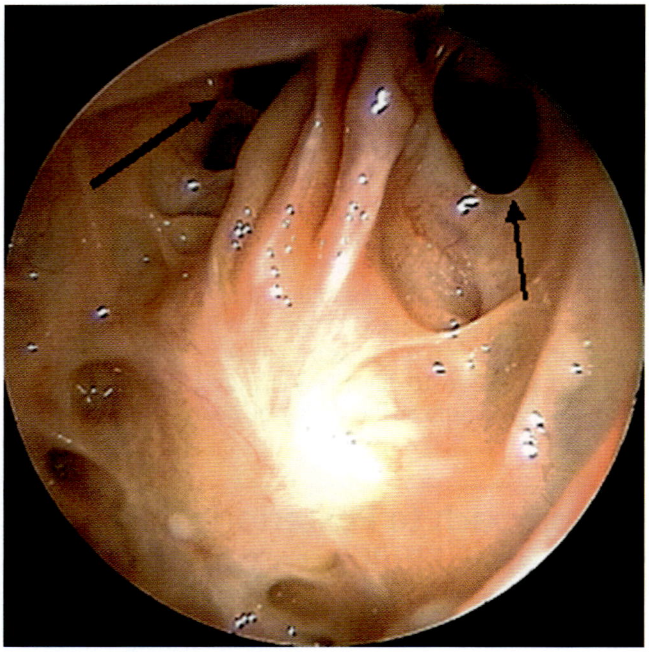

Fig. 13.10 Postoperative view of the both frontal sinus ostia (*black arrows*) and the residual intervening nasal septum after removal of a posterior based meningioma.

The exposure and clearance of the frontal ostia is necessary, as the entire skull base up to and including the frontal ostia needs to be visualized during resection of the posterior skull base. Leaving the anterior ethmoids cells intact reduces the visibility of the region of the skull base to be removed, and if these cells are left, the narrow mucosal spaces of the frontal sinus drainage may be compromised with stenosis or occlusion of the frontal ostia in the postoperative period. The posterior part of the nasal septum is removed.

Osteotomies are made around the tumor, allowing the skull base to drop into the nasal cavity. The tumor is removed and the defect repaired using a multilayer closure with fascia lata, pedicled septal flap, fibrin glue, and Gelfoam. The approach differs in tumors that do not extend past the planum sphenoidale (**Fig. 13.3**).

In tumors located in the suprasellar region without anterior extension past the planum, the frontal sinus does not need to be dissected.

References

1. Lothrop HA. Frontal sinus suppuration: the establishment of permanent nasal drainage; the closure of external fistulae; epidermization of sinus. Ann Surg 1914;59:937–957
2. Draf W. Endonasal micro-endoscopic frontal sinus surgery, the Fulda concept. Oper Tech Otolaryngol–Head Neck Surg 1991;2:225–234
3. Gross WE, Gross CW, Becker D, Moore D, Phillips D. Modified transnasal endoscopic Lothrop procedure as an alternative to frontal sinus obliteration. Otolaryngol Head Neck Surg 1995;113:427–434
4. Tran KN, Beule AG, Singal D, Wormald PJ. Frontal ostium restenosis after theendoscopicmodifiedLothropprocedure.Laryngoscope2007;117:1457–1462
5. Hadad G, Bassagasteguy L, Carrau RL, et al. A novel reconstructive technique after endoscopic expanded endonasal approaches: vascular pedicle nasoseptal flap. Laryngoscope 2006;116:1882–1886

14 Sphenoid Sinus in Skull Base Surgery

Aldo Cassol Stamm, Shirley S.N. Pignatari, Daniel Timperley, Fernando Oto Balieiro, and Fábio Pires Santos

Tips and Pearls

- The sphenoid sinuses have a critical role in ventral skull base surgery due to their central strategic location and their close relationship with vital neurovascular structures of the central nervous system.
- Access to the sphenoid sinus is the first step in endoscopic transsphenoidal skull base surgery, as it provides access and orientation to the ventral skull base and neurovascular structures.
- A good understanding of the anatomy of the sphenoid sinus and surrounding structures and a detailed preoperative evaluation are essential before transsphenoidal skull base surgery.
- CT excels at evaluating fine bone detail and fibro-osseous lesions. MRI is better for soft tissue evaluation, particularly differentiating neoplastic or inflammatory tissue and retained secretions, and for aggressive lesions and perineural spread. The two modalities are complementary and are used together for many skull base lesions.
- Angiographic studies (magnetic resonance, angio-CT, and conventional angiography) are useful in assessing the internal carotid and vertebrobasilar systems.
- Wide exposure of the sphenoid enhances visualization and facilitates two-surgeon access.

Introduction

In recent years, the evolution of imaging methods (mainly computed tomography [CT], magnetic resonance imaging [MRI], and endoscopic-assisted transnasal surgery) have contributed to the progress that has been made in the ability to access the skull base via the nasal cavity.

The sphenoid sinuses are the starting point for approaches to the ventral skull base, providing access and orientation to relevant neurovascular structures.[1] The privileged location and anatomical relationships in the skull base make it possible to treat transsphenoidally a wide variety of skull base lesions traditionally approached transcranially.

Several transnasal approaches to the skull base have been developed. The appropriate technique depends on the nature, anatomic location, and extent of the lesion, the instrumentation, and the surgeon's skills and experience.

The endoscopic-assisted transsphenoidal (EAT) approach is a commonly used technique in skull base surgery to reach the clivus, sellar and parasellar region, cavernous sinus, and even the petrous apex.[2]

Approaches to the Sphenoid Sinuses

Access to the sphenoid sinus is the first step in EAT skull base surgery. Multiple endoscopic approaches have been described, including transseptal, transnasal, transethmoidal, transmaxillary/transpterygoid, and transnasal with removal of the posterior nasal septum. Recently, Stamm and Pignatari[2] described a novel endoscopic transseptal/transnasal approach without posterior nasal septal perforation and using a posterior nasal septal mucosal flap based on the sphenopalatine artery, which is discussed further in Chapter 19 (**Fig. 14.1**). The approach used depends on the anatomic extent of the pathology, and combinations are often used, for example, transnasal on one side combined with transethmoid or transpterygoid on the other. Regardless of the choice of approach, the reconstruction should be considered at this stage of the procedure. If a vascularized flap is required, the flap and its pedicle must be preserved, usually by raising the flap at the start of the procedure and storing it in the nasopharynx or maxillary sinus.[3]

Transseptal Approach (Fig. 14.2)

This is the classic microscopic neurosurgical approach; however, it can also be performed under endoscopic visualization. Classically an anterior septoplasty incision is performed; alternatively, the approach may be modified to use a posterior septal incision. Mucoperichondrial/periosteal flaps are elevated and the posterior bony septum resected, preserving the superior attachment of the quadrangular cartilage to the perpendicular plate of the ethmoid to prevent nasal saddling. The flaps are elevated over the sphenoid rostrum to identify the natural ostia, and the rostrum is removed using an osteotome, Kerrison rongeurs, or a drill.[4] The advantages of this approach are that it is a midline approach and usually avoids septal perforation. However, the exposure is limited compared with that of other approaches, and access is via one nostril, severely limiting the ability to use bimanual or two-surgeon techniques.

Direct Transnasal Approach (Fig. 14.3)

The sphenoid sinus ostium lies medial to the attachment of the superior turbinate. The middle turbinate is usually

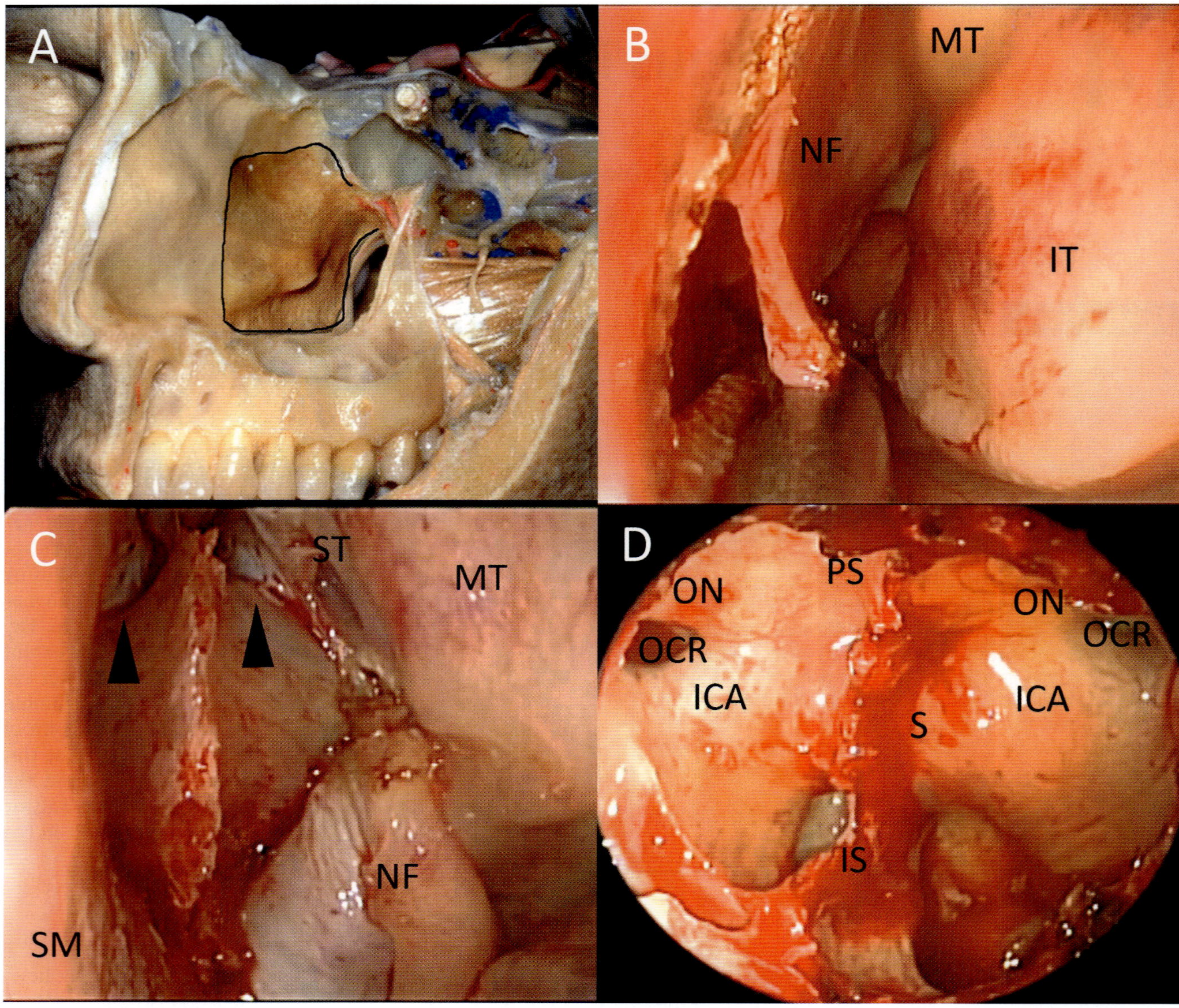

Fig. 14.1 Modified transeptal (bi-nostril) approach. **(A)** A hemitransfixion incision is made, usually on the right, and a nasoseptal flap will be developed on the contralateral side (outlined). **(B)** Following elevation of bilateral mucoperichondrial/mucoperiosteal flaps and resection of the posterior bony septum, the nasoseptal flap is developed. Monopolar diathermy is used to outline the flap, and the incisions are completed as necessary using scissors. **(C)** The flap is placed in the nasopharynx. Access is via the hemitransfixion incision on the right and via the nasal cavity on the right. The sphenoid rostrum and sphenoid sinus ostia are exposed (*arrowheads*). The sinus is opened as in the standard transeptal approach using an osteotome, Kerrison rongeurs, or a drill. **(D)** Wide exposure of the sphenoid sinus is obtained. ICA: internal carotid artery; IS: intersinus septum; IT: inferior turbinate; MT: middle turbinate; NF: nasoseptal flap; OCR: opticocarotid recess; ON: optic nerve; PS: planum sphenoidale; S: sella turcica; SM: right septal mucoperiosteum; ST: superior turbinate.

lateralized and the inferior half of the superior turbinate resected. If access is narrow, the posterior portion of the middle turbinate is also removed. The sphenoid ostium is identified and opened using a Kerrison rongeur. Bilateral access can be obtained by creating a posterior septal window and removal of the sphenoid rostrum.[4] This approach has the advantage of being familiar to otorhinolaryngology (ORL) surgeons and simple to perform, providing a wide exposure of the sphenoid when performed bilaterally. The main disadvantages are the potential for nasal synechiae formation and the need for a posterior septal perforation.

Transethmoidal Approach (Fig. 14.4)

The transethmoidal approach involves resection of the ethmoid sinuses. The middle turbinate is usually partially or completely removed, and a posterior septectomy facilitates binasal access. Uncinectomy, middle meatal antrostomy, and removal of the ethmoid bulla enable identification of the orbital floor, lamina papyracea, and the posterior wall of the maxillary sinus. The ground lamella of the middle turbinate is opened and the superior turbinate identified. Resection of the inferior half of the superior turbinate reveals the sphenoid

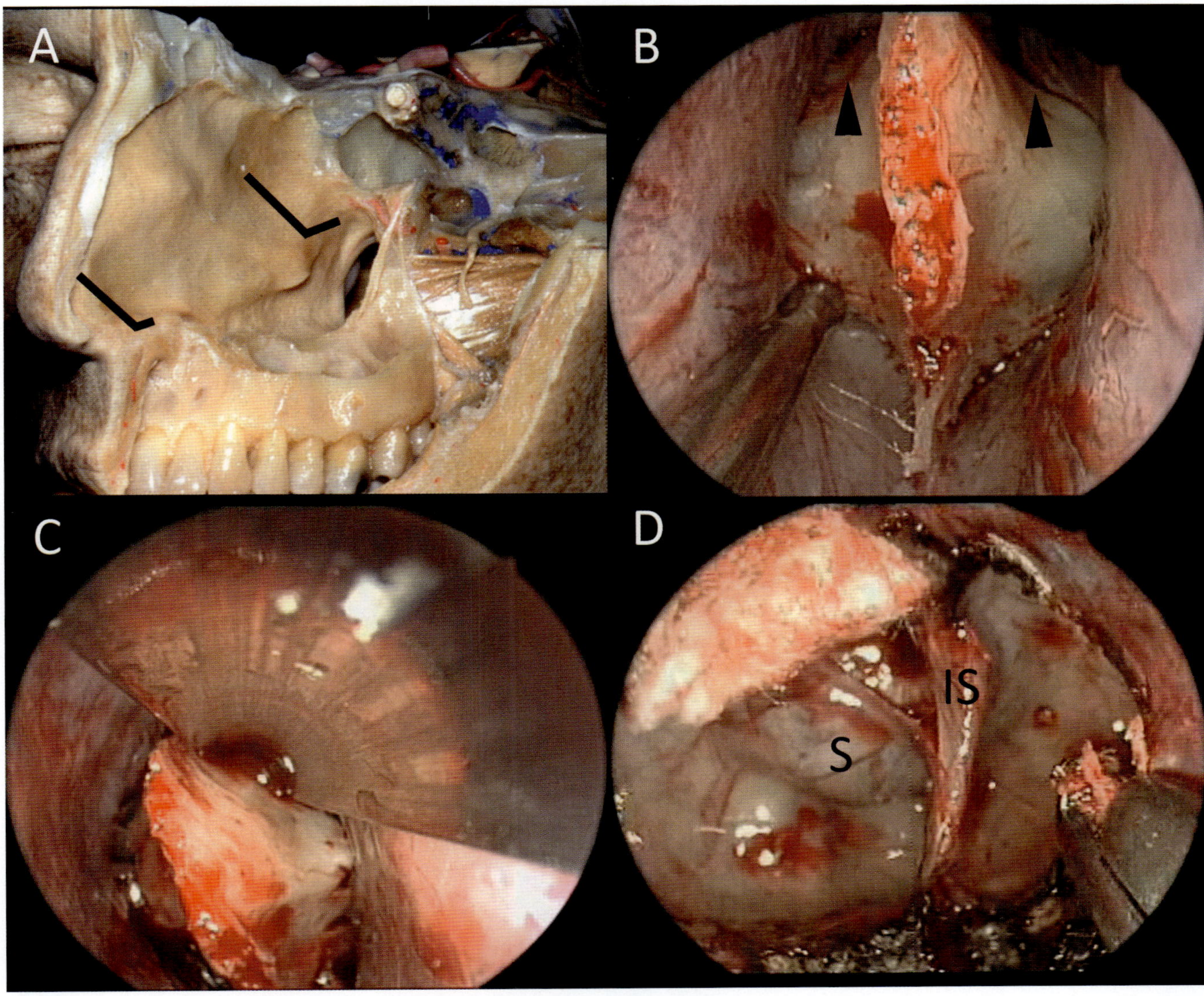

Fig. 14.2 Transseptal approach. **(A)** Traditionally an anterior septal incision is used; however, the technique may be modified to use a posterior incision. **(B)** Bilateral mucoperichondrial/mucoperiosteal flaps have been elevated and the posterior bony septum removed to expose the sphenoid rostrum. The flaps are elevated to identify the sphenoid sinus ostia (*arrowheads*). **(C)** Bony incisions are made using the osteotome. Vertical incisions are made from the natural ostia through the choanal rim. The vertical incisions are then joined with horizontal incisions inferiorly and superiorly between the ostia. **(D)** Following removal of the sphenoid rostrum, the sella is visible. The opening may be enlarged using a Kerrison rongeur. IS: intersinus septum; S: sella turcica.

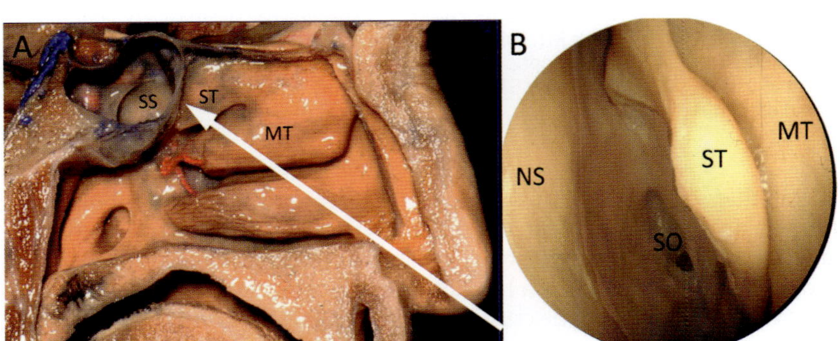

Fig. 14.3 Direct transnasal approach (left). The superior turbinate is lateralized or partially resected to reveal the sphenoid ostium medial and posterior to the superior (or supreme) turbinate. **(A)** Cadaver dissection of the left nasal cavity demonstrates the trajectory of the direct transnasal approach (*arrow*). **(B)** The superior turbinate has been lateralized to reveal the left sphenoid sinus ostium. MT: middle turbinate; NS: nasal septum; SO: sphenoid sinus ostium; SS: sphenoid sinus; ST: superior turbinate.

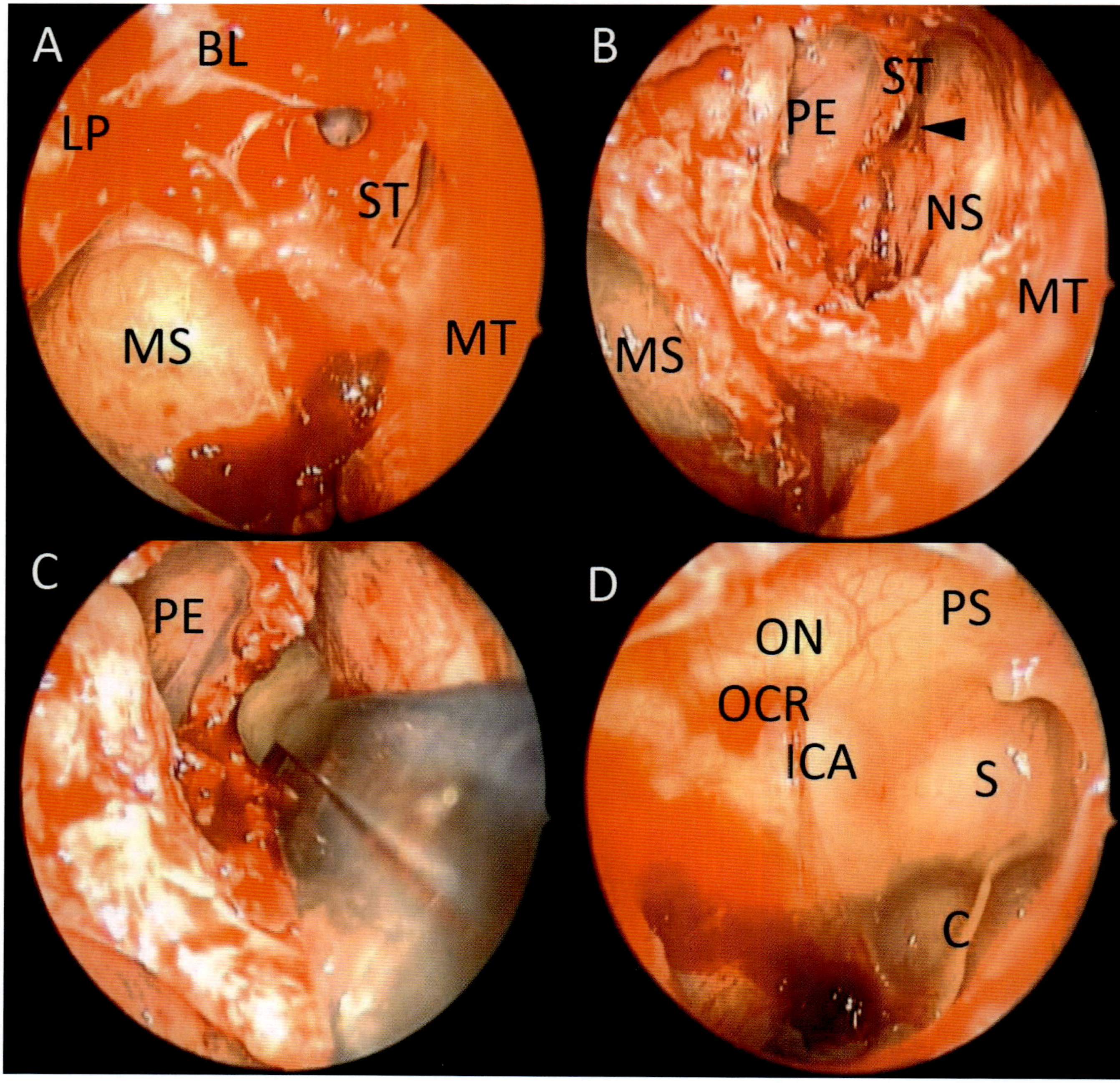

Fig. 14.4 Transethmoidal approach (right). **(A)** Uncinectomy, wide middle meatal antrostomy, and anterior ethmoidectomy have been performed with identification of the lamina papyracea, orbital floor, and posterior wall of the maxillary sinus. The basal lamella of the middle turbinate has been opened, revealing the superior turbinate. **(B)** Resection of the inferior part of the superior turbinate reveals the sphenoid ostium (*arrowhead*) lying medial to its attachment. **(C)** The sphenoid ostium is opened using a Kerrison rongeur. **(D)** Wide access to the sphenoid is achieved. BL: basal lamella of the middle turbinate (cut); C: clivus; ICA: internal carotid artery; LP: lamina papyracea; MS: maxillary sinus (posterior wall); MT: middle turbinate; NS: nasal septum; OCR: opticocarotid recess; ON: optic nerve; PE: posterior ethmoid; PS: planum sphenoidale; S: sella turcica; ST: superior turbinate.

ostium lying medial to its attachment. The ostium can then be widely opened and the skull base identified. The remaining ethmoid cells are then removed as required.[4] The advantage of this approach is the creation of a large cavity, facilitating the movement of instruments and improved lateral access. This approach is more technically demanding and time-consuming than the transseptal or transnasal approaches, although it should be familiar to ORL surgeons. Provided that the mucosa has not been stripped, healing is usually rapid, with little crusting or risk of adhesion formation.

Transpterygoid Approach (Fig. 14.5)

The transpterygoid approach is used in conjunction with a transethmoidal approach to gain access to the lateral sphenoid recess, cavernous sinus, Meckel's cave, and petrous apex. A wide middle meatal antrostomy is performed, opening the maxillary sinus from the natural ostium to the posterior wall and from the orbital floor to either the inferior turbinate or the nasal floor (as a modified medial maxillectomy). The mucoperiosteum is then elevated from the vertical plate of the palatine bone to identify the sphenopalatine foramen lying behind the crista ethmoidalis. The distal jaw of a 2-mm Kerrison rongeur can be introduced into the foramen, pushing the periosteum posteriorly, and the bone is removed. Alternatively, the posterior maxillary wall can be opened directly using either a drill or curette, and then the opening is enlarged in a subperiosteal plane using the Kerrison rongeur. The maxillary artery and branches are displaced or ligated and divided to gain access to the pterygoid process, which is then removed as required with rongeurs or a drill.[5] Care is taken where possible to preserve the maxillary nerve, the vidian nerve, and the pterygopalatine ganglion and its branches. The vidian nerve can be followed posteriorly and is a useful landmark for the foramen lacerum and petrous carotid artery.

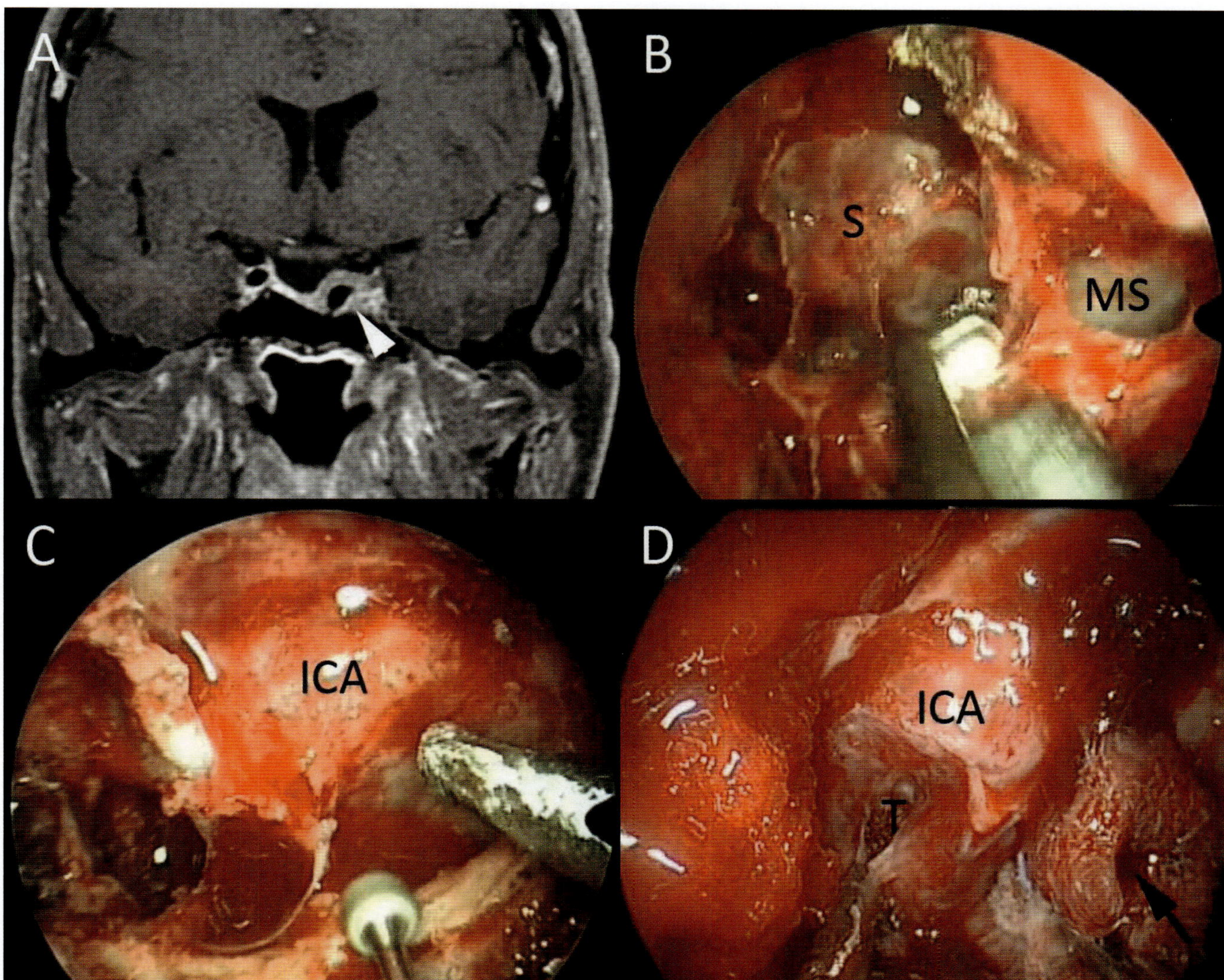

Fig. 14.5 Transpterygoid approach (left). **(A)** Coronal magnetic resonance imaging (MRI) demonstrates a sella tumor surrounding the left internal carotid artery (*arrowhead*). Empty sella is also noted. **(B)** The posterior wall of the maxillary sinus is removed using the Kerrison rongeurs, starting at the sphenopalatine foramen. **(C)** The pterygoid process is partially removed using the drill. **(D)** Access to the cavernous sinus, both medial and lateral to the internal carotid artery, is achieved. ICA: internal carotid artery; MS: maxillary sinus; S: sella turcica; T: tumor extending posterior to ICA.

Modified Transseptal (Bi-Nostril) Approach (Fig. 14.1)

The bi-nostril approach is performed as a transseptal approach initially. Following elevation of the mucoperichondrial/mucoperiosteal flaps and removal of the posterior bony nasal septum, a nasoseptal flap is developed on the contralateral side to the septal incision and placed into the nasopharynx. Access is therefore via the septal incision on one side (usually the right) and via the nasal cavity on the other. This approach has the advantages of providing excellent bilateral access, avoiding septal perforation, and including the routine harvesting of a vascularized nasoseptal flap.[2] The bi-nostril approach is discussed further in Chapter 25.

The common feature of these approaches is entry into the sphenoid sinus to provide access to the skull base. Regardless of the approach used, the anterior face of the sphenoid should be opened widely to facilitate access with the endoscope and up to three instruments simultaneously. Panoramic visualization of surgical landmarks aids orientation during the surgical procedure, and wide openings enable two surgeons to operate simultaneously without criss-crossing of instruments.[6] In contrast, small openings restrict visualization and restrict the ability to use a two-surgeon technique, encouraging the use of curettes and blind scraping techniques rather than sharp capsular dissection and limiting the ability to control bleeding.

Anatomy

A good understanding of the anatomy of the sphenoid sinus and adjacent structures is essential before undertaking EAT skull base surgery.

The sphenoid bone is located at the base of the skull, anterior to the temporal and occipital bones and posterior to the ethmoid sinuses. The sphenoidal (sphenoid) sinuses, contained within the body of the sphenoid bone, are extremely variable in size and shape and in their relationship to the sella.

The degree of pneumatization is highly variable and can be classified as postsellar, presellar, or conchal. Postsellar sinuses are well pneumatized with bulging of the sellar floor into the sinus. In presellar sinuses, pneumatization does not extend beyond the perpendicular plate of the tuberculum sellae. In the conchal type, the sphenoid sinus is not pneumatized and the area below the sella is a solid block of bone.[7]

The sphenoid sinuses are usually divided by one or more vertical septa that are often asymmetric. Sometimes, parasagittal minor septa (accessory septa) are inserted into the bony bulge over the optic nerve or the internal carotid artery (respectively 7% and 40%),[7] requiring care during removal to avoid internal carotid artery (ICA) injury.

In some patients, posterior ethmoid cells may pneumatize above the sphenoid sinus, forming an anatomic variation known as the Onodi cell. This variant should be recognized on the preoperative CT scan because the optic nerve and even the ICA may run through the Onodi cell[7–9] (**Fig. 14.6**).

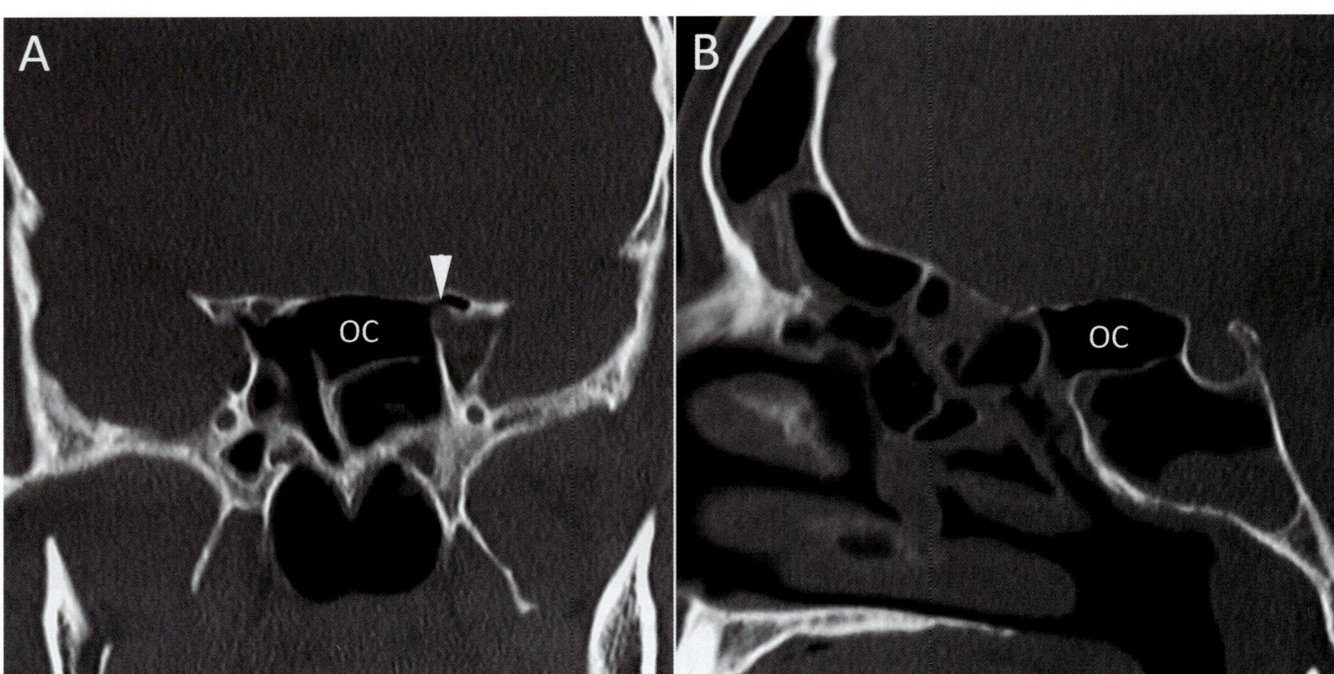

Fig. 14.6 A computed tomography (CT) scan demonstrates a large left Onodi cell (OC). **(A)** Coronal scan. The left optic nerve lies within the Onodi cell and there is a bony dehiscence (*arrowhead*). **(B)** Sagittal scan showing Onodi cell extending above the sphenoid sinus.

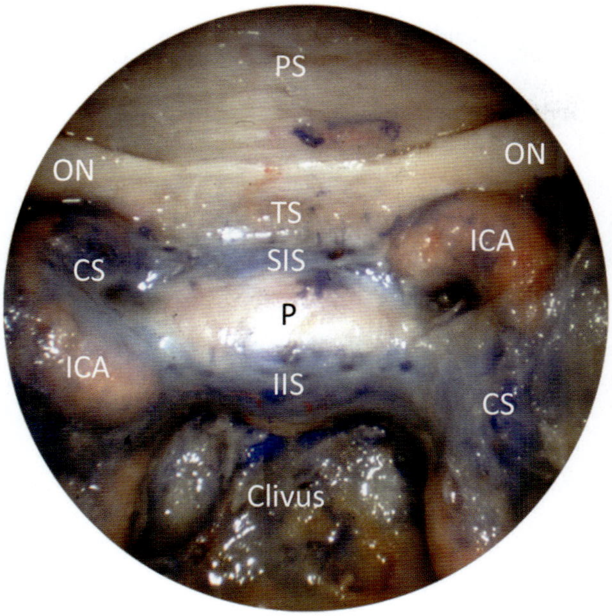

Fig. 14.7 Endoscopic view of sphenoid sinus dissection. CS: cavernous sinus; ICA: internal carotid artery; IIS: inferior intercavernous sinus; ON: dura overlying optic nerve; P: pituitary gland; PS: planum sphenoidale; SIS: superior intercavernous sinus; TS: tuberculum sellae.

The anterior surface of the sinus contains its natural ostium, located in the sphenoethmoidal recess, medial to the superior or supreme nasal turbinates. The natural sphenoid ostium varies in size from 1 to 4 mm and lies approximately 15 mm above the upper margin of the choana.[8]

In a well-developed sphenoid sinus and from an EAT approach, its lateral wall is the cavernous sinus medial wall. The cavernous sinus is formed by the dura splitting and is immediately lateral to the sella in the parasellar space. It contains the internal carotid artery and cranial nerves III, IV, V_1, and, most medially, VI. The paired cavernous sinuses are joined by intercavernous sinuses (superior and inferior), forming the circular venous sinus (**Fig. 14.7**). Laterally, posteroinferiorly and adjacent to the inferior aspect of the cavernous sinus, lies Meckel's cave with the trigeminal ganglion on the superior surface of the petrous apex.[10]

The intracavernous portion of the ICA is the most medial structure within the cavernous sinus, and it may produce a serpiginous bony bulge called the carotid prominence. The carotid prominence is divided into presellar, infrasellar, and retrosellar segments.[11]

The optic canal is often partially encircled by the sphenoid sinus (**Fig. 14.8**) and creates a bony bulge in the anterosuperior portion of its lateral wall. The bony depression between the optic canal and the presellar segment of the carotid prominence is called the optic-carotid recess, which varies in depth and represents pneumatization of the anterior clinoid process[10] (**Fig. 14.9**).

The bony lateral sphenoid sinus wall over the ICA and the optic nerve is usually very thin and may be absent in some areas. Although Lang[8] observed that the canal of the optic

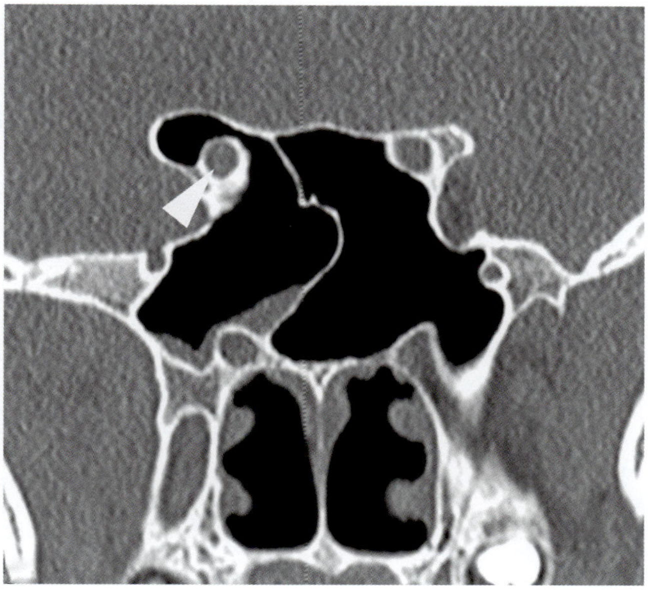

Fig. 14.8 Coronal CT demonstrates the optic canal (*arrowhead*) partially encircled by the sphenoid sinus.

nerve was dehiscent in 6% of cases, Seibert[12] found that 57% of the optic nerves bulged into the sphenoid sinus and 1% had no bony canal. Seibert also noted that the horizontal portion of the intracavernous carotid artery extended prominently into the sphenoid sinus in 67% of cases and its bony covering was dehiscent in 6%. In his series the maxillary nerve was

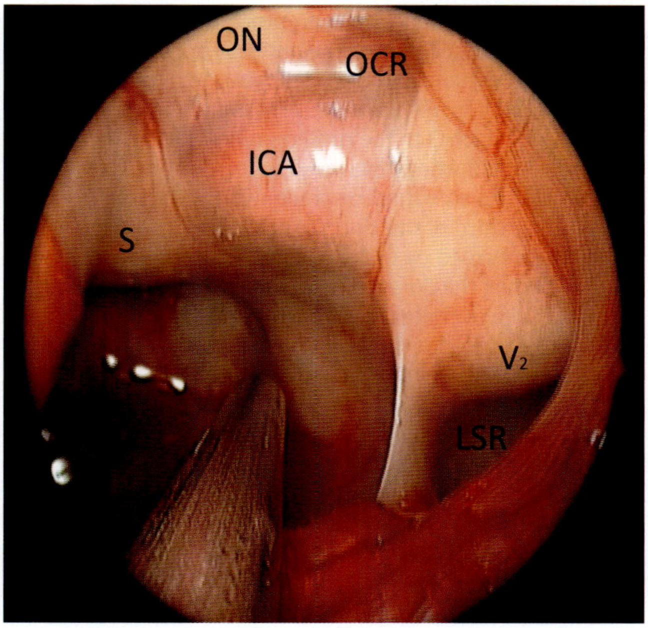

Fig. 14.9 Intraoperative view of the left sphenoid sinus demonstrates the relationships between the internal carotid artery and the optic and maxillary nerves. ICA: internal carotid artery; LSR: lateral sphenoid recess; OCR: opticocarotid recess; ON: optic nerve; S: sella; V2: maxillary nerve.

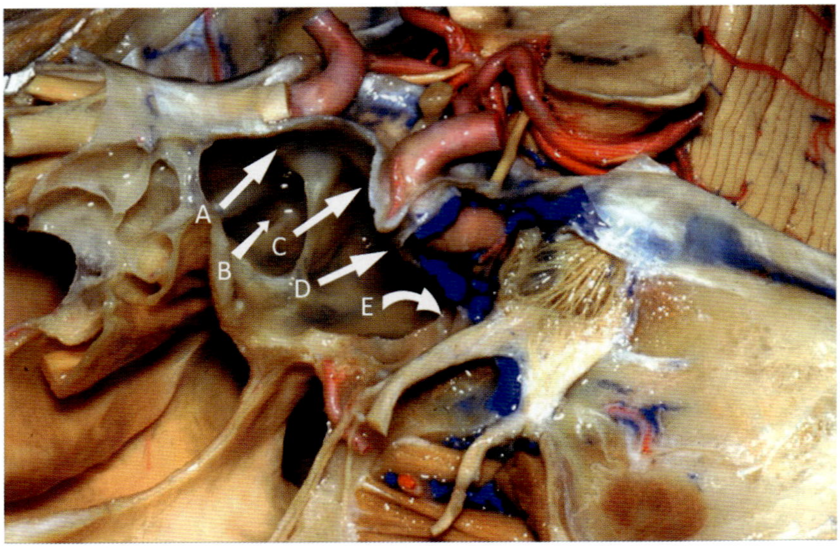

Fig. 14.10 Cadaver dissection (oblique view) illustrating transsphenoidal approaches: A, transplanum; B, cavernous sinus; C, sellar; D, transclival; E, petrous apex (posterior to internal carotid artery).

prominent in the sphenoid sinus in 48% of specimens, and dehiscent in 5%, and the pterygoid nerve (vidian) was prominent 18% of the time (**Fig. 14.9**).

The roof of the sphenoid sinus is the planum sphenoidale, and the junction of the roof with the pituitary fossa has an indentation known as the tuberculum sellae. Just below the tuberculum sellae where they are closest to each other, the average distance between the left and right internal carotid arteries is 13.9 mm (range, 10 to 17 mm). At the anterior wall of the sella the carotid arteries are separated by 20 mm (range, 13 to 26.5 mm), and at the level of the clivus the distance between them is 17.4 mm (range, 10.5 to 26.5 mm).[11]

The sella turcica contains the anterior and posterior lobes of the pituitary gland and the distal portion of pituitary stalk. It is covered by a reflection of dura mater, the diaphragma sella, which attaches to the clinoid processes, and has a small dehiscence facilitating transmission of the pituitary infundibulum and its surrounding arachnoid.

The upper third of the clivus is at the level of the sphenoid sinus and is formed by the posterior portion of the sphenoid body, including the dorsum sella (basisphenoid) and the basilar part of the occipital bone (basiocciput).[4]

From the above description it can be seen that the sphenoid sinus provides access to multiple areas: posteriorly to the clivus and posterior fossa, posterosuperiorly to the sella, superiorly to suprasellar structures, and laterally to the cavernous sinus, trigeminal ganglion, and petrous apex (**Fig. 14.10**). It therefore can be considered the gateway to these areas, and the ability to obtain adequate exposure within the sinus is fundamental to endoscopic skull base surgery.

Indications

Endoscopic-assisted transsphenoidal skull base surgery is indicated for pituitary tumors, sphenoidal mucoceles, meningoencephaloceles, clival region lesions, meningiomas, petrous apex cholesterol granulomas, optic nerve decompression, craniocervical junction pathologies, and cavernous sinuses disease, among others.

Contraindications

Endoscopic-assisted transsphenoidal approaches (at this time) may not be suitable for large lesions with anterior suprasellar extension or large lateral extension into the cavernous sinus, conchal-type sphenoid sinuses, and large retroclival lesions.

Diagnostic Workup

An extensive and detailed preoperative endoscopic examination and radiologic evaluation of sphenoid sinuses, skull base anatomy, and its boundaries are imperative for planning the transsphenoidal route and intraoperative guidance. CT and MRI provide complementary information.

Radiologic evaluation should include coronal, axial, and sagittal reconstructions of CT sections of the sinuses and skull base as essential parts of the assessment of all skull base lesions. CT enables assessment of critical anatomic information, such as the presence and extent of erosion of the skull base; integrity and degree of aeration of the sphenoid sinuses; location and presence of intersinus septa; position of the ICA, optic nerves, and cavernous sinuses; and the presence of an Onodi cell. When used in conjunction with an image guidance system, CT can also facilitate three-dimensional reconstruction of the patient's skull base region during surgery.[4] CT excels at evaluating fine bone detail, and fibro-osseous lesions are usually better assessed with this modality.[13]

Magnetic resonance imaging is important in showing the morphology of the soft tissues and the presence of fluid, but is not helpful in assessing bony architecture. MRI is better for distinguishing neoplastic or inflammatory tissue and retained secretions and to clarify the diagnosis of a skull base malformation, such as a meningoencephalocele. Aggressive lesions and perineural spread are best imaged with MRI, and it is also valuable in patients who have erosion of the lateral sphenoid wall.[4,13] MRI and CT provide complementary information and are used together in evaluation of many skull base lesions.

Magnetic resonance angiography assesses the structure of medium to large arteries and should be considered for visualizing the relationship between the basilar and ICAs in patients with lateral and posterior sphenoid walls erosion.

Angio-CT provides simultaneous visualization of bony and vascular structures and is especially useful in assessing the internal carotid and vertebrobasilar systems. Venous structures of particular surgical interest are the cavernous sinus, inferior and superior intercavernous sinuses, and the basilar venous plexus. This technology is particularly helpful in procedures involving the parasphenoidal regions and the anterior skull base.[4]

Conventional angiography provides essential information in a lesion involving, impinging on, or displacing the ICA, particularly when the transnasal transsphenoidal approach is contemplated. Although it is not routinely performed, it is also helpful for verifying the functional integrity of the circle of Willis and determining the extent of a carotid artery narrowing or occlusion.[4]

Conclusion

The sphenoid sinuses have a critical role in ventral skull base surgery due to their central and strategic location in the skull base and close relationship with vital neurovascular structures of the central nervous system.

Thus, thorough knowledge of the complex anatomy combined with preoperative imaging enable the recognition of landmarks and anatomic variations that are essential for surgical planning and avoiding intraoperative complications. In addition, advanced endoscopic surgery training and experience are vital for a successful outcome.

References

1. Zanation AM, Snyderman CH, Carrau RL, Gardner PA, Prevedello DM, Kassam AB. Endoscopic endonasal surgery for petrous apex lesions. Laryngoscope 2009;119:19–25
2. Stamm AC, Pignatari S, Vellutini E, Harvey RJ, Nogueira JF Jr. A novel approach allowing binostril work to the sphenoid sinus. Otolaryngol Head Neck Surg 2008;138:531–532
3. Harvey RJ, Nogueira JF Jr, Schlosser RJ, Patel SJ, Vellutini E, Stamm AC. Closure of large skull base defects after endoscopic transnasal craniotomy. Clinical article. J Neurosurg 2009;111:371–379
4. Stamm AC, Pignatari SS, Vellutini E. Transnasal endoscopic surgical approaches to the clivus. Otolaryngol Clin North Am 2006;39:639–656, xi
5. Bolger WE, Osenbach R. Endoscopic transpterygoid approach to the lateral sphenoid recess. Ear Nose Throat J 1999;78:36–42
6. Stamm AC, Vellutini E, Harvey RJ, Nogeira JF Jr, Herman DR. Endoscopic transnasal craniotomy and the resection of craniopharyngioma. Laryngoscope 2008;118:1142–1148
7. Sethi DS, Stanley RE, Pillay PK. Endoscopic anatomy of the sphenoid sinus and sella turcica. J Laryngol Otol 1995;109:951–955
8. Lang J. Clinical Anatomy of the Nose, Nasal Cavity, and Paranasal Sinuses. Stuttgart, New York: Thieme Medical Publishers; 1989
9. Elwany S, Elsaeid I, Thabet H. Endoscopic anatomy of the sphenoid sinus. J Laryngol Otol 1999;113:122–126
10. Stamm AM. Transnasal endoscopy-assisted skull base surgery. Ann Otol Rhinol Laryngol Suppl 2006;196:45–53
11. Fujii K, Chambers SM, Rhoton AL Jr. Neurovascular relationships of the sphenoid sinus. A microsurgical study. J Neurosurg 1979;50:31–39
12. Seibert DR. Estudo Anatômico de Seios Esfenoidais em Brasileiros Adultos. Thesis presented at the Universiy of Sao Paulo, Sao Paulo, Brazil, 1992.
13. Branstetter BF IV, Weissman JL. Role of MR and CT in the paranasal sinuses. Otolaryngol Clin North Am 2005;38:1279–1299, x

IV Tips and Pearls in Orbital and Optic Nerve Surgery

15 Anatomy of the Orbit and Related Structures

Helder Tedeschi and Albert L. Rhoton, Jr.

Tips and Pearls

- Perform a thorough preoperative radiologic investigation of the orbital walls, as excessive bony thickness can preclude the chosen surgical approach.
- Accessing intraconal lesions endonasally requires manipulation of the extraocular muscles. The nerve branches that supply the oculomotor muscles run in the medial surface of the muscles. Thus, try to avoid excessive retraction of the extraocular muscles to avoid inadvertent muscle paresis.
- The orbital fat is divided into distinct compartments by connective tissue septa. Although it is difficult, to preserve the integrity of the fat, try to dissect around these connective tissue septa.
- The orbital fat content usually diminishes as the intraconal apex region is approached, but the space also tightens.
- Pay special attention to the central retinal artery when operating on more posterior and medial lesions, as usually the artery arises at the ventral aspect of the optic nerve and then runs below its inferior surface before penetrating it at a short distance from the orbital apex.

Introduction

Endoscopy has inaugurated a new era in the treatment of lesions located at the skull base. The concept of minimally invasive surgery has been broadened by the use of the endoscope, and many of the so-called surgically inaccessible areas can now be safely reached with considerably lower morbidity. New techniques of reconstruction have also substantially lessened the surgical complications. Being in close proximity with the nose and the paranasal sinuses, the optic canal and the medial and inferior walls of the orbit can be surgically approached with the aid of the surgical endoscope.

This chapter thoroughly describes the microsurgical anatomy of the orbital contents, which is important to the various surgical approaches directed to the orbit.

Anatomy of the Orbit

The orbit is a complexly organized group of neural, vascular, muscular, ligamentous, and osseous structures that opens onto the face and external world to collect and provide binocular visual information to the brain.

Nearly all of the bones forming the anterior and middle cranial base contribute to the formation of the orbit's walls. The orbit communicates posteriorly with the anterior and middle cranial fossae and inferiorly with the pterygopalatine and infratemporal fossa. The nerves and vessels entering and exiting the orbit pass through the optic canal and superior orbital fissure, which are partially surrounded by an annular tendon, from which the recti muscles arise.

The fact that many of the neural and vascular structures entering the orbit pass through not only an osseous channel but also through the annular tendon creates an added complexity when considering approaches to the orbit, and especially those involving the orbital apex. The orbit can be approached surgically from anteriorly through the face and conjunctivae or through any of its walls and from intracranially. The most common neurosurgical approaches are directed through the superior and lateral walls to lesions located deep in the orbit, near the apex or involving the optic canal, superior orbital fissure, and adjacent areas.[1–3] Endoscopic approaches are somewhat restricted to the structures of the orbit that are related to the paranasal sinuses, which include the optic canal and the medial and inferior walls of the orbit.

Osseous Relationships

The walls of the orbit are formed by seven bones: frontal, zygomatic, sphenoid, lacrimal, ethmoid, and palatine bones and the maxilla (**Fig. 15.1**). The upper border of the orbital opening is formed by the frontal bone, which is notched or is the site of one or several small foramina that transmit the supraorbital and supratrochlear nerves and vessels. The lateral border of the orbital opening is formed by the frontal process of the zygomatic bone, except for the upper part, which is formed by the zygomatic process of the frontal bone. The lower margin of the orbital opening is formed laterally by the zygomatic bone and medially by the maxilla. The upper part of the medial border is formed by the frontal bone, and the lower part is formed by the frontal process of the maxilla. The medial part of the upper border contains the frontal sinus. The anterior part of the orbital roof is formed by the orbital plate of the frontal bone, and the posterior part is formed by the lesser wing of the sphenoid bone, which

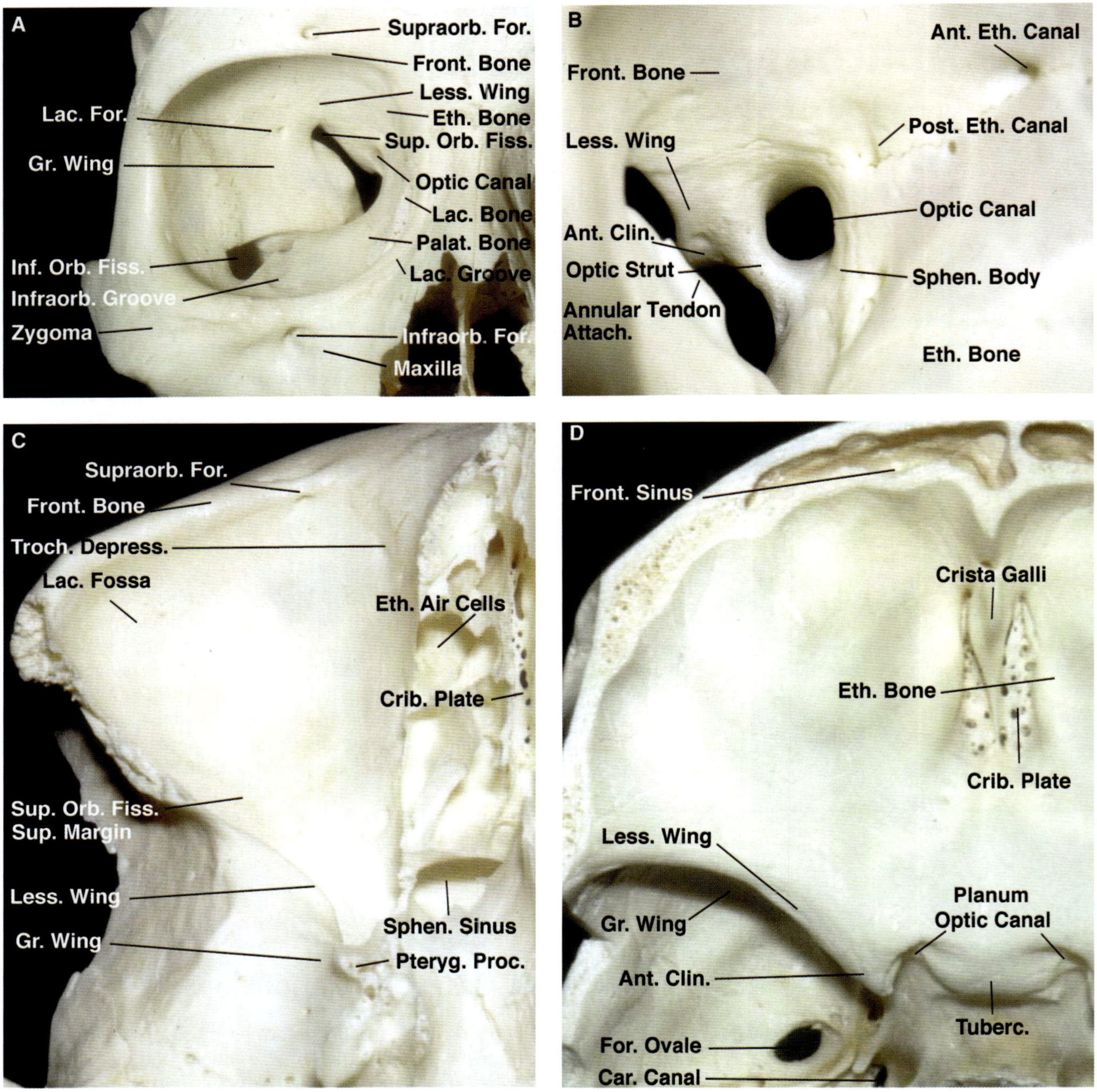

Fig. 15.1 Osseous relationships of the orbit. **(A)** Anterior view of the right orbit. **(B)** Anterior aspect of the right optic canal. **(C)** Roof of the right orbit viewed from below. **(D)** Superior aspect of the floor of the anterior cranial fossae that forms the roof of both orbits.

also forms most of the sphenoid ridge (**Figs. 15.1** and **15.2**). The sphenoid and ethmoid bones are interposed between the orbital roofs. The ethmoid bone is the site of the cribriform plate and the upward-projecting crista galli to which the falx attaches. Anteriorly, the frontal bone splits into two laminae, which enclose the frontal sinuses. The lacrimal fossa, the depression in which the lacrimal gland rests, is located below the anterolateral part of the roof.

Another small depression in the anteromedial part of the roof, the trochlear fossa, serves as the attachment for the trochlea of the superior oblique muscle. The floor of the orbit is formed by the orbital plate of the maxilla, the orbital surface of zygomatic bone, and the orbital process of the palatine bone. The orbital floor, which is very thin, forms the roof of the maxillary sinus. The floor is continuous with the medial wall, except in the most anterior part, where the floor is

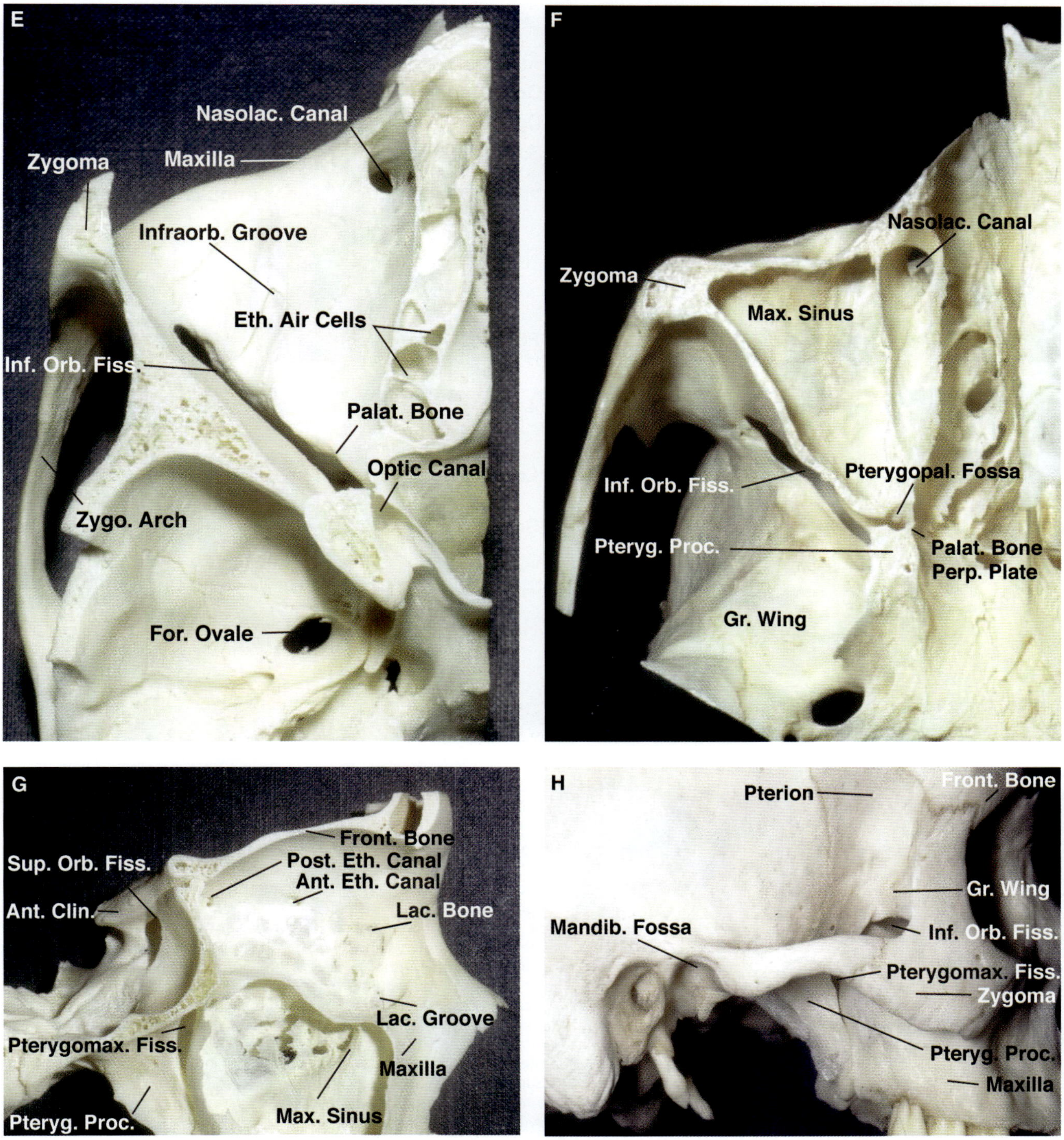

Fig. 15.1 *(Continued)* **(E)** Floor of the right orbit viewed from above. **(F)** Inferior aspect of the roof of the maxillary sinus, which also forms the floor of the orbit. **(G)** Lateral view of the medial wall of the right orbit. **(H)** Lateral aspect of the lateral wall of the r ght orbit. *(continued on next page)*

perforated by the nasolacrimal canal. The anterior part of the floor is continuous with the lateral wall, but posteriorly, the floor and lateral wall are separated by the inferior orbital fissure. The infraorbital groove, which transmits the infraorbital branch of the maxillary nerve, leads forward out of the inferior orbital fissure to cross the floor to reach the infraorbital canal, which ends below the lower orbital rim in the infraorbital foramen. The lateral wall consists predominantly of the greater sphenoid wing and the frontal process of the zygomatic bone. The greater sphenoid wing also forms much of the middle fossa floor and the roof of the infratemporal fossa. Superiorly, the anterior part of the lateral orbital wall

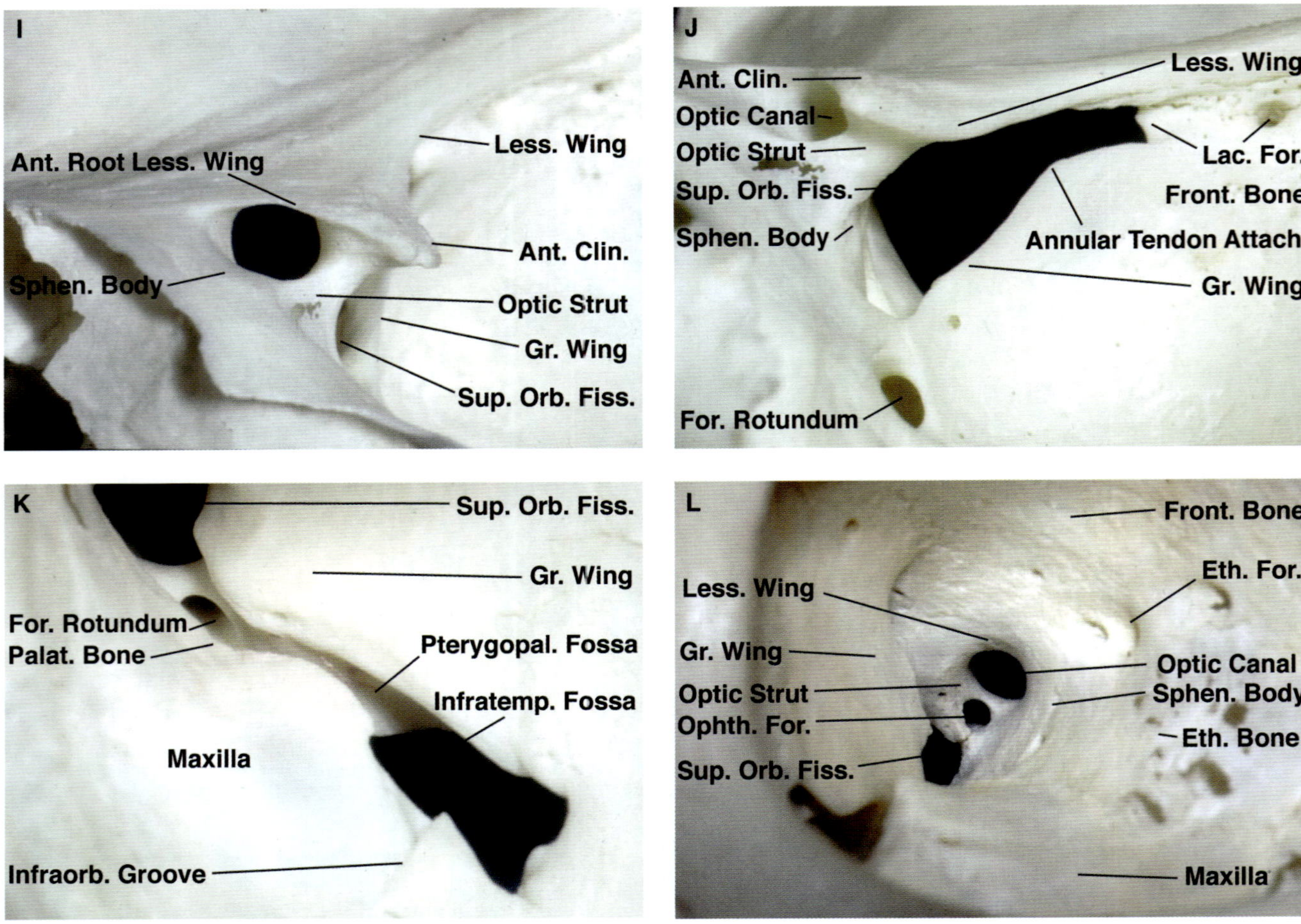

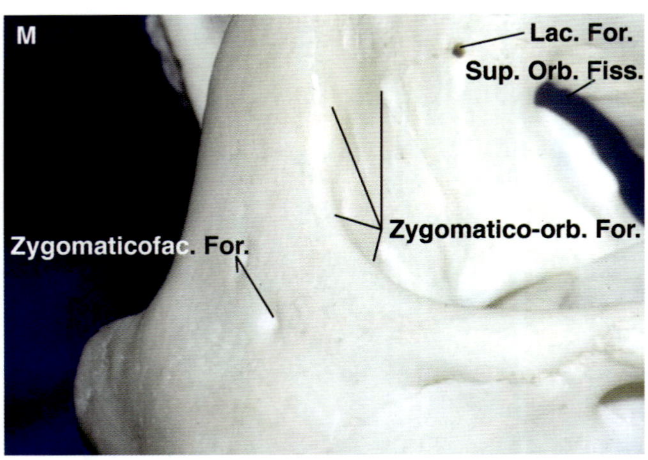

Fig. 15.1 (*Continued*) **(I)** Intracranial aspect of the right optic canal. **(J)** Intracranial aspect of the right superior orbital fissure. **(K)** Orbital aspect of the right inferior orbital fissure. **(L)** Anterior aspect of the right optic canal and an anomalous ophthalmic foramen. **(M)** Anterolateral view of the right zygomaticofacial foramina. Ant.: anterior; Attach.: attachment; Car.: carotid; Clin.: clinoid; Crib.: cribriform; Depress.: depression; Eth.: ethmoid: ethmoidal; Fiss.: fissure; For.: foramen; Front.: frontal; Gr.: greater; Inf.: inferior; Infraorb.: infraorbital; Infratemp.: infratemporal; Lac.: lacrimal; Less.: lesser; Mandib.: mandibular; Max.: maxillary; Nasolac.: nasolacrimal; Ophth.: ophthalmic; Orb.: orbital; Palat.: palatine; Perp.: perpendicular; Post.: posterior; Proc.: process; Pteryg.: pterygoid; Pterygomax.: pterygomaxillary; Pterygopal.: pterygopalatine; Sphen.: sphenoidal; Sup.: superior; Supraorb.: supraorbital; Troch.: trochlear; Tuberc.: tuberculum; Zygo.: zygomatic; Zygomaticofac.: zygomaticofacial; Zygomatico-orb.: zygomatico-orbital.

is continuous with the roof, but the posterior part of the lateral wall is separated from the roof by the superior orbital fissure.

The lacrimal foramen, which transmits the recurrent meningeal branch of the ophthalmic artery, is located anterior to the superior orbital fissure along the superior edge of the lateral wall. The zygomatico-orbital foramina on the anterolateral part of the intraorbital surface of the lateral wall transmits the zygomaticofacial and zygomaticotemporal nerves, which exit the external surface of the zygoma at the zygomaticofacial and zygomaticotemporal foramina to reach the skin of the cheek and temple. The medial wall is formed, from anterior to posterior, by the frontal process of the maxilla, the lacrimal bone, the orbital plate of the ethmoid bone, and the body of the sphenoid bone. The medial wall is extremely thin, especially in the area of the orbital plate of the

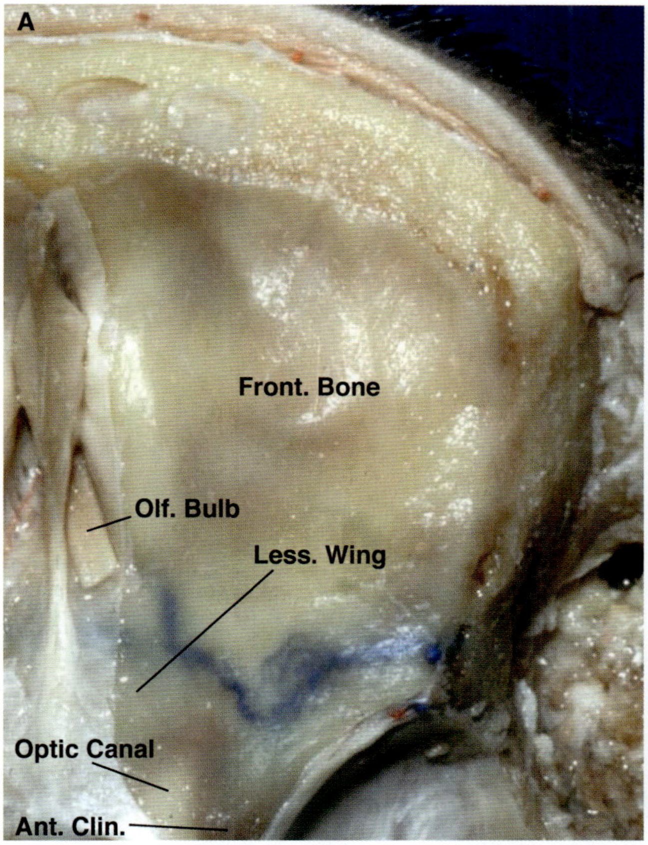

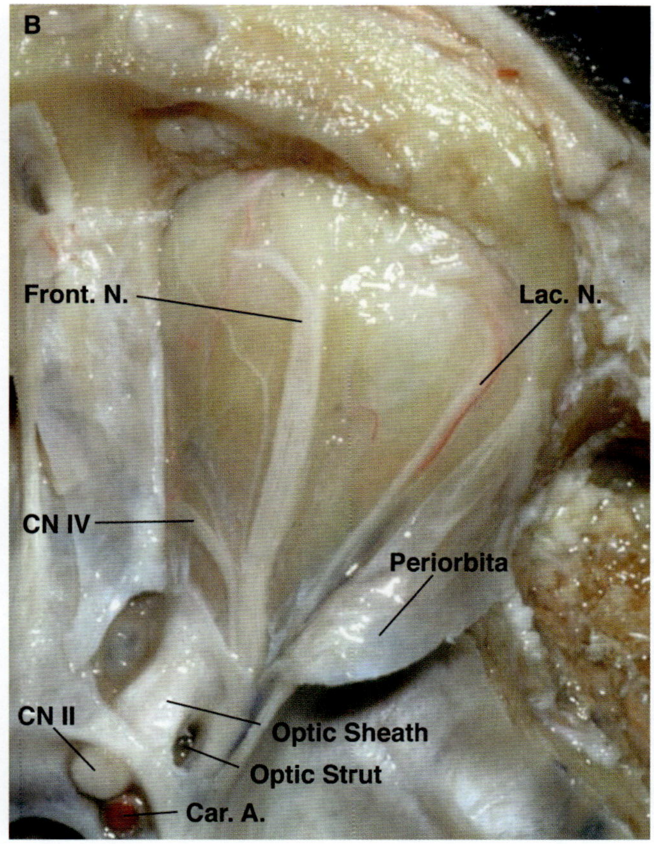

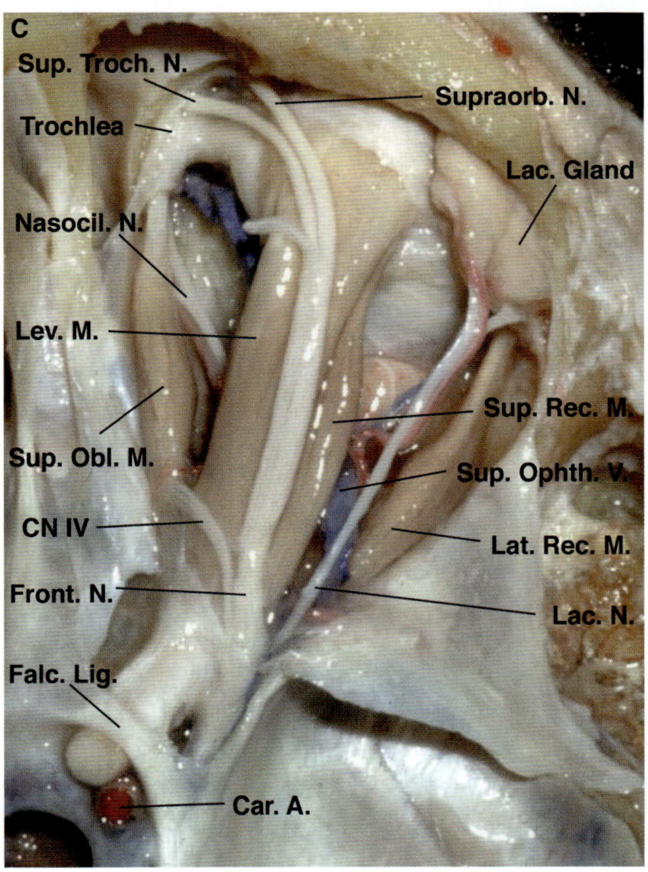

Fig. 15.2 Superior view of a stepwise dissection of the neural structures in the orbit and superior orbital fissure. **(A)** The dura has been removed from the part of the frontal and sphenoid bones forming the orbital roof. **(B)** The orbit and optic canal have been unroofed, the anterior clinoid process removed, and the periorbita opened to expose the trochlear, frontal, and lacrimal nerves coursing in the orbital fat just beneath the periorbita. **(C)** The orbital fat has been removed. (*continued on next page*)

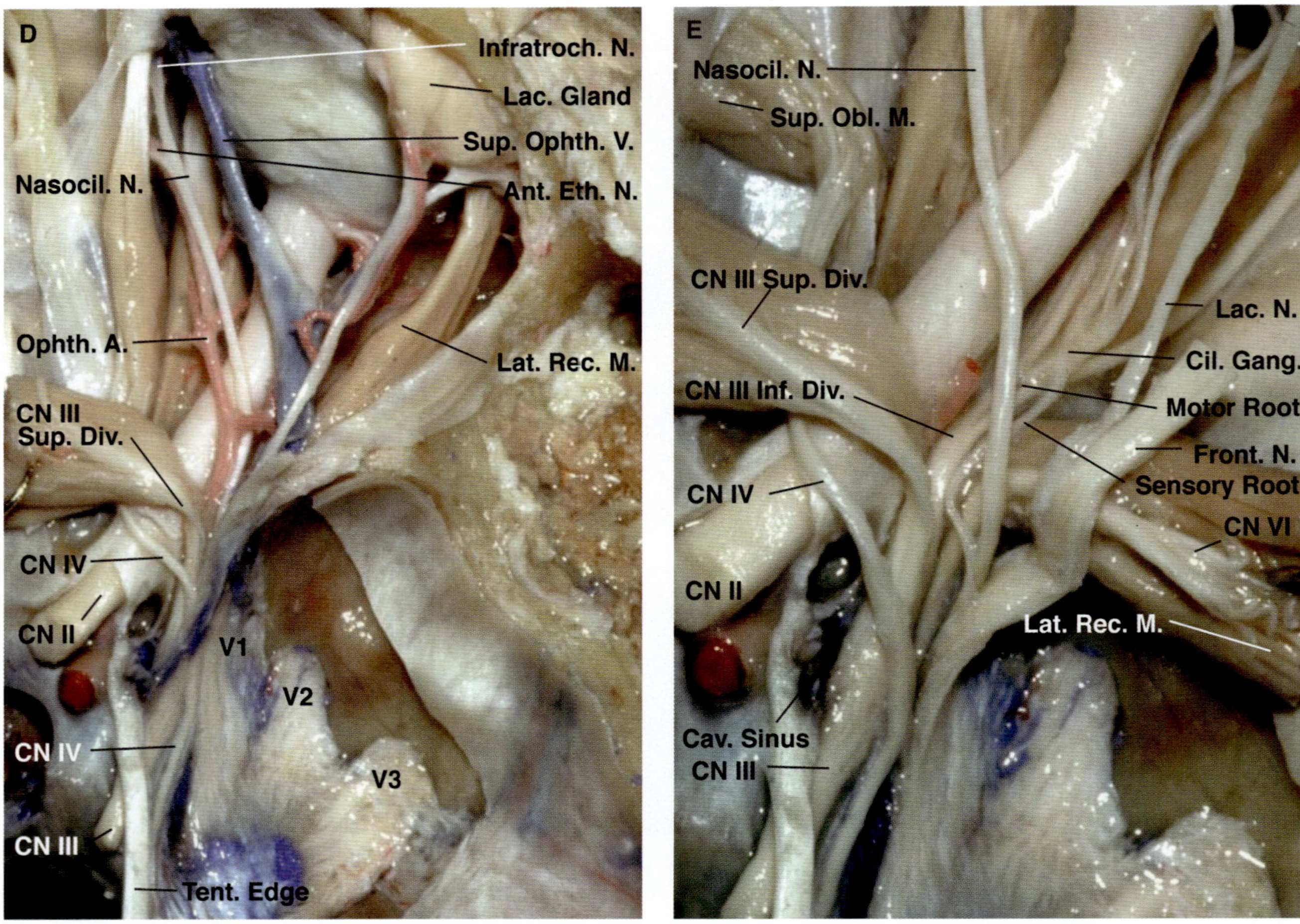

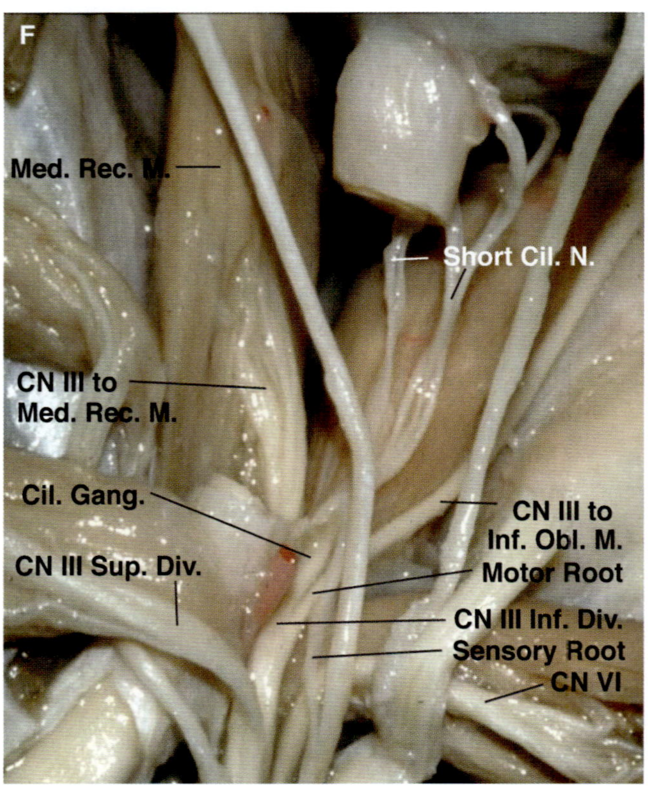

Fig. 15.2 (*Continued*) **(D)** The frontal nerve and the levator and superior rectus muscles have been divided and reflected to expose the superior ophthalmic vein, ophthalmic artery, and nasociliary nerve as they pass above the optic nerve. **(E)** The annular tendon has been divided in the interval between the origin of the superior and lateral rectus muscles. **(F)** A segment of the orbital portion of the optic nerve has been removed. This exposes the branch of the inferior division of the oculomotor nerve, which passes below the optic nerve and enters the medial rectus muscle. A.: artery; Ant.: anterior; Car.: carotid; Cav.: cavernous; Cil.: ciliary; Clin.: clinoid; CN: cranial nerve; Div.: division; Eth.: ethmoidal; Falc.: falciform; Front.: frontal; Gang.: ganglion; Inf.: inferior; Infratroch.: infratrochlear; Lac.: lacrimal; Lat.: lateral; Less.: lesser; Lev.: levator; Lig.: ligament; M.: muscle; Med.: medial; N.: nerve; Nasocil.: nasociliary; Obl.: oblique; Olf.: olfactory; Ophth.: ophthalmic; Rec.: rectus; Sup.: superior; Supraorb.: supraorbital; Sup. Troch.: supratrochlear; Tent.: tentorial; Troch.: trochlear; V.: vein.

ethmoid bone, which separates the orbit and ethmoid air cells. The lacrimal sac, which sits in the lacrimal groove formed by the frontal process of the maxilla anteriorly and the lacrimal bone posteriorly, opens into the nasal cavity through the nasolacrimal canal. The anterior and posterior ethmoidal foramina, which transmit the anterior and posterior ethmoidal branches of the ophthalmic artery and the nasociliary nerve, are located at the junction of the roof and medial wall of the orbit and pass through the frontoethmoidal suture or the adjacent part of the frontal bone and open into the anterior cranial fossa along the lateral edge of the cribriform plate.

The optic canal, through which the optic nerve and ophthalmic artery pass, opens into the superomedial corner of the orbital apex at the junction of the roof and medial wall. The optic canal is situated at the junction of the lesser wing with the body of the sphenoid bone. It is separated from the superior orbital fissure by the optic strut, a bridge of bone, also referred to as the posterior root of the lesser wing, which extends from the lower margin of the base of the anterior clinoid process to the sphenoid body. The tendinous ring (annular tendon) from which the superior, inferior, medial, and lateral rectus muscles arise is attached to the upper, lower, and medial margin of the optic canal. The anterior clinoid process projects backward from the lesser wing of the sphenoid bone into the interval between where the optic nerve enters the optic canal and where the oculomotor nerve enters the superior orbital fissure. The intracranial end of the optic canal has an ovoid shape with a slightly greater diameter in the mediolateral than in the superior-inferior dimension. It is situated medial to the anterior clinoid process and optic strut.

The medial margin is formed by the body of the sphenoid bone. The upper margin is formed by the anterior root of the lesser wing of the sphenoid bone. The lateral margin is formed by the optic strut. The lower margin of the foramen is formed by the optic strut and the adjacent part of the body of the sphenoid bone. The optic strut blends superolaterally into the base of the anterior clinoid process and inferiorly and medially into the body of the sphenoid bone. The anterior bend of the intracavernous segment of the internal carotid artery rests against the posterior surface of the optic strut and ascends on the medial side of the anterior clinoid process. The body of the sphenoid bone contains the sphenoid sinus. The chiasmatic sulcus is a shallow groove situated on the intracranial surface of the sphenoid formed by the lateral surface of the optic strut, and the lower part is formed by the body of the sphenoid bone. The anterior part of the carotid sulcus, the shallow groove marking the course of the intracavernous segment of the carotid artery, is situated just inside and behind the medial edge of the fissure and continues upward along the posterior margin of the optic strut and the medial side of the anterior clinoid process. The lower margin of the fissure is formed by the junction of the greater wing with the sphenoid body and is located at the level of the lower edge of the cavernous sinus and the floor of the middle fossa. The lower edge of the fissure is separated from the foramen rotundum by a narrow bridge of bone, referred to as the maxillary strut. The lower end of the superior orbital fissure is located above and blends into the medial end of the inferior orbital fissure. The inferior orbital fissure is a narrow crevasse with long anterior and posterior borders and narrow medial and lateral ends. The long posterior edge is formed by the greater wing of the sphenoid bone. The long anterior wall is formed by the orbital surface of the maxilla, except for a short segment formed by the orbital process of the palatine bone. The narrow lateral end is formed by the zygomatic bone, and the narrow medial end is formed by the sphenoid body. The posteromedial part of the fissure communicates below with the pterygopalatine fossa and the anterolateral part communicates with the infratemporal fossa, which is located below the greater sphenoid wing. The structures passing through the fissure are the zygomatic and the infraorbital and zygomatic branches of the maxillary nerve, some branches of the internal maxillary artery, and the branches of the inferior ophthalmic vein, which communicate with the pterygoid plexus. The orbital smooth muscle spans the upper part of the fissure. The pterygomaxillary fissure is the narrow cleft between the posterior surface of the maxilla and the anterior surface of the pterygoid process of the sphenoid bone. The pterygomaxillary fissure opens into the pterygopalatine fossa, which is located below and communicates through the medial part of the inferior orbital fissure with the orbital apex. The upper part of the pterygoid process is penetrated by the foramen rotundum, through which the maxillary nerve passes to reach the pterygopalatine fossa, where it gives rise to the infraorbital and zygomatic nerves, which course in the floor and lateral orbital wall. The ostium of the vidian canal, which transmits the vidian nerve, is located below the foramen rotundum. The medial wall of the pterygopalatine fossa is formed by the perpendicular plate of the palatine bone.

Periorbita, Dura, and Annular Tendon

At the superior orbital fissure, the dura covering the middle fossa and cavernous sinus blends into the periorbita of the orbital apex and into the annular tendon from which the recti muscles arise (**Fig. 15.3**). The annular tendon surrounds the orbital end of the optic foramen and the adjacent part of the superior orbital fissure. The fibrous components, which blend together to form the annular tendon, are the periorbita covering the orbital apex, the dura lining the superior orbital fissure and optic canal, and the optic sheath. The annular tendon is attached along the upper, medial, and lower margins of the optic canal, and to a bony prominence at the midportion of the lateral edge of the superior orbital fissure, at the junction of the fissure's narrow lateral and larger medial parts. The annular tendon does not surround the whole superior orbital fissure, but encompasses only the upper-medial portion, which is situated lateral to the optic strut and optic foramen. The lower portion of the annular tendon, the site of origin of the inferior rectus muscle, extends horizontally from the sphenoid body below the optic strut and optic foramen to an attachment on the lateral edge of the fissure.

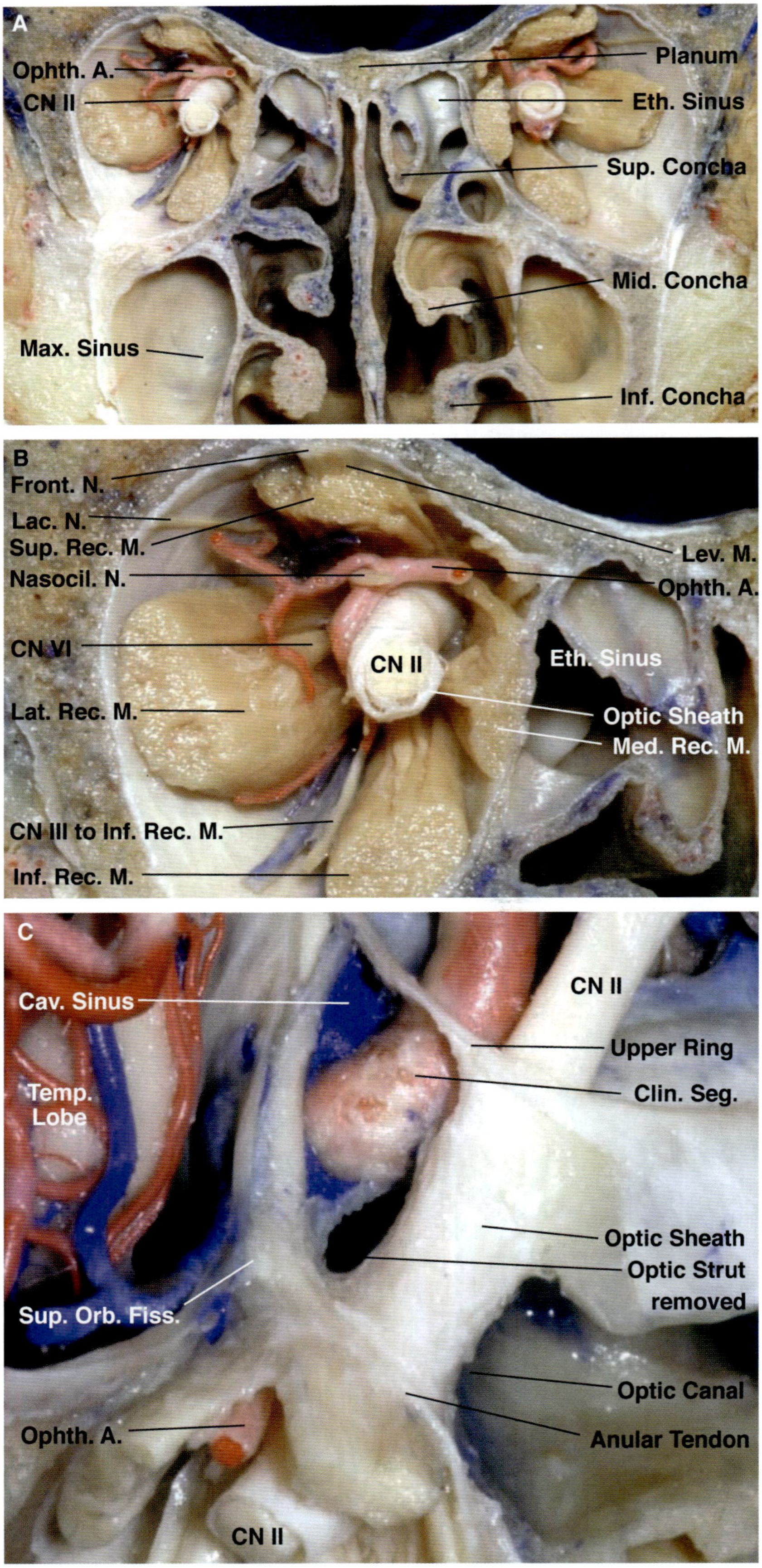

Fig. 15.3 **(A)** Coronal section of orbits and cranial base anterior to the orbital apex. **(B)** Enlarged view of right side shown in **A.** **(C)** Anterosuperior view showing the relationship of the orbital apex to the optic strut, optic canal, and superior orbital fissure.

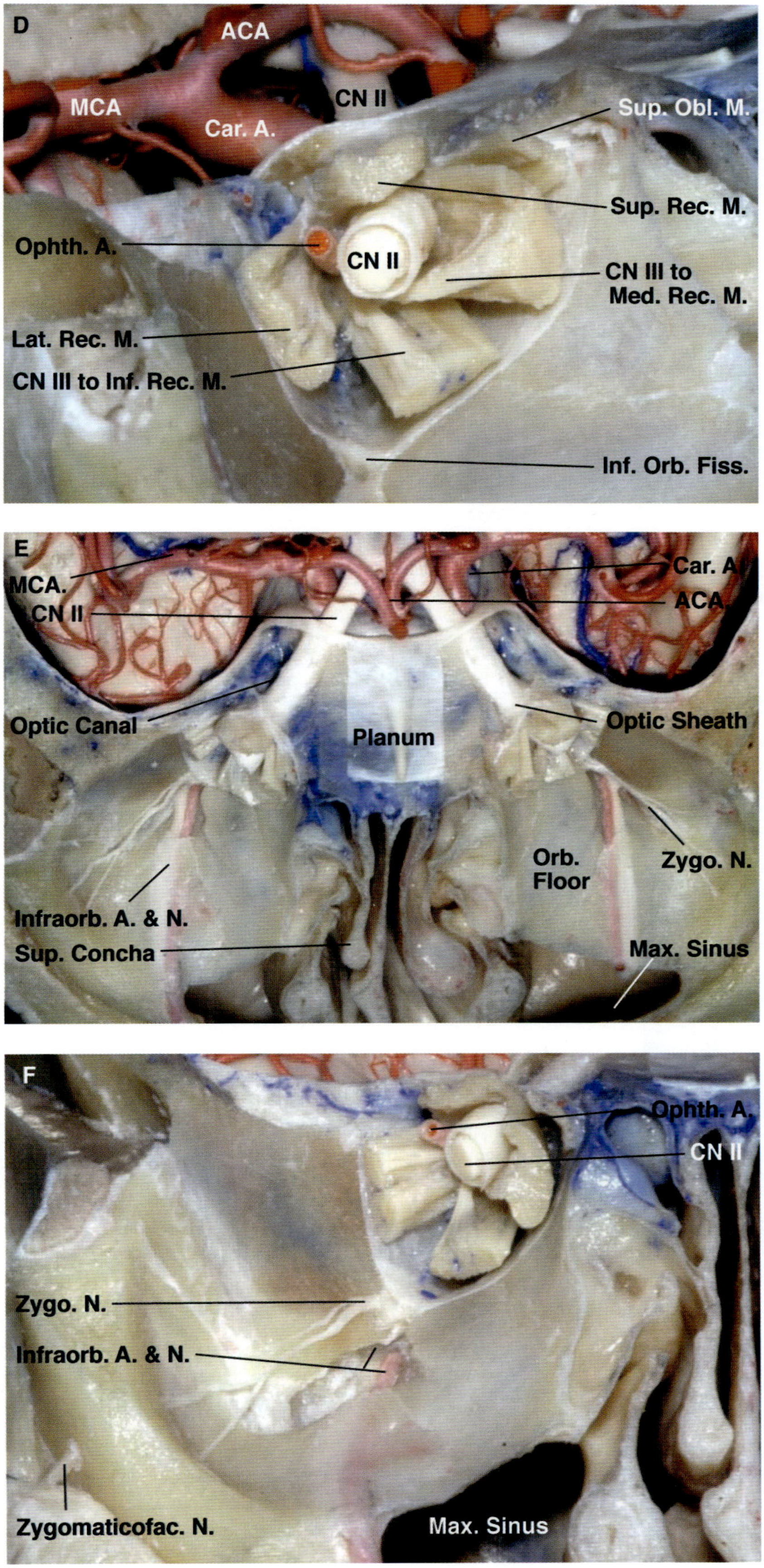

Fig. 15.3 (*Continued*) **(D)** Cross section of right orbit just in front of the orbital apex. **(E)** Superior view of the floor of both orbits. The roof of the maxillary sinus forms the orbital floors. **(F)** Enlarged view of the right orbit showing the course along the orbital walls taken by the zygomaticofacial, zygomaticotemporal, and infraorbital nerves. (*continued on next page*)

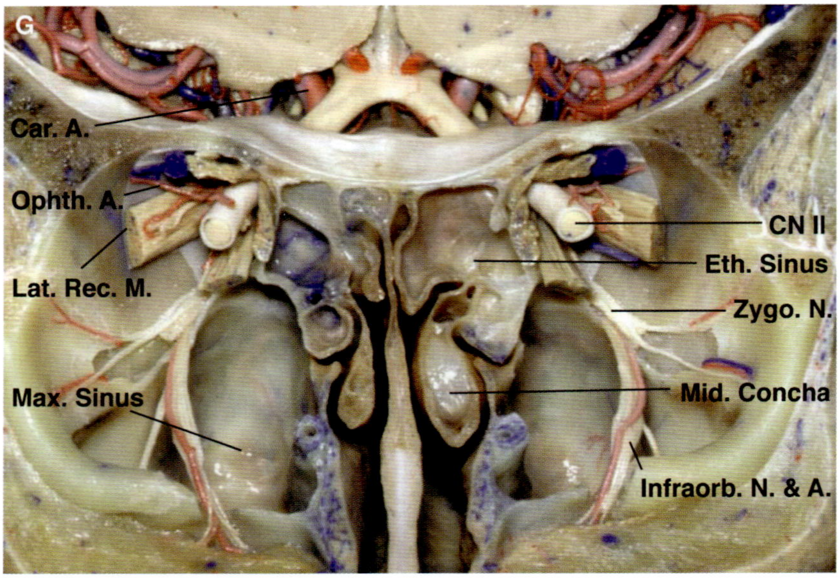

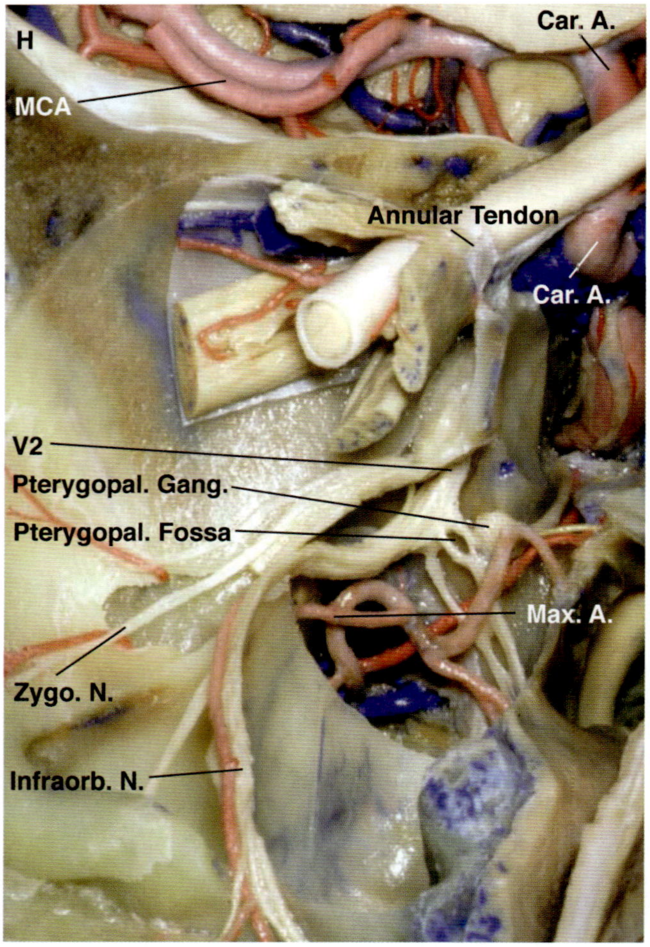

Fig. 15.3 (*Continued*) **(G)** Anterior view of both orbits in another specimen. A portion of the floor of both orbits has been removed to expose the maxillary sinus while preserving the infraorbital and zygomatic nerves. **(H)** Enlarged view. Some of the posterior wall of the maxillary sinus has been removed to expose the pterygopalatine fossa and the origin of the infraorbital and zygomatic nerves from the maxillary nerve. A.: artery; ACA: anterior cerebral artery; Car.: carotid; Cav.: cavernous; Clin.: clinoid; CN: cranial nerve; Eth.: ethmoid; Fiss.: fissure; Front.: frontal; Gang.: ganglion; Inf.: inferior; Infraorb.: infraorbital; Lac.: lacrimal; Lat.: lateral; Lev.: levator; M.: muscle; Max.: maxillary; MCA: middle cerebral artery; Med.: medial; Mid.: middle; N.: nerve; Nasocil.: nasociliary; Obl.: oblique; Ophth.: ophthalmic; Orb.: orbital; Pterygopal.: pterygopalatine; Rec.: rectus; Seg.: segment; Sup.: superior; Temp.: temporal; Zygo.: zygomatic; Zygomaticofac.: zygomaticofacial.

From its attachment to the greater wing, the annular tendon is directed upward to blend into the periorbita and dura, which meet on the lower margin of the lesser sphenoid wing. The segment of the annular tendon passing from the greater to the lesser wing separates the narrow lateral part of the fissure from the larger medial part and serves as the site of origin of the lateral rectus muscle. The annular tendon and the connective tissue layer extending backward divide the superior orbital fissure into three sectors: lateral, central, and inferior. The lateral sector is quite narrow, being bounded above by the lesser wing of the sphenoid bone, below by the part of the greater wing lateral to the site of attachment of the annular tendon, and medially by the annular tendon and the origin of the lateral rectus muscle.

The lateral sector transmits the trochlear, frontal, and lacrimal nerves, all of which pass through the fissure outside the annular tendon. The lacrimal nerve occupies the most lateral part of the fissure; the frontal nerve is more medial. The trochlear nerve passes through the fissure on the superomedial margin of the frontal nerve. The superior ophthalmic vein also passes through this sector by coursing along the lower side of the lacrimal and frontal nerves to reach the cavernous sinus. The central sector of the superior orbital fissure, referred to as the oculomotor foramen because it is the part of the fissure through which the oculomotor nerve passes, is bounded above by the annular tendon and the adjacent part of the lesser wing, medially by the optic strut and sphenoid body, laterally by the annular tendon and the prominence on the lateral margin of the fissure to which the annular tendon attaches, and below by the segment of the annular tendon spanning the interval between the sphenoid body and the bony prominence on the lateral edge of the fissure. The inferior rectus muscle arises from the annular tendon at the lower margin of this sector. The oculomotor, nasociliary, and abducens nerves and the sensory and sympathetic roots of the ciliary ganglion pass through this sector. The optic nerve and ophthalmic artery pass medially to the oculomotor foramen through the part of the annular tendon attached to the upper, lower, and medial margins of the optic foramen. The connective tissue membrane, which extends posteriorly from the annular tendon, separates the nerves passing through the lateral and central sectors of the fissure. This connective tissue extends backward from the annulus between the frontal branch of the ophthalmic nerve, which passes through the lateral sector outside the annular tendon, and the nasociliary nerve, which passes through the central sector and the annular tendon.

The inferior sector of the superior orbital fissure is situated below the annular tendon. It is bounded below by the junction of the body and greater wing of the sphenoid bone, above by the annular tendon, laterally by the part of the greater wing below the attachment of the annular tendon, and medially by the sphenoid body. The inferior rectus muscle arises from the annular tendon at the upper margin of this sector. Orbital fat extends backward below the inferior rectus muscle into this part of the fissure. The lower margin of this sector contains a posterior extension of the orbital smooth muscle, which spans the upper margin of the inferior orbital fissure. The orbital fat extends backward between the inferior rectus muscle and the orbital smooth muscle and medial to the segment of the abducens and nasociliary nerves passing through the fissure. Removal of this fat exposes the fine branches of the carotid sympathetic plexus entering the orbit, some of which form the sympathetic root of the ciliary ganglion.

Neural Relationships

Optic Nerve

The optic nerve is divided into four parts: intraocular, intraorbital, intracanalicular, and intracranial (**Figs. 15.2, 15.3, 15.4,** and **15.5**). The intracanalicular part, located in the optic canal, and the intraorbital portions of the optic nerve are surrounded by dura and arachnoid. The subarachnoid space surrounding the intracranial part of the nerve extends forward from and communicates with the subarachnoid space around the intracanalicular and intraorbital portions of the

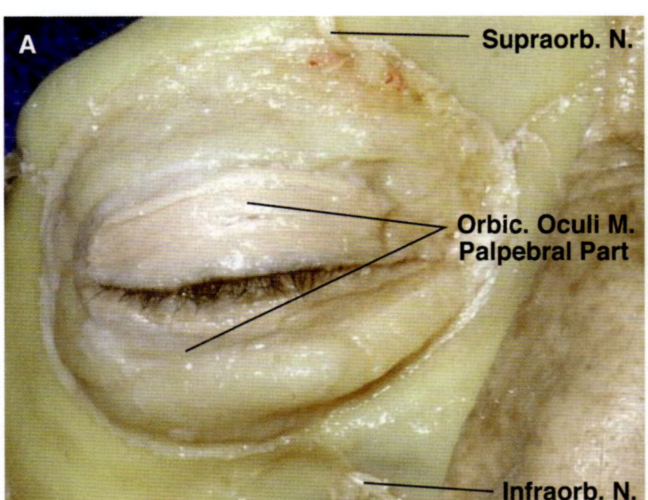

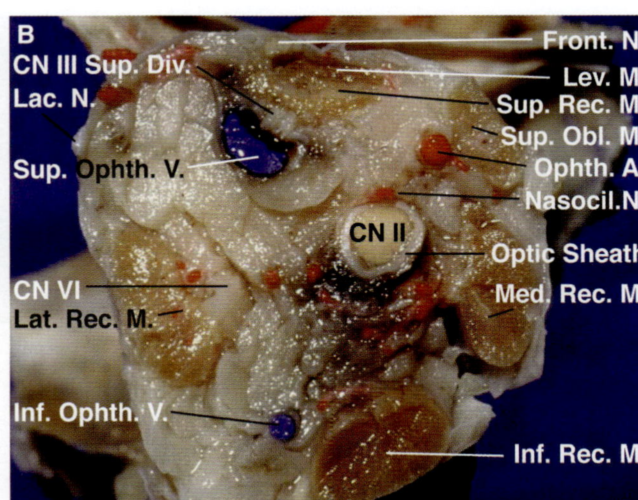

Fig. 15.4 **(A)** The orbital part of the orbicularis oculi muscle has been removed and the palpebral part preserved. **(B–H)** Anterior views of cross sections of the orbit at progressively deeper levels. **(B)** Anterior aspect of a coronal section through the right orbit just posterior to the globe and the inferior oblique muscle. (*continued on next page*)

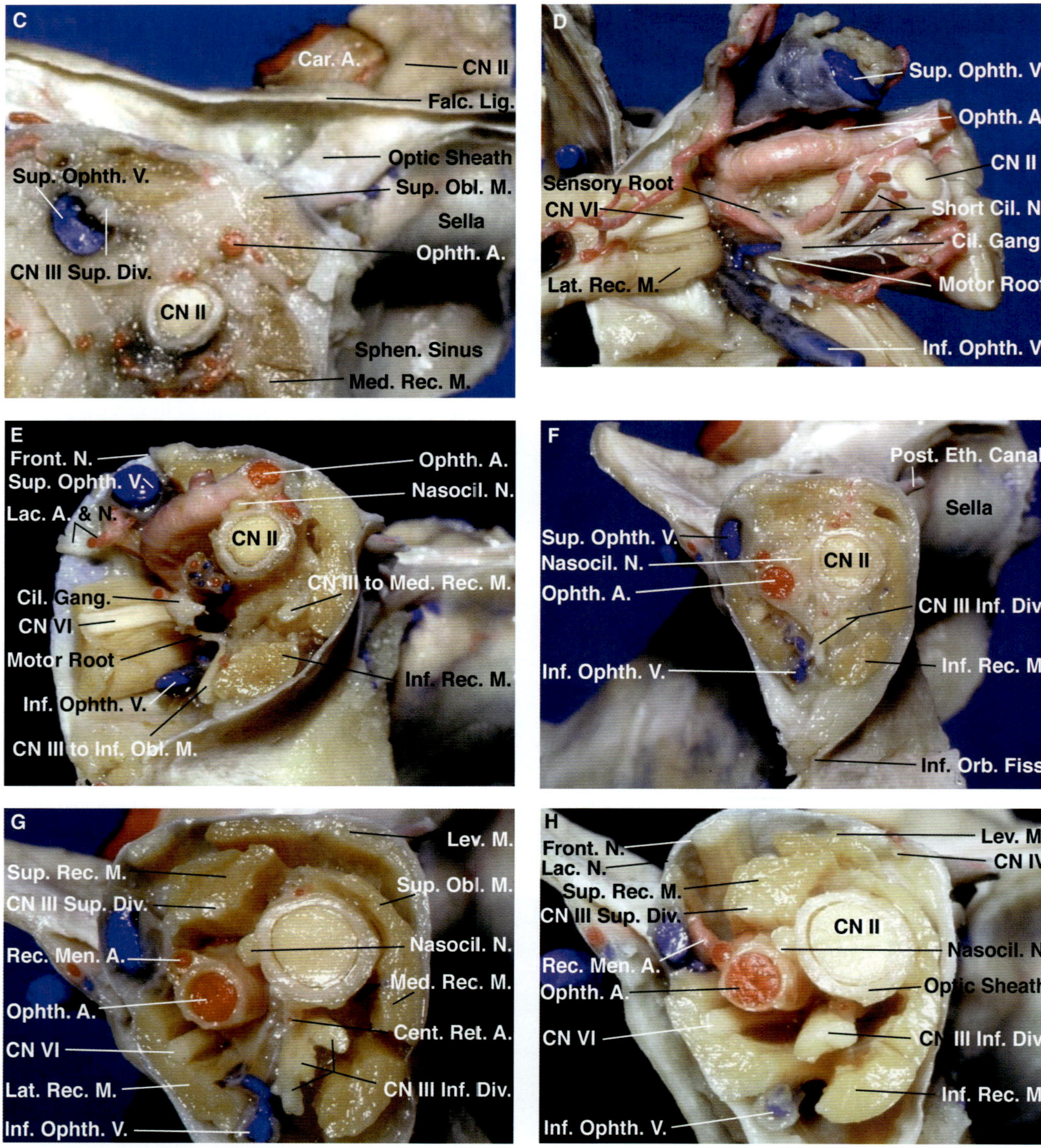

Fig. 15.4 *(Continued)* **(C)** Enlarged view of **B** to show the relationship of the cisternal and canalicular segments of the optic nerve to the intraorbital part. **(D)** The orbital fat has been removed and the lateral rectus muscle has been reflected to expose the ciliary ganglion, which is located inferolateral to the optic nerve. **(E)** Anterior aspect of a coronal section at the level of the ciliary ganglion. **(F)** Section located just anterior to the lateral end of superior orbital fissure at the level of the posterior ethmoidal canal. At this level, the ophthalmic artery courses on the lateral side of the optic nerve and the nasociliary nerve courses between the optic nerve and ophthalmic artery. **(G)** Enlarged view of the section shown in **F** after removal of the orbital fat. At this level, the oculomotor nerve has split into a superior division that supplies the superior rectus and levator muscles and an inferior division that innervates the inferior rectus, medial rectus, and inferior oblique muscles. **(H)** Section through the orbital apex immediately in front of the superior orbital fissure. A.: artery; Car.: carotid; Cent.: central; Cil.: ciliary; CN: cranial nerve; Div.: division; Falc.: falciform; Front.: frontal; Gang.: ganglion; Inf.: inferior; Infraorb.: infraorbital; Lac.: lacrimal; Lat.: lateral; Lev.: levator; Lig.: ligament; M.: muscle; Med.: medial; Men.: meningeal; N.: nerve; Nasocil.: nasociliary; Obl.: oblique; Ophth.: ophthalmic; Orbic.: orbicularis; Rec.: rectus: recurrent; Ret.: retinal; Sphen.: sphenoidal; Sup.: superior; Supraorb.: supraorbital; V.: vein.

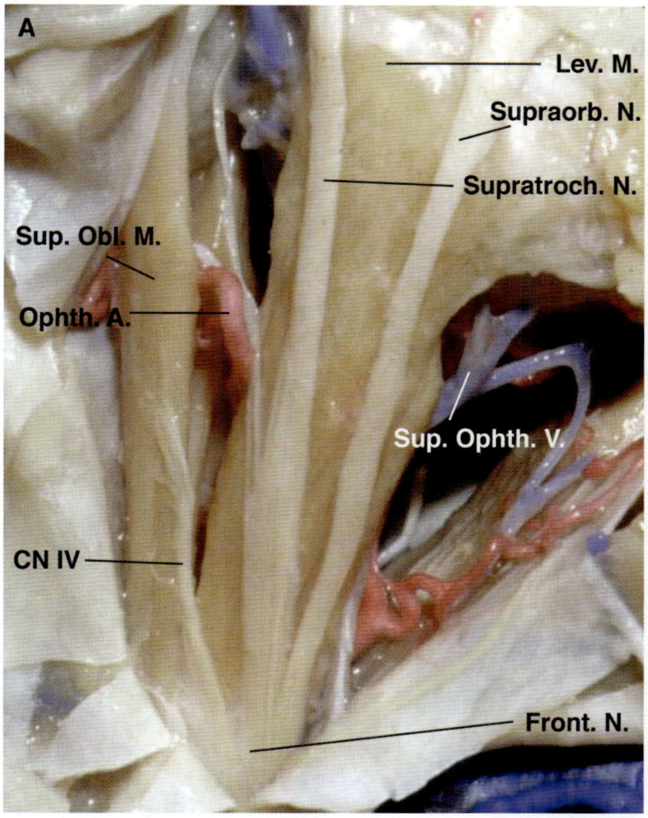

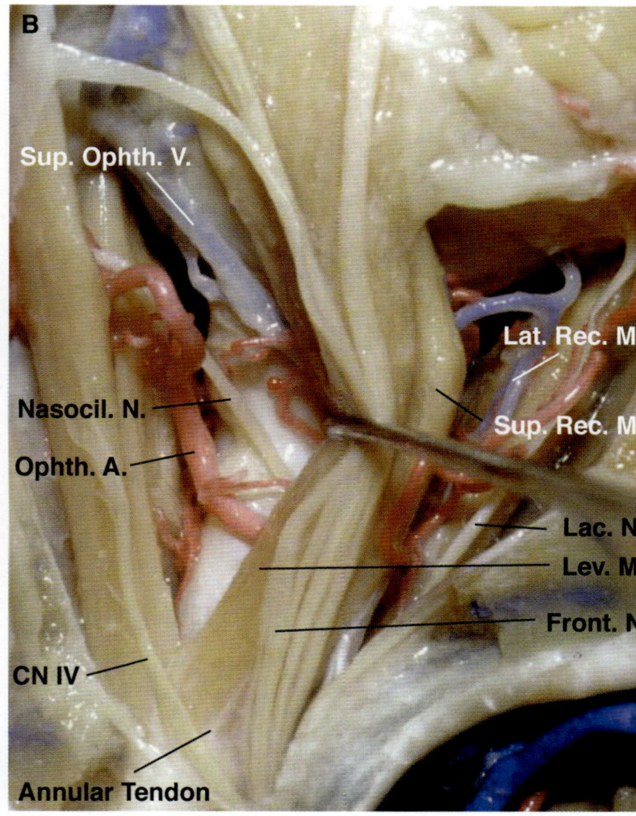

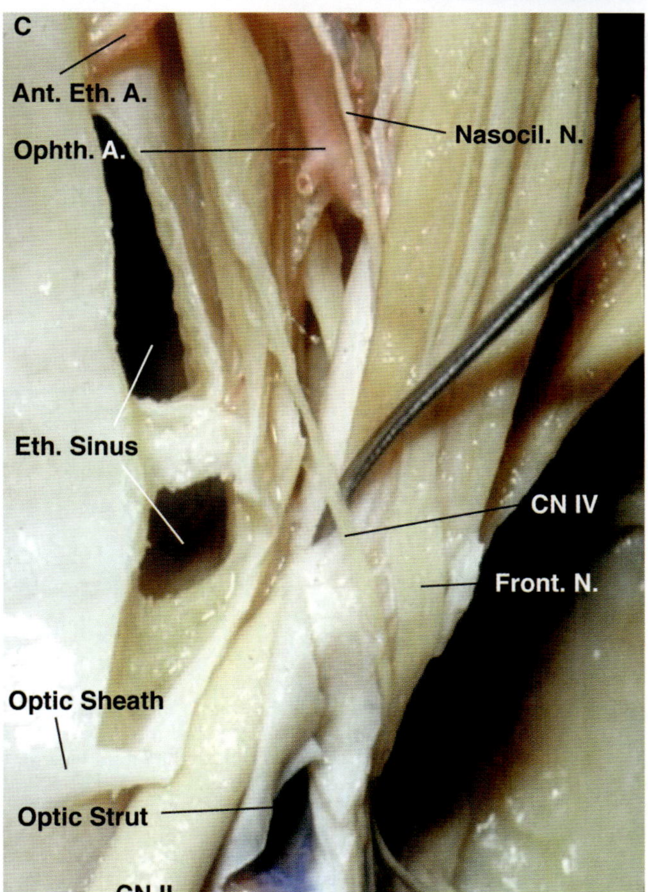

Fig. 15.5 Superior view of the right orbit. **(A)** The periorbita has been opened and the orbital fat removed to expose the trochlear nerve, the supraorbital and supratrochlear branches of the frontal nerve, and the levator and superior oblique muscles. **(B,C)** Medial route to the optic nerve. **(B)** The medial approach is directed through the interval between the superior oblique and the levator muscles. **(C)** An incision has been extended backward through the annular tendon between the superior and medial rectus muscles and through the optic sheath to expose the full length of the optic nerve. (*continued on next page*)

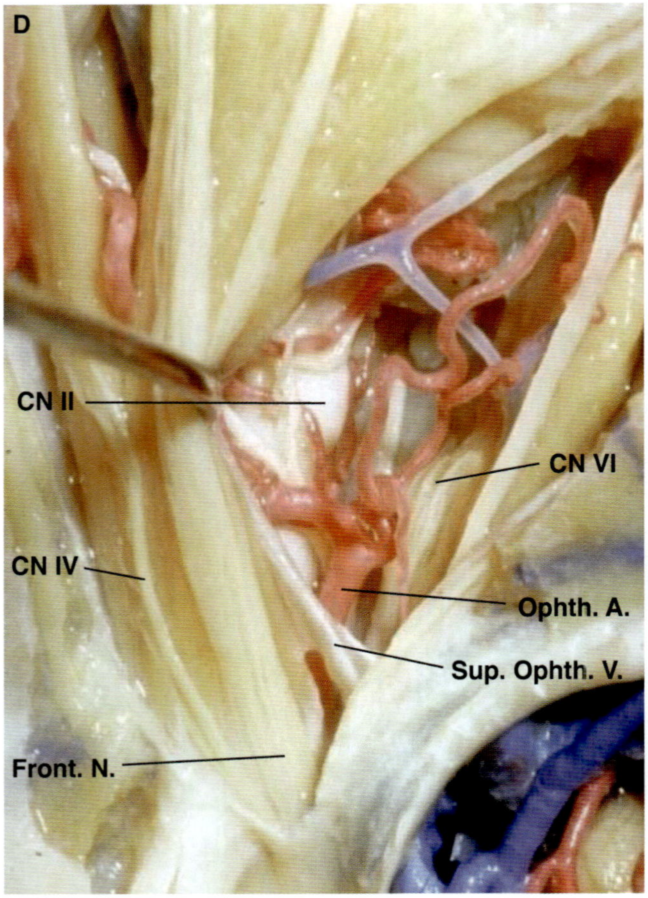

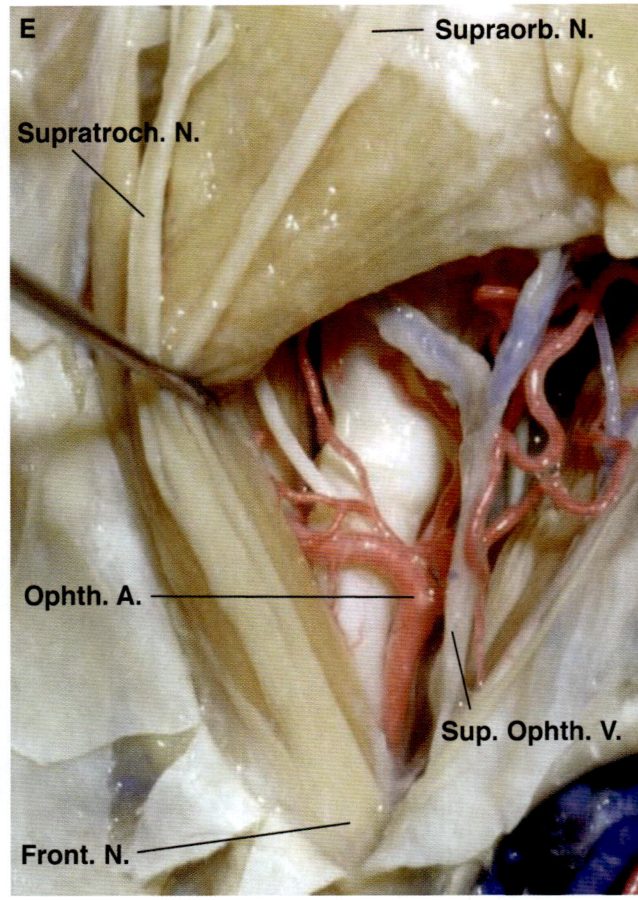

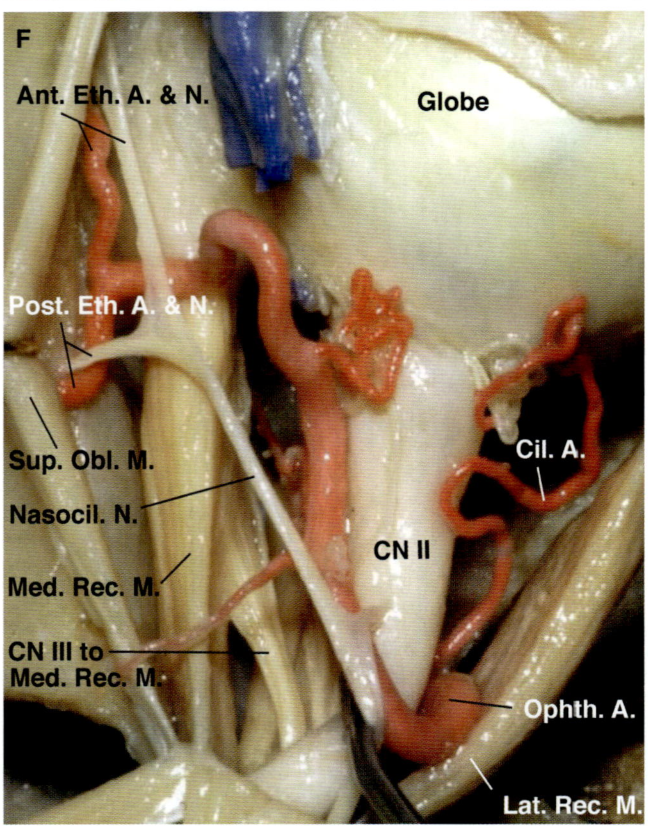

Fig. 15.5 (*Continued*) **(D,E)** Lateral route to the intraconal and apical area. **(D)** The levator and superior rectus muscles and the superior ophthalmic vein have been retracted medially to expose the intraorbital part of the optic nerve. **(E)** The superior ophthalmic vein has been displaced laterally to expose the deep apical area. **(F)** The levator, superior rectus, and superior oblique muscles have been reflected to expose the ophthalmic artery coursing above the optic nerve. Inf.: inferior; Lat.: lateral; Lev.: levator; M.: muscle; Med.: medial; Obl.: oblique; Orbic.: orbicularis; Rec.: rectus; Sup.: superior.

nerve. The optic nerve passes through the medial part of the annular tendon and below the levator and superior rectus muscles. The dural sheath around the optic nerve blends smoothly into the periorbita at the anterior end of the optic canal. After passing through the optic canal, which forms a prominence in the upper part of the sphenoid sinus immediately in front of the sella turcica and along the medial aspect of the anterior clinoid process, the intracranial portion of the nerve is directed posterior, superiorly, and medially toward the optic chiasm. The intraocular portion of the optic nerve, which includes the optic disc, lies within the sclera. The intraorbital portion of the optic nerve is surrounded by orbital fat and follows a slightly tortuous course. The ciliary nerves and arteries pierce the sclera in the area around the optic nerve. The ophthalmic artery enters the orbit on the lateral side of the nerve and passes above the nerve to reach the medial sides of the orbit. The superior ophthalmic vein arises in the anteromedial part of the orbit and crosses above the nerve to reach the orbital apex. Both the artery and vein course between the superior rectus muscle and the optic nerve. The branch of the inferior division of the oculomotor nerve to the medial rectus muscle passes below the optic nerve at about the same level that the ophthalmic artery and nasociliary nerve pass above the optic nerve.

Oculomotor, Trochlear, and Abducens Nerves

The oculomotor nerve enters the orbit by passing through the medial part of the fissure on the lateral surface of the optic strut (**Fig. 15.2**). At the level of the posterior margin of the fissure, in the area medial to the trochlear and nasociliary nerves, the oculomotor nerve splits into superior and inferior divisions that course one above the other as they pass through the central sector of the fissure and the oculomotor foramen on the medial side of the branches of the ophthalmic nerve. The superior division of the oculomotor nerve enters the orbit below the attachment of the superior rectus muscle to the annular tendon and sends its branches upward lateral to the optic nerve to reach the lower surface of the superior rectus and levator muscles. The inferior division courses inferiorly and medially as it proceeds through the fissure on the medial side of the nasociliary and abducens nerves. At the orbital apex, it splits into three individual branches: two are directed forward to reach the inferior rectus and inferior oblique muscles, and one passes medially below the optic nerve to enter the medial rectus muscle. In addition, the branch to the inferior oblique muscle gives rise to the motor (parasympathetic) root to the ciliary ganglion. The parasympathetic fibers synapse in the ciliary ganglion, which gives rise to the short ciliary nerves that pierce the sclera to reach the ciliary body and iris.

The trochlear nerve courses in the lateral wall of the cavernous sinus below the oculomotor nerve and above the ophthalmic nerve. It passes through the upper edge of the narrow lateral part of the superior orbital fissure outside the annular tendon and passes medially above the frontal nerve and the levator muscle to reach the superior oblique muscle.

The abducens nerve travels forward in the cavernous sinus on the medial side of the ophthalmic nerve and shifts laterally below the nasociliary nerve as it passes through the superior orbital fissure and annular tendon to enter the medial surface of the lateral rectus muscle. At the apex of the orbit, the nasociliary nerve and the inferior division of the oculomotor nerve curve medially as the abducens nerve shifts laterally to enter the medial surface of the lateral rectus muscle. Some fibers of the carotid sympathetic plexus pass to and course within the abducens nerve in the cavernous sinus.

Trigeminal Nerve

The ophthalmic branch of the trigeminal nerve is the smallest of the three trigeminal divisions (**Figs. 15.2** and **15.5**). It is inclined upward as it passes forward near the medial surface of the dura forming the lower part of the lateral wall of the cavernous sinus to reach the superior orbital fissure. It is flattened in the wall of the cavernous sinus, but at the superior orbital fissure it takes on an oval configuration. The ophthalmic nerve splits into the lacrimal, frontal, and nasociliary nerves as it approaches the superior orbital fissure. The lacrimal nerve arises at the level of or just behind the superior orbital fissure from the lateral edge of the ophthalmic nerve and passes through the lateral edge of the fissure on the lateral side of the frontal nerve and above the superior ophthalmic vein. On entering the orbit, the lacrimal nerve courses along the superior margin of the lateral rectus muscles, where it receives secretory fibers conveyed initially in the zygomatic nerve from the pterygopalatine ganglion and distributed through the lacrimal nerve to the lacrimal gland. The lacrimal nerve conveys sensation from the area in front of the lacrimal gland.

The remainder of the ophthalmic nerve splits into the frontal nerve, which passes through the lateral sector of the fissure, and the nasociliary nerve, which passes through the central sector on the medial side of the origin of the lateral rectus muscle from the annular tendon. The frontal branch of the ophthalmic nerve arises in the lateral wall of the cavernous sinus and passes through the narrow lateral part of the superior orbital fissure on the medial side of the lacrimal nerve and superior ophthalmic vein and below the trochlear nerve. The frontal nerve courses outside and superolateral to the annular tendon and divides into the supratrochlear and supraorbital nerves within the orbit. The supratrochlear nerve runs anteriorly above the trochlea of the superior oblique muscle with the supratrochlear artery. The supraorbital nerve courses above the levator muscle with the supraorbital artery. It conveys sensation from the upper eyelid and forehead and may also carry some sympathetic fibers to the globe and pupillary dilator. The nasociliary nerve arises from the medial side of the ophthalmic nerve and is situated above and lateral to the abducens nerve in the anterior part of the cavernous sinus.

Both the abducens and the nasociliary nerves course medial to the part of the ophthalmic nerve from which the lacrimal and frontal nerves arise. At the level of the fissure, the nasociliary nerve gently ascends laterally to the inferior division of the oculomotor nerve and then crosses medially between the two divisions of the oculomotor nerve and above the optic nerve to reach the medial part of the orbit, where it gives rise to the anterior and posterior ethmoidal and infratrochlear nerves. The sensory root of the ciliary ganglion arises from the lower edge of the nasociliary nerve during passage through the lateral wall of the cavernous sinus or within the fissure. The sensory root may infrequently arise as far forward as the anterior margin of the fissure. Within the fissure, it courses between the abducens nerve laterally and the inferior oculomotor division medially and passes forward to join the posterior edge of the ciliary ganglion. The fibers from the sensory root are distributed to the globe with the short ciliary nerves and convey sensation from the cornea and globe. The nasociliary nerve also gives rise to the long ciliary nerves that enter the sclera around the optic nerve with the short ciliary nerves. The long ciliary nerve conveys sympathetic fibers to the globe and pupillary dilator and may also carry some sensation from the globe and cornea.

The maxillary nerve passes through the foramen rotundum to enter the pterygopalatine fossa, where it gives rise to the infraorbital and zygomatic nerves and communicating rami to the sphenopalatine ganglion. The infraorbital and zygomatic branches pass through the inferior orbital fissure to course within the orbit. The infraorbital nerve courses along the orbital floor in the infraorbital groove and canal to reach the infraorbital foramen, where its branches are distributed to the cheek. The zygomatic branch passes through the inferior orbital fissure and courses just inside the lateral wall of the orbit, where it divides into zygomaticofacial and zygomaticotemporal branches. These branches enter the zygomatico-orbital foramina on the intraorbital surface of the zygoma and exit the zygoma at the zygomaticofacial and zygomaticotemporal foramina to reach the skin of the cheek and temple, respectively.

Ciliary Ganglion

The ciliary ganglion is situated on the inferolateral aspect of the optic nerve and on the medial side of the lateral rectus muscle (**Figs. 15.2** and **15.4**). It receives three branches: the motor (parasympathetic) root from the inferior division of the oculomotor nerve, the sensory root from the nasociliary nerve, and sympathetic fibers from the plexus around the internal carotid artery. The sympathetic fibers sometimes blend with the sensory root in the orbit. The parasympathetic fibers synapse in the ciliary ganglion. The sympathetic fibers arise in the cervical sympathetic ganglia and pass through the ciliary ganglion without synapsing. The short ciliary nerves pass from the ganglion to the globe.

Sympathetic Fibers

Sympathetic fibers ascend on the surface of the internal carotid artery, pass through the medial part of the superior orbital fissure and the oculomotor foramen, and course with the abducens and ophthalmic nerves in the cavernous sinus and also with the ophthalmic artery. Some of these fibers collect together to form the sympathetic root of the ciliary ganglion, which courses as an independent branch surrounded by orbital fat. The fibers forming the sympathetic root run forward and upward along the medial margin of the abducens nerve to reach the area lateral to the inferior division of the oculomotor nerve, where they pass through the central sector of the superior orbital fissure. Some sympathetic fibers join the ophthalmic division and are distributed to the pupil in the long ciliary and sensory root of the ciliary ganglion, both of which arise from the nasociliary nerve. Others pass directly through the fissure and orbit to the globe. Some sympathetic fibers from the carotid plexus accompany the ophthalmic artery.

Vidian Nerve and Pterygopalatine Ganglion

The vidian nerve, formed by the union of the greater petrosal branch of the facial nerve and the deep petrosal nerve from the carotid plexus, exits the vidian canal and enters the posterior aspect of the sphenopalatine ganglion in the pterygopalatine fossa. Parasympathetic fibers are conveyed in the greater petrosal nerve and sympathetic fibers are conveyed in the deep petrosal nerve. Communicating branches, typically two in number, arise from the inferior portion of the maxillary nerve and descend to join the sphenopalatine ganglion, which is located anterior to the aperture of the vidian canal. The parasympathetic fibers synapse in the ganglion, and the sympathetic fibers pass through the ganglion without synapse. Fibers exiting the ganglion join the nasal, nasopalatine, and palatine nerves to convey secretory impulses to the nasal and palatine glands. The secretory fibers to the lacrimal gland pass from the ganglion via the maxillary nerve to join the zygomatic nerve, which sends a communication to the gland via the lacrimal nerve. In addition, sensory fibers, which pass through the pterygopalatine ganglion, reach the maxillary nerve and convey sensation from the ethmoidal and sphenoid sinuses, nasal cavity, nasal septum, hard palate, and roof of the pharynx.

■ Arterial Relationships

Internal Carotid Artery

The anterior bend of the intracavernous segment of the internal carotid artery courses along the posterior edge of the medial margin of the superior orbital fissure and rests against the posterior surface of the optic strut (**Fig. 15.3**). After ascending along the posterior margin of the optic strut, the artery turns upward along the medial margin of the anterior clinoid process to reach the subarachnoid space. The segment of the artery coursing along the medial margin of the clinoid process is referred to as the clinoid segment.

Ophthalmic Artery

The ophthalmic artery usually arises just above the cavernous sinus from the medial half of the superior aspect of the anterior bend of the internal carotid artery (**Figs. 15.3, 15.4, 15.5,** and **15.6**). Its origin is located under the medial part of the optic nerve, just behind the optic canal. In the optic canal, the ophthalmic artery courses within the optic sheath below the optic nerve and through the annular tendon. It exits the optic canal and penetrates the optic sheath to enter the orbital apex on the inferolateral aspect of the optic nerve. In the optic canal, the ophthalmic artery sometimes gives a recurrent branch to the intracranial segment of the optic nerve. Approximately 8% of ophthalmic arteries arise in the cavernous sinus rather than in the subarachnoid space.[4] Those ophthalmic arteries arising in the cavernous sinus pass through the superior orbital fissure, rather than the optic canal, to reach the orbit.

In some cases in which the larger ophthalmic artery passes through the superior orbital fissure, a second, smaller or hypoplastic ophthalmic artery may arise in the supraclinoid area and course in the usual manner through the optic foramen to reach the orbit. In other cases, with a normal-sized ophthalmic artery passing through the optic foramen, a smaller artery that arises from the intracavernous carotid may pass through the fissure, usually supplying the territory normally supplied by the lacrimal artery. The ophthalmic artery may also arise as duplicate arteries of nearly equal size.[3] The upper duplicate artery usually arises from the supraclinoid portion of the internal carotid artery and passes through the optic canal to enter the orbital apex on the lateral side of the optic nerve. The lower duplicate artery usually arises from the internal carotid artery in the cavernous sinus and passes through the superior orbital fissure between the oculomotor nerve laterally and the abducens and ophthalmic nerves medially. Both usually cross the optic nerve, one above and one below, to reach the medial part of the orbit. The ophthalmic artery may infrequently arise from the clinoid segment, in which case it passes through the superior orbital fissure to reach the orbit. A few will pass through an accessory foramen, called the ophthalmic foramen, which pierces the optic strut (**Fig. 15.1L**). It may also infrequently arise as a branch of the middle meningeal artery.[5]

The ophthalmic artery, after passing through the optic foramen and annular tendon and reaching the lateral aspect of the optic nerve, may give rise to a recurrent meningeal artery that passes backward through the superior orbital fissure to reach the dura. The ophthalmic artery passes above the optic nerve in approximately 85% of orbits. In the remainder, it passes below the nerve. After passing the optic nerve, the artery courses between the superior oblique and the medial rectus muscles, where it gives rise to the anterior and posterior ethmoidal arteries that pass through the anterior and posterior ethmoidal canals with the anterior and posterior ethmoidal nerves. The ophthalmic artery gives rise to the central retinal, lacrimal, long and short ciliary, supraorbital, medial palpebral, infratrochlear, supratrochlear, and dorsal nasal arteries, plus muscular branches to the extraocular muscles and meningeal branches that pass through the ethmoidal or lacrimal foramina or superior orbital fissure to reach the meninges. The palpebral branches of the ophthalmic artery plus the supratrochlear, infratrochlear, supraorbital, dorsal nasal, and lacrimal branches supply the skin and soft tissues of the eyelids and area around the orbital rim. The central retinal artery, which is the first and one of the smallest branches of the ophthalmic artery, arises medial to the ciliary ganglion, pierces the lower surface of the nerve, and courses a short distance inside the dural sheath of the nerve before passing to the center of the nerve and forward to the retina in the center of the nerve. The central retinal artery is a terminal branch without anastomotic connections. Its loss results in blindness.

The lacrimal artery, one of the largest and earliest branches of the ophthalmic artery, accompanies the lacrimal nerve and is distributed to the lacrimal gland and the lateral part of the eyelids and conjunctiva. A recurrent branch may also arise from the lacrimal artery or adjacent part of the ophthalmic artery and pass through the superior orbital fissure to reach the dura, only to return to the periorbita by passing through the lacrimal foramen located lateral to the superior orbital fissure on the greater sphenoid wing. The supraorbital artery arises from the ophthalmic artery as it crosses the optic nerve and runs along the medial side of the levator and superior rectus muscles to course with the supraorbital nerves. The supratrochlear artery courses with the supratrochlear nerve. The short and long posterior ciliary arteries arise from the ophthalmic artery, course with the short and long ciliary nerves, pierce the sclera around the optic nerve, and supply the choroidal coat and ciliary processes. The anterior ciliary arteries are derived from the branches to the extraocular muscles and run to the front of the globe with the tendons of the extraocular muscles, where they pierce the sclera and end in the greater arterial circle of the iris. The anterior and posterior ethmoidal branches of the ophthalmic artery, of which the anterior is the larger, arise beneath the superior oblique muscle and pass through the anterior and posterior ethmoidal canal to reach the dura beside the cribriform plate (**Figs. 15.2** and **15.5**). The anterior ethmoidal artery crosses near the anterior edge of the cribriform plate. The posterior ethmoidal artery crosses near the posterior edge of the cribriform plate a few millimeters anterior to the orbital end of the optic canal. As the anterior ethmoidal artery passes across the floor of the anterior cranial fossa near the cribriform plate, it gives rise to the anterior falx artery, which runs between and supplies the anterior portion of the falx and walls of the superior sagittal sinus. The anterior and posterior ethmoidal arteries then pass through the cribriform plate area to supply the ethmoidal sinuses, the infundibulum of the frontal sinus, the anterior nasal cavity, and the skin over the cartilaginous part of the nose. Arteries that supply the margins of the superior orbital fissure and may be recruited to supply tumors in the region include the anterior branch of the middle meningeal artery, the recurrent meningeal branches of the ophthalmic and lacrimal arteries, the meningeal branches of the internal carotid artery, the tentorial branch of the meningohypophyseal trunk, the anterior

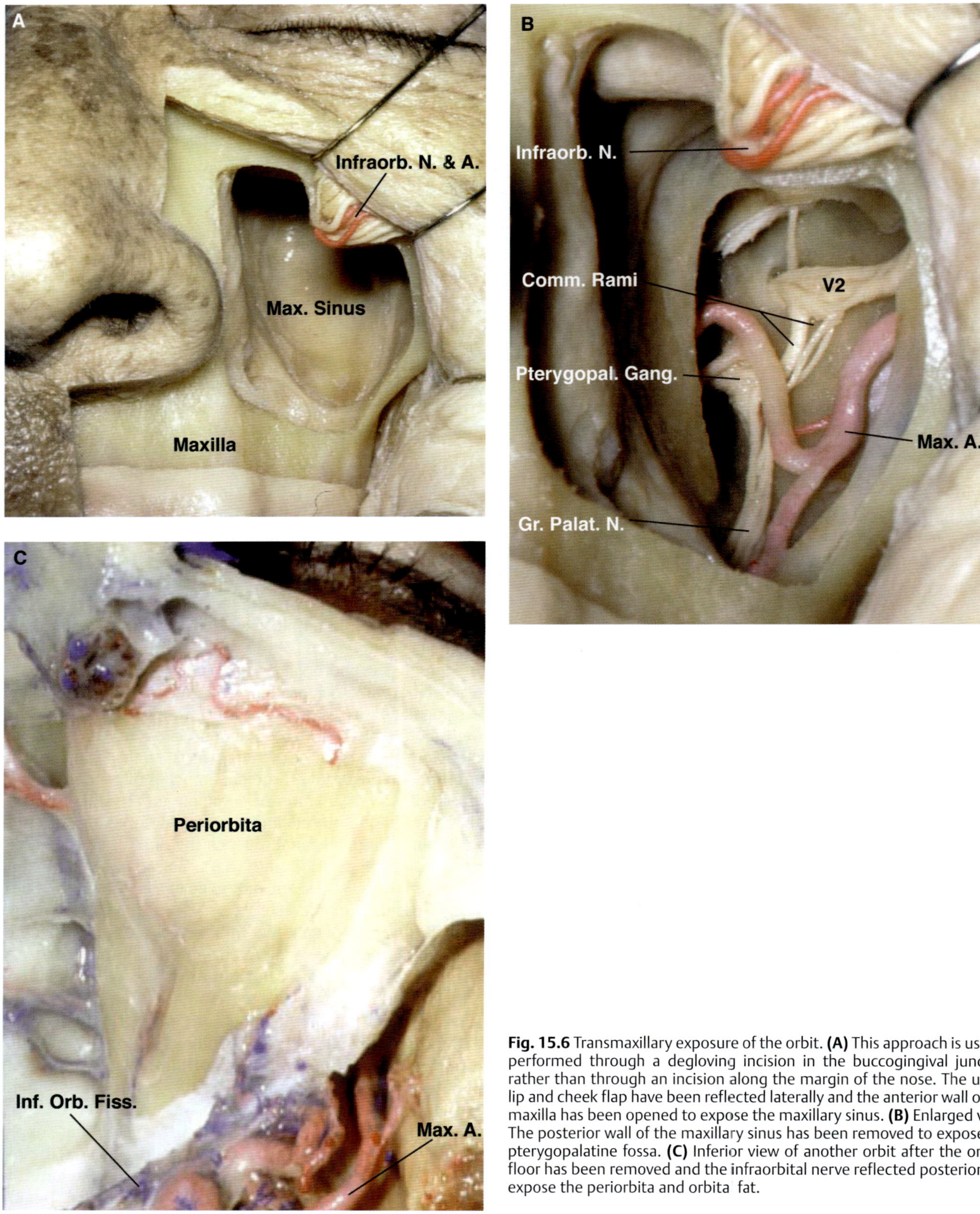

Fig. 15.6 Transmaxillary exposure of the orbit. **(A)** This approach is usually performed through a degloving incision in the buccogingival junction rather than through an incision along the margin of the nose. The upper lip and cheek flap have been reflected laterally and the anterior wall of the maxilla has been opened to expose the maxillary sinus. **(B)** Enlarged view. The posterior wall of the maxillary sinus has been removed to expose the pterygopalatine fossa. **(C)** Inferior view of another orbit after the orbital floor has been removed and the infraorbital nerve reflected posteriorly to expose the periorbita and orbita fat.

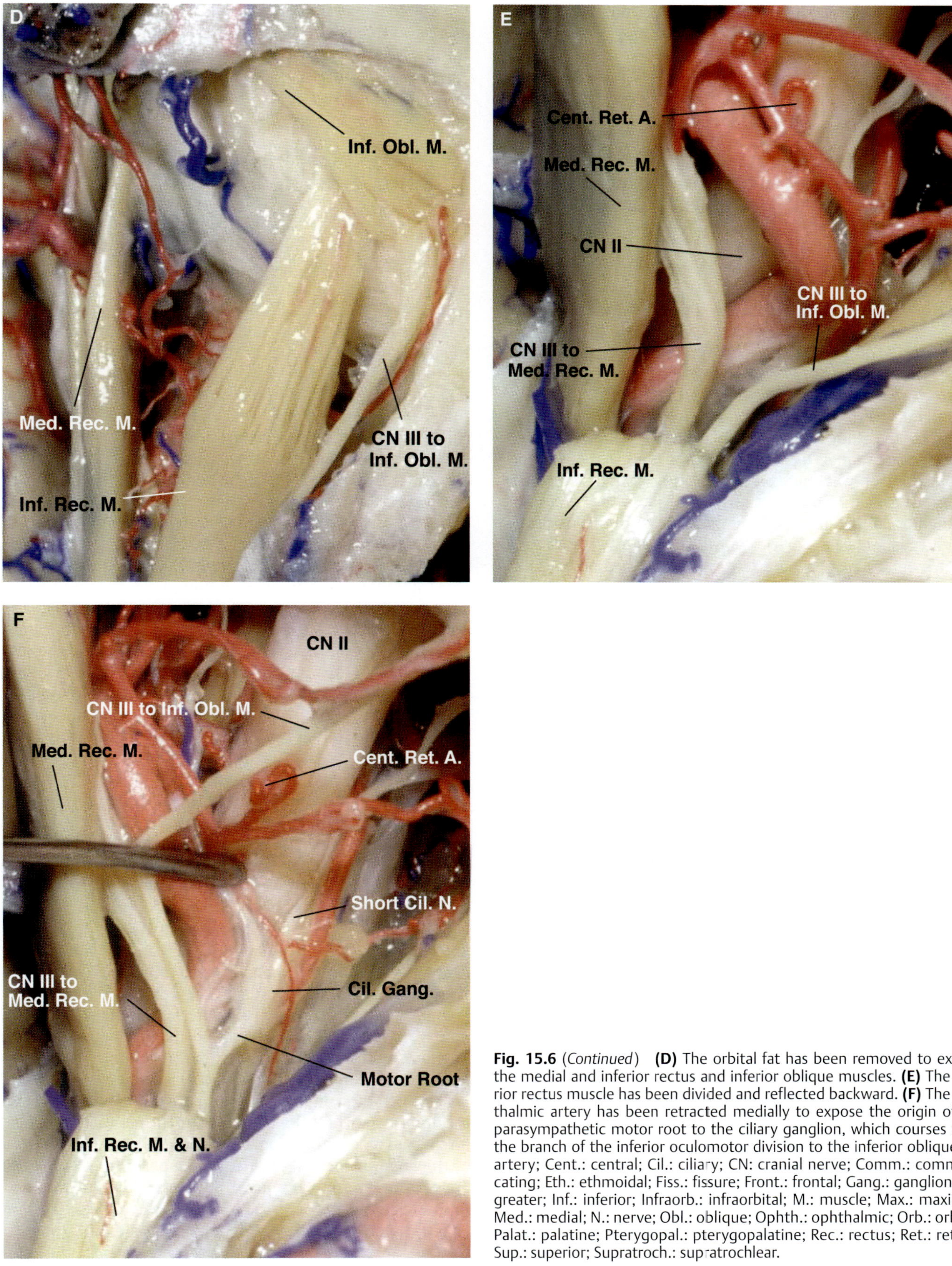

Fig. 15.6 (*Continued*) **(D)** The orbital fat has been removed to expose the medial and inferior rectus and inferior oblique muscles. **(E)** The inferior rectus muscle has been divided and reflected backward. **(F)** The ophthalmic artery has been retracted medially to expose the origin of the parasympathetic motor root to the ciliary ganglion, which courses from the branch of the inferior oculomotor division to the inferior oblique. A.: artery; Cent.: central; Cil.: ciliary; CN: cranial nerve; Comm.: communicating; Eth.: ethmoidal; Fiss.: fissure; Front.: frontal; Gang.: ganglion; Gr.: greater; Inf.: inferior; Infraorb.: infraorbital; M.: muscle; Max.: maxillary; Med.: medial; N.: nerve; Obl.: oblique; Ophth.: ophthalmic; Orb.: orbital; Palat.: palatine; Pterygopal.: pterygopalatine; Rec.: rectus; Ret.: retinal; Sup.: superior; Supratroch.: supratrochlear.

branch of the inferolateral trunk, and the terminal branches of the internal maxillary artery.

Venous Relationships

The venous spaces of the cavernous sinus fill the posterior margin of the superior orbital fissure and may extend forward along the medial and lower edges of the fissure (**Fig. 15.2**). The veins passing through the fissure empty into the cavernous sinus. The dural sinuses into which the sylvian veins empty commonly pass below the sphenoid ridge and along the intracranial edge of the lateral margin of the superior orbital fissure to reach the cavernous sinus. These sinuses are encountered in exposures directed through the lateral margin of the fissure. The superior ophthalmic vein arises from tributaries in the superomedial part of the orbit, and the inferior ophthalmic vein arises from tributaries in the inferolateral part of the orbit (**Figs. 15.2** and **15.4**). These veins are connected along the anterior margin of the orbit by large anastomotic channels formed by the facial and angular veins. This inferior ophthalmic vein may empty directly into the cavernous sinus, but more commonly, joins the superior ophthalmic vein to form a common stem that drains into the cavernous sinus. The superior ophthalmic vein arises in the upper medial part of the orbit, passes backward on the lateral side of the superior oblique muscle, and crosses above the optic nerve to reach the lateral part of the orbit. It exits the muscle cone by passing between the heads of the superior and lateral rectus muscles and outside the annular tendon, through the narrow lateral part of the superior orbital fissure. It passes downward along the lateral margin of the annular tendon at the level of the superior orbital fissure, where it is commonly joined by the inferior ophthalmic vein to form a common trunk that enters the anteroinferior part of the cavernous sinus.

Both the superior ophthalmic vein and the ophthalmic artery course along the superolateral aspect of the optic nerve in the orbital apex, but the vein passes outside the annular tendon and through the narrow lateral part of the superior orbital fissure, whereas the artery passes through the annular tendon and the optic foramen. The superior ophthalmic vein is anchored in the lateral corner of the superior orbital fissure by several fibrous bands that form a hammock around the vein, creating an obstacle to approaches to the lateral part of the orbital apex. The inferior ophthalmic vein originates from tributaries on the anterior part of the floor and lateral wall of the orbit. It drains the inferior rectus and inferior oblique muscles, the lacrimal sac, and eyelids. It courses medially and posteriorly between the lateral and inferior rectus muscles with the branch of the oculomotor nerve to the inferior oblique muscle. It communicates with the pterygoid venous plexus through the inferior orbital fissure. It exits the muscle cone by passing between the origin of the lateral and inferior rectus muscles and the orbit, coursing below the annular tendon and through the inferior sector of the superior orbital fissure. It commonly joins the superior ophthalmic vein on the lateral aspect the annular tendon as it passes through the superior orbital fissure. The common trunk passes backward to enter the anteroinferior part of the cavernous sinus.

Muscular and Tendinous Relationships

The orbicularis oculi muscle surrounds the circumference of the orbit and spreads out on the temple and cheek (**Fig. 15.7**). It has orbital, palpebral, and lacrimal parts. The orbital part spreads in a wide band around the margin of the orbit. The palpebral part is located in the margins of the eyelids. The orbital part arises from the nasal process of the frontal bone, the frontal process of the maxilla, and the medial palpebral ligament. On the lateral side, it blends with the occipitofrontalis and the corrugator muscles. Many of the upper orbital fibers are inserted into the skin and subcutaneous tissues of the eyebrow. The palpebral part arises from the medial palpebral ligament and the bone above and below the ligament. Some of its fibers lie close to the margin of the eyelid behind the eyelashes. The lacrimal part extends behind the lacrimal sac and attaches to the lacrimal bone. The orbital part is the sphincter muscle of the eyelids. The palpebral portion closes the eyelids. The actions of the lacrimal part are important in tear transport. The tarsi are two thin plates of dense fibrous tissue situated deep to the palpebral part of the orbicularis oculi muscle. The tarsi are placed in and give support and shape to each eyelid. Some of the fibers of the levator muscle are attached to the upper tarsus. The medial ends of the tarsi are attached by a tendinous band, the medial palpebral ligament, to the upper part of the lacrimal crest and the adjoining part of the frontal process of the maxilla in front of the lacrimal crest. The lateral ends of the tarsi are attached by a band, the lateral palpebral ligament, to a tubercle on the zygomatic bone immediately within the orbital margin.

The orbital septum is a membranous sheet attached to the orbital margin where it is continuous with the periosteum along the anterior edge of the orbit. It separates the facial from the orbital structures. In the upper eyelid, the septum blends with the superficial part of the aponeurosis of the superior levator, and in the lower eyelid, it blends with the anterior surface of the tarsus. The medial and lateral cheek ligaments are fibrous expansions extending from sheaths of the lateral and medial rectus muscles that attach to the zygomatic and lacrimal bone, respectively. The cheek ligaments limit the actions of the lateral and medial rectus muscles. The four rectus muscles arise from the annular tendon and form a cone around the neural and vascular structures passing through the annulus. The annular tendon is adherent to the dural sheath of the optic nerve and the periosteum above, below, and medial to the optic canal and to the lateral margin of the superior orbital fissure. The superior rectus muscle arises from the annular tendon, passes forward, and attaches to the sclera posterior to the margin of the cornea. The line of attachment is slightly oblique and curved. The superior oblique muscle arises from the periorbita covering the body

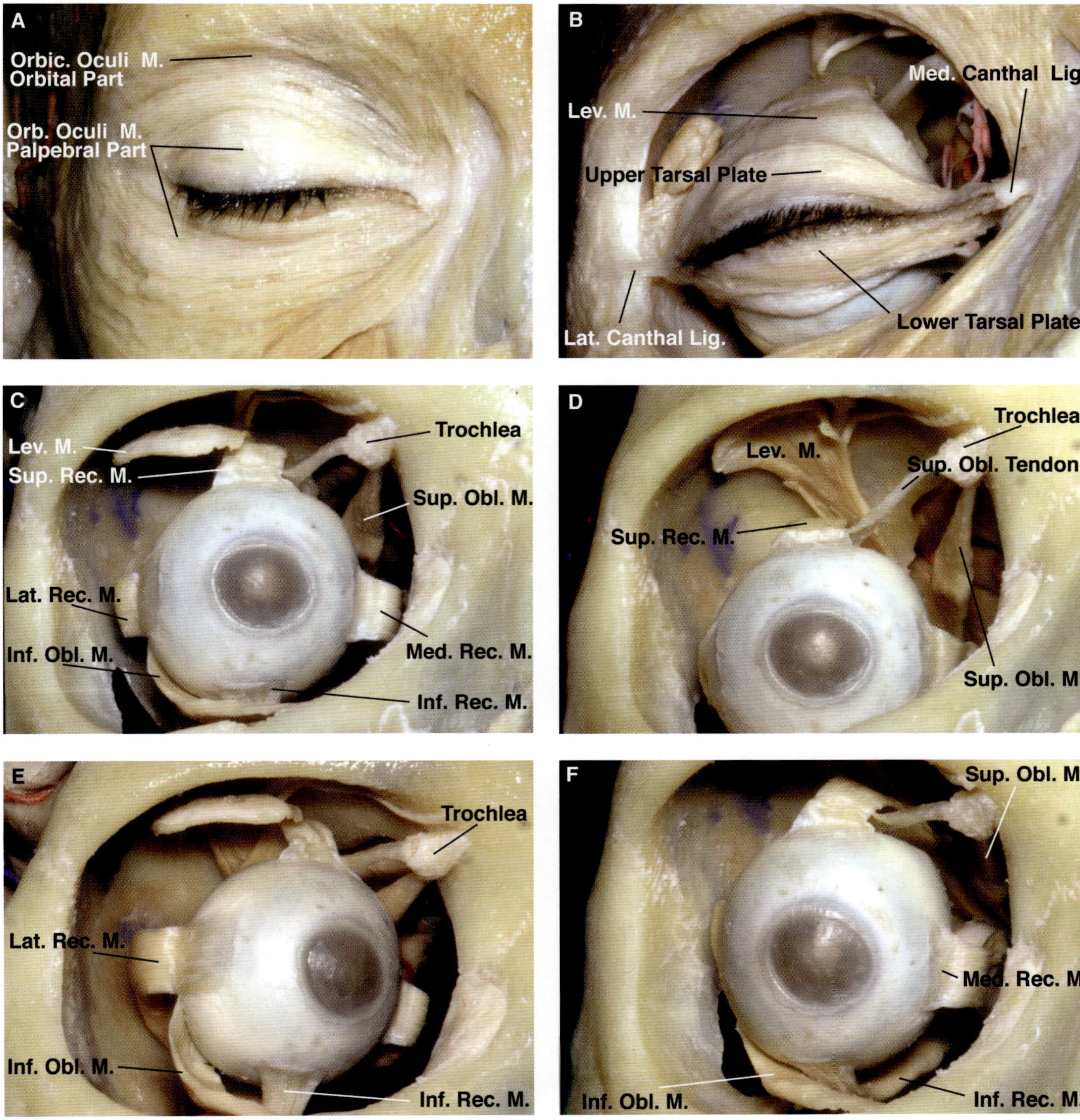

Fig. 15.7 Anterior view of orbit and extraocular muscles. **(A)** The skin around the right orbit has been removed to expose the orbicularis oculi muscle. **(B)** The orbicular muscle has been removed to expose the upper and lower tarsi, thin plates of dense fibrous tissue situated deep to the palpebral part of the orbicularis oculi muscle. **(C)** The globe and the optic nerve are surrounded by the four rectus, the levator, and two oblique muscles. **(D)** Globe depressed to show the insertion of the superior rectus muscle and the trochlea and distal tendon of the superior oblique muscle. **(E)** Globe adducted to show the insertion of the lateral rectus muscle. **(F)** Globe positioned to show the relationship of the inferior rectus and inferior oblique muscles. Inf.: inferior; Lat.: lateral; Lev.: levator; Lig.: ligament; M.: muscle; Med.: medial; Obl.: oblique; Orb.: orbit; Rec.: rectus; Sup.: superior.

of the sphenoid bone superomedial to the optic canal and runs forward, ending in a tendon that loops through the trochlea, a round tendon that attaches to the trochlear fossa of the frontal bone. After looping through the trochlea, the tendon passes laterally and posteriorly below the superior rectus muscle to insert on the sclera between the superior and lateral rectus muscles. The lateral rectus muscle arises from the annular tendon and adjacent part of the greater wing of the sphenoid bone and has a vertical line of attachment to the sclera posterior to the margin of the cornea. The inferior rectus muscle arises from the annular tendon and has an oblique line of attachment, with the medial side slightly anterior to the lateral side of the attachment. The inferior oblique muscle arises from the part of the orbital floor formed by the orbital surface of the maxilla in the area just lateral to the nasolacrimal duct, not from the orbital apex. It runs laterally and posteriorly, passing between the inferior rectus muscle and the orbital floor, and then between the lateral rectus muscle and the globe, to insert into the sclera between the superior and lateral rectus muscles near the insertion of the superior oblique muscle. The medial rectus muscle arises from the annular tendon, runs forward, and has a vertical line of attachment to the sclera. The orbital smooth muscle (Müller's muscle) spans the upper margin of the inferior orbital fissure, and blends into the periorbita, the periosteum of the maxillary bone, and the perineurium of the infraorbital nerve.

■ Surgical Considerations

The earliest reports of surgery for orbital lesions involved approaches directed through the lateral wall of the orbit.[6,7] The first report of a transcranial approach to the orbit was published in 1922 by Dandy.[8] Since then, both extra- and intracranial routes to orbital lesions have been developed.[9–11] The transcranial approach is commonly selected for tumors located in the orbital apex and/or optic canal, or involving both the orbit and adjacent intracranial areas.[8,12,13] Tumors confined within the periorbita in the anterior two thirds of the orbit can often be approached extracranially, but those located in the apical area, and especially those on the medial side of the optic nerve, often require a transcranial approach. An approach directed through the lateral orbital wall, involving an osteotomy of lateral rim and wall, is commonly selected for tumors confined to the superior, lateral, or inferior compartment of the orbit and those in the lateral part of the apex.[6,7] An approach directed along the medial orbital wall may be used for tumors located medial to the optic nerve that are not located deep in the apex.[7,14,15] The transcranial surgical approaches to the orbit may be arbitrarily divided into two types based on whether the orbital rim is or is not elevated in exposing the orbital lesion. Early approaches involved removal of a frontal or frontotemporal bone flap, with preservation of the supraorbital rim, and opening of the orbit behind the rim.[10,16–22] The transcranial approach can be tailored to the site of the lesion. For limited lesions, an approach directed through a small frontal craniotomy or frontotemporal craniotomy, with removal of the orbital roof and/or lateral wall, will provide access. However, for larger lesions, it is advantageous to elevate the orbital rim with the bone flap as is performed in the orbitofrontal or orbitozygomatic approach. In the orbitofrontal approach, only the upper rim of the orbit is elevated, and in the orbitozygomatic approach, the superior and lateral parts of the orbital rim are elevated. The orbitofrontal craniotomy would be selected for lesions involving the optic canal and orbital apex. The orbitozygomatic craniotomy would be selected for orbital lesions involving the middle fossa or superior orbital fissure, in addition to the orbit.

The Medial Orbitofrontal Approach

The medial approach is directed through the space between the superior oblique muscle, which is retracted medially, and the levator and superior rectus muscles, both of which are retracted laterally (**Fig. 15.5B**). This approach exposes the optic nerve throughout the interval from the globe to the optic canal. It is the most direct surgical approach to the apical part of the optic nerve.

The following structures are on the medial side of the optic nerve: anteriorly near the globe, the ophthalmic artery, the nasociliary nerve, and the superior ophthalmic vein; and posteriorly near the orbital apex, the trochlear nerve and the posterior ethmoidal artery. The interval between the anteriorly and posteriorly situated structures is free of important structures, thus providing a route to the optic nerve. The medial approach is selected for lesions located superomedial to the optic nerve or for cases in which there is a need to expose the optic nerve from the optic canal to the globe. It is the approach most commonly selected for tumors of the optic sheath or optic nerve. The medial approach is not suitable for lesions located on the lateral side of the optic nerve or for those involving the superior orbital fissure and the cavernous sinus.

The Central and the Lateral Orbitofrontal Approaches

In the central approach, the levator muscle is retracted medially and the superior rectus muscle is retracted laterally. The central approach, which is the least used of the three approaches directed through an orbitofrontal craniotomy, is the most direct and shortest way to the midportion of the intraorbital segment of the optic nerve (**Fig. 15.5**).

For the lateral approach, the optic nerve is approached between the lateral rectus muscle, which is retracted laterally, and the superior rectus and levator muscles, both of which are retracted medially. The lateral approach provides a wider working space than the medial or central approach. The wider angle of access allows the approach to be directed through all parts of the orbitofrontal exposure. It is the best of the three orbitofrontal routes for exposing the deep apical area on the lateral side of the optic nerve.

Transmaxillary Approach

The transmaxillary approach, directed through the orbital floor, is most commonly performed using a sublabial incision in the gingivobuccal margin rather than through an incision on the face.[23,24] Soft tissues are elevated to expose the anterior surface of the right maxilla (**Figs. 15.6** and **15.8**). The approach can be completed without dividing the infraorbital nerve at the infraorbital foramen, but if divided, it can be resutured at the time of closing. Removing the anterior wall of the maxillary sinus exposes the infraorbital canal in the roof of the sinus, which forms the orbital floor. Opening the orbital floor exposes the periorbita covering the orbital floor and the infraorbital artery and nerve. Structures that may be exposed include the inferior and medial rectus and inferior oblique muscles, the inferior division of the oculomotor nerve and its branches, the ciliary ganglion and its roots, plus short ciliary nerves that arise in the ciliary ganglion and pierce the sclera around the optic nerve and the central retinal artery. This approach may be used to reconstruct the orbital floor after trauma or to open the floor for orbital decompression.

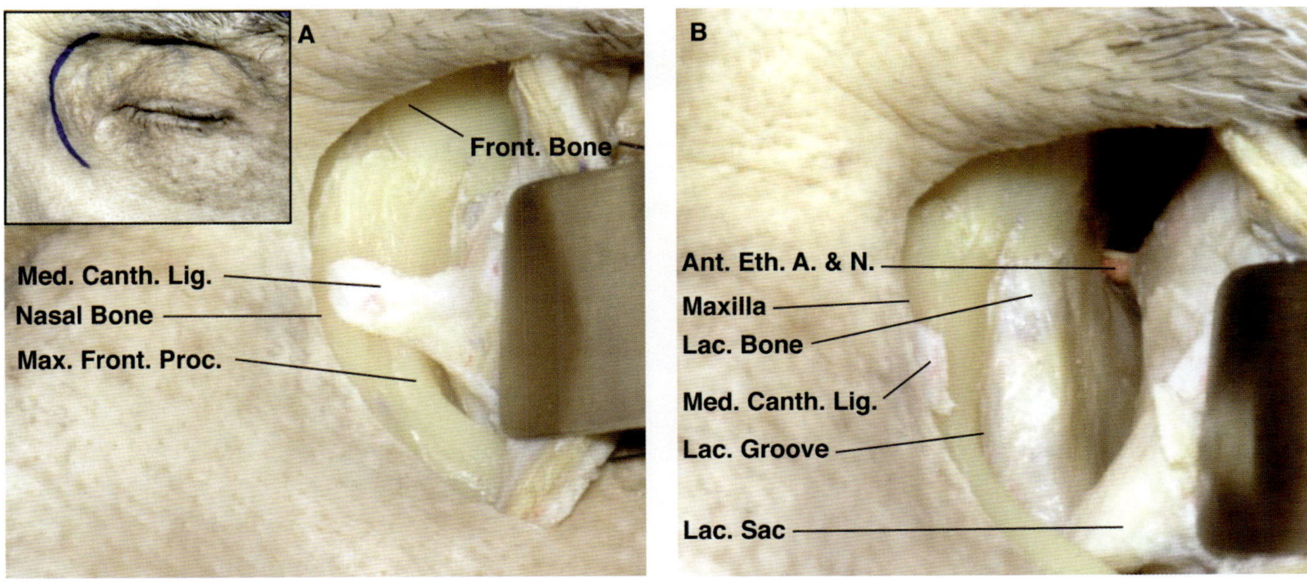

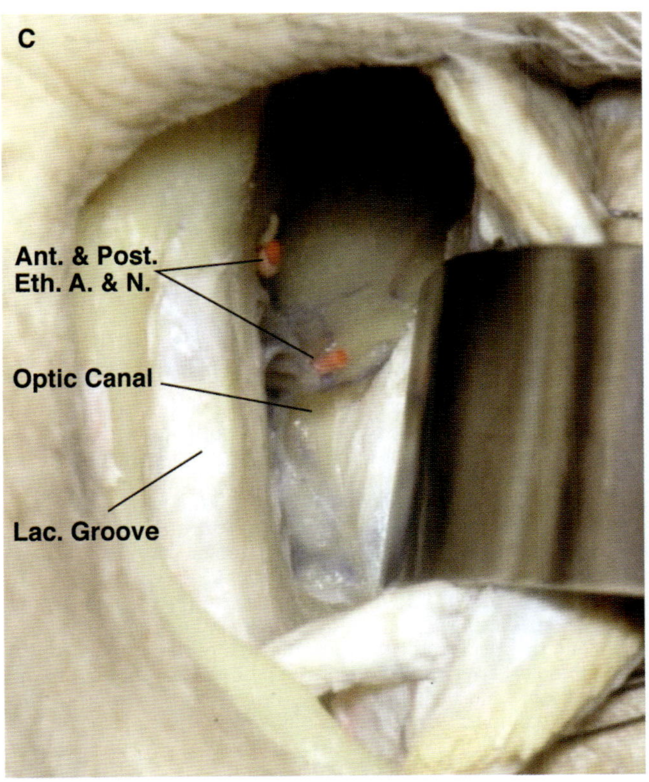

Fig. 15.8 Medial orbital approach. **(A–C)** Medial orbital exposure. **(A)** The medial orbital incision on the left side is shown in the inset. The approach exposes the medial orbital wall, ethmoid air cells, and sphenoid sinus back to the level of the optic canal. The periorbita has been elevated from the frontal process of the maxillary bone and adjacent frontal bone forming the medial part of the orbital rim to expose the medial canthal ligament, which, if divided, should be reapproximated at the end of the procedure to maintain canthal balance. **(B)** The medial palpebral ligament has been divided and the edges of the divided ligament have been preserved for reapproximation at the end of the procedure. The lacrimal sac has been retracted laterally. The exposure extends backward along the lacrimal and ethmoid bones to the level where the anterior ethmoidal artery enters the anterior ethmoidal canal. **(C)** The exposure has been extended backward along the ethmoid, lacrimal, and frontal bones, past the level where the anterior and posterior ethmoidal arteries enter the anterior and posterior ethmoidal canal to the orbital apex and anterior end of the optic canal. The medial ethmoid air cells and adjacent part of the sphenoid sinus can be removed to expose the optic nerve in the optic canal. This approach is sometimes used to decompress the optic canal. (*continued on next page*)

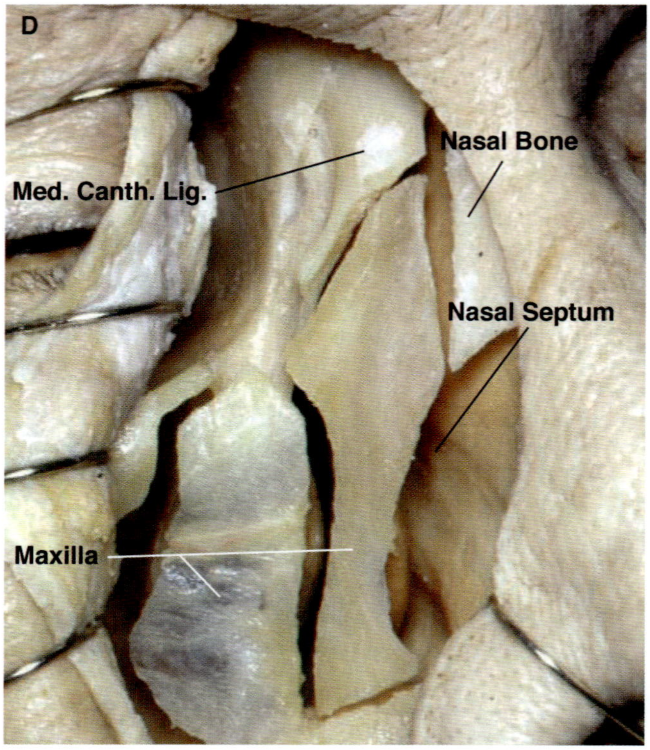

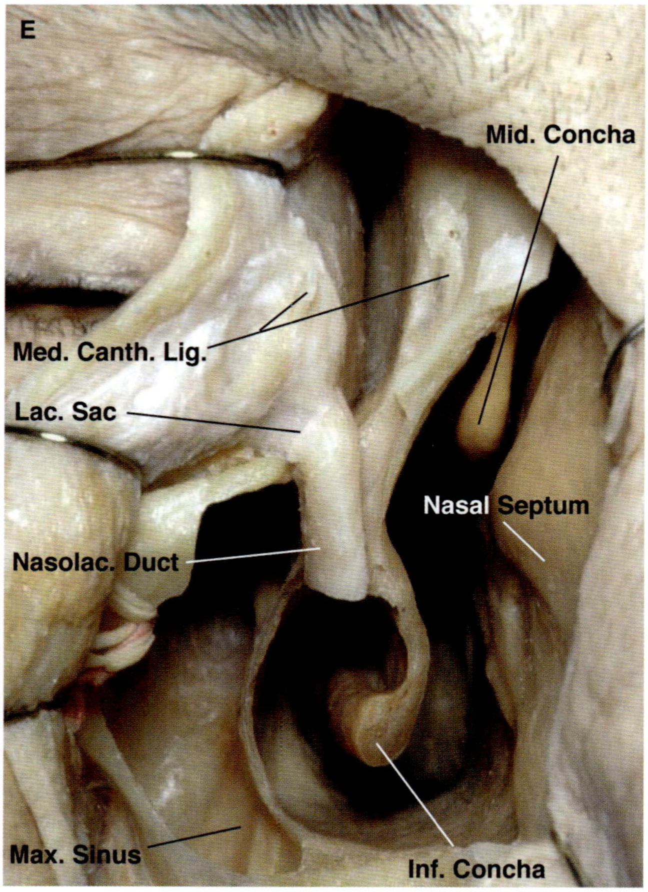

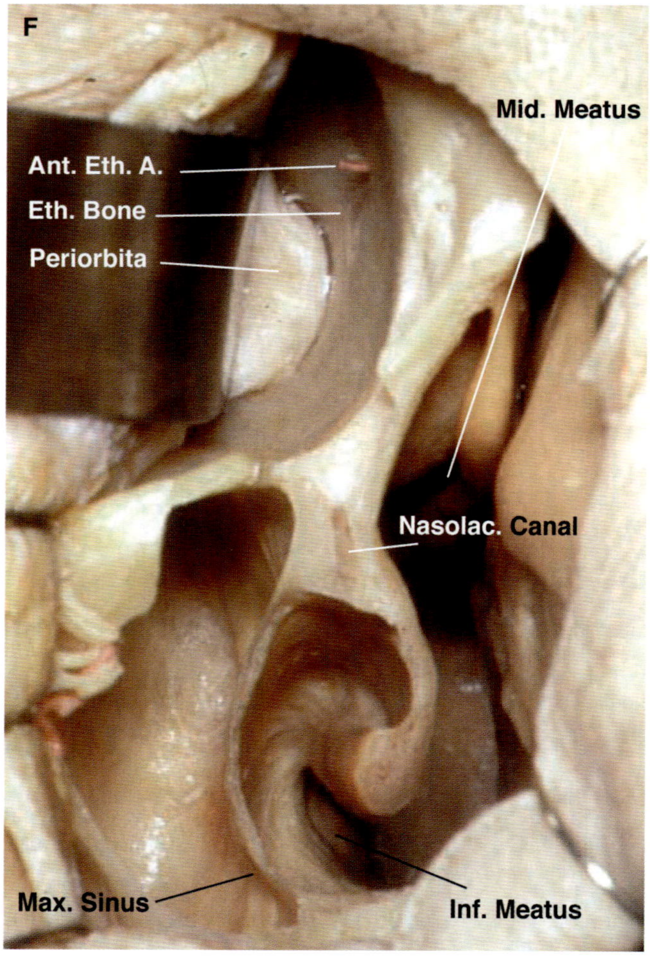

Fig. 15.8 *(Continued)* **(D–F)** Combined medial orbital and maxillary exposures. **(D)** The exposure includes not only the medial orbital wall, but also the adjacent part of the floor. Two small maxillary osteotomies have been completed. The medial one includes the part of the maxilla forming the anterior wall of the nasal cavity. The lateral osteotomy exposes the anterior part of the maxillary sinus. The medial palpebral ligament has been divided to expose the medial wall of the orbit. **(E)** Removing the medial osteotomy fragment exposes the nasal cavity and the nasal septum and inferior and middle conchae. Removing the lateral osteotomy fragment exposes the maxillary sinus, medial part of the orbital floor, and the nasolacrimal duct, which courses along the medial maxillary wall and opens below the inferior concha into the inferior meatus. **(F)** The nasolacrimal duct and lacrimal sac have been retracted laterally and the exposure extended along the medial orbital wall to the area posterior to where the anterior ethmoidal artery was divided. The posterior part of the osseous nasolacrimal canal has been exposed. A.: artery; Ant.: anterior; Canth.: canthal; Eth.: ethmoidal; Front.: frontal; Inf.: inferior; Lac.: lacrimal; Lig.: ligament; Max.: maxillary; Med.: medial; Mid.: middle; N.: nerve; Nasolac.: nasolacrimal; Post.: posterior; Proc.: process.

Medial Orbital and Transethmoidal Approaches

The medial orbital incision can be used to provide access to the area lateral to the lacrimal and ethmoid bones back to the orbital apex, and with removal with some of the ethmoid air cells and sphenoid sinus facing the orbit, the optic canal can be exposed or decompressed (**Fig. 15.8**).[23,24] The medial orbital incision extends between the medial orbit and nose along the frontal process of the maxillary bone. The exposure is extended using subperiosteal and subperiorbital dissection except at the medial canthal ligament, which is attached to the anterior and posterior margins of the lacrimal groove, and which should be divided or elevated in such a way that it can be preserved and reapproximated if divided. The lacrimal sac, which sits in the lacrimal groove, can usually be elevated. Behind this, the anterior ethmoidal branch of the ophthalmic artery is encountered as it penetrates the periorbita to enter the anterior ethmoidal canal. This artery is divided if a more posterior exposure is needed. As the exposure proceeds, posteriorly along the orbital plate of the ethmoid, the posterior ethmoidal artery is encountered entering the posterior ethmoidal canal. It passes medially along the planum sphenoidale and can be divided. The optic canal is found approximately 7 mm behind the posterior ethmoidal canal.[24] Removing some of the ethmoid plate and adjacent part of the sphenoid sinus will expose the optic nerve in the optic canal. Extending the medial orbital incision downward, lateral to the nose, provides access to the anterior part of the maxilla. Removing the medial part of the anterior wall of the maxillary sinus bordering the nasal cavity provides access to the medial orbital floor.

References

1. Natori Y, Rhoton AL Jr. Transcranial approach to the orbit: microsurgical anatomy. J Neurosurg 1994;81:78–86
2. Natori Y, Rhoton AL Jr. Microsurgical anatomy of the superior orbital fissure. Neurosurgery 1995;36:762–775
3. Rhoton AL Jr, Natori Y. The Orbit and Sellar Region: Microsurgical Anatomy and Operative Approaches. New York: Thieme Medical Publishers, 1996:3–25
4. Harris FS, Rhoton AL Jr. Anatomy of the cavernous sinus. A microsurgical study. J Neurosurg 1976;45:169–180
5. Liu Q, Rhoton AL Jr. Middle meningeal origin of the ophthalmic artery. Neurosurgery 2001;49:401–406, discussion 406–407
6. Krönlein RU. Zur Pathologie und operativen Behandlung der Dermoidcysten der Orbita. Beitr Klin Chir 1889;4:149–163
7. Maroon JC, Kennerdell JS. Surgical approaches to the orbit. Indications and techniques. J Neurosurg 1984;60:1226–1235
8. Dandy WE. Prechiasmal intracranial tumors of the optic nerves. Am J Ophthalmol 1922;5:169–188
9. Al-Mefty O, Fox JL. Superolateral orbital exposure and reconstruction. Surg Neurol 1985;23:609–613
10. Housepian EM. Surgical treatment of unilateral optic nerve gliomas. J Neurosurg 1969;31:604–607
11. Jane JA, Park TS, Pobereskin LH, Winn HR, Butler AB. The supraorbital approach: technical note. Neurosurgery 1982;11:537–542
12. Hassler W, Eggert HR. Extradural and intradural microsurgical approaches to lesions of the optic canal and the superior orbital fissure. Acta Neurochir (Wien) 1985;74:87–93
13. Housepian EM. Microsurgical anatomy of the orbital apex and principles of transcranial orbital exploration. Clin Neurosurg 1978;25:556–573
14. Kelman SE, Heaps R, Wolf A, Elman MJ. Optic nerve decompression surgery improves visual function in patients with pseudotumor cerebri. Neurosurgery 1992;30:391–395
15. Niho S, Niho M, Niho K. Decompression of the optic canal by the transethmoidal route and decompression of the superior orbital fissure. Can J Ophthalmol 1970;5:22–40
16. Frazier CH. I. An Approach to the hypophysis through the anterior cranial fossa. Ann Surg 1913;57:145–150
17. Hamby WB. Pterional approach to the orbits for decompression or tumor removal. J Neurosurg 1964;21:15–18
18. Jackson H. Orbital tumours. Proc R Soc Med 1945;38:587–594
19. Love JG, Benedict WL. Transcranial removal of intraorbital tumors. JAMA 1945;129:777–784
20. MacCarty CS, Brown DN. Orbital tumors in children. Clin Neurosurg 1964;11:76–93
21. McArthur LL. An aseptic surgical access to the pituitary body and its neighborhood. JAMA 1912;LVIII:2009–2011
22. Naffziger HC. Progressive exophthalmos following thyroidectomy: Its pathology and treatment. Ann Surg 1931;94:582–586
23. Hitotsumatsu T, Rhoton AL Jr. Unilateral upper and lower subtotal maxillectomy approaches to the cranial base: microsurgical anatomy. Neurosurgery 2000;46:1416–1452, discussion 1452–1453
24. Hitotsumatsu T, Matsushima T, Rhoton AL Jr. Surgical anatomy of the midface and the midline skull base. In: Spetzler RF, ed. Operative Techniques in Neurosurgery, vol. 2. Philadelphia: WB Saunders, 1999: 160–180

16 Endoscopic Periorbital and Optic Nerve Surgery and Intraorbital Resections

Richard J. Harvey, Raymond Sacks, Aldo Cassol Stamm, and João Flávio Nogueira

Tips and Pearls

- Finding the orbital axis, via the orbital floor, in a wide sphenoidotomy with lateral wall identification, is essential.
- Pathology lateral to the neural axis (lateral to the optic and infraorbital nerves) usually requires an external approach.
- Preservation of the frontal recess and very wide antrostomy is important to ensure normal postoperative sinonasal function.
- The medial rectus lies closer to the periorbita posteriorly.
- The ophthalmic artery is inferior in the canal when incising the optic nerve sheath.
- Defining and dividing the ethmoidal arteries, whether transorbital or transethmoidal, is critical for access to the orbital roof.

Introduction

External approaches to the orbit are essential in managing pathology lateral to the optic nerve and globe (the neural axis). For those lesions that are medial to the neural axis or displace the neural structures laterally, endoscopic approaches offer an incision-free approach. Additionally, there is preservation of sinonasal physiology in the approach for orbital and periorbital pathology. Endoscopic approaches also include endoscopic-assisted transcaruncular, transconjunctival[1,2] (to the floor), transblepharoplasty[3] (to the roof) approaches to the orbit, and transsupraorbital craniotomy.[4] However, this chapter focuses on the endoscopic transnasal/sinus surgery.

Endoscopic techniques rely on the presence of an operative cavity in which to work. Distensible spaces are created in laparoscopic surgery, and, similarly, sinus cavities provide the operative field in sinus surgery. However, the intraorbital fat precludes easy operative working space in the orbit. Distension of the intraconal tissues is limited due to the bony confines of the orbit. Although lateral orbitotomy can be performed to allow temporary lateral shift of intraorbital structures,[5] significant limitations remain in the ability to create a working space within orbital fat.

Utilizing the maxillary, ethmoid, and sphenoid sinuses to define the orbital axis and create a working space is a fundamental part of our endoscopic orbital surgery (**Fig. 16.1**). Further subperiosteal (subperiorbital) dissection can occur both superior and inferior around the orbital contents to access pathology. Once the periorbita is opened, however, prior displacement of orbital fat by pathology is important to have a workable operative field. Orbital fat can be displaced, removed, or ablated to reach pathology, but the conal muscles and neurovascular structures within the orbit make this a challenging exercise. The lack of dead space due to the intermuscular septations and ubiquitous fat will always obscure visualization if not previously displaced.

Indications and Advantages

Posterior access to pathology near the orbital apex is excellent via an endoscopic approach. The near vision view allows

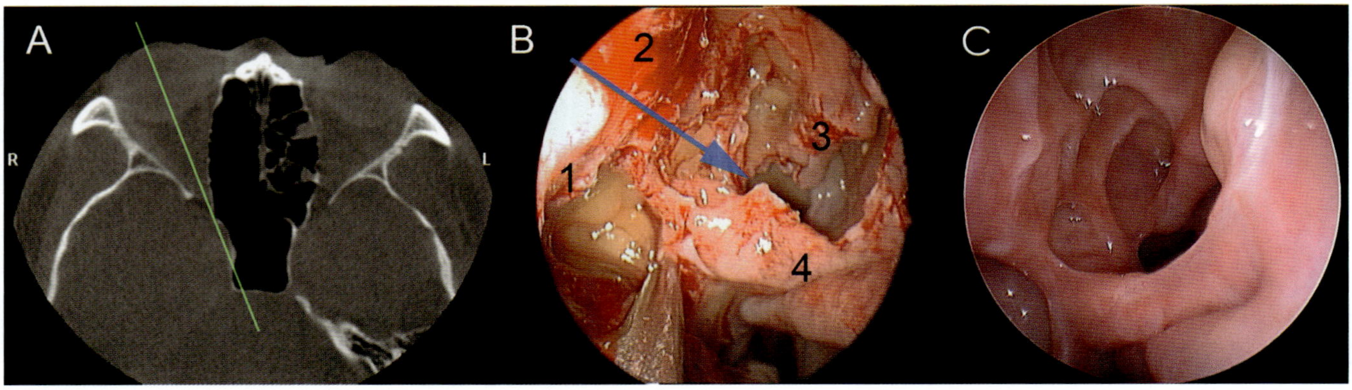

Fig. 16.1 The orbital axis. Defining the line of the orbit in endoscopic surgery is important **(A,B)**. It also allows easy postoperative surveillance **(C)**.

easy identification of the optic nerve transition to the orbit apex and fibrous annulus. Endoscopic approaches also avoid disruption of the orbicularis oculi, lacrimal pump, or canthal ligament disruption. The final access to any orbital pathology will ultimately need to be customized to the patient and the lesion. However, the final goal should always be to preserve ocular function and effectively treat the pathology. The combined efforts of both the ophthalmologist and the rhinologist are essential to ensure an optimal outcome for extended endoscopic orbital surgery.[5–7]

A summary of common indications for endoscopic orbital surgery is presented below. Thyroid eye disease and inflammatory conditions, such as subperiosteal abscess, are not discussed in this chapter.[8,9] However, the surgical management of these lesions utilizes the same principles discussed for managing more extended pathology. Absolute contraindications to the endoscopic approach are pathology lateral to the neural axis and a lack of specialized equipment and expertise. A relative contraindication is the presence of acute or subacute sinusitis. These conditions should be managed medically if possible prior to any intervention. Chronic rhinosinusitis is not a contraindication, as many of the persistent mucosal changes in this condition are inflammatory rather than infective. Chronic mucosal disease is often present in managing these lesions because sinonasal dysfunction often occurs from the local effects of large masses.

Common Indications

Extraconal Pathology

Neoplastic
- Meningioma[10]
- Osteoma[11]
- Inverted papilloma[12]
- Solitary fibrous tumor[13]
- Malignant disease[14]
- Chondrosarcoma
- Optic nerve trauma (sheath excision)[15–17]
- Fibro-osseous[18]

Intraconal Pathology

Hemangioma[19,20]
Schwannoma
Removal of foreign body[21]

Diagnostic Workup

Radiologic Assessment

Orbital evaluation is based on the combination of magnetic resonance imaging (MRI) and computed tomography (CT). The use of fat-suppression sequences in MRI greatly assists delineation of intraorbital pathology.

Ophthalmology Assessment

Formal visual acuity and visual field assessment is required to delineate any deficit, including papilledema. Formal visual assessment is performed with an ophthalmologist. Other cranial neuropathies need to be documented.

Surgery

Instruments

There are several instruments beyond the standard endoscopic sinus surgery setup that are required to manage orbital pathology. These include a diamond burr; a bipolar, sharp right-angle knife; and suction dissection elevator.

The diamond burr is essential for three areas. First, the junction of the medial orbital wall to the lateral wall of the sphenoid results in a thick buttress of bone (optic tubercle[22]). Controlled removal of bone and subsequent exposure of the optic canal in the lateral sphenoid wall is required. The optic canal is too narrow for rongeurs to be used for bone removal. Second, the medial orbital wall is commonly too thick to simply fracture and discover the periorbita. Thinning down of the bone prior to removal is important to preserve the periorbita and allow further dissection. Small amounts of fat exposed into the surgical field will have little functional significance but dramatically change the conditions of the surgical field. Fat protruding will obscure the view and increase the chance of further trauma from instruments (drills/debriders). Third, the bone around the upper lacrimal sac is often too thick to be removed with a rongeur alone. Full exposure of the lacrimal apparatus is often required in both access and reconstruction during orbital surgery.

The bipolar forceps is essential to control intraorbital vessels, especially the anterior and posterior ethmoidal arteries and control periorbital vasculature. Standard neurosurgical bayonets are often not appropriate via the long surgical corridor of endoscopic skull base surgery. Specialized bipolar instrumentation is essential. The availability of hemostatic materials and techniques are important, but the principles of hemostasis in endoscopic surgery differ little from those of open surgery. Prevention of bleeding is obviously the best solution. Tumor debulking, extracapsular sharp dissection, and countertraction using gentle suction still form the foundation of vascular control.[23]

Carefully incising the periorbita, lacrimal sac, or optic nerve sheath requires a sharp blade. Simple nasal sickle knives are often not sufficient, and No. 11 surgical blades may be too big and not allow enough freedom of movement to make angled cuts. Straight and right-angled keratome blades, dedicated dacrocystorhinostomy (DCR) blades, or beaver blades are usually required. Finally, dissection in the subperiosteal space of the orbita is often facilitated by a suction or malleable suction dissector. As the periorbita is elevated, the exposed bony haversian channels initially provide a bloody narrow surgical field that will eventually resolve. Suction instruments can be of value in the initial elevation.

Preparation

Endoscopic transnasal craniotomy is performed under general controlled hypotensive anesthesia without Mayfield fixation. Total intravenous anesthesia is associated with better mucosal hemostasis.[24,25] Cotton pledgets containing adrenaline 1:1000 are placed in the nasal cavity over the areas of surgical access for 10 minutes before the surgical procedure. The lateral nasal wall and septum are infiltrated with 1% Naropin with adrenaline 1:100.000.

Approach

Extraconal Lesions

An uncinectomy, wide antrostomy combined with anterior and posterior ethmoidectomy is performed. The antrostomy is widened superiorly to ensure that the maxillary sinus roof can be easily seen. This defines the orbital floor, allows easier skeletonization of the medial orbital wall, places the infraorbital canal on view, and is an important landmark for defining the level of the skull base posteriorly. A parallel line to the nasal floor from the maxillary sinus roof facilitates safe debulking of tumor and access to the sphenoid sinus (**Fig. 16.2**). The inferior half of the superior turbinate is resected to give access to the entire front wall of the sphenoid. The maximum amount of the front wall is then removed by commencing at the sphenoid ostium. The sphenoid sinus is key for orientation, as the roof defines the skull base and the lateral wall defines the optic nerve canal.

Prior to any pathology removal, the full axis of the orbit is usually defined (**Fig. 16.1**). Division of the sphenopalatine artery may be required to assist with hemostasis. Additional access to the orbital floor can be achieved using further access routes. A maxillary trephine through the intersection of the midpupillary point and the transverse line extending from the nasal sill allow an additional port for an endoscope or other instrument. Dental or anterior superior alveolar nerve injury is minimal using these landmarks.[26–28] The modified medial maxillectomy[29] was originally described to manage recalcitrant inflammatory disease[30,31] but has become a useful technique to increase access to the maxillary sinus and orbital floor.

Access above the orbital contents and the bony roof of the orbit is limited by the frontoethmoidal suture line and the neurovascular structures traversing it.[32] The anterior and posterior ethmoidal arteries need to be exposed either from their bony canal (**Fig. 16.3**) or on the orbital side to allow further lateral dissection on the orbital roof.[33]

Involvement of the Lacrimal System by Tumor

Anteriorly, orbital pathology may involve the lacrimal system. Depending on the extent of the involvement of the lacrimal system by the tumor, various reconstructive options are available. When tumor involves nasolacrimal duct, the duct can be completely resected along with the tumor and typically no formal reconstruction is required. After the surgical margin is defined, the remaining duct can simply be marsupialized. Should the remaining duct be less than 5 mm, then a formal DCR is preferred (**Fig. 16.4A**). For tumor involving the lacrimal sac, a formal endoscopic DCR with wide bone removal is required. The medial sac wall can be safely sacrificed and the DCR completed as per standard techniques. Occasionally the lateral sac mucosa will need to be resected, and reconstruction will need to be achieved by the placement

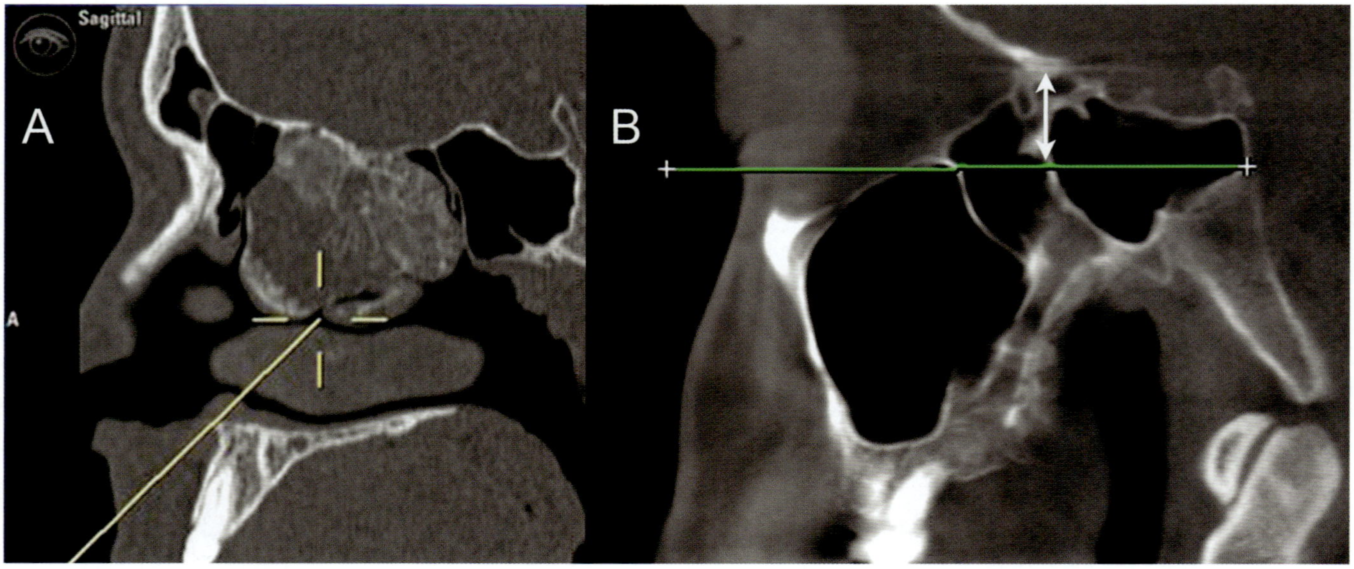

Fig. 16.2 The orbital floor. **(A)** Intraoperative orientation is important with large pathology such as this chondrosarcoma of the ethmoid. **(B)** A line from the maxillary sinus roof (parallel with reference to the nasal floor) enables safe identification of the skull base posteriorly and provides an entry to the sphenoid sinus. Discovery of the entire lateral sphenoid wall in orbital surgery is essential.

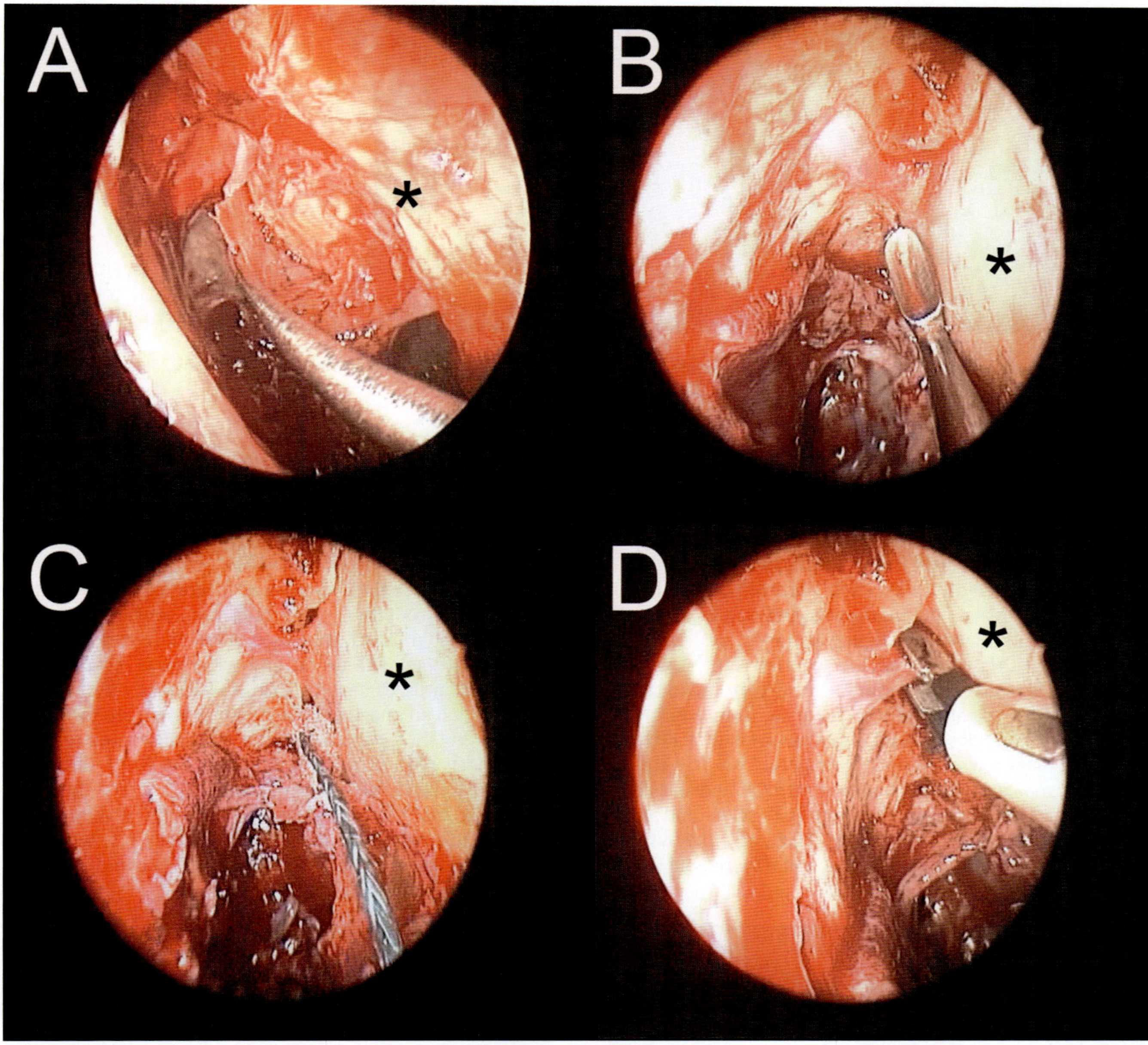

Fig. 16.3 Anterior ethmoid artery (AEA) control: ligation of the left AEA. **(A)** Removal of the medial orbital wall (*, *periorbita*). **(B)** Removal of the bony AEA canal with a curette or diamond drill. **(C)** Mobilization of a long segment, which **(D)** enables clips or bipolar forceps to control the vessel.

of a free mucosal graft. A 3-mm punch biopsy cutter is used on a Blakesley forceps to preserve the common canaliculus opening and mucosa. The remaining lateral sac is removed. A central perforation of the graft is created with the same 3-mm punch biopsy instrument. The graft is placed to provide nearly complete mucosal apposition, preserving the common canaliculus. Stenting is used, and then a Gelfoam "donut" dressing is used to secure the graft (**Fig. 16.4B**). Finally, when a tumor involves the common canaliculus, the entire sac and common canaliculus need to be resected, and reconstruction will be required by the insertion of a glass Jones tube through the medial canthus (**Fig. 16.4C**). This is best performed in combination with an ocular plastic surgeon and an endoscopic surgeon.

Intraconal Lesions

Intraconal lesions are more challenging due to the limitations of the working field, and among those lesions the cavernous hemangiomas (CHs) are the most common intraorbital tumors in adults.[34] Other lesions, such as orbital pseudotumors, can also be found. Although histologically benign, these tumors can encroach on intraorbital or adjacent structures and

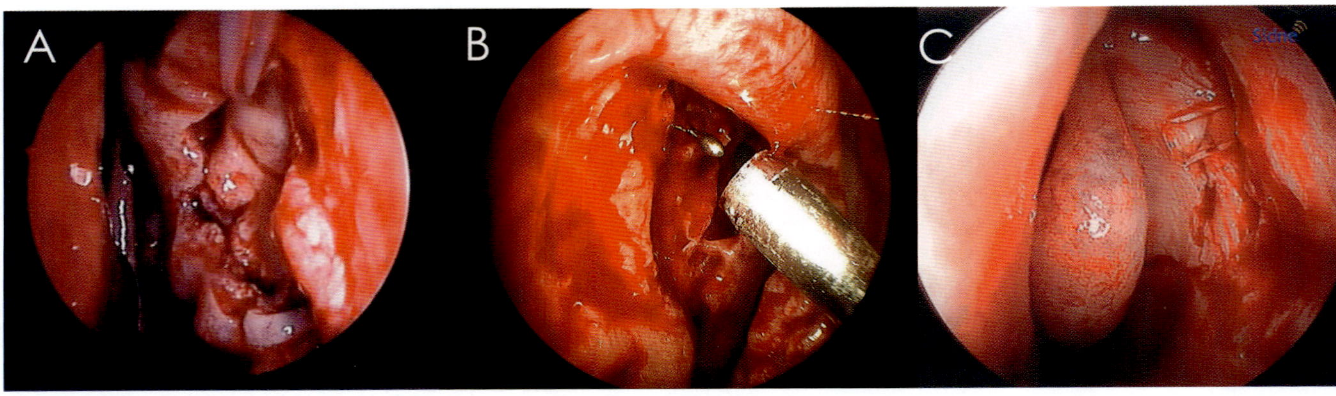

Figs. 16.4 Lacrimal management. **(A)** Left formal dacrocystorhinostomy. **(B)** Removal of entire right sac except the common canaliculus by biopsy punch. **(C)** Left Jones tube in situ.

be considered anatomically or positionally malignant.[34,35] Most of these tumors are unilateral and can increase intraorbital volume with a resultant mass effect. Visual acuity or field compromise, diplopia, and extraocular muscle or pupillary dysfunction can result from compression of intraorbital contents. The morbidity associated with orbital CH is the threat of compressive optic neuropathy, extraocular muscle dysfunction, and cosmetic disfigurement.[34,35]

Most orbital CHs require no intervention, but, especially when there is visual compromise, the surgery is indicated. The approach is dictated by the tumor location within the orbit. The typically described approaches are lateral orbitotomy, transconjunctival, or frontotemporal.[34–36] The totally endoscopic management can be performed for medial lesions, confirmed by computed tomography (CT) scans and magnetic resonance imaging (MRI) (**Fig. 16.5**), and the surgery usually starts as described previously, and if there is an Onodi cell, special care has to be taken to identify the optic nerve channel.

After large exposure, the internal carotid artery, orbital nerve, optic-carotid recess, and papyracea lamina all must be identified. A diamond burr may be used to remove the bone and better expose these structures. Attention should be given to the heat produced by the burr, and constant irrigation with saline solution must be used. After those steps, the periorbita is opened. Orbital fat and the medial rectus muscle must be identified; in some cases this identification may be difficult, and an image guidance system will need to be used. After careful dissection, the lesion is identified and removed with sharp cutting instruments (**Fig. 16.6**). If the nerve sheath is to be incised, the position of the artery should be noted (**Fig. 16.7**). The nasal cavity is packed with hemostatic reabsorbable material. The patient is usually discharged the next day. Nasal cleanings are performed to avoid any nasal

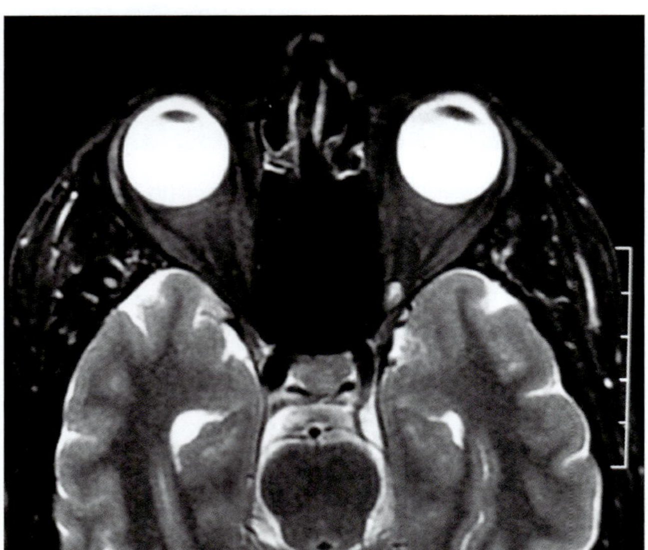

Fig. 16.5 Cavernous hemangioma. T2-weighted magnetic resonance imaging, axial view, demonstrates a hyperintense mass at the orbital apex.

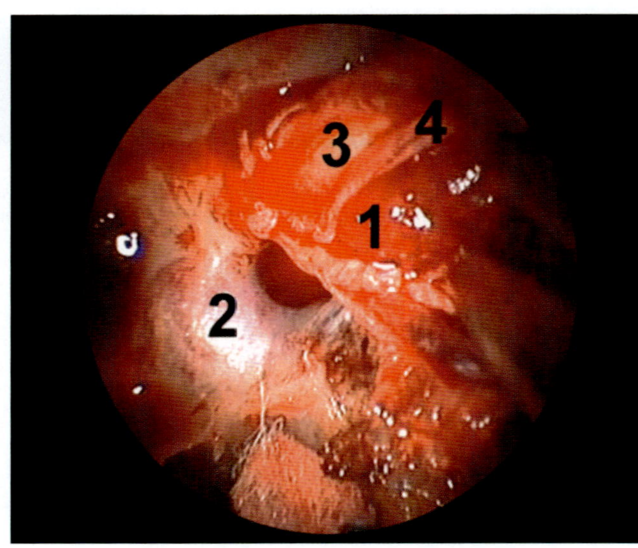

Fig. 16.6 Endoscopic resection of cavernous hemangioma. Endoscopic view with a 0-degree, 5-mm endoscope of the surgical field: 1, orbital cavernous hemangioma; 2, left internal carotid artery; 3, exposed optic nerve; 4, medial rectus muscle.

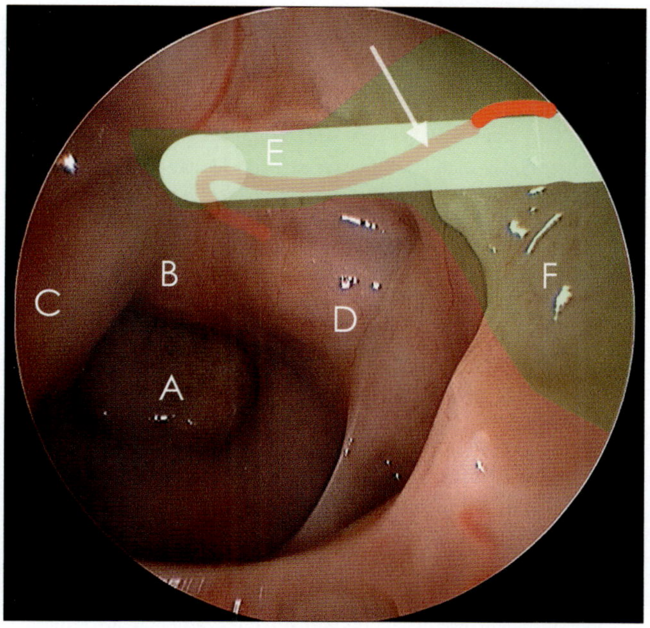

Fig. 16.7 Ophthalmic artery anatomy: A, clivus; B, sella; C, sphenoid intersinus septum; D, clival internal carotid; E, left optic canal; F: orbital apex. Arrow, position of artery.

obstruction or infection. Another eye campimetry must be performed 1 week after surgery to determine the possible recovery of the visual acuity.

Patients who present with clinically significant CH usually are middle-aged and the main complaint is of a change in visual acuity.[34] A careful clinical history and review of symptoms are paramount to formulate the differential diagnoses, which must include meningioma, fibrous histiocytoma, and hemangiopericytoma, among other orbital tumors. The radiologic and clinical features are the most important keys to provide a preoperative diagnosis idea.[34,35] Progressive and total homogeneous filling of an orbital mass on gadolinium-enhanced MRI is a pathognomonic sign of CH.[35] Most CHs are found between the optic nerve and extraocular muscles within the intraconal space, classically within the medial aspect of the orbit. They are traditionally approached through an upper eyelid or a transcaruncular-based medial orbitotomy. Endoscopic approaches can also be performed; however, this surgery requires extensive anatomical knowledge and endoscopic surgical skills.

After adequate exposure, a well-circumscribed, purple, encapsulated lesion is seen with distinct vessels on its surface. Gentle dissection allows for en-bloc removal after all vessels have been identified and cauterized with bipolar cautery.[36–38] Although external approaches provide direct exposure of the lesion, they are associated with significant morbidity. The transnasal totally endoscopic resection of intraorbital tumors is feasible and may offer some advantages when compared with the traditional approaches. However, it is paramount to have specialized instruments, such as long hand-piece drills, a good camera system, and long bipolar forceps, as well as an experienced endoscopic surgeon, especially to control vascular lesions and potential life-threatening complications.

Postoperative Care

Gelfoam or Surgiflo is used to cover exposed bone. This enhances granulation and remucosalization of these raw surfaces and reduces crusting. When the periorbita remains intact, high-volume saline irrigations improve the postoperative surgical field. They remove debris and mucus, which are inherently static during the period of postoperative mucociliary dysfunction. However, when the orbit is open, a simple saline spray is used to keep the cavity moist and prevent nose blowing. The potential for extrusion of saline and air into the orbital cavity is much greater.[39–41] After 1 to 2 weeks, high-volume positive pressure irrigation is used as discussed previously. Oral antibiotics, usually Augmentin, are utilized for 2 weeks postoperatively due to the disturbance of normal sinonasal function. If the lacrimal system is reconstructed, then dexamethasone and antibiotic ocular drops are used. Paraffin and petroleum-based ointments are avoided in the open orbital cavity due to the risk of foreign-body inflammatory reactions.[42–44]

Conclusion

Extended resections of the orbital pathology are possible via transnasal endoscopic approaches. Good surgical exposure and hemostasis are key principles in successful surgery. Defining the full length of the orbital access is a fundamental step in all cases.

References

1. Pillai P, Lubow M, Ortega A, Ammirati M. Endoscopic transconjunctival surgical approach to the optic nerve and medial intraconal space: a cadaver study. Neurosurgery 2008;63(4, Suppl 2)204–208, discussion 208–209
2. Sillers MJ, Cuilty-Siller C, Kuhn FA, Porubsky ES, Morpeth JF. Transconjunctival endoscopic orbital decompression. Otolaryngol Head Neck Surg 1997;117:S137–S141
3. Knipe TA, Gandhi PD, Fleming JC, Chandra RK. Transblepharoplasty approach to sequestered disease of the lateral frontal sinus with ophthalmologic manifestations. Am J Rhinol 2007;21:100–104
4. Düz B, Secer HI, Gonul E. Endoscopic approaches to the orbit: a cadaveric study. Minim Invasive Neurosurg 2009;52:107–113
5. Tsirbas A, Kazim M, Close L. Endoscopic approach to orbital apex lesions. Ophthal Plast Reconstr Surg 2005;21:271–275
6. Lund VJ. Extended applications of endoscopic sinus surgery—the territorial imperative. J Laryngol Otol 1997;111:313–315
7. Rose GE. Endoscopic removal of periorbital lesions - where next? Orbit 2002;21:261–262
8. Leong SC, Karkos PD, Macewen CJ, White PS. A systematic review of outcomes following surgical decompression for dysthyroid orbitopathy. Laryngoscope 2009;119:1106–1115
9. Lund VJ, Larkin G, Fells P, Adams G. Orbital decompression for thyroid eye disease: a comparison of external and endoscopic techniques. J Laryngol Otol 1997;111:1051–1055

10. Lund VJ, Rose GE. Endoscopic transnasal orbital decompression for visual failure due to sphenoid wing meningioma. Eye (Lond) 2006;20: 1213–1219

11. Pletcher SD, Metson R. Endoscopic optic nerve decompression for nontraumatic optic neuropathy. Arch Otolaryngol Head Neck Surg 2007; 133:780–783

12. Golub JS, Parikh SL, Budnick SD, Bernardino CR, DelGaudio JM. Inverted papilloma of the nasolacrimal system invading the orbit. Ophthal Plast Reconstr Surg 2007;23:151–153

13. Miller NR, Agrawal N, Sciubba JJ, Lane AP. Image-guided transnasal endoscopic resection of an orbital solitary fibrous tumor. Ophthal Plast Reconstr Surg 2008;24:65–67

14. Gerencer RZ, Patel U, Hunter C, Heffernan JT. The role of endoscopic sinus surgery in the diagnosis and treatment of metastatic orbital carcinoid tumors. Ear Nose Throat J 2007;86:157–161

15. Li H, Zhou B, Shi J, Cheng L, Wen W, Xu G. Treatment of traumatic optic neuropathy: our experience of endoscopic optic nerve decompression. J Laryngol Otol 2008;122:1325–1329

16. Luxenberger W, Stammberger H, Jebeles JA, Walch C. Endoscopic optic nerve decompression: the Graz experience. Laryngoscope 1998;108: 873–882

17. Pletcher SD, Sindwani R, Metson R. Endoscopic orbital and optic nerve decompression. Otolaryngol Clin North Am 2006;39:943–958

18. Naraghi M, Kashfi A. Endonasal endoscopic resection of ethmoido-orbital osteoma compressing the optic nerve. Am J Otolaryngol 2003; 24:408–412

19. Karaki M, Kobayashi R, Mori N. Removal of an orbital apex hemangioma using an endoscopic transethmoidal approach: technical note. Neurosurgery 2006;59(1 Suppl 1): 159–160; discussion 159–160

20. Herman P, Lot G, Silhouette B, et al. Transnasal endoscopic removal of an orbital cavernoma. Ann Otol Rhinol Laryngol 1999;108:147–150

21. Feichtinger M, Zemann W, Kärcher H. Removal of a pellet from the left orbital cavity by image-guided endoscopic navigation. Int J Oral Maxillofac Surg 2007;36:358–361

22. Wormald PJ. Endoscopic Sinus Surgery: Anatomy, Three-Dimensional Reconstruction, and Surgical Technique. New York: Thieme Medical Publishers; 2005

23. Kassam A, Snyderman CH, Carrau RL, Gardner P, Mintz A. Endoneurosurgical hemostasis techniques: lessons learned from 400 cases. Neurosurg Focus 2005;19:E7

24. Eberhart LH, Folz BJ, Wulf H, Geldner G. Intravenous anesthesia provides optimal surgical conditions during microscopic and endoscopic sinus surgery. Laryngoscope 2003;113:1369–1373

25. Wormald PJ, van Renen G, Perks J, Jones JA, Langton-Hewer CD. The effect of the total intravenous anesthesia compared with inhalational anesthesia on the surgical field during endoscopic sinus surgery. Am J Rhinol 2005;19:514–520

26. Sathananthar S, Nagaonkar S, Paleri V, Le T, Robinson S, Wormald P-J. Canine fossa puncture and clearance of the maxillary sinus for the severely diseased maxillary sinus. Laryngoscope 2005;115:1026–1029

27. Robinson SR, Baird R, Le T, Wormald PJ. The incidence of complications after canine fossa puncture performed during endoscopic sinus surgery. Am J Rhinol 2005;19:203–206

28. Robinson S, Wormald P-J. Patterns of innervation of the anterior maxilla: a cadaver study with relevance to canine fossa puncture of the maxillary sinus. Laryngoscope 2005;115:1785–1788

29. Harvey RJ, Sheahan PO, Schlosser RJ. Surgical management of benign sinonasal masses. Otolaryngol Clin North Am 2009;42:353–375, x

30. Cho D-Y, Hwang PH. Results of endoscopic maxillary mega-antrostomy in recalcitrant maxillary sinusitis. Am J Rhinol 2008;22:658–662

31. Woodworth BA, Parker RO, Schlosser RJ. Modified endoscopic medial maxillectomy for chronic maxillary sinusitis. Am J Rhinol 2006;20: 317–319

32. Floreani SR, Nair SB, Switajewski MC, Wormald PJ. Endoscopic anterior ethmoidal artery ligation: a cadaver study. Laryngoscope 2006;116: 1263–1267

33. Pletcher SD, Metson R. Endoscopic ligation of the anterior ethmoid artery. Laryngoscope 2007;117:378–381

34. Cohen AJ, Mercandetti M, Weinberg DA. Hemangioma, cavernous. http://emedicine.medscape.com/article/1218120-overview. 2009

35. Wilms G, Raat H, Dom R, et al. Orbital cavernous hemangioma: findings on sequential Gd-enhanced MRI. J Comput Assist Tomogr 1995;19: 548–551

36. Scheuerle AF, Steiner HH, Kolling G, Kunze S, Aschoff A. Treatment and long-term outcome of patients with orbital cavernomas. Am J Ophthalmol 2004;138:237–244

37. Cheng JW, Wei RL, Cai JP, Li Y. Transconjunctival orbitotomy for orbital cavernous hemangiomas. Can J Ophthalmol 2008;43:234–238

38. Kiratli H, Bulur B, Bilgiç S. Transconjunctival approach for retrobulbar intraconal orbital cavernous hemangiomas. Orbital surgeon's perspective. Surg Neurol 2005;64:71–74

39. Rodriguez MJ, Dave SP, Astor FC. Periorbital emphysema as a complication of functional endoscopic sinus surgery. Ear Nose Throat J 2009; 88:888–889

40. Rubinstein A, Riddell CE, Akram I, Ahmado A, Benjamin L. Orbital emphysema leading to blindness following routine functional endoscopic sinus surgery. Arch Ophthalmol 2005;123:1452

41. Tzifa KT, Skinner DW. Peri-orbital surgical emphysema following functional endoscopic sinus surgery, during extubation. J Laryngol Otol 2001;115:916–917

42. Castro E, Seeley M, Kosmorsky G, Foster JA. Orbital compartment syndrome caused by intraorbital bacitracin ointment after endoscopic sinus surgery. Am J Ophthalmol 2000;130:376–378

43. Keefe MA, Bloom DC, Keefe KS, Killian PJ. Orbital paraffinoma as a complication of endoscopic sinus surgery. Otolaryngol Head Neck Surg 2002;127:575–577

44. Rosner M, Kurtz S, Shelah M, Rosen N. Orbital lipogranuloma after sinus surgery. Eur J Ophthalmol 2000;10:183–186

V Tips and Pearls in the Transcribriform Approach

17 Endoscopic Endonasal Approach for Anterior Skull Base Meningiomas

Amin B. Kassam, Daniel M. Prevedello, Paul A. Gardner, Juan C. Fernandez-Miranda, Ricardo L. Carrau, and Carl H. Snyderman

Tips and Pearls

- Endoscopic endonasal approaches (EEAs) can provide adequate access for the management of meningiomas located at the median skull base (from the crista galli to the clivus and cervicomedullary junction).
- A significant advantage of EEAs for the treatment of meningiomas is that they provide early tumor devascularization, arising from the ligation of the ethmoidal arteries, removal of the median skull base, and coagulation of the dura at the base of the tumor.
- The lateral limits of EEAs are the internal carotid arteries (ICAs) and optic nerves in the suprasellar space, and the midorbital plane in the anterior fossa (anterior to the planum sphenoidale).
- Access to anterior fossa tumors that extend laterally, up to the midorbital plane, require the removal of the lamina papyracea. This enables the displacement of the orbital soft tissues.
- Meningiomas that originate at the tuberculum sella and planum sphenoidale can extend into the optic canal. Their most common extension is to the medial aspect of the optic nerve canal. This medial extension is better accessed with an EEA than with an anterolateral craniotomy, as it does not require retraction or displacement of the optic nerve.
- The EEAs for meningioma are associated with <5% risk of postoperative visual deterioration.
- The technical complexity and morbidity of EEAs for the removal of a meningioma are determined by its relationship to the surrounding vessels (anterior cerebral artery).
- Meningiomas that are associated with a cuff of cerebral cortex protecting the vasculature are the simplest and safest tumors to manage with EEAs.
- Tumors in direct dorsal contact with the vasculature are more complex, and safe dissection of their capsule requires a higher level of skill and experience of the endoscopic surgical team.
- Tumors with vascular encasement (anterior cerebral artery) are the most complicated and imply the highest risk. These require a very experienced EEA team to safely access, dissect, and control these critical vessels.
- Reconstruction following EEA for a meningioma is best accomplished with a vascularized flap such as the pedicled nasoseptal flap.

Introduction

Treatment for skull base tumors has significantly evolved[1–4] since Dandy[5] first described the removal of a cranial base/orbital tumor via a craniotomy in 1941. This early effort was followed by Smith et al's[6] description of a combined transfacial-transcranial approach for the removal of a skull base tumor originating in the frontal sinus. However, it was not until the 1960s that Ketcham et al[7,8] described the first craniofacial resection using a coronal incision and craniotomy combined with facial incisions for removal of sinonasal tumors. Over the subsequent decades, surgical techniques were refined, but the field of skull base surgery changed slowly. In 1997, Yuen et al[9] described an endoscopic-assisted craniofacial resection applying the principles and instruments developed for inflammatory endoscopic sinus surgery to surgically address a malignant neoplasm. In 1999, Stammberger et al[10] described the endoscopic resection of an esthesioneuroblastoma. Since then, multiple case series have reported good results following endoscopic resection of esthesioneuroblastomas and other neoplasms of the skull base.[11–15]

Transsphenoidal approaches followed a similar evolution. Guiot et al[16] in 1963 proposed using the endoscope for transsphenoidal procedures, and Apuzzo et al[17] revisited this concept in 1977. In 1984, Griffith and Veerapen[18] utilized the pure endonasal technique to approach the sella for excision of a pituitary adenoma. Jho and Carrau[19] decisively established this as a purely endoscopic technique in 1997, and, subsequently, De Divitiis and Cappabianca's group[20,21] expounded on the advantages the nuances of such an approach. In 2001, Jho[22] reported the first patient to undergo an endoscopic, endonasal resection of an intracranial meningioma compressing the optic nerve. Kelly's group,[23] in 2004, reported on three patients in whom the endonasal route with endoscopic support was used to resect suprasellar meningiomas, achieving good short-term results.

The goals of a skull base resection, endoscopic or open, remain the same: complete tumor extirpation with negative margins for oncologic cases, and separation of the cranial cavity and sinonasal tract.[24] Regardless of the approach, when dealing with benign disease, such as meningiomas, the surgeon must minimize surgical morbidities such as neurologic sequelae, visual dysfunction, or cognitive impairment. Cosmesis, although not the primary goal, is an important concern, especially when undergoing extensive open procedures. Advanced endoscopic techniques facilitate extensive resections without the need for external incisions.[25–27]

Currently, the literature lacks a systematic review comparing open techniques to endoscopic techniques for meningiomas. A recent systematic review compared endoscopic and open techniques for treatment of sinonasal inverting papillomas.[28] In patients treated endoscopically, the recurrence rate was significantly lower than for those treated nonendoscopically (12% versus 20%). Casler et al[29] compared endoscopic and open techniques for pituitary surgery in a cohort study, and noted that patients undergoing transsphenoidal endoscopic resection of adenomas experienced less pain, less blood loss, fewer complications, and shorter length of stay in the intensive care unit and hospital. Additional benefits include superior visualization, lack of incisions, a reduction in swelling, and decreased pain and bleeding.[30,31] However, the surgical indications for endoscopic and open approaches are not necessarily the same, and comparing these heterogeneous groups of patients may yield misleading conclusions. Nonetheless, we believe that there is a critical advantage for endonasal resection of tumors such as meningiomas that originate in the median skull base and do not extend laterally to involve critical neurovascular structures.

Indications and Advantages

Anterior skull base meningiomas, including those originating at the olfactory groove, planum sphenoidale, and tuberculum sellae, are challenging tumors despite well-described transcranial approaches. These tumors are often associated with significant cerebral edema and distortion of the optic apparatus, thereby requiring some degree of frontal lobe retraction and manipulation of the optic apparatus for their access and resection. Furthermore, these tumors originate at the base of the skull base, and as such they are always in direct contact with the roof of the sinuses. The endoscopic endonasal approach (EEA) takes advantage of this anatomic relationship to enable resection of the meningioma without brain retraction.[32]

Once the approach is performed, these skull base tumors are managed in a manner similar to that used for convexity meningiomas. The tumor's main blood supply is coagulated before the dissection. For olfactory groove meningiomas, the anterior and posterior ethmoidal arteries are coagulated or ligated early during exposure, and the dura mater is broadly coagulated before the dural opening. McConnell's arteries are coagulated before accessing tuberculum sellae meningiomas. In summary, there is decreased neurologic tissue manipulation, and the tumors are devascularized early during the endonasal approach (**Figs. 17.1, 17.2,** and **17.3**).[25]

Contraindications

The endoscopic endonasal route approaches the anterior skull base pathology from a medial, anterior, and inferior trajectory; therefore, there are potential surgical limits laterally, posteriorly, and superiorly. In reality, these limitations can be minimized as long as safety and vascular control are maintained.

The lateral limit of resection for olfactory groove meningiomas is the midorbital plane (**Figs. 17.1A,B** and **17.2A**). Removal of the lamina papyracea enables the displacement of the orbital soft tissues to provide access to the orbital roof laterally. Lesions that present a lateral extension beyond the midorbit meridian should not be accessed with a pure endonasal approach.

The posterior limit for an EEA is essentially the same as for any anterior skull base approach—the optic chiasm and anterior cerebral circulation. Meningiomas tend to displace the optic nerves laterally, the chiasm posteriorly, and, in most of the cases, the anterior cerebral and communicating arteries are displaced superiorly and posteriorly (**Fig. 17.2B**). Tumors lateral to the optic nerves should not be resected from a midline endonasal approach.

Very tall tumors can be difficult to access and care must be taken not to remove too much of the inferior and anterior capsule before the apex of the tumor has been debulked. The frontal lobes can descend into the field, obscuring the view. Sometimes these tumors need to be resected in stages, after a significant initial debulking allows descent of the tumor. The surgical team needs to be comfortable with the use of angle endoscopes. Commonly, most of the delicate dissection of an anterior fossa meningioma is performed with a 45-degree endoscope.

Diagnostic Workup

The physical examination should include a neurologic assessment with special focus on cranial nerve function. Olfaction is compromised by most olfactory groove meningiomas, but its function must be documented preoperatively. Endoscopic assessment of the nasal cavity is recommended to visualize any nasal lesions and document septal integrity, septal deviations, and any other anatomical findings. A complete ophthalmologic examination is mandatory for anterior fossa

Fig. 17.1 (*opposite*) Moderate-size olfactory groove meningioma. **(A)** Preoperative T1-weighted magnetic resonance imaging (MRI) coronal section at the level of the cribriform plate. **(B)** Preoperative T1-weighted coronal section at the anterior level of the planum sphenoidale. **(C)** Six-months postoperative T1-weighted coronal section showing complete resection of the tumor and removal of the cribriform plate and crista galli. Note the natural enhancement of the nasoseptal flap used for reconstruction of the anterior skull base defect. **(D)** Postoperative T1-weighted coronal section showing complete resection of the tumor and minimal encephalomalacia. The tumor has been removed without any need for brain retraction or manipulation. **(E)** Preoperative fluid-attenuated inversion recovery (FLAIR) sequence axial section showing significant signal change at the right frontal lobe. **(F)** Postoperative FLAIR sequence axial section showing nearly complete resolution of the signal changes. Nasosept.: nasoseptal.

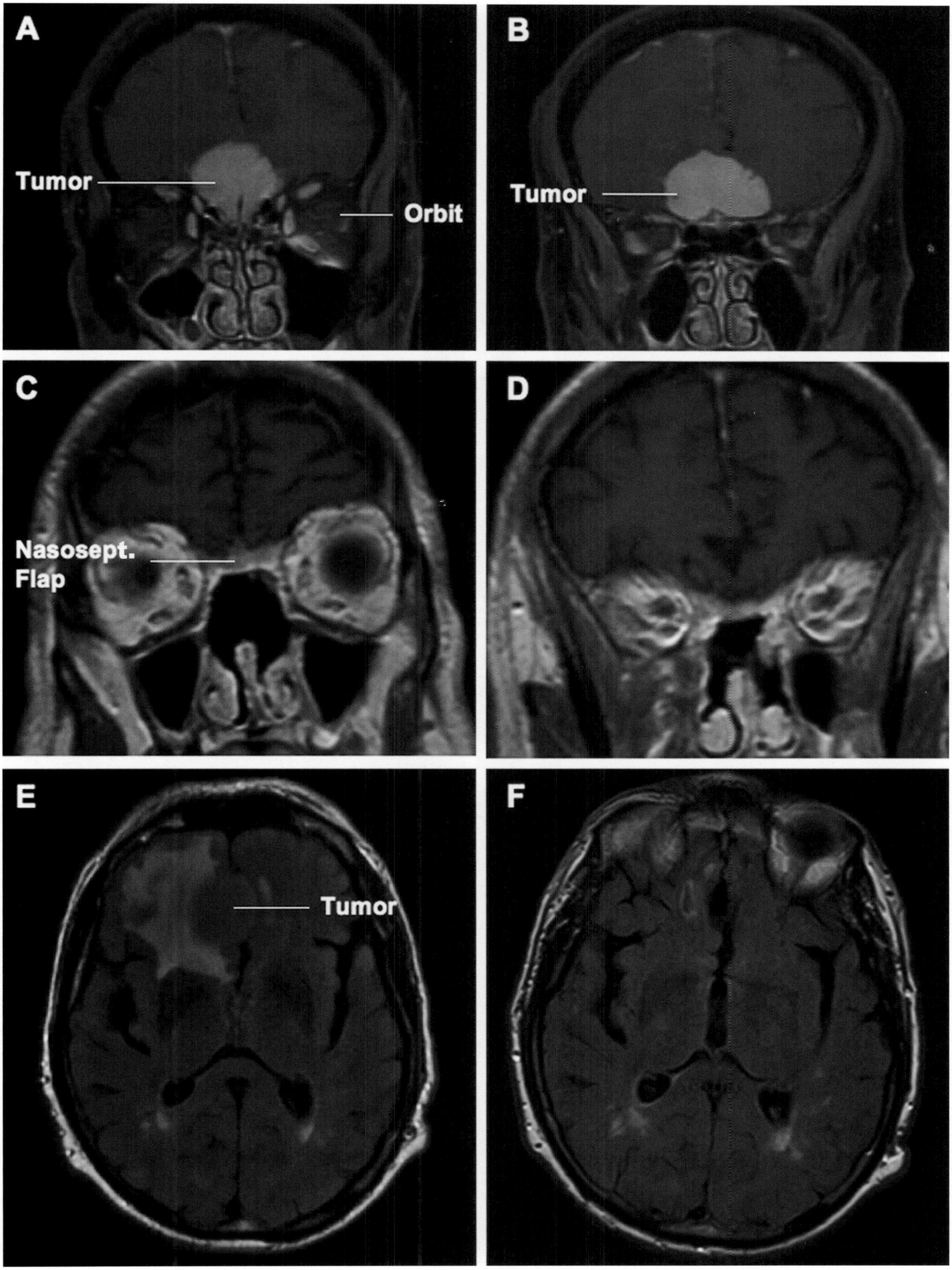
A
Tumor
Orbit
B
Tumor
C
Nasosept.
Flap
D
E
Tumor
F

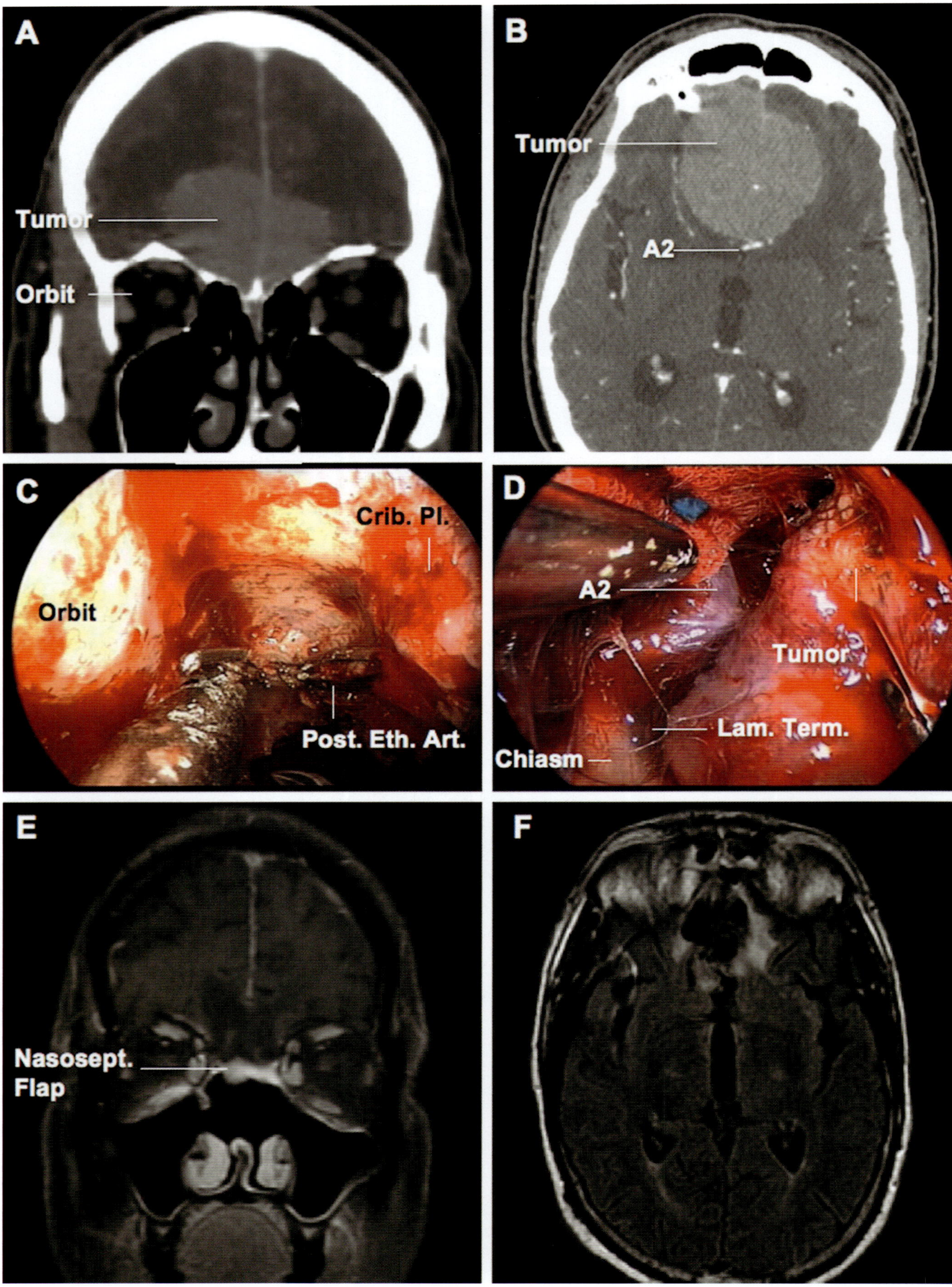
A
Tumor
Orbit
B
Tumor
A2
C
Crib. Pl.
Orbit
Post. Eth. Art.
D
A2
Tumor
Lam. Term.
Chiasm
E
Nasosept.
Flap
F

meningiomas and must include visual fields examination. Signs of intracranial hypertension detected by papilledema should be addressed preoperatively. These cases frequently require preoperative cerebrospinal fluid (CSF) diversion with external ventricular drainage (EVD) or ventriculoperitoneal (VP) shunt to control the pressure and for vision protection.

Imaging

Patients undergo a preoperative computed tomographic angiography (CTA) and magnetic resonance imaging (MRI), which are fused for frameless stereotactic image guidance during the procedure (Stryker-Leibinger Corp., Kalamazoo, MI).

Surgery

Instrumentation

Appropriate instrumentation is vital for the endoscopic endonasal approach to the anterior fossa. Critical equipment includes high-quality rod lens endoscopes (0-, 45-, and 70-degree); video equipment (camera and monitor); extended endoscopic bipolar forceps; extended and delicate high-speed drills including 3- and 4-mm hybrid burrs; extended dissection instruments; and hemostatic materials.

Operative Setup

Following orotracheal intubation the patient is placed in a three-pin head holder positioned with the head turned to the right and slightly tilted to the left. This maneuver helps to move the patient's body away, providing extra space for the surgeons.

Preparation

The nose is decongested with topical 0.05% oxymetazoline applied using ½" × 3" cottonoids. A povidone solution is applied to the perinasal and periumbilical areas (in the event that an autologous fat-free graft is necessary for reconstruction).

Nasal Corridor

Reconstruction following removal of a meningioma via an endoscopic endonasal approach requires a reconstruction using vascularized tissue. A pedicled vascularized flap reliably separates the cranial cavity from the sinonasal tract, thus avoiding a postoperative CSF leak and its associated infectious complications. Harvesting of the reconstructive nasoseptal flap needs to be performed as the first step of the exposure. Its pedicle is based on the posterior nasal artery, and if not elevated at the beginning of the procedure, it would be damaged during the sphenoidotomies or posterior septectomy. Once harvested, the flap is stored in the nasopharynx.[33–35]

For suprasellar meningiomas, wide sphenoidotomies and partial bilateral posterior ethmoidectomies are performed. For olfactory groove meningiomas, opening the surgical corridor involves bilateral uncinectomies, maxillary antrostomies, anterior and posterior ethmoidectomies, and in some instances bilateral frontal sinusotomies (Draf III). Unilateral or bilateral middle turbinate resection(s) can be performed as needed.

For complete anterior skull base exposure, the nasofrontal recesses are identified and an endoscopic Lothrop procedure (Draf III) is performed. This involves removal of the frontal intersinus septum, its floor, and the superior nasal septum.[25,36,37] A portion of the superior nasal septum is removed from the anterior wall of the frontal sinus to the rostrum of the sphenoid posteriorly.

Ligation of the ethmoidal arteries (**Fig. 17.2C**) decreases the tumor blood supply, which in turn diminishes bleeding during dissection. The partial removal of the lamina papyracea is recommended to facilitate identification of the ethmoidal arteries and to enable further resection of the orbital roof and enhanced lateral exposure. The ethmoidal arteries are coagulated with bipolar cautery or ligated with surgical clips.[25]

After achieving appropriate exposure, the skull base osteotomies are tailored to the extent of disease with the help of image guidance. In general, for suprasellar, diaphragmatic, and tuberculum sellae meningiomas, the face of the sella, the tuberculum sellae, and the posterior aspect of the planum sphenoidale are drilled out exposing the dura. Olfactory groove meningiomas, however, require the removal of the fovea ethmoidalis and the cribriform plate.

Fig. 17.2 (*opposite*) Large olfactory groove meningioma. **(A)** Preoperative thin-sliced CT-angiogram scan (coronal section). **(B)** Axial section showing intimate relation of the posterior border of the tumor with both anterior cerebral arteries at the proximal A2 segment. **(C)** Intraoperative picture. The right lamina papyracea has been removed to expose the periorbita and provide access to the orbital roof. The anterior and posterior ethmoidal arteries are coagulated and sectioned to expose the anterior skull base and provide early devascularization of the tumor. **(D)** Intraoperative picture. Once the tumor has been extensively debulked, gentle extracapsular dissection is performed. The tumor is adherent to the anterior cerebral arteries and needs to be sharply dissected using meticulous microsurgical technique. The optic chiasm has been pushed down by the tumor, facilitating identification of the lamina terminalis. **(E)** Postoperative T1-weighted MRI (coronal section) showing complete resection of the tumor, cribriform plate, and crista galli. The anterior skull base has been reconstructed with the nasoseptal flap. **(F)** Postoperative FLAIR sequence MRI (axial section) showing nearly complete resolution of the signal changes and minimal encephalomalacia. A2: anterior cerebral artery; Art.: artery; Crib.: cribriform; Eth.: ethmoidal; Lam.: lamina; Nasosept.: nasoseptal; Pl.: plate; Post.: posterior; Term.: terminalis.

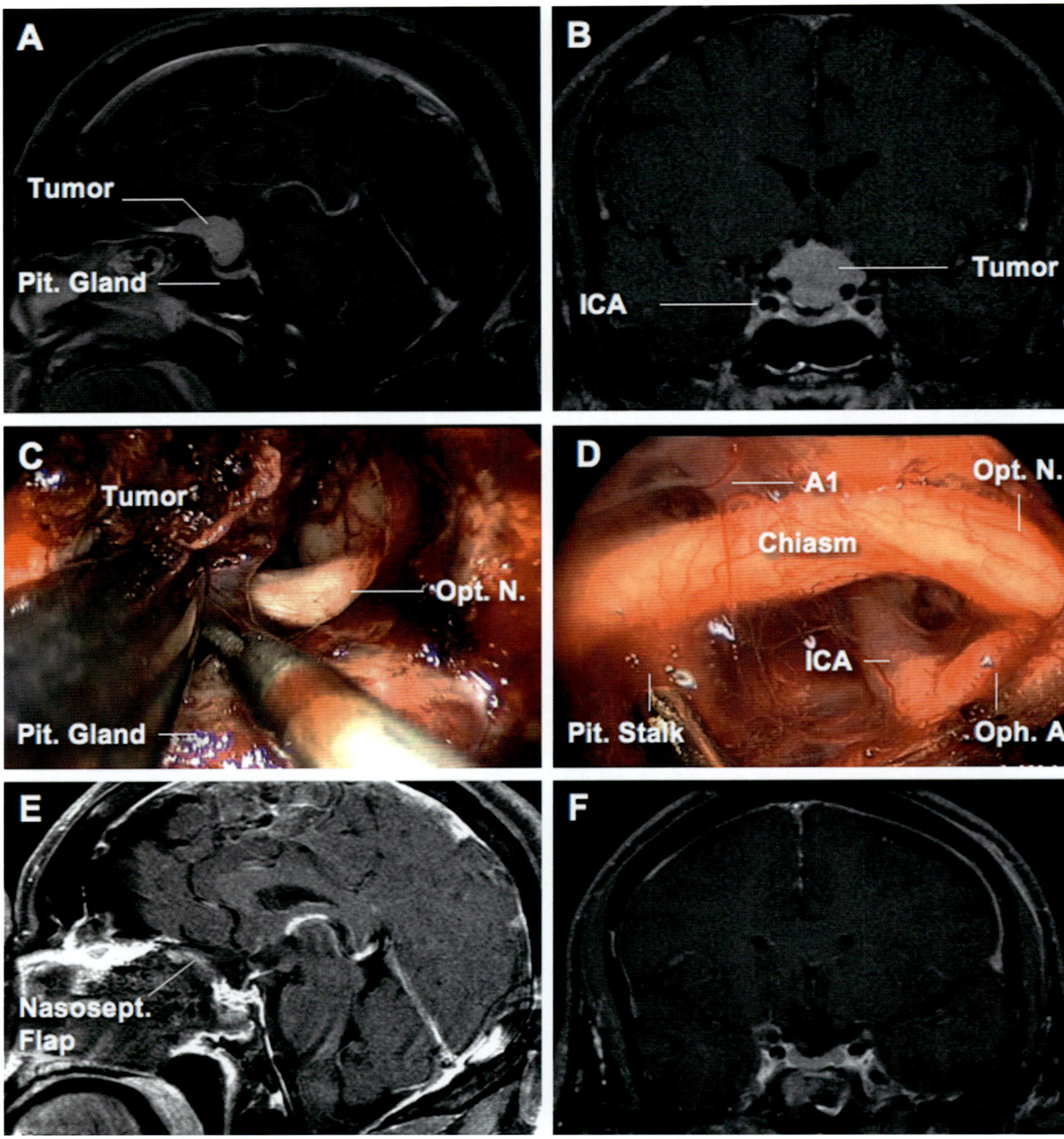

Fig. 17.3 Tuberculum sellae meningioma. **(A)** Preoperative T1-weighted MRI sagittal section. **(B)** Coronal section. **(C)** Intraoperative picture. After tumor debulking, the extracapsular dissection is pursued. The first step is the internal carotid artery and optic nerve identification. **(D)** Intraoperative picture. The optic nerve is followed until the chiasm is found. After complete resection, the optic nerves and chiasm, pituitary stalk, superior hypophyseal arteries, anterior cerebral arteries, internal carotid arteries, and ophthalmic arteries (if medially located, as in the presented case) are identified. Note the preservation of the arachnoid membranes that form the suprasellar and chiasmatic cisterns. **(E)** Postoperative T1-weighted MRI (sagittal section) showing complete resection of the tumor and reconstruction of the skull base opening with the nasoseptal flap. **(F)** Postoperative T1-weighted MRI (coronal section). A.: anterior cerebral artery; ICA.: internal carotid artery; N.: nerve; Nasosept.: nasoseptal; Oph.: ophthalmic; Opt.: optic; Pit.: pituitary.

Tumor Resection

The principles of tumor resection via EEA are identical to those of a standard microsurgical approach. The tumor is internally debulked prior to careful extracapsular dissection using standard microsurgical techniques. There are some modifications of instrumentation required to provide extended reach, including microscissors, bipolars, and dissectors.

Once the dura is coagulated to further decrease vascular supply to the tumor, then the dura is opened. For olfactory groove meningiomas, debulking begins by opening the dura on either side of the falx and internally debulking the tumor up to the falx bilaterally. The small, falcine arterioles that feed the tumor can be coagulated. Sacrificing these early in the dissection provides further tumor devascularization. Once the falx is isolated from both sides, it can be bipolar-coagulated and carefully cut with scissors or through-cutting instruments at its most anterior aspect. This is repeated sequentially deeper into the tumor until the falx is transected anteriorly. Care should be taken to ensure the A2's and their branches are not adhered to the surface of the tumor overlying the falx. The tumor should not be detached anteriorly before all of the internal debulking is complete, as the frontal lobe may descend and interfere with the visualization. This is especially true for tumors that extend in the vertical dimension (tall tumors).

Once the capsule is disconnected from the falx anteriorly, it can be dissected from the overlying cortex and associated structures as such as the anterior cerebral arteries (ACAs) and optic apparatus (**Fig. 17.2D**). The tumor and capsule are debulked as they are sequentially exposed using a combination of blunt and sharp dissection and using the same technique as that of the microsurgical approaches.

Resection of large anterior fossa meningiomas can be staged without increasing morbidity. During second-stage surgery, the nasoseptal flap is easily elevated from the skull base, providing direct tumor access within a few minutes. Interestingly, the flap can be reutilized for the reconstruction. A staged surgery provides time for tall and wide tumors to descend or fill in the tumor cavity, which can facilitate a complete resection.

The anterior communicating and anterior cerebral arteries are often intricately associated or even encased by meningiomas that grow in the suprasellar area (**Fig. 17.3**). The ability to avoid and control a major arterial injury during an endoscopic endonasal approach is critical. For an experienced surgical team, this situation can be managed endonasally as effectively as it can be via an open approach. In suprasellar tumors, special care should be taken when dissecting the tumor from the superior hypophyseal arteries, as they supply the cisternal component of the optic nerves. Dissection following a careful microsurgical technique using gentle countertraction combined with sharp dissection helps to avoid this injury.

To prevent arterial injuries, a careful understanding of the preoperative imaging and tumor/vessel relationships is critical. Image guidance using CTA is ideal for this purpose (**Fig. 17.2B**). Early identification of the optic nerves, ICAs, ACAs, and their branches is essential during extracapsular dissection (**Fig. 17.3C,D**).

Repair

The reconstruction should be planned before approaching the tumor. Our preference is to use vascularized tissue, most commonly in the form of a nasoseptal flap, which is raised at the beginning of the procedure. The flap is stored in the nasopharynx until the end of the tumor dissection.

The reconstruction starts with an inlay layer of a collagen matrix membrane. This yields a significant decrease in CSF flow through the defect.

Unlike the reconstruction of EEA for sinonasal tumors, the septal mucosa is not invaded by the meningioma and preservation of olfaction is not an issue; thus, the full extent of the septal mucosa can be elevated and used for the reconstruction. In cases that involve the exposure of the entire anterior cranial fossa, we often need to supplement the nasoseptal flap. Some alternatives include the use of a free fat graft for obliteration of the sphenoid sinus, allowing the placement of the nasoseptal flap over the fat graft to then cover the anterior fossa, and the use of membrane grafts as fascia lata or acellular dermis to augment the area covered by the flap.

■ Complications

From our first 400 patients with anterior skull base meningiomas, 5% of the patients suffered postoperative worsening of their vision. One patient suffered an intraoperative injury to A2 and despite obtaining adequate control with no immediate consequences, it eventually led to a subsequent pseudoaneurysm bleeding associated with permanent neurologic deficits. We encountered no mortality at 30 days.

The most common postoperative complication was a CSF leak. CSF leak rates decreased significantly from an initial rate of around 40% to rates of less than 6% once a vascularized nasoseptal flap became routine for reconstruction.[33] Other complications encountered in 124 patients who underwent EEA for meningioma resections, included pulmonary embolus/deep venous thrombosis (4.8%), seizures (5.6%), pituitary dysfunction (3.2%), new cranial nerve deficit (other than vision, 1.6%), bacterial meningitis (1.6%), and myocardial infarction (0.8%).

■ Postoperative Care

Seventy percent of patients who presented with vision compromise preoperatively had significant improvement in visual function, defined as improvement of two or more lines of Snellen visual acuity, or improvement of the visual field defect.

Our policy is to take patients back to the operating room for exploration and CSF leak repair, if necessary, upon any suspicion for a CSF leak during the postoperative period. In our series, the use of a lumbar drain with the hope that the CSF leak would cease spontaneously, proved to increase the risk of meningitis early. With the use of vascularized tissue for reconstruction and our aggressive exploration and repair policy, we have been able to decrease the rate of postoperative meningitis to less than 1%.

Conclusion

The endoscopic endonasal approach for the resection of anterior skull base/olfactory groove meningiomas is a feasible and safe approach. It holds the potential for reduction of vision complications and perhaps even neurocognitive deficits. Adequate selection of cases is critical, as issues such as vascular control, maintenance of visualization for microsurgical dissection, and reconstruction can be daunting for some meningiomas. The surgical team should have experience in both endoscopic endonasal and standard approaches to offer the best possible corridor for each specific tumor and to meet the needs of the patient.

References

1. Har-El G, Casiano RR. Endoscopic management of anterior skull base tumors. Otolaryngol Clin North Am 2005;38:133–144, ix ix.
2. Lund VJ, Howard DJ, Wei WI, Cheesman AD. Craniofacial resection for tumors of the nasal cavity and paranasal sinuses—a 17-year experience. Head Neck 1998;20:97–105
3. Patel SG, Singh B, Polluri A, et al. Craniofacial surgery for malignant skull base tumors: report of an international collaborative study. Cancer 2003;98:1179–1187
4. Shah JP, Kraus DH, Arbit E, Galicich JH, Strong EW. Craniofacial resection for tumors involving the anterior skull base. Otolaryngol Head Neck Surg 1992;106:387–393
5. Dandy W. Orbital Tumour: Results Following the Transcranial Operative Attack. New York: Oskar Priest; 1941:168–188
6. Smith RR, Klopp CT, Williams JM. Surgical treatment of cancer of the frontal sinus and adjacent areas. Cancer 1954;7:991–994
7. Ketcham AS, Hoye RC, Van Buren JM, Johnson RH, Smith RR. Complications of intracranial facial resection for tumors of the paranasal sinuses. Am J Surg 1966;112:591–596
8. Ketcham AS, Wilkins RH, Vanburen JM, Smith RR. A combined intracranial facial approach to the paranasal sinuses. Am J Surg 1963;106:698–703
9. Yuen AP, Fung CF, Hung KN. Endoscopic cranionasal resection of anterior skull base tumor. Am J Otolaryngol 1997;18:431–433
10. Stammberger H, Anderhuber W, Walch C, Papaefthymiou G. Possibilities and limitations of endoscopic management of nasal and paranasal sinus malignancies. Acta Otorhinolaryngol Belg 1999;53:199–205
11. Snyderman CH, Carrau RL, Kassam AB, et al. Endoscopic skull base surgery: principles of endonasal oncological surgery. J Surg Oncol 2008;97:658–664
12. Snyderman CH, Pant H, Carrau RL, Prevedello D, Gardner P, Kassam AB. What are the limits of endoscopic sinus surgery?: the expanded endonasal approach to the skull base. Keio J Med 2009;58:152–160
13. Casiano RR, Numa WA, Falquez AM. Endoscopic resection of esthesioneuroblastoma. Am J Rhinol 2001;15:271–279
14. Folbe A, Herzallah I, Duvvuri U, et al. Endoscopic endonasal resection of esthesioneuroblastoma: a multicenter study. Am J Rhinol Allergy 2009;23:91–94
15. Castelnuovo PG, Delù G, Sberze F, et al. Esthesioneuroblastoma: endonasal endoscopic treatment. Skull Base 2006;16:25–30
16. Guiot J, Rougerie J, Fourestier M, et al. [Intracranial endoscopic explorations.]. Presse Med 1963;71:1225–1228
17. Apuzzo ML, Heifetz MD, Weiss MH, Kurze T. Neurosurgical endoscopy using the side-viewing telescope. J Neurosurg 1977;46:398–400
18. Griffith HB, Veerapen R. A direct transnasal approach to the sphenoid sinus. Technical note. J Neurosurg 1987;66:140–142
19. Jho HD, Carrau RL. Endoscopic endonasal transsphenoidal surgery: experience with 50 patients. J Neurosurg 1997;87:44–51
20. Cappabianca P, Alfieri A, Colao A, et al. Endoscopic endonasal transsphenoidal surgery in recurrent and residual pituitary adenomas: technical note. Minim Invasive Neurosurg 2000;43:38–43
21. Cappabianca P, Cavallo LM, Colao A, et al. Endoscopic endonasal transsphenoidal approach: outcome analysis of 100 consecutive procedures. Minim Invasive Neurosurg 2002;45:193–200
22. Jho HD. Endoscopic endonasal approach to the optic nerve: a technical note. Minim Invasive Neurosurg 2001;44:190–193
23. Cook SW, Smith Z, Kelly DF. Endonasal transsphenoidal removal of tuberculum sellae meningiomas: technical note. Neurosurgery 2004;55:239–244, discussion 244–246
24. Kaplan MJ, Fischbein NJ, Harsh GR. Anterior skull base surgery. Otolaryngol Clin North Am 2005;38:107–131, ix ix.
25. Gardner PA, Kassam AB, Thomas A, et al. Endoscopic endonasal resection of anterior cranial base meningiomas. Neurosurgery 2008;63:36–52, discussion 52–54
26. Kassam AB, Prevedello DM, Carrau RL, et al. The front door to Meckel's cave: an anteromedial corridor via expanded endoscopic endonasal approach—technical considerations and clinical series. Neurosurgery 2009;64(3, Suppl):71–82, discussion 82–83
27. Prevedello DM, Fernandez-Miranda JC, Gardner P, et al. The transclival endoscopic endonasal approach (EEA) for prepontine neuroenteric cysts: report of two cases. Acta Neurochir (Wien) 2010;152:1223–1229
28. Busquets JM, Hwang PH. Endoscopic resection of sinonasal inverted papilloma: a meta-analysis. Otolaryngol Head Neck Surg 2006;134:476–482
29. Casler JD, Doolittle AM, Mair EA. Endoscopic surgery of the anterior skull base. Laryngoscope 2005;115:16–24
30. Krouse JH. Endoscopic treatment of inverted papilloma: safety and efficacy. Am J Otolaryngol 2001;22:87–99
31. Baruah P, Deka RC. Endoscopic management of inverted papillomas of the nose and paranasal sinuses. Ear Nose Throat J 2003;82:317–320
32. Prevedello DM, Doglietto F, Jane JA Jr, Jagannathan J, Han J, Laws ER Jr. History of endoscopic skull base surgery: its evolution and current reality. J Neurosurg 2007;107:206–213
33. Zanation AM, Carrau RL, Snyderman CH, et al. Nasoseptal flap reconstruction of high flow intraoperative cerebral spinal fluid leaks during endoscopic skull base surgery. Am J Rhinol Allergy 2009;23:518–521
34. Pinheiro-Neto CD, Prevedello DM, Carrau RL, et al. Improving the design of the pedicled nasoseptal flap for skull base reconstruction: a radioanatomic study. Laryngoscope 2007;117:1560–1569
35. Kassam AB, Thomas A, Carrau RL, et al. Endoscopic reconstruction of the cranial base using a pedicled nasoseptal flap. Neurosurgery 2008;63(1, Suppl 1):ONS44–ONS52, discussion ONS52–ONS53
36. Prevedello DM, Thomas A, Gardner P, Snyderman CH, Carrau RL, Kassam AB. Endoscopic endonasal resection of a synchronous pituitary adenoma and a tuberculum sellae meningioma: technical case report. Neurosurgery 2007;60(4, Suppl 2):E401, discussion E401
37. Fernandez-Miranda JC, Gardner PA, Prevedello DM, Kassam AB. Expanded endonasal approach for olfactory groove meningioma. Acta Neurochir (Wien) 2009;151:287–288, author reply 289–290

18 Endoscopic Management of Anterior Skull Base Meningoencephalocele

Daniel Timperley, Rodney J. Schlosser, and Richard J. Harvey

Tips and Pearls

- Clinical and radiographic signs of benign intracranial hypertension should be sought in patients with spontaneous meningoencephaloceles, and appropriate management instituted.
- A large meningoencephalocele sac should be opened to both provide visualization of potential vascular loops and to enable part of the sac wall to be used in the repair.
- The reconstruction should be considered prior to beginning the approach so that pedicled flaps can be preserved if necessary.
- Frontal recess involvement should be managed as part of the repair, and secondary frontal recess surgery avoided.
- Lumbar drains are unnecessary for the successful closure of even very large defects in the anterior cranial fossa. They may still have a role in benign intracranial hypertension (BIH) or postradiotherapy.
- Endoscopic repair may allow for quick recovery, but the potential for serious intracranial complications remains the same as when performed by an open approach.

Introduction

Anterior skull base meningoencephaloceles are herniations of brain and meningeal tissue into the nose or paranasal sinuses. There has been an evolution in management of these lesions from open to transnasal endoscopic approaches. The endoscopic approach is effective[1–3] with the potential for lower morbidity[4] and shorter hospital stay[5] than the traditional open approaches.

Etiology

Meningoencephaloceles may be congenital or acquired as a result of increased intracranial pressure (ICP) or surgical or accidental trauma.

Congenital

Frontoethmoidal meningoencephaloceles originate between the frontal and ethmoid bones at or anterior to the foramen cecum and present externally on the face from the glabella to the columella, often in association with nasal dermoid cysts. Basal types present intranasally and may occur in any location, with 14% of ethmoid bones demonstrating bony dehiscences in anatomic studies.[6] The most common sites clinically have been reported as the cribriform adjacent to the middle turbinate attachment and from the superior and lateral walls of the sphenoid (**Fig. 18.1**).[6,7] Transsphenoidal encephaloceles are associated with other midline abnormalities.[6,8] The optimum timing of repair has yet to be determined and is a balance between growth of the child to improve surgical access and the risk of meningitis or cosmetic deformity. The risk of meningitis before the age of 5 years in the absence of a cerebrospinal fluid (CSF) leak seems to be low, so the indications for early repair are cosmetic deformity or CSF leak, and successful endoscopic repair has been reported in a 23-month-old.[9]

Increased Intracranial Pressure and Benign Intracranial Hypertension

The majority of spontaneous or idiopathic meningoencephaloceles are associated with evidence of increased ICP and are now thought to be a clinical manifestation of raised intracranial hypertension on a spectrum from benign intracranial hypertension (BIH) to pseudotumor cerebri.[10–12]

Patients with BIH are typically obese middle-aged women, and they may present with headache, pulsatile tinnitus, balance problems, and visual disturbance. However, in the presence of an active CSF leak, ICP may be artificially lowered. These symptoms may only manifest following closure of the leak with a subsequent increase in ICP.[12–14]

The postulated mechanism is erosion of the skull base at points of inherent structural weakness due to constant pulsatile pressure.[12] Common sites for spontaneous encephaloceles are the cribriform plate and the lateral pneumatized sphenoid recess. Those in the lateral sphenoid recess typically occur lateral to the foramen rotundum (**Fig. 18.2**) and vidian canal in patients with extensive pneumatization of the sphenoid.[15] Some authors have described these lesions as occurring though the lateral craniopharyngeal (Sternberg's) canal, but this was described posteromedial to the foramen rotundum and it is argued that the skull base defect is due to the effects of increased ICP on a thin skull base.[12,16]

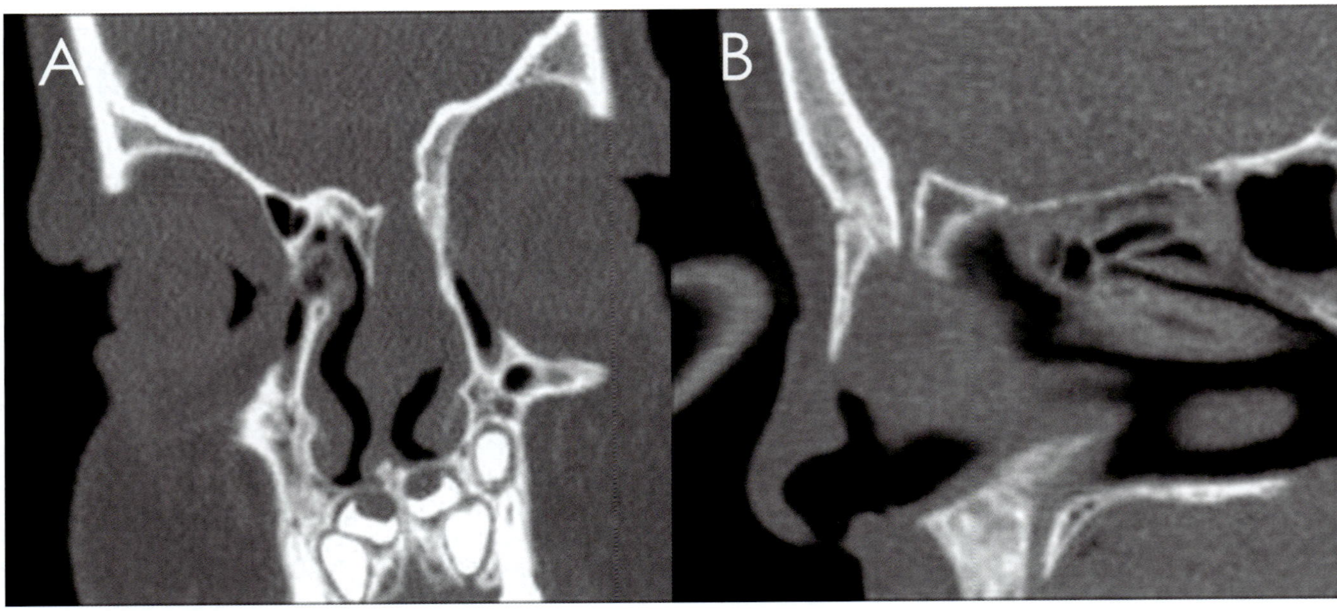

Fig. 18.1 Congenital meningoencephalocele of the right fonticulus frontalis defect type. **(A)** Coronal view. **(B)** Sagittal view.

Diagnostic Workup

Laboratory Investigations

In patients who present with a suspicion of CSF rhinorrhea, the diagnosis should be confirmed by testing a sample of the nasal discharge. β_2-transferrin is formed by desialization of β_1-transferrin by cerebral neuraminidase in CSF. It is found only in CSF, vitreous humor, and perilymph, and testing can be performed on as little as 0.5 mL of fluid.[17]

β-trace protein is prostaglandin D synthase found in CSF and is an alternative marker for CSF, which has been used mainly in parts of Europe. It requires a larger sample than

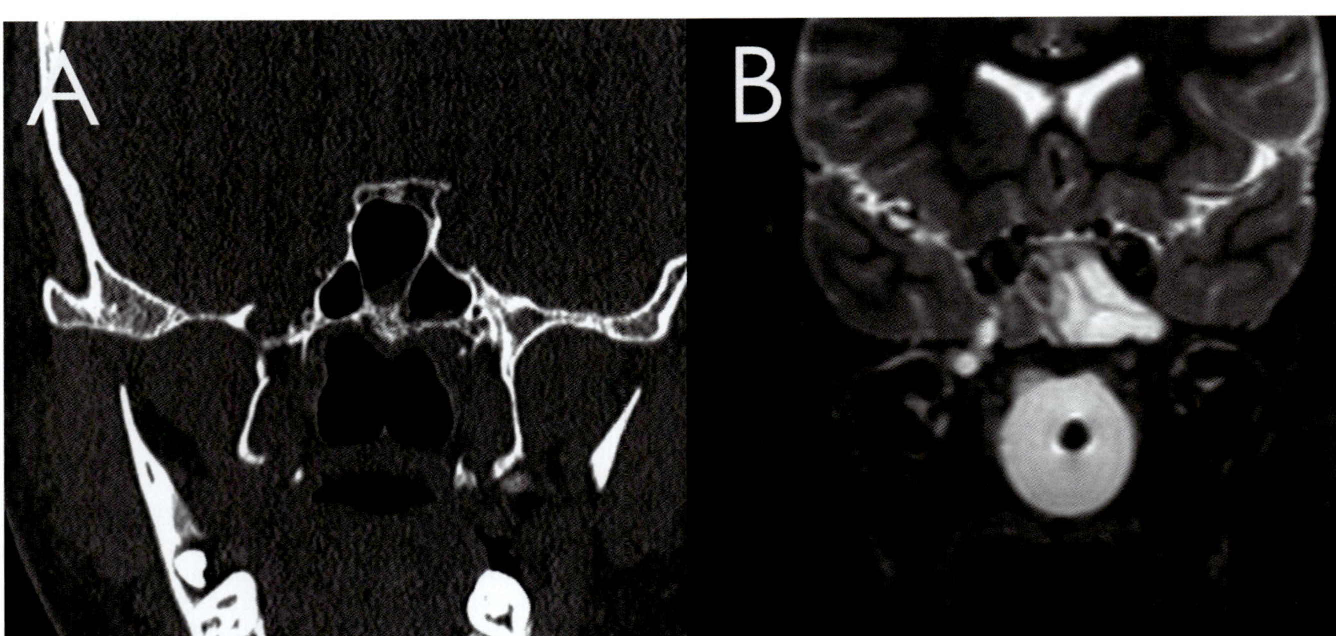

Fig. 18.2 Pits and small diverticulum within the right V2 and foramen rotundum. **(A)** Computed tomography (CT). **(B)** T2-weighted magnetic resonance imaging (MRI).

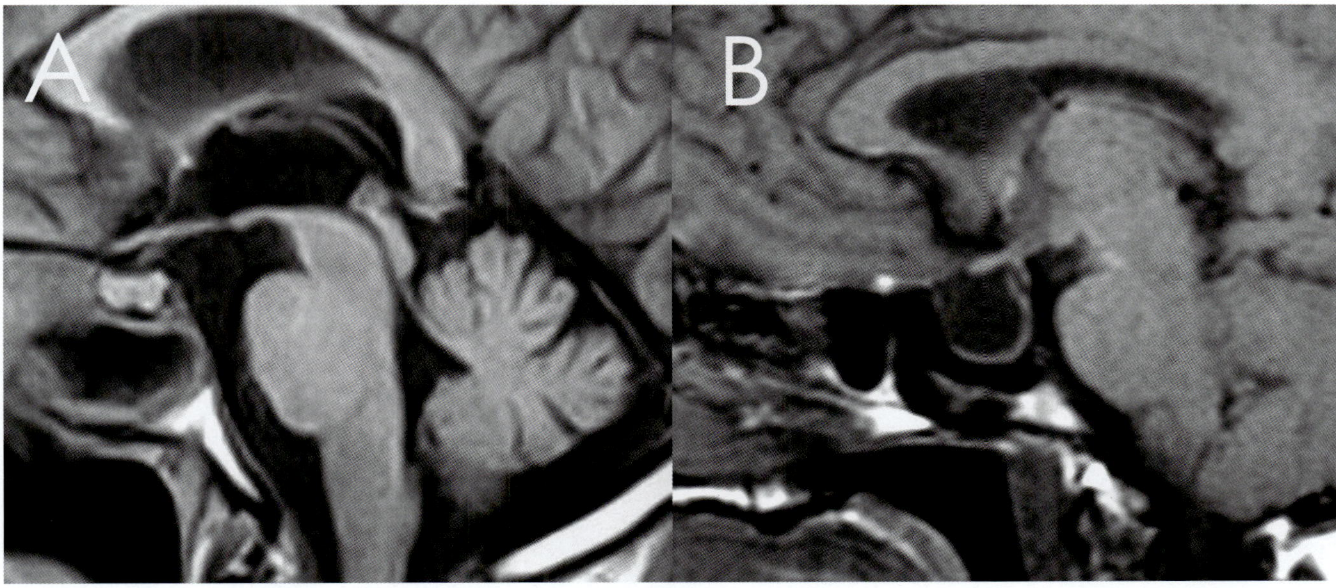

Fig. 18.3 The normal sella **(A)** and the empty sella **(B)** on T1-weighted MRI.

β_2-transferrin but has a lower processing cost, and the assay is more rapid (15 to 20 minutes).[13] In those with spontaneous leaks, a lumbar puncture for opening pressures (normal range, 5 to 195 mm H_2O)[18]) may be useful preoperatively to guide perioperative management. However, several large series has shown excellent results with only postoperative management of increased ICP.[1,12,19]

Imaging

Coronal, axial, and parasagittal bone window computed tomography (CT) images of the paranasal sinuses and skull base are essential in defining the bony defect and the anatomy for surgery, but cannot distinguish the encephalocele from nasal polyp or secretions.

Magnetic resonance imaging (MRI) and MRI cisternography (using highly T2-weighted images without intrathecal contrast) are useful in determining the contents of the sac, differentiating the sinus mucosa and mucus from the meningoencephalocele and demonstrating signs of increased ICP.[20] Radiographic evidence of increased ICP include a totally or partially empty sella; optic complex abnormalities; dural ectasia, most commonly at Meckel's cave; and arachnoid pits, which are small pits in the skull base hypothesized to occur at the site of arachnoid granulations due to increased CSF pressure (**Figs. 18.2** and **18.3**). The optic complex abnormalities are vertical tortuosity of the optic nerve, increased subarachnoid space around the optic nerve (total width of CSF greater than the diameter of the nerve), and scleral flattening. Meningoencephalocele formation, especially multiple (**Fig. 18.4**), in itself is considered a sign of BIH.[11,12,14,21] CT angiography or magnetic resonance angiography (MRA) may be used, particularly in large lesions to show vessels within the sac (**Fig. 18.5**).

CT cisternography can help define the meningoencephalocele and can show the site of an active CSF leak when there is the need for further diagnostic information (**Fig. 18.6**).[20,21]

■ Endoscopic Approach

Indications and Advantages

Repair is indicated to separate the cranial and nasal cavities. The rate of intracranial complications in nonleaking meningoencephaloceles is unknown. However if there is an associated CSF leak, the risk is high, with 13.9 to 41% of patients reported to have had an intracranial complication in different series, dropping to <1% following successful repair.[1] The endoscopic approach allows treatment of the meningoencephalocele without brain retraction or external incisions. Olfaction is usually preserved and sequelae of brain retraction such as postoperative epilepsy avoided.

Contraindications

Active acute or subacute bacterial sinusitis is the main contraindication and should be treated prior to repair. Chronic inflammatory sinus changes do not prevent successful closure, but management should be optimized prior to surgery. Lesions in the lateral frontal sinus (lateral to the medial orbital wall) or supraorbital ethmoid cells can be difficult to access transnasally and may require an ancillary frontal trephine or an open approach. The lack of a multidisciplinary team and specialized equipment should be considered a contraindication.

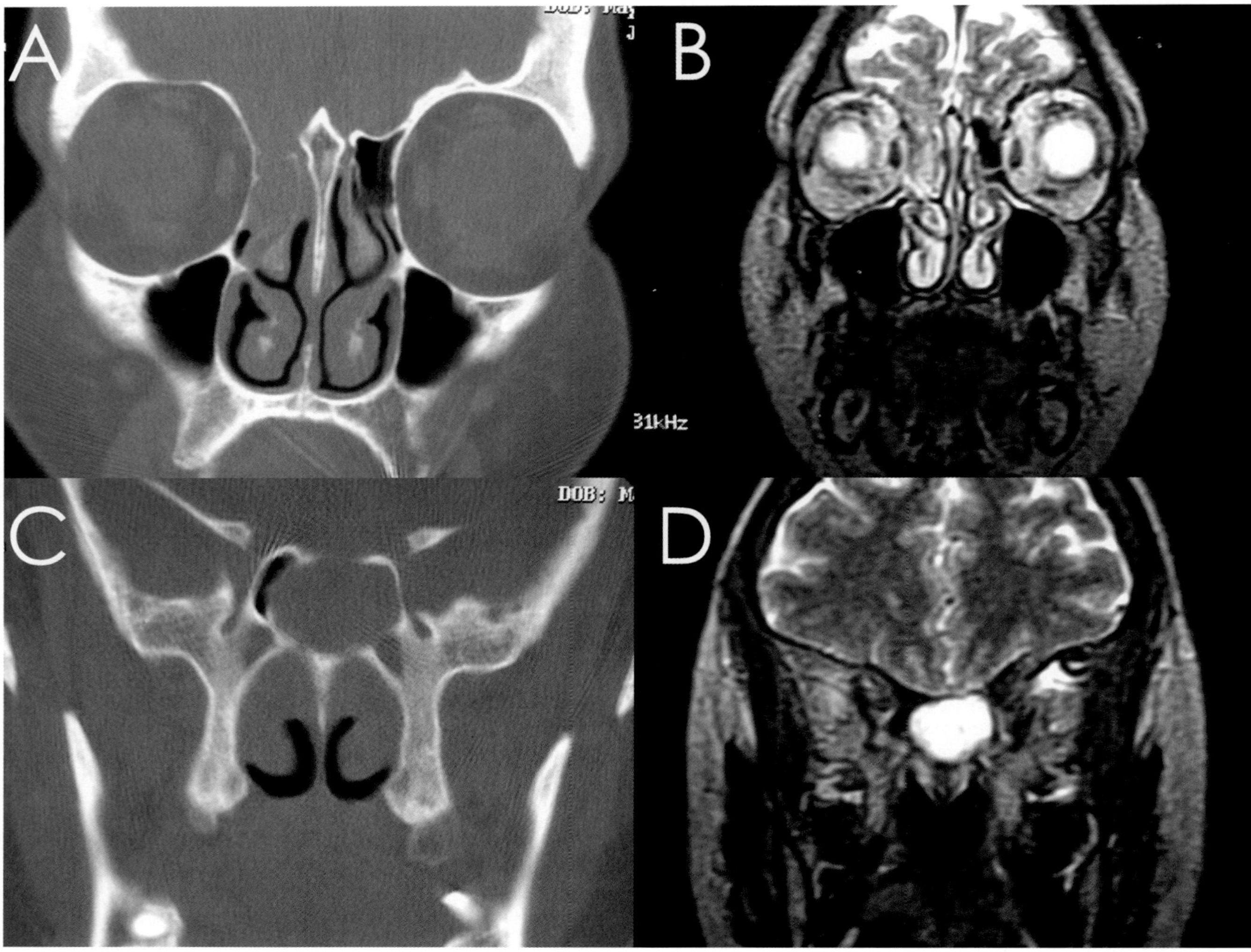

Fig. 18.4 Multiple meningoencephaloceles are a hallmark for benign intracranial hypertension. CT **(A,C)** and MRI **(B,D)** of right cribriform defect in the same patient with a sphenoid defect.

A 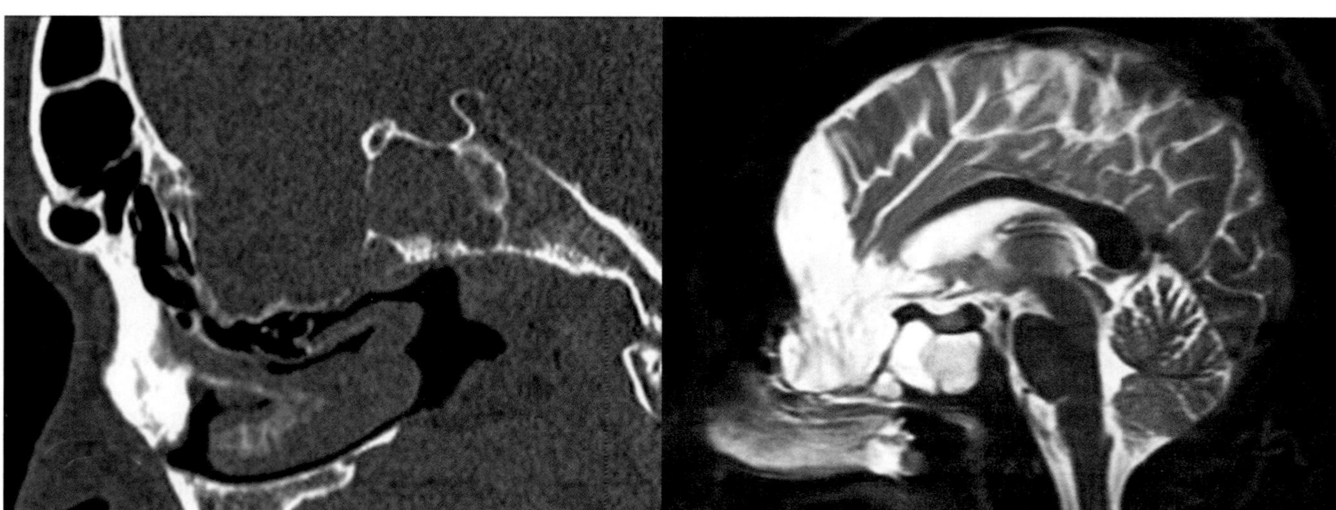 B

Fig. 18.5 Large vascular loop may be part of the sac contents for very large defects and should be evaluated with both CT **(A)** and MRI **(B)**.

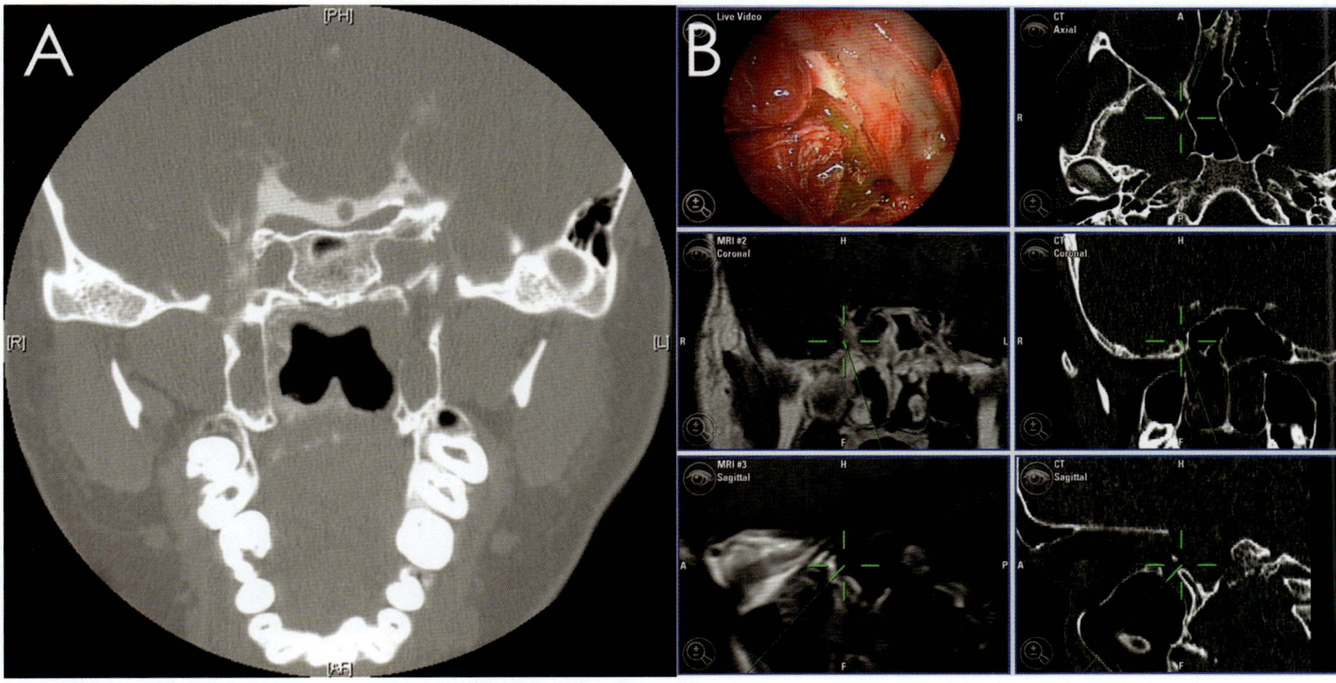

Fig. 18.6 Contrast cisternography **(A)** and intrathecal fluorescein **(B)** can be very helpful in identifying unusual cerebrospinal fluid (CSF) leaks. In this patient, contrast and CSF leaked into the nasopharynx from a right foramen rotundum defect.

Surgery

Instrumentation

A standard endoscopic setup is required. The bipolar forceps and frontal instruments (when required) are the essential additions to this setup. Image guidance systems, although not essential in every case, are extremely useful as the approach becomes more complex.

Operative Setup

The patient is placed supine in the reverse Trendelenburg position with the head turned slightly toward the surgeon. Intravenous antibiotic such as cefazolin is given at induction of anesthesia. Total intravenous hypotensive, bradycardic anesthesia is preferred to reduce bleeding, typically with remifentanil and propofol infusions.[22,23] Topical epinephrine 1:1000 is applied on cottonoids for 10 minutes before the start of the procedure, but ceased once dura is reached.

A lumbar cistern catheter enables measurement of CSF opening pressure, instillation of fluorescein, and postoperative lumbar drainage if required. Intrathecal fluorescein in the setting of an encephalocele can be useful in identifying a difficult leak site (**Fig. 18.6**), confirming closure of the CSF leak, and showing other leaks if multiple defects are present (**Fig. 18.4**). A dose of 0.1 mL of 10% fluorescein diluted into 10 mL of CSF instilled over 10 minutes is safe, although not approved by the Food and Drug Administration (FDA).[21,24,25]

Approach

Prior to beginning the approach, the nature of the planned repair should be determined so that local flaps can be preserved if necessary.

Frontal Sinus

A frontal recess approach may be sufficient or a modified endoscopic Lothrop procedure may be required both to gain access for the repair and to ensure adequate frontal sinus drainage postoperatively to prevent subsequent mucocele formation. For frontal sinus defects lateral to the medial orbital wall, a frontal trephine may be required as an adjunctive procedure, or an osteoplastic flap may be required.[26] Obliteration and ablative approaches should be avoided as the risk of long-term sequelae is very high. The potential for creating a mucocele in this setting is significant.[27,28] This may sentence a patient to a life of chronic frontal sinusitis, headaches, intracranial complications, and cosmetic deformities of the forehead. Unfortunately, these iatrogenic conditions only reveal themselves 8 to 10 years[29] after the obliteration. Where possible, maintenance of frontal sinus ventilation should be performed. Defects involving the frontal sinus can

Table 18.1 Frontal Sinus Defect and Cerebrospinal Fluid Leak Classification

• Type A	Defects wholly within the frontal sinus (medial or lateral to the lamina papyracea)
• Type B	Defects that involve any part of the frontal recess
• Type C	Defect not within the frontal recess but anatomically adjacent to the frontal recess.

be classified into three important management groups based on anatomic localization that impacts the surgical approach (**Table 18.1**).[26]

Ethmoid Roof/Cribriform Plate

An ethmoidectomy provides access to the ethmoid roof and lateral lamella, and, combined with middle turbinate resection, the cribriform plate. If the middle turbinate is resected, it should be taken as high as possible to enable the graft to sit flat on the skull base and to prevent lateralization and frontal recess obstruction. Typically, the cribriform bone is very thin and fragmented. It is common to create a final bony defect much greater than the original neck of the meningoencephalocele to define the boundaries of the repair.

Sphenoid

Lesions located close to the midline can be addressed using a transnasal or transethmoidal approach with a wide sphenoidotomy, with or without posterior septectomy and removal of the intersinus septum. The lateral recess usually requires a transpterygoid approach (**Fig. 18.7**). An ethmoidectomy, removal of the entire front face of the sphenoid, and a wide middle meatal antrostomy are performed and the sphenopalatine foramen identified. The posterior wall of the maxillary sinus is removed, exposing the pterygopalatine and infratemporal fossa. The maxillary artery and its branches are identified, clipped, and divided or transposed inferiorly to allow access to the pterygoid root. The remaining front face of the sphenoid laterally is removed to expose the defect. Care is taken to preserve the maxillary nerve, pterygopalatine ganglion, and branches, particularly the descending palatine nerves, which are at risk during this approach. The vidian nerve and its parasympathetic fibers that join V2 are preserved if possible to prevent the risk of postoperative dry eye.[11,30,31]

Resection and Preparation

The encephalocele is carefully resected back to the skull base defect using bipolar diathermy. Alternatively, the sac can be opened and the defect defined from within. The surrounding

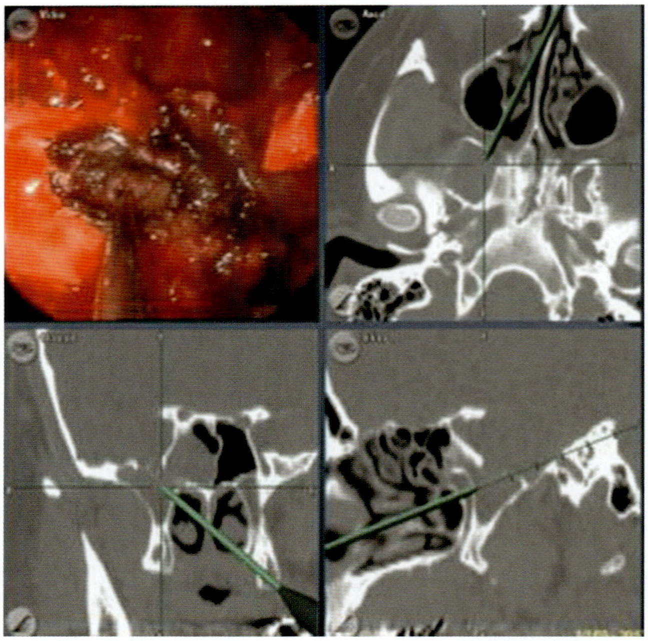

Fig. 18.7 Very lateral sphenoid defects are often best repaired via a transptyergoid approach. This access takes a direct route through the back of the maxillary sinus rather than using angled endoscopes and instruments via a sphenoidotomy.

mucoperiosteum is removed to prepare the graft site. In the cribriform plate, this is often not possible, and the mucosa is instead ablated.[15] The ascending olfactory fascicles prevent simple stripping of the mucosa. If a lumbar drain is used, removal of 10 to 15 mL of CSF with an ongoing drainage of 5 to 10 mL/hour can facilitate reduction of the encephalocele intracranially.[13,21] Most underlay grafts are subdural, but the edges of the dura can be carefully elevated for a few millimeters around the defect if an intracranial extradural layer is required.

Repair

A wide variety of materials and techniques have been described for repair of skull base defects with good results. Our preference is for a multilayer repair with an underlay graft within the subdural space and an overlay graft or flap in the nasal cavity.[1,2,32] The cribriform fossa represents a difficult area for underlay grafting.[15] The crista galli prevents easy medial placement and support for an underlay graft. Grafts in this area are carefully positioned to follow the crista and falx cerebri dura. Graft materials used include fat, temporalis fascia or fascia lata, bone, Alloderm (LifeCell [LifeCell Corp., Branchburg, NJ], acellular human dermis), and Duragen (Integra Lifesciences, Plainsboro NJ, bovine-derived collagen sponge). Mucosa should not be used intracranially due to the risk of intracranial mucocele formation and meningitis.[21]

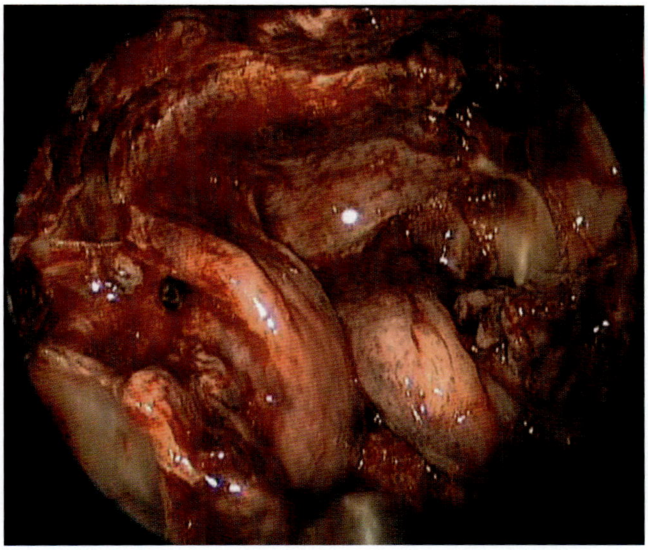

Fig. 18.8 Large pedicled septal flaps now form the basis of most of our large defect repairs. Bilateral flaps are used to cover a 4-cm defect or larger of the sphenoid planum and cribriform.

For small defects (<1 cm), the defect is plugged with Duragen or fat.[33] A free mucosal graft is then placed and supported with multiple layers of Gelfoam.

For high-pressure leaks, some authors advocate using bone from the septum, mastoid, or turbinate as an underlay to provide rigidity, although others have not found improved success rates or suggest that the bone interferes with obtaining a watertight seal.[12,13,34,35]

For larger defects (1 cm or more) or postradiotherapy, we prefer to use a vascularized flap to cover the underlay graft. The nasoseptal flap is the most versatile and is able to cover almost any defect of the anterior skull base (**Fig. 18.8**).[1,2,32,36–38] Alternatives include the posterior pedicle inferior turbinate flap, contralateral septal flap, middle turbinate flap, pericranial flap, and the transpterygoid temporoparietal flap.[2,39–41] Duraseal (Confluent Surgical Inc., Waltham MA) is a two-component synthetic glue that forms an absorbable polyethylene glycol hydrogel when mixed by the supplied applicator. It can be stored at room temperature and has a long shelf life. Tisseel (Baxter Healthcare, Deerfield, IL) is a two-component human-derived fibrin glue that is stored frozen and must be thawed prior to use. Large amounts of glue between layers of the repair may prevent the graft material from coming into contact with the wound bed, leading to subsequent leak.[21] We apply the fibrinogen component to the final flap and then place Gelfoam soaked in the thrombin solution to tack down the edges of the flap.

Nasal packing is used in layers to provide support for the repair. Packing does not provide sufficient compression to prevent CSF leakage, so it does not replace the need for a robust, watertight repair. We use multiple layers of Gelfoam with support from a Merocel sponge or a balloon such as a Foley catheter or Epistat (Xomed Inc., Jacksonville, FL). In the sphenoid, fat packing is avoided as it is usually impossible to remove all the mucosa and obliterate the sinus.[21]

Table 18.2 Indications for Lumbar Drain/Diversion Use at the Authors' Institution

- Raised intracranial pressure
- Post radiotherapy
- Early postoperative leak in the first 2 to 3 days

Postoperative Care

Antibiotics are used in our practice because of the extensive use of absorbable packing, the resultant sinus dysfunction, and the exposed secondary healing of the graft site, rather than for the prevention of intracranial complications. Our practice is to continue antibiotics after removal of the nonabsorbable nasal packs for 14 days.

Patients who do not have lumbar drains are nursed in a 30-degree head-up position and are instructed to avoid breath holding and Valsalva maneuvers. Laxatives and cough suppressants may be used. Gentle mobilization is started on day 2, and the patient can resume normal activity at 6 weeks.

Postoperative lumbar drainage is unnecessary.[1,2,19,32,42] Traditionally, many authors used it routinely for the first 24 to 48 hours.[7,43,44] However, modern practice has suggested that lumbar drainage is required in only specific settings (**Table 18.2**).

In patients with increased ICP or suspected BIH, good results have been shown using lumbar drainage for monitoring CSF pressure in conjunction with acetazolamide, a carbonic anhydrase inhibitor that reduces CSF production. In addition, long-term medical or surgical management of increased ICP may help prevent recurrent leaks from other skull base sites.[12,43]

Complications

Failure of repair usually presents with CSF leakage in the first 24 hours, but delayed leakage can occur, especially in those with BIH who may develop leaks from other sites. Other early complications include intracranial or nasal bleeding or infection. Longer-term complications are typically related to the approach and include cranial nerve injuries, particularly of the olfactory, V2, and vidian nerves; nasal synechiae; crusting; and mucoceles. Complication rates of meningitis, brain abscess, and subdural hematoma are all less than 1%, and late complications are rare.[1,3]

Reported success rates for closure of CSF leak are 90 to 98%, although most studies do not differentiate between patients with or without encephalocele.[1,3,19,42,45–47] Secondary repair, the presence of pneumocephalus, and spontaneous leaks, which are more likely to be associated with encephalocele formation, have a lower success rate, but a rate of 95% has been reported in a large series with careful perioperative management of ICP.[1,12,19,42]

Conclusion

Endoscopic management of anterior skull base encephaloceles is effective and safe, and is the treatment of choice in the majority of cases. The evaluation and management of elevated intracranial pressure is important, particularly in spontaneous cases.

References

1. Harvey RJ, Smith JE, Wise SK, Patel SJ, Frankel BM, Schlosser RJ. Intracranial complications before and after endoscopic skull base reconstruction. Am J Rhinol 2008;22:516–521
2. Harvey RJ, Nogueira JF, Schlosser RJ, Patel SJ, Vellutini E, Stamm AC. Closure of large skull base defects after endoscopic transnasal craniotomy. Clinical article. J Neurosurg 2009;111:371–379
3. Hegazy HM, Carrau RL, Snyderman CH, Kassam A, Zweig J. Transnasal endoscopic repair of cerebrospinal fluid rhinorrhea: a meta-analysis. Laryngoscope 2000;110:1166–1172
4. Batra PS, Citardi MJ, Worley S, Lee J, Lanza DC. Resection of anterior skull base tumors: comparison of combined traditional and endoscopic techniques. Am J Rhinol 2005;19:521–528
5. Casler JD, Doolittle AM, Mair EA. Endoscopic surgery of the anterior skull base. Laryngoscope 2005;115:16–24
6. Woodworth BA, Schlosser RJ, Faust RA, Bolger WE. Evolutions in the management of congenital intranasal skull base defects. Arch Otolaryngol Head Neck Surg 2004;130:1283–1288
7. Lund VJ. Endoscopic management of cerebrospinal fluid leaks. Am J Rhinol 2002;16:17–23
8. Locatelli D, Rampa F, Acchiardi I, Bignami M, Pistochini A, Castelnuovo P. Endoscopic endonasal approaches to anterior skull base defects in pediatric patients. Childs Nerv Syst 2006;22:1411–1418
9. Woodworth B, Schlosser RJ. Endoscopic repair of a congenital intranasal encephalocele in a 23 months old infant. Int J Pediatr Otorhinolaryngol 2005;69:1007–1009
10. Schlosser RJ, Bolger WE. Significance of empty sella in cerebrospinal fluid leaks. Otolaryngol Head Neck Surg 2003;128:32–38
11. Schlosser RJ, Bolger WE. Management of multiple spontaneous nasal meningoencephaloceles. Laryngoscope 2002;112:980–985
12. Woodworth BA, Prince A, Chiu AG, et al. Spontaneous CSF leaks: a paradigm for definitive repair and management of intracranial hypertension. Otolaryngol Head Neck Surg 2008;138:715–720
13. Bleier B, Govindaraj S, Palmer JN. State of the art cerebrospinal fluid leak and encephalocele repair. Oper Tech Otolaryngol 2006;17:49–57
14. Silver RI, Moonis G, Schlosser RJ, Bolger WE, Loevner LA. Radiographic signs of elevated intracranial pressure in idiopathic cerebrospinal fluid leaks: a possible presentation of idiopathic intracranial hypertension. Am J Rhinol 2007;21:257–261
15. Woodworth BA, Bolger WE, Schlosser RJ. Nasal cerebrospinal fluid leaks and encephaloceles. Oper Tech Otolaryngol 2006;17:111–116
16. Barañano CF, Curé J, Palmer JN, Woodworth BA. Sternberg's canal: fact or fiction? Am J Rhinol Allergy 2009;23:167–171
17. Papadea C, Schlosser RJ. Rapid method for beta2-transferrin in cerebrospinal fluid leakage using an automated immunofixation electrophoresis system. Clin Chem 2005;51:464–470
18. Han CY, Backous DD. Basic principles of cerebrospinal fluid metabolism and intracranial pressure homeostasis. Otolaryngol Clin North Am 2005;38:569–576
19. Wise SK, Harvey RJ, Neal JG, Patel SJ, Frankel BM, Schlosser RJ. Factors contributing to failure in endoscopic skull base defect repair. Am J Rhinol Allergy 2009;23:185–191
20. Lund VJ, Savy L, Lloyd G, Howard D. Optimum imaging and diagnosis of cerebrospinal fluid rhinorrhoea. J Laryngol Otol 2000;114:988–992
21. Schlosser RJ, Bolger WE. Endoscopic management of cerebrospinal fluid rhinorrhea. Otolaryngol Clin North Am 2006;39:523–538, ix
22. Eberhart LHJ, Folz BJ, Wulf H, Geldner G. Intravenous anesthesia provides optimal surgical conditions during microscopic and endoscopic sinus surgery. Laryngoscope 2003;113:1369–1373
23. Wormald PJ, van Renen G, Perks J, Jones JA, Langton-Hewer CD. The effect of the total intravenous anesthesia compared with inhalational anesthesia on the surgical field during endoscopic sinus surgery. Am J Rhinol 2005;19:514–520
24. Tabaee A, Placantonakis DG, Schwartz TH, Anand VK. Intrathecal fluorescein in endoscopic skull base surgery. Otolaryngol Head Neck Surg 2007;137:316–320
25. Keerl R, Weber RK, Draf W, Wienke A, Schaefer SD. Use of sodium fluorescein solution for detection of cerebrospinal fluid fistulas: an analysis of 420 administrations and reported complications in Europe and the United States. Laryngoscope 2004;114:266–272
26. Woodworth BA, Schlosser RJ, Palmer JN. Endoscopic repair of frontal sinus cerebrospinal fluid leaks. J Laryngol Otol 2005;119:709–713
27. Chandra RK, Kennedy DW, Palmer JN. Endoscopic management of failed frontal sinus obliteration. Am J Rhinol 2004;18:279–284
28. Weber R, Draf W, Keerl R, et al. Osteoplastic frontal sinus surgery with fat obliteration: technique and long-term results using magnetic resonance imaging in 82 operations. Laryngoscope 2000;110:1037–1044
29. Bockmühl U, Kratzsch B, Benda K, Draf W. Surgery for paranasal sinus mucocoeles: efficacy of endonasal micro-endoscopic management and long-term results of 185 patients. Rhinology 2006;44:62–67
30. Woodworth BA, Neal JG, Schlosser RJ. Sphenoid sinus cerebrospinal fluid leaks. Oper Tech Otolaryngol 2006;17:37–42
31. Schwartz TH, Fraser JF, Brown S, Tabaee A, Kacker A, Anand VK. Endoscopic cranial base surgery: classification of operative approaches. Neurosurgery 2008;62:991–1002, discussion 1002–1005
32. Stamm AC, Vellutini E, Harvey RJ, Nogeira JF Jr, Herman DR. Endoscopic transnasal craniotomy and the resection of craniopharyngioma. Laryngoscope 2008;118:1142–1148
33. Wormald PJ, McDonogh M. 'Bath-plug' technique for the endoscopic management of cerebrospinal fluid leaks. J Laryngol Otol 1997;111:1042–1046
34. Zweig JL, Carrau RL, Celin SE, et al. Endoscopic repair of cerebrospinal fluid leaks to the sinonasal tract: predictors of success. Otolaryngol Head Neck Surg 2000;123:195–201
35. Wormald PJ. Cerebrospinal fluid leak closure. In: Endoscopic Sinus Surgery—Anatomy, Three Dimensional Reconstruction, and Surgical Technique. New York: Thieme Medical Publishers; 2005:109–119
36. Hadad G, Bassagasteguy L, Carrau RL, et al. A novel reconstructive technique after endoscopic expanded endonasal approaches: vascular pedicle nasoseptal flap. Laryngoscope 2006;116:1882–1886
37. Kassam AB, Thomas A, Carrau RL, et al. Endoscopic reconstruction of the cranial base using a pedicled nasoseptal flap. Neurosurgery 2008;63(1, Suppl 1):ONS44–ONS52, discussion ONS52–ONS53
38. Pinheiro-Neto CD, Prevedello DM, Carrau RL, et al. Improving the design of the pedicled nasoseptal flap for skull base reconstruction: a radioanatomic study. Laryngoscope 2007;117:1560–1569
39. Harvey RJ, Sheahan PO, Schlosser RJ. Inferior turbinate pedicle flap for endoscopic skull base defect repair. Am J Rhinol Allergy 2009;23:522–526
40. Fortes FSG, Carrau RL, Snyderman CH, et al. The posterior pedicle inferior turbinate flap: a new vascularized flap for skull base reconstruction. Laryngoscope 2007;117:1329–1332
41. Carrau RL, Snyderman CH, Kassam AB. The management of cerebrospinal fluid leaks in patients at risk for high-pressure hydrocephalus. Laryngoscope 2005;115:205–212

42. Wise SK, Harvey RJ, Patel SJ, Frankel BM, Schlosser RJ. Endoscopic repair of skull base defects presenting with pneumocephalus. J Otolaryngol Head Neck Surg 2009;38:509–516

43. Schlosser RJ, Wilensky EM, Grady MS, Palmer JN, Kennedy DW, Bolger WE. Cerebrospinal fluid pressure monitoring after repair of cerebrospinal fluid leaks. Otolaryngol Head Neck Surg 2004;130:443–448

44. Casiano RR, Jassir D. Endoscopic cerebrospinal fluid rhinorrhea repair: is a lumbar drain necessary? Otolaryngol Head Neck Surg 1999;121: 745–750

45. Banks CA, Palmer JN, Chiu AG, O'Malley BW Jr, Woodworth BA, Kennedy DW. Endoscopic closure of CSF rhinorrhea: 193 cases over 21 years. Otolaryngol Head Neck Surg 2009;140:826–833

46. Kirtane MV, Gautham K, Upadhyaya SR. Endoscopic CSF rhinorrhea closure: our experience in 267 cases. Otolaryngol Head Neck Surg 2005; 132:208–212

47. Schick B, Ibing R, Brors D, Draf W. Long-term study of endonasal duraplasty and review of the literature. Ann Otol Rhinol Laryngol 2001; 110:142–147

VI Tips and Pearls in the Transplanum Approach

19 Endoscopic Transnasal Craniectomy and the Resection of Extensive Craniopharyngiomas

Richard J. Harvey, Aldo Cassol Stamm, Daniel Timperley, and Eduardo Vellutini

Tips and Pearls

- The most important hemostatic technique, especially in venous bleeding, may be patience.

Introduction

Craniopharyngioma is an uncommon benign tumor, accounting for 2 to 5% of all intracranial neoplasms.[1] Distribution by age is bimodal, with the peak incidence in children at 5 to 14 years of age and in adults at 65 to 74 years of age, with an incidence of 0.14 to 2 per 100,000.[2,3] Although total surgical removal is the aim of the treatment, craniopharyngioma is a difficult tumor to excise completely. Morbidity from an intrapial tumor adherent to the pituitary stalk, hypothalamus, and anterior cerebral vessels has always dictated the completeness of resection. Tumor involvement of these structures combined with poor surgical access, limited instrumentation for sharp dissection, and limited visualization of the anatomical relationships has often hindered dissection regardless of the approach. The use of endoscopes in surgery for these lesions has been particularly successful, allowing minimal operative morbidity, direct access to pathology, and detailed visual assessment of anatomy and resection limits (Harvey laryngoscope). For craniopharyngioma, effective and safe treatment of lesions involving the skull base is still a challenging problem.

Debate exists regarding the histologic description of craniopharyngiomas. Currently, three theories are widely accepted, and from these, the adamantinomatous, squamous papillary, and mixed variants have been derived. They are as follows:

- Embryogenetic theory: the adamantinomatous type ("adamantinoma") arises from epithelial remnants of the Rathke pouch or the precursors to the adenohypophysis and infundibulum migrate. Rests can occur from the pharynx to the sella turcica and third ventricle.
- Metaplastic theory: the squamous papillary type results secondary to metaplasia of squamous epithelial cell rests that arise from squamous cell nests of the pituitary stalk and pars distalis junction.
- Variant of midline congenital cyst: the variant is a midline congenital tumor not fundamentally different from an epidermoid cyst.

Craniopharyngiomas are usually composed of both solid and cystic components. Cyst walls are lined with stratified squamous epithelium with pearly keratin formations. An outer layer is columnar epithelium. Calcifications occur 90% of children and 40% in adults. A "motor oil" description is often given to the cystic fluid.

Subfrontal and pterional craniotomies have been the traditional approaches to extensive craniopharyngioma with suprasellar extension.[4] The transsphenoidal route had been previously reserved for purely intrasellar tumors. The extended transsphenoidal transplanum endoscopic[5] approach may benefit patients with extensive craniopharyngioma (**Fig. 19.1**), facilitating direct access to pathology, minimizing brain retraction, and reducing manipulation of the optic chiasm, the hospital stay,[6] and morbidity.[7]

Morbidity from the open approaches may be significant, especially when surgical resection is subtotal. The balance of surgical morbidity and long-term control is a decision for the patient and the operative team. Karavitaki et al[8] recently

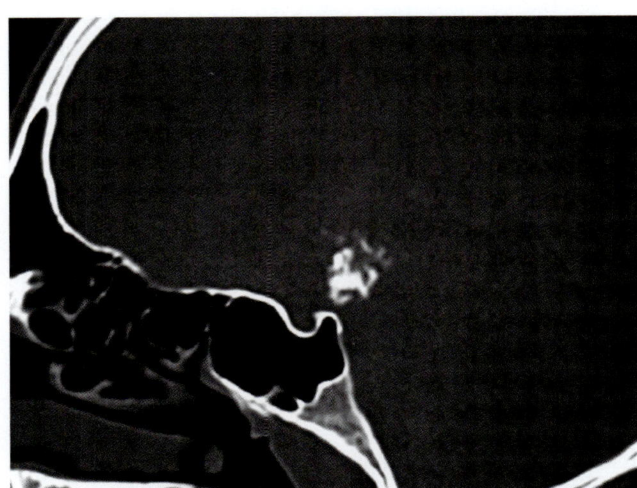

Fig. 19.1 Extensive suprasellar craniopharyngioma on computer tomography (CT). Sagittal view. Note calcification, which is common within large tumors.

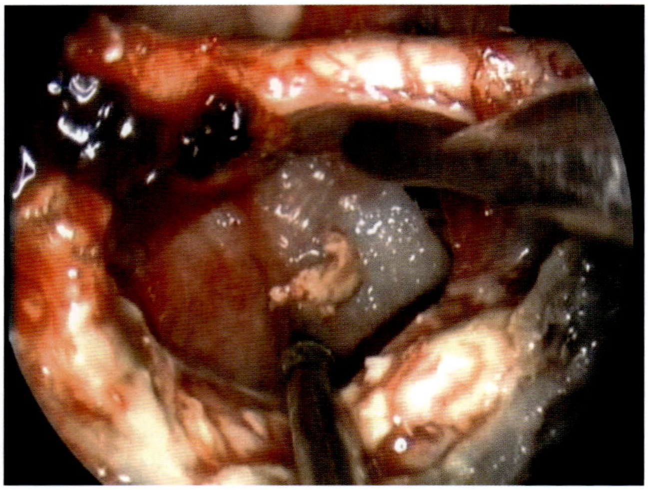

Fig. 19.2 Visualization via the endoscopic transnasal craniectomy. Two-surgeon dissection is performed. Note optic chiasma and residual tumor being removed.

reviewed the literature on the long-term outcomes in craniopharyngioma. Accepted 10-year recurrence-free survival rates were 74 to 81% after gross total resection, 41 to 42% after partial removal, and 83 to 90% after surgery (defined as partial or minimal resection) and radiotherapy. The aggressiveness of craniopharyngioma in adults compared with children has been debated. There appears to be little evidence supporting a substantial difference in behavior from larger cohorts.[8–10]

The extended transsphenoidal approach has been described with microsurgical dissection,[11–17] and extensive nonadenomatous tumors have been managed with these techniques.[13] The use of an extended sellar opening by removing the sphenoid planum and tuberculum sellae is described in these series.[13] This route is often the first option even for suprasellar lesions.[17] Transsphenoidal approaches have gained wide acceptance because they offer direct access to the tumor site and avoid the morbidity of transcraniectomy surgery.[17] Subsequently, the transsphenoidal approach has evolved to a totally endoscopic transnasal surgery.[18] A large transnasal craniectomy is not hampered by a long narrow surgical corridor, which previously combined both vision and surgical instruments (**Fig. 19.2**). Visualization can be superior with an endoscopic approach compared with the microsurgical access.[19]

Indications and Advantages

Broadly, the goals of transnasal craniectomy for craniopharyngioma should include the following:

- Removal of disease and prevention of regrowth
- Relief of hydrocephalus
- Decompression of the optic nerve and chiasm
- Minimal functional loss
    - o Vision
    - o Other cranial nerve integrity
    - o Pituitary/hypothalamic function
    - o Orbital function

An understanding of the significant complications associated with surgery, whether neurologic, orbital, endocrine, or infectious, is paramount for an informed discussion with a patient considering craniopharyngioma resection.

Contraindications

Contraindications include the following:

- Acute/subacute sinusitis
- No multidisciplinary team available
- Lack of specialized equipment

Relative situations that may lead to poor outcomes include tumor size >4 cm, patient age <5 years, severe hypothalamic dysfunction preoperatively, and a surgical approach that is overly focused on total resection without balancing the impact of morbidity.

Diagnostic Workup

Radiologic Assessment

Tumor classification is based on magnetic resonance imaging (MRI), computed tomography (CT), and intraoperative findings. The size, position relative to the optic chiasm (pre- or postchiasmatic), and the vertical extension is recorded. The extension vertically is defined as a combination of sellar, suprasellar, or ventricular. The suprasellar or intracranial extension can be categorized as C, D, E, or F by the Yasargil[20] classification.

Endocrinologic Assessment

All patients should undergo assessment by an endocrinologist, which should include the following:

- Adrenocorticotropic hormone (ACTH or corticotropin)
- Growth hormone (GH) and insulin growth factor (IGF-1)
- Cortisol
- Prolactin
- Thyrotropin (thyroid-stimulating hormone [TSH])
- Triiodothyronine (T_3)
- Thyroxine (T_4)
- Luteinizing hormone (LH)
- Follicle-stimulating hormone (FSH)

The diagnosis of preoperative diabetes insipidus should be made with serum sodium levels and osmolarity, together with urine specific gravity and osmolarity. Hypothalamic injury, including appetite dysfunction and violent behavior, should be assessed. Any abnormalities should be corrected preoperatively, but, at the very least, low cortisol levels and diabetes insipidus should be treated prior to any surgical procedure.

Ophthalmology Assessment

Visual acuity and visual field assessment are required to delineate any deficit, including papilledema. Formal visual assessment is performed by an ophthalmologist. Other cranial neuropathies need to be documented.

■ Surgery

A large transnasal craniectomy forms the basis of our intradural endoscopic procedure. It provides optimal visualization of pathology (**Fig. 19.3**) and critical anatomy, and entails less manipulation of brain tissue and easy access for several instruments. This is fundamentally different from the small sellar floor openings that are described in most adenomatous pituitary surgery.[21] The wider approach also enables two surgeons to work concomitantly binasally without constant criss-crossing of instruments. The endoscopic route may also provide unoperated surgical planes when multiple previous open approaches have been performed.

Instruments

Endoscopic craniopharyngioma is highly dependent on specialized instrumentation, and its absence is an absolute contraindication to surgery. Dissection instruments and drills that are appropriately long enough to perform dissection beyond the sphenoid are essential. Similarly, high-quality endoscopes and video equipment is required. It is not appropriate to perform endoscopic skull base surgery (SBS) without camera equipment. The operative team needs to be visually informed of the state of surgery. A second surgeon, for bimanual dissection, and the operating room staff should be actively involved. The ability to maintain hemostasis and a workable operative field during prolonged surgery is a demanding aspect of extended endoscopic surgery. Long endoscopic bipolar forceps and hemostatic materials such as Surgicel or Avitene are essential to this process.[22]

This surgery should not be performed with simple pituitary curette instrumentation. Sharp dissection needs to be performed to remove the tumor without vascular injury.

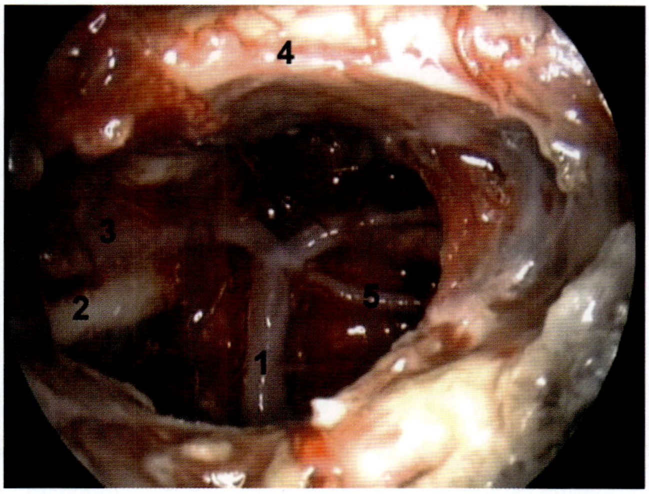

Fig. 19.3 Large transnasal craniectomy. 1, basilar artery; 2, third cranial nerve; 3, posterior cerebral artery; 4, optic chiasm; 5, superior cerebellar artery.

Preparation

An endoscopic transnasal craniectomy is performed with the patient under general controlled hypotensive anesthesia without Mayfield fixation. Total intravenous anesthesia is associated with better mucosal hemostasis.[23,24] Cotton pledgets containing adrenaline 1:1000 are placed in the nasal cavity over the areas of surgical access for 10 minutes before the surgical procedure. The septum is infiltrated with lidocaine with adrenaline 1:100,000.

The availability of hemostatic materials and techniques is important. The principles of hemostasis in endoscopic surgery differ little from those of the microsurgical era. Prevention of bleeding is obviously the best solution. Tumor debulking, extracapsular sharp dissection, and countertraction using gentle suction still form the foundation of cerebrovascular control.[22] Standard neurosurgical bayonets are often not appropriate via the long surgical corridor of endoscopic skull base surgery. Specialized bipolar instrumentation is essential.

Approach

An uncinectomy, wide antrostomy with anterior and posterior ethmoidectomy is performed. The inferior half of the superior turbinate is resected to give access to the entire front wall of the sphenoid. The maximum amount of the front wall is then removed by commencing at the sphenoid ostium. At this stage, a posterior pedicled mucoperiosteal flap based on the septal branch of the sphenopalatine artery is usually developed bilaterally (**Fig. 19.4**). A posterior septectomy is then performed. The same exposure is then repeated on the contralateral side.

The mucosa of the posterior sphenoid wall is then displaced laterally. Drilling of the thick tuberculum sellae bone and the sella is then performed (**Fig. 19.5**). An area the entire intercarotid width is thinned down to eggshell thickness with a high-speed drill and then removed. A Kerrison rongeur may be used for additional bone removal. This is a much wider and higher area that the one exposed in standard pituitary surgery. Bone removal continues along the sphenoid planum. The intercavernous sinus is then coagulated or ligated.

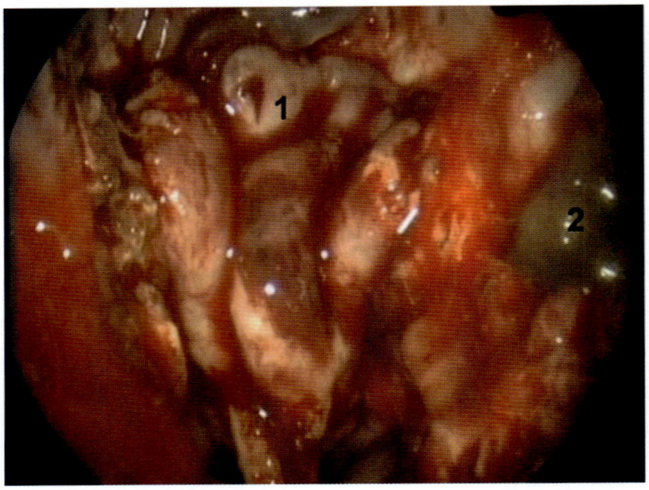

Fig. 19.4 A pedicled mucoperiosteal flap based on the septal branch of the sphenopalatine artery (1). 2, maxillary sinus.

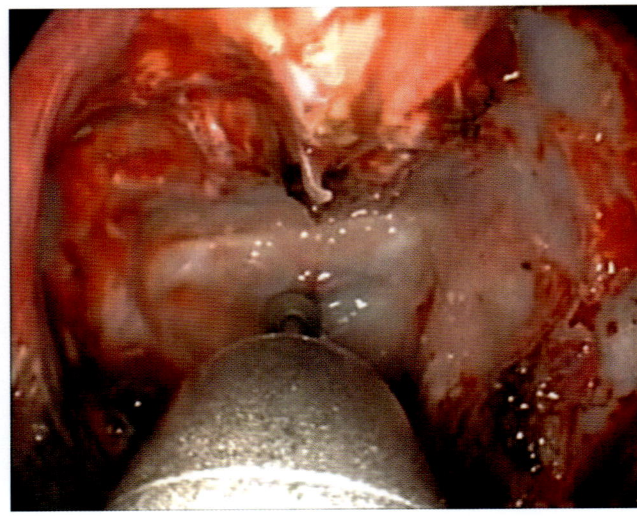

Fig. 19.5 Drilling of the thick tuberculum sellae bone.

The dura is opened above and below the intercavernous sinus, exposing the suprasellar region and optic chiasm. Sharp extraarachnoid dissection of the tumor proceeds with a two-surgeon technique (**Fig. 19.6**).

Even with the best preoperative imaging, the relationship of tumor to intracranial structures can be difficult to demonstrate. It is still extremely difficult to evaluate before surgery whether some tumors are extraarachnoidal, extrapial-subarachnoidal, or partially intraparenchymal-subpial.[25] This weighs heavily on considerations to obtain complete resection. Suprasellar pathologies such as craniopharyngiomas may often encase the pituitary stalk or involve the hypothalamus. Resection of the pituitary stalk carries considerable morbidity, with hormone replacement and reproductive dysfunction for adults and even greater impact on the growth and development for children. Hypothalamic injury may result in severe, crippling, and life-threatening sequelae, such as adipsia, morbid obesity, sleep disturbances, and behavioral and cognitive disorders.[26] The decision to attempt complete tumor removal, when resection or injury to these structures is inevitable, should be discussed with the patient prior to surgery and not left to an intraoperative dilemma when such circumstances arise.[27]

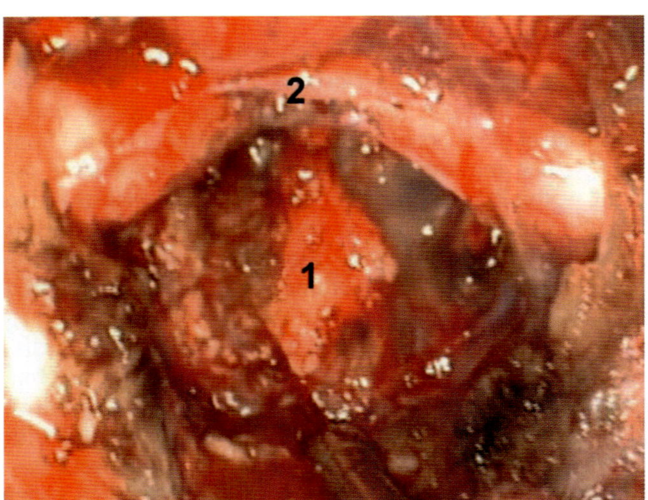

Fig. 19.6 Exposing and dissection the tumor. 1, craniopharyngioma; 2, optic chiasma.

Revision Surgery

Revision endoscopic surgery may be necessary, and for pituitary adenoma it is almost the standard of care in many centers.[28] There are three important implications of previous surgery in this area. First, the optic chiasm may lie superior or inferior to its original position and will often have fat from a previous repair adherent in the prechiasmatic position. Second, the anterior cerebral vessels may be adherent to the previous repair of a transplanum approach. If the arteries are adherent to fat or fascia, it may be prudent to leave an island of scar tissue on the vessel rather than attempt dissection. Finally, the vasculature of the pituitary may be easily damaged if there is scar tissue involving the stalk. Most importantly, a recurrent superior hypophyseal artery may lie within the vasculature of the pituitary stalk, and injury can result in optic nerve or pituitary injury.[29,30]

Repair

A rotation pedicled mucoperiosteal flap forms the foundation for repair of the defect that has been made in the central skull base.[31,32] This flap is raised from the septum and based on the septal branch of the sphenopalatine artery. The flap is

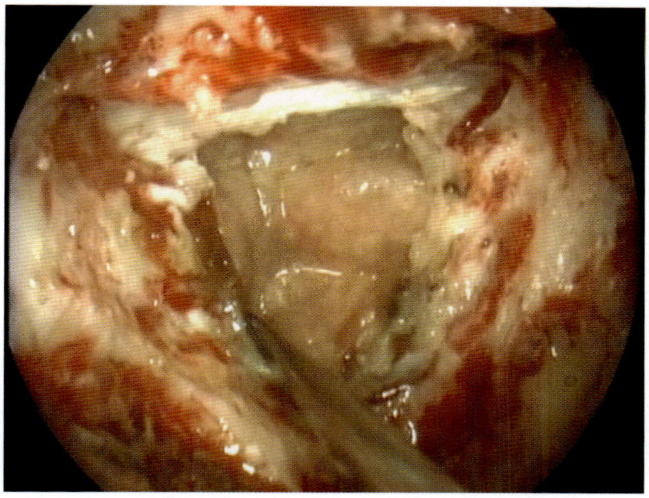

Fig. 19.7 Duragen is used to fill dead space and form a buttress.

raised unilaterally or bilaterally at the beginning of the surgery. The flap is then guarded from subsequent trauma by relocating it to the ipsilateral maxillary sinus or in the nasopharynx until later reconstruction.

Duragen is used to fill dead space and form a buttress for the graft (**Fig. 19.7**). Fibrin tissue glue is used to secure the repair. Gelfoam is layered to the area with or without gauze packing. The packing is supported by a Foley or Epistat balloon catheter.

Complications

Endocrine recovery has not been widely reported after resection and is likely to be extremely rare.[8] The compressive or vascular effects on the pituitary and on the hypothalamus may be potentially irreversible, and much of the long-term sequelae might be predetermined prior to surgical intervention. Published rates of hyperphagia/excessive weight gain and manifestations of severe hypothalamic injury at 10 years are approximately 39%.[8] Even though the endoscopic visualization of the relationship between the tumor and critical anatomy can be precise, careful preoperative assessment with an endocrinologist, within a multidisciplinary team, for pituitary and hypothalamic dysfunction is essential in the operative planning for these patients.[26,33,34] Visual deterioration postresection should be avoided and represents vascular disruption to the chiasmic vasculature.

Major complications include the following:

- Death
- Infection (meningitis, ventriculitis, subdural abscess)
- Intracranial bleeding (arachnoid or subdural)
- Endocrine disturbances (diabetes insipidus, pituitary)
- Neurologic (cranial nerve deficits, cerebrovascular accidents, epilepsy, hypothalamic dysfunction)
- Pneumocephalus

Postoperative Care

Recovery entails neurologic observation with the patient in high dependency status. CT is performed at our institution on the first postoperative day, scanning for evidence of hemorrhage. Antibiotics are used perioperatively and continued postoperatively while nasal packing remains in situ. Packing is left in place for 3 to 7 days, as most grafts are adherent to bone in 1 week.[35] The onset of diabetes insipidus is monitored with serum and urine sodium/osmolality measurements. Patients are confined to bed for 48 hours, with 30-degree head elevation, and avoid straining, Valsalva maneuvers, and nose blowing. Compression stockings are used. Lumbar drains are not used unless there is an additional comorbidity such as raised intracranial hypertension or prior radiotherapy. Discharge usually occurs at 3 to 5 days postoperatively, and an MRI is done early for baseline assessment. This is important, as postsurgical MRI signaling is often difficult to interpret.[36]

Conclusion

The ability to robustly close large skull base defects endoscopically has greatly improved the feasibility of the endoscopic approach for extensive craniopharyngioma.[31,32] There should not be an attempt to work through a small sella opening with curette techniques, but rather widely display the anatomical field and sharply remove disease as is done with open techniques. Direct assessment of vascular, pituitary, and hypothalamic involvement should reduce morbidity with this approach. Although data supporting a shift will be slow to appear, the type of approach for extensive disease should rely on the skill and resources of the treatment team. The results for recurrent craniopharyngioma vary greatly, depending on the philosophy of the surgical team.[8]

References

1. Nelson JS, Parisi JE, Schochet SS. Principles and Practice of Neuropathology. St. Louis: Mosby; 1993
2. Garrè ML, Cama A. Craniopharyngioma: modern concepts in pathogenesis and treatment. Curr Opin Pediatr 2007;19:471–479
3. Haupt R, Magnani C, Pavanello M, Caruso S, Dama E, Garrè ML. Epidemiological aspects of craniopharyngioma. J Pediatr Endocrinol Metab 2006;19(Suppl 1):289–293
4. de Divitiis E, Cavallo LM, Cappabianca P, Esposito F. Extended endoscopic endonasal transsphenoidal approach for the removal of suprasellar tumors: Part 2. Neurosurgery 2007;60:46–58, discussion 58–59
5. Snyderman C, Kassam A, Carrau R, Mintz A, Gardner P, Prevedello DM. Acquisition of surgical skills for endonasal skull base surgery: a training program. Laryngoscope 2007;117:699–705
6. Casler JD, Doolittle AM, Mair EA. Endoscopic surgery of the anterior skull base. Laryngoscope 2005;115:16–24
7. Batra PS, Citardi MJ, Lanza DC. Isolated sphenoid sinusitis after transsphenoidal hypophysectomy. Am J Rhinol 2005;19:185–189
8. Karavitaki N, Brufani C, Warner JT, et al. Craniopharyngiomas in children and adults: systematic analysis of 121 cases with long-term follow-up. Clin Endocrinol (Oxf) 2005;62:397–409
9. Petito CK, DeGirolami U, Earle KM. Craniopharyngiomas: a clinical and pathological review. Cancer 1976;37:1944–1952

10. Manaka S, Teramoto A, Takakura K. The efficacy of radiotherapy for craniopharyngioma. J Neurosurg 1985;62:648–656

11. Dumont AS, Kanter AS, Jane JA Jr, Laws ER Jr. Extended transsphenoidal approach. Front Horm Res 2006;34:29–45

12. Chakrabarti I, Amar AP, Couldwell W, Weiss MH. Long-term neurological, visual, and endocrine outcomes following transnasal resection of craniopharyngioma. J Neurosurg 2005;102:650–657

13. Couldwell WT, Weiss MH, Rabb C, Liu JK, Apfelbaum RI, Fukushima T. Variations on the standard transsphenoidal approach to the sellar region, with emphasis on the extended approaches and parasellar approaches: surgical experience in 105 cases. Neurosurgery 2004;55: 539–547, discussion 547–550

14. Dusick JR, Esposito F, Kelly DF, et al. The extended direct endonasal transsphenoidal approach for nonadenomatous suprasellar tumors. J Neurosurg 2005;102:832–841

15. König A, Lüdecke DK, Herrmann HD. Transnasal surgery in the treatment of craniopharyngiomas. Acta Neurochir (Wien) 1986;83:1–7

16. Kouri JG, Chen MY, Watson JC, Oldfield EH. Resection of suprasellar tumors by using a modified transsphenoidal approach. Report of four cases. J Neurosurg 2000;92:1028–1035

17. Maira G, Anile C, Albanese A, Cabezas D, Pardi F, Vignati A. The role of transsphenoidal surgery in the treatment of craniopharyngiomas. J Neurosurg 2004;100:445–451

18. Stamm AM. Transnasal endoscopy-assisted skull base surgery. Ann Otol Rhinol Laryngol Suppl 2006;196:45–53

19. Catapano D, Sloffer CA, Frank G, Pasquini E, D'Angelo VA, Lanzino G. Comparison between the microscope and endoscope in the direct endonasal extended transsphenoidal approach: anatomical study. J Neurosurg 2006;104:419–425

20. Yaşargil MG, Curcic M, Kis M, Siegenthaler G, Teddy PJ, Roth P. Total removal of craniopharyngiomas. Approaches and long-term results in 144 patients. J Neurosurg 1990;73:3–11

21. Sethi DS, Leong JL. Endoscopic pituitary surgery. Otolaryngol Clin North Am 2006;39:563–583, x

22. Kassam A, Snyderman CH, Carrau RL, Gardner P, Mintz A. Endoneurosurgical hemostasis techniques: lessons learned from 400 cases. Neurosurg Focus 2005;19:E7

23. Eberhart LH, Folz BJ, Wulf H, Geldner G. Intravenous anesthesia provides optimal surgical conditions during microscopic and endoscopic sinus surgery. Laryngoscope 2003;113:1369–1373

24. Wormald PJ, van Renen G, Perks J, Jones JA, Langton-Hewer CD. The effect of the total intravenous anesthesia compared with inhalational anesthesia on the surgical field during endoscopic sinus surgery. Am J Rhinol 2005;19:514–520

25. Frank G, Pasquini E, Doglietto F, et al. The endoscopic extended transsphenoidal approach for craniopharyngiomas. Neurosurgery 2006; 59(1, Suppl 1):ONS75–ONS83, discussion ONS75–ONS83

26. Spoudeas HA, Saran F, Pizer B, Spoudeas HA, Saran F, Pizer B. A multimodality approach to the treatment of craniopharyngiomas avoiding hypothalamic morbidity: a UK perspective. J Pediatr Endocrinol Metab 2006;19(Suppl 1):447–451

27. Frank G, Sciarretta V, Calbucci F, Farneti G, Mazzatenta D, Pasquini E. The endoscopic transnasal transsphenoidal approach for the treatment of cranial base chordomas and chondrosarcomas. Neurosurgery 2006; 59(1, Suppl 1):ONS50–ONS57, discussion ONS50–ONS57

28. Carrau RL, Kassam AB, Snyderman CH. Pituitary surgery. Otolaryngol Clin North Am 2001;34:1143–1155, ix

29. van Overbeeke J, Sekhar L. Microanatomy of the blood supply to the optic nerve. Orbit 2003;22:81–88

30. Krisht AF, Barrow DL, Barnett DW, Bonner GD, Shengalaia G. The microsurgical anatomy of the superior hypophyseal artery. Neurosurgery 1994;35:899–903, discussion 903

31. Harvey RJ, Nogueira JF, Schlosser RJ, Patel SJ, Vellutini E, Stamm AC. Closure of large skull base defects after endoscopic transnasal craniotomy. Clinical article. J Neurosurg 2009;111:371–379

32. Stamm AC, Vellutini E, Harvey RJ, Nogeira JF Jr, Herman DR. Endoscopic transnasal craniotomy and the resection of craniopharyngioma. Laryngoscope 2008;118:1142–1148

33. Puget S, Garnett M, Wray A, et al. Pediatric craniopharyngiomas: classification and treatment according to the degree of hypothalamic involvement. [see comment] J Neurosurg 2007;106(1, Suppl)3–12

34. May JA, Krieger MD, Bowen I, Geffner ME. Craniopharyngioma in childhood. Adv Pediatr 2006;53:183–209

35. Schlosser RJ, Bolger WE. Endoscopic management of cerebrospinal fluid rhinorrhea. Otolaryngol Clin North Am 2006;39:523–538, ix

36. Anand VK, Arrowood JP Jr, Patel RB, Leonetti JP, al-Mefty O. Significance of MRI changes after surgery of the skull base. Otolaryngol Head Neck Surg 1993;109:35–45

20 Transplanum, Transtuberculum Approach

Gurston G. Nyquist, Vijay K. Anand, and Theodore H. Schwartz

Tips and Pearls

- Common lesions of the suprasellar region include giant pituitary macroadenomas, Rathke cleft cysts, craniopharyngiomas, and meningiomas of the tuberculum sellae or planum sphenoidale.
- The transtuberculum, transplanum approach provides the most direct route to midline lesions of the suprasellar cistern, does not place critical neurovascular structures between the surgeon and the lesion, obviates the need for brain retraction, and allows the surgeon to interrupt the blood supply early in the operation and perform bilateral decompression of the optic canals.
- Limitations of this approach include limited ability to remove pathology lateral to the internal carotid arteries.
- The bone opening of the tuberculum and planum sphenoidale is facilitated by outlining the margins of the lesion via stereotactic image guidance.
- Sharp extracapsular dissection helps to ensure a safe and complete surgical resection.

Introduction

Extended endoscopic transsphenoidal approaches have been adapted to address a variety of lesions beyond intrasellar pathologies (**Fig. 20.1**).[1–6] The suprasellar cistern is a region located above the diaphragma sellae, and midline lesions of this area are especially amenable to an endoscopic transsphenoidal, transplanum, transtuberculum approach. The extended application of the transsphenoidal approach to manage suprasellar pathologies represents the next step in the development of an endoscopic skull base practice after the surgeon has mastered the transsphenoidal, transsellar approach.

It is imperative to clearly define the surgical objectives preoperatively, and this largely depends on the biologic characteristics of the lesion. Rathke cleft cysts are benign congenital lesions derived from remnants of Rathke's pouch. The local mass effect of these lesions can produce headaches, pituitary dysfunction from compression on the pituitary gland or stalk, and visual impairment secondary to optic chiasm compression. Although complete excision of the cyst is possible, the surgical goal is usually decompression of the cyst for symptomatic relief and to obtain a biopsy of the cyst wall.[7]

Craniopharyngioma is a slow-growing, epithelial-squamous, calcified cystic tumor arising from remnants of the craniopharyngeal duct and/or Rathke cleft (**Fig. 20.1B**). Craniopharyngiomas are dysontogenic tumors with benign histology and malignant behavior, as they have a tendency to invade surrounding structures. Craniopharyngioma usually presents as a single large cyst or multiple cysts filled with a turbid, proteinaceous material of brownish-yellow color owing to the high content of floating cholesterol crystals. It most frequently arises in the pituitary stalk and projects into the hypothalamus and third ventricle.

Management options for craniopharyngioma include gross total tumor resection or cyst decompression for symptomatic relief followed by radiotherapy. Inflammatory reactions make the tumor adherent to critical neurovascular structures, and attempts at complete resection may significantly damage the hypothalamic-pituitary axis. Serious psychosocial deficits are also possible with hypothalamic injury, and preservation of hypothalamic function is imperative. Goals for surgery include gross tumor resection when possible, preservation of the patient's ability to maintain independent social functioning, prevention of symptomatic recurrence, and survival.

Pituitary macroadenomas often extend into the suprasellar cistern; however, these lesions can often be removed with a wide opening of the bony sella (**Fig. 20.1A**). Thorough, systematic removal of sellar portions of the adenoma facilitates descent of the diaphragma and suprasellar portions of the tumor into the operative field. However, complete removal of suprasellar tumor may require a transplanum, transtuberculum approach. Lastly, meningiomas arise from arachnoidal cap cells and are commonly located along the planum sphenoidale (**Fig. 20.1C**) and tuberculum sellae (**Fig. 20.1D**). Surgical goals for these tumors are to achieve maximal resection and decompress critical structures (optic nerves) while causing minimal morbidity.

Diagnostic Workup

A detailed history and physical examination is necessary, including a cranial nerve examination, ophthalmologic evaluation along with visual field testing, assessment of cognitive function, comprehensive endocrine workup, and endoscopic examination of the nasal cavity. Computed tomography (CT) images provide important information about the bony anatomy of the paranasal sinuses and skull base, and magnetic resonance imaging (MRI) is essential to demonstrate

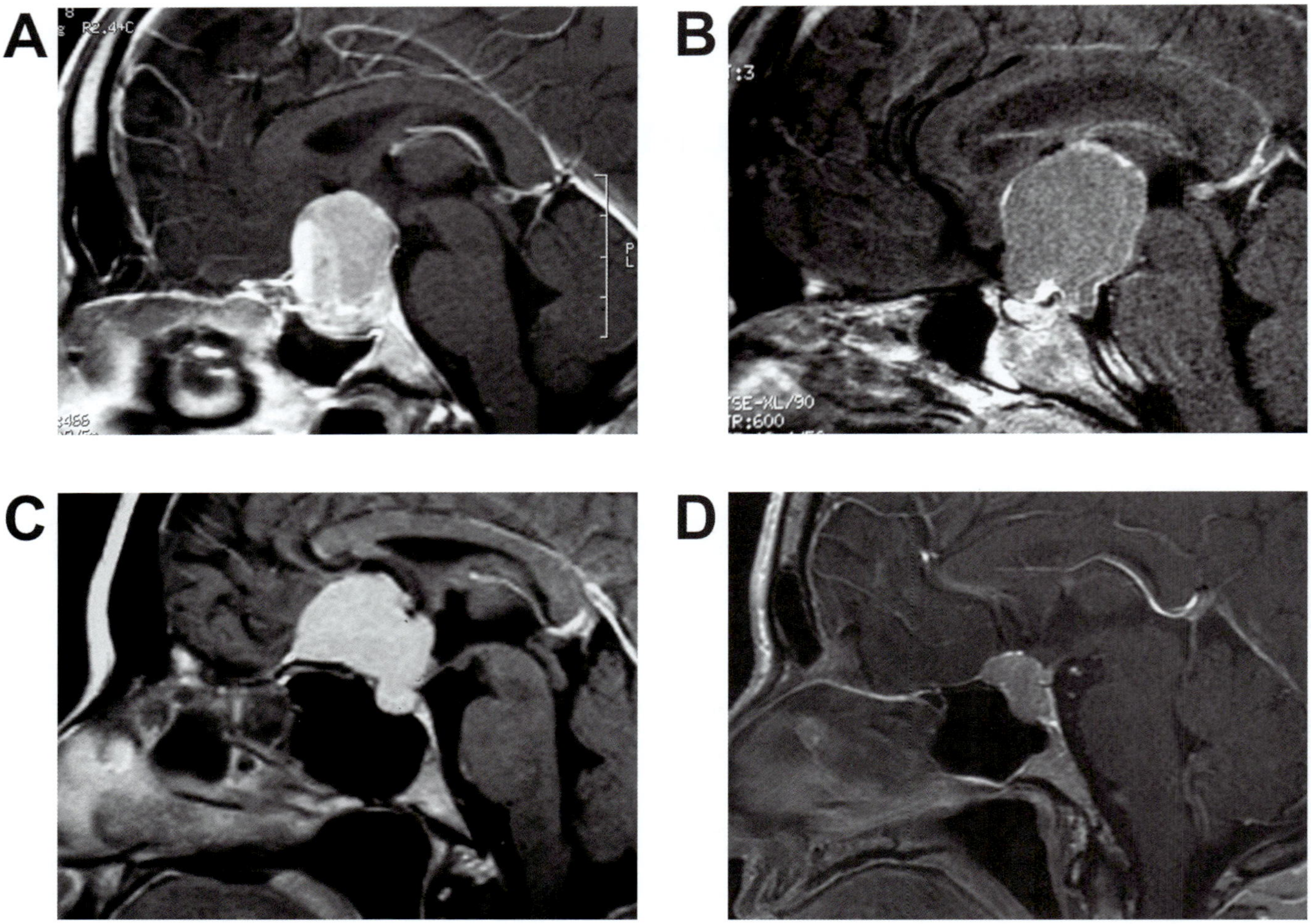

Fig. 20.1 Examples of pathology amenable to extended endonasal endoscopic transsphenoidal surgery that requires removal of the tuberculum sellae and planum sphenoidale. **(A)** Pituitary macroadenoma with significant suprasellar extension. **(B)** Craniopharyngioma with large suprasellar cyst above a normal sized sella. **(C)** Meningioma of the planum sphenoidale. **(D)** Meningioma of the tuberculum sellae.

the morphology of the soft tissues. Angiography may be indicated preoperatively if carotid artery compromise is suspected or the functional integrity of the circle of Willis requires assessment. CT or MR angiography generally provides sufficient information about the vascular anatomy for surgical planning.

■ Advantages and Indications

The transplanum, transtuberculum approach is well suited to address midline suprasellar lesions, including giant pituitary macroadenomas, Rathke cleft cysts, craniopharyngiomas, meningiomas of the planum sphenoidale or tuberculum sellae, and rare tumors like hemangioblastomas, epidermoids, germinomas, gliomas, and malignant pituitary tumors. More important than the histopathology of the lesion is its location and lateral extension.

The transplanum, transtuberculum approach provides a direct route to these lesions that obviates the need for brain retraction. Also, unlike a transcranial approach, it does not place critical neurovascular structures such as the optic nerves and carotid arteries between the surgeon and the tumor. The transplanum, transtuberculum approach facilitates complete, bilateral optic canal decompression without manipulation of a compressed optic nerve. Moreover, approaching these tumors from below enables the surgeon to remove bone at the base of the tumor, which is a common site for meningioma recurrence, and to interrupt the dural vascular supply early in the operation. This enables a relatively bloodless dissection.

The use of angled endoscopes enables a panoramic view and the ability to inspect around corners to ensure a complete resection. In the case of craniopharyngiomas, the entire third ventricle may be visualized through the endoscope, which is not possible in the transcranial approach. Lastly, the transnasal approach does not require external incisions.

Contraindications and Considerations

Patient comorbidities that preclude prolonged anesthesia are general contraindications to any extended transsphenoidal approach. Next, the lateral extent of the tumor must be carefully assessed. The width of the planum sphenoidale, between the laminae papyracea, has been measured in cadaver studies at 26 ± 4 mm, which narrows to 16 ± 3 mm at the posterior aspect of the tuberculum sellae.[8] Tumor just lateral to this area can be mobilized into the surgical field; however, significant lateral extension should be approached via a craniotomy if complete resection is the goal. The extended transsphenoidal approach is the preferred corridor when tumor is medial to these structures and optimally exposes the medial aspect of the optic canal. Encasement of critical neurovascular structures such as the optic nerve, internal carotid artery (ICA), and anterior communicating artery (ACA) complex is not an absolute contraindication to this approach. Much like the transcranial approach, the surgeon must judge his or her ability to safely dissect tumor from these structures and must have a plan to address a surgical emergency such as an ICA injury.

The bony pneumatization of the sphenoid sinus is another consideration. In patients with a presellar or conchal-type sinus, bony landmarks for the optic nerves and ICAs are not easily identifiable, and the risk of injury is elevated. In addition, if the sella is small or the distance between internal carotid arteries is narrow, the surgeon may not have adequate surgical access with the transsphenoidal approach. Lastly, patients with poor wound healing capabilities may not tolerate successful skull base reconstruction and are at risk for a persistent cerebrospinal fluid leak. This includes patients with osteoradionecrosis or who suffer from systemic diseases like poorly controlled diabetes mellitus or immunosuppression.

Approach

A nasal septal flap can be elevated at the outset of the procedure and tucked in the nasopharynx until the extirpative portion of the procedure is complete. The sphenoid ostia are identified bilaterally and opened widely with a mushroom punch. Next, the posterior third of the bony septum is resected and a piece of vomeric bone is harvested as a rigid buttress for reconstruction of the skull base. The sphenoid rostrum is opened widely with a high-speed cutting drill, and bilateral posterior ethmoidectomies are performed. Mucosa of the sphenoid sinus is removed, and identification of the sella, optic nerves, and ICA is verified with frameless stereotactic image guidance (**Fig. 20.2**). A 0-degree, 30-cm, rigid 4-mm endoscope is introduced into the left nostril by the assisting surgeon while the primary operating surgeon works bimanually from the right nostril or through both nostrils.

The tuberculum sellae is thinned with a high-speed diamond drill under constant irrigation. The opening extends between the medial clinoids bilaterally. The inferior extent of bony removal continues halfway down into the sella unless mobilization of the pituitary is necessary. The thinned bone is removed with a curette and Kerrison rongeur. Bone removal is continued along the planum sphenoidale until

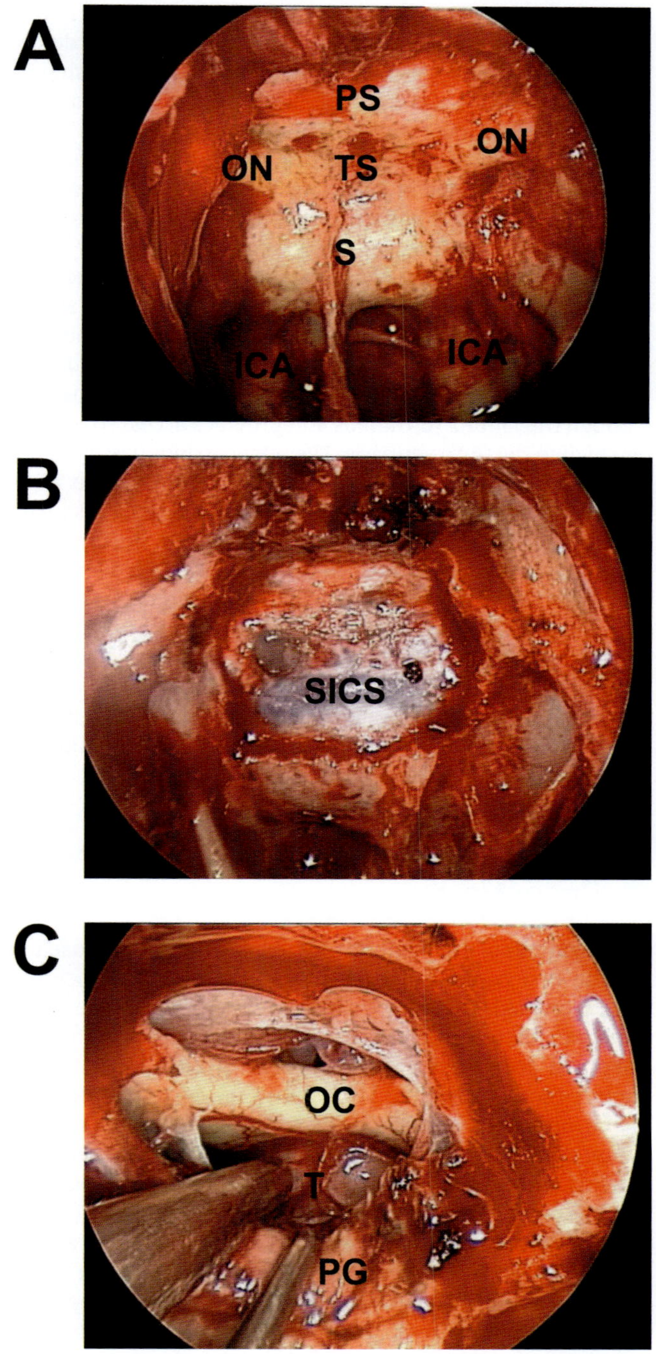

Fig. 20.2 **(A–C)** Endoscopic views of the suprasellar approach. Within the sphenoid sinus one can see the bone impressions of the internal carotid arteries (ICA), sella (S), tuberculum sellae (TS), planum sphenoidale (PS), and optic nerves (ON). OC: optic chiasm; PG: pituitary galnd; SICS: superior intercavernous sinus.

adequate access for complete tumor identification is obtained. The use of stereotactic image guidance helps determine the size of the bony opening. Additional bone should be removed along the optic nerves for meningiomas with intracanalicular involvement.

The dura above and below the superior intercavernous sinus (SICS) is opened in a cruciate fashion with a sickle knife (**Fig. 20.2**). The SICS is then isolated, cauterized with a bipolar cautery, and transected. Four corridors are now available to address lesions of the suprasellar cistern. The first corridor passes in front of the optic chiasm and is well suited for meningiomas of the planum and tuberculum sellae. The second corridor is a prechiasmal approach to the third ventricle. This approach passes between the chiasm and the ACA through the lamina terminalis and provides access to pathology high in the third ventricle. The next corridor passes below the chiasm and above the pituitary gland. If the stalk is midline, it can be gently displaced laterally for access. This is the preferred method for cystic lesions arising from the infundibulum that extend into the third ventricle. The fourth corridor passes beneath the pituitary gland and requires superior mobilization of the gland. The bony anterior face and floor of the sellae along with the dorsum sellae, superior clivus, and often the posterior clinoids have to be removed. This corridor provides access to lesions such as craniopharyngiomas, chordomas, and petroclival meningiomas located behind the pituitary gland and infundibulum.

Resection

Meningiomas of the planum and tuberculum are approached via the first corridor and immediately visualized once the dura is opened. The dura is cauterized to interrupt the blood supply to the tumor. Dural and bony attachments of the meningioma are resected to prevent recurrence. Internal decompression is performed often with the assistance of a Cavitron ultrasonic surgical aspirator or Ellman cautery. The tumor capsule is then sharply dissected away methodically, starting with the optic nerve (**Fig. 20.3**). The ICA is identified just lateral and inferior to the optic nerve and tumor is then traced to the chiasm, along the contralateral optic nerve until the associated ICA is identified and free of tumor. An ultrasound Doppler is extremely valuable in mapping the course of vascular structures like the ICA. For tuberculum sellae meningiomas, the diaphragm sella must also be removed (**Fig. 20.3**). Important structures such as the ACA complex, recurrent artery of Heubner, subchiasmal perforating vessels, optic nerves, and pituitary stalk are preserved by sharp dissection off the tumor capsule. Arteries that may appear to be encased can often be dissected free of the tumor (**Fig. 20.4**). The resection bed is examined using angled endoscopes, with special attention paid to ensuring that the optic nerves and canals are free of tumor. The optic canals and sheath can be opened to remove intracanalicular tumor (**Fig. 20.4**).

Postchiasmal cystic tumors, either craniopharyngiomas or Rathke cleft cysts, arise from the pituitary stalk. The most common approach to these lesions is through a corridor above the pituitary gland and below the optic chiasm. If the cyst is small enough, dissection around the capsule is initiated. Otherwise, the anterior cyst wall is opened sharply and the cyst is drained to facilitate extracapsular dissection. The stalk is identified at the level of the diaphragma and sharp dissection of the lesion from the stalk is performed (**Fig. 20.5**). If the lesion is transinfundibular or retroinfundibular, it may require working on either side of the stalk to dissect the cyst wall free. This maneuver is facilitated by division of the SICS and a wide bony opening of the sella to facilitate manipulation of the pituitary gland. Sharp and blunt dissection is used to free tumor from the optic chiasm, carotid arteries, ACA complex, and hypothalamic and chiasmal perforating arteries. In most cases, the lesion extends into the third ventricle, and careful dissection here and along the hypothalamus is critical to prevent injury. Although not always possible, stalk preservation is the goal of surgery (**Fig. 20.5**). Although complete resection of the tumor is the optimal outcome, in some situations, such as in children or in young women with normal pituitary function who desire to get pregnant, tumor biopsy within the stalk can be followed by fractionated radiation (**Fig. 20.6**).

Repair

Reconstruction begins with obliteration of the dead space with fat to prevent pooling of cerebrospinal fluid (CSF) at the bony defect. The exception is patients in whom the third ventricle is widely opened, as there is increased risk of fat migration and obstructive hydrocephalus. Next, a "gasket-seal" closure is performed.[9] This reconstruction technique consists of a soft tissue graft (fascia lata, Alloderm) centered over the defect with the edges of the graft exceeding the bony defect circumferentially (**Fig. 20.3**). Next, a piece of rigid material (vomer, Medpore) is fashioned to be roughly the size of the bony defect. The rigid graft is centered over the soft tissue graft so that there is excess soft tissue graft circumferentially around the rigid graft. The rigid graft is gently countersunk into the bony defect, forming a watertight gasket seal around the rigid graft. A nasoseptal flap is then rotated to cover the defect, and a tissue sealant (DuraSeal) is used to secure the multilayer graft in place (**Fig. 20.3**).

Complications

Potential intraoperative complications include arterial (internal carotid artery, ophthalmic artery) or venous bleeding, cranial nerve injury, and damage to the pituitary gland, stalk, or hypothalamus. Expedient identification and treatment of postoperative complications such as CSF leak, meningitis, hematoma formation, sinusitis, and synechia formation is mandatory.

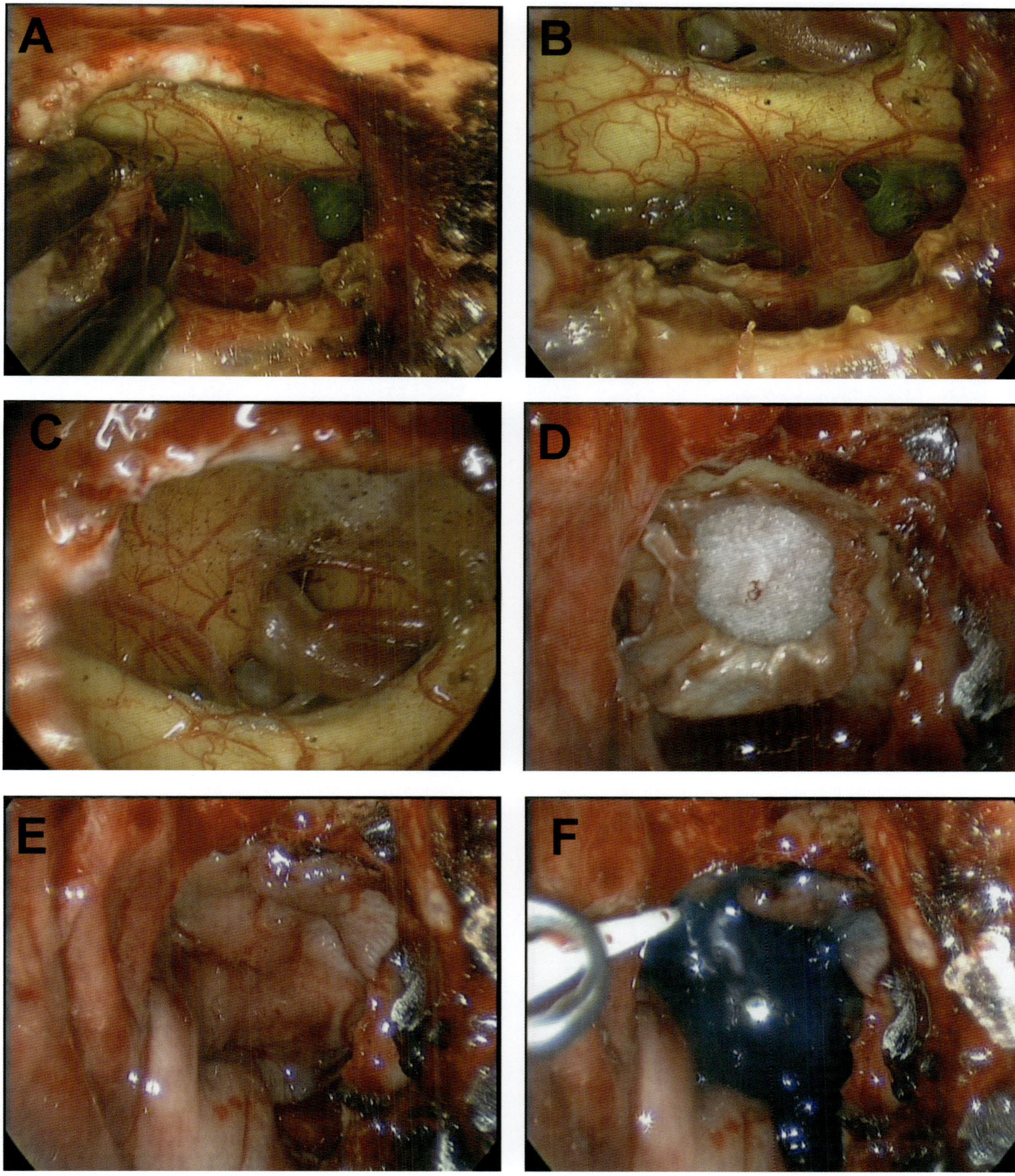

Fig. 20.3 Meningioma resection and skull base repair. **(A)** The tumor is dissected off the optic chiasm and nerves. Usually there is an arachnoid plane. The diaphragm sellae is sharply removed. **(B)** The chiasm and stalk should be completely free of tumor. **(C)** Looking above the chiasm, the anterior cerebral arteries are preserved as well as gyrus rectus. **(D)** Closure is performed with the gasket-seal technique using fascia lata and Medpore. **(E)** A nasoseptal flap, harvested at the start of the operation, covers the gasket-seal closure. **(F)** DuraSeal is used to keep the flap in place during the early healing process.

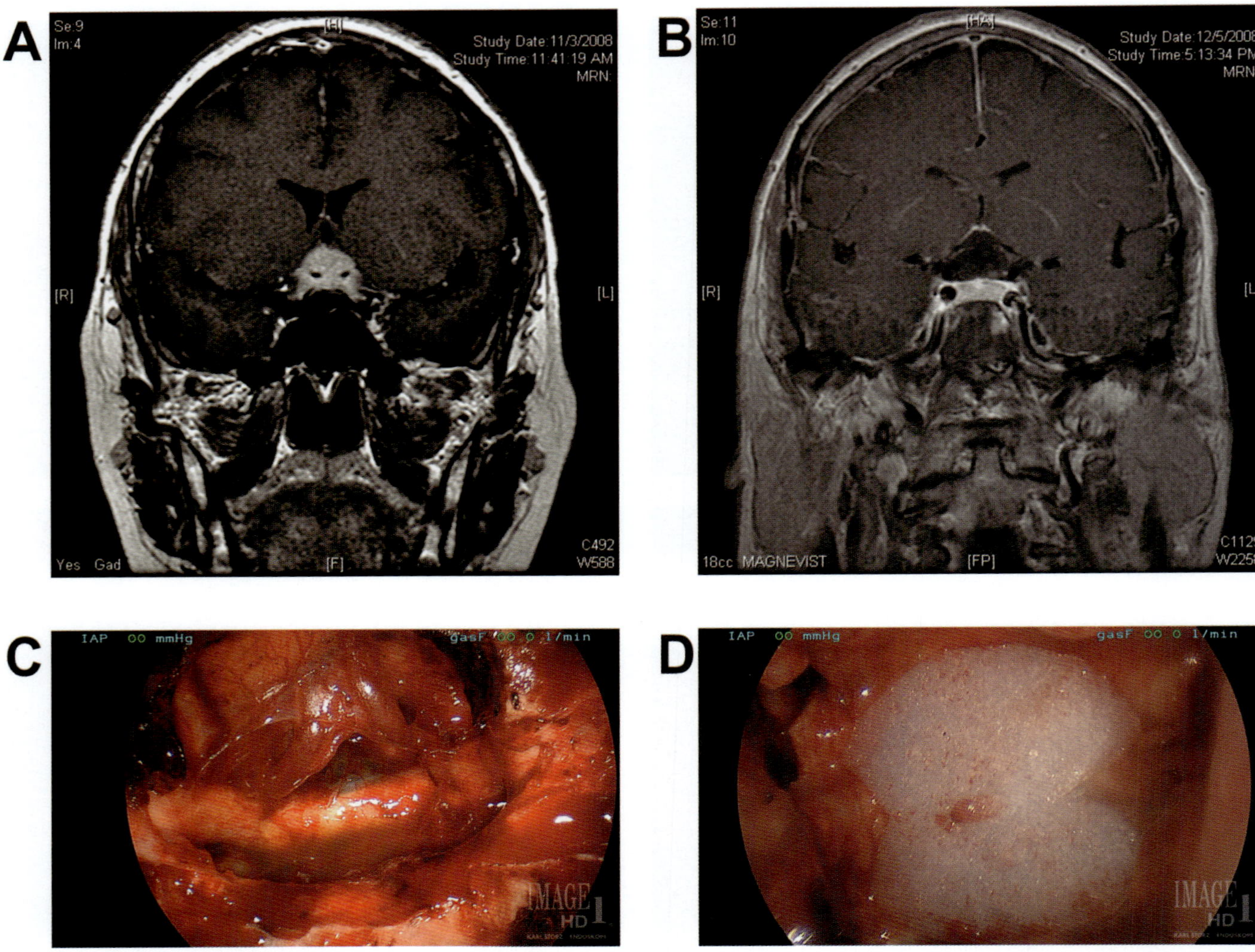

Fig. 20.4 Meningiomas may invade the optic canals and encase vessels. **(A)** Contrast-enhanced coronal magnetic resonance imaging (MRI) scan preoperatively shows the anterior cerebral arteries (ACAs) encased by the tumor as well as invasion in the optic canals. **(B)** Postoperatively the tumor is completely removed. **(C)** Intraoperative image shows the postresection bed following opening of the optic canals and removal of the intracanalicular tumor from within the sphenoid sinus, and shows the ACAs free of tumor. **(D)** The gasket seal can still be used in this situation, but the Medpore must be cut so as not to compress the optic nerves. In this image the Medpore is sitting over the fascia lata but has not yet been countersunk into the cavity.

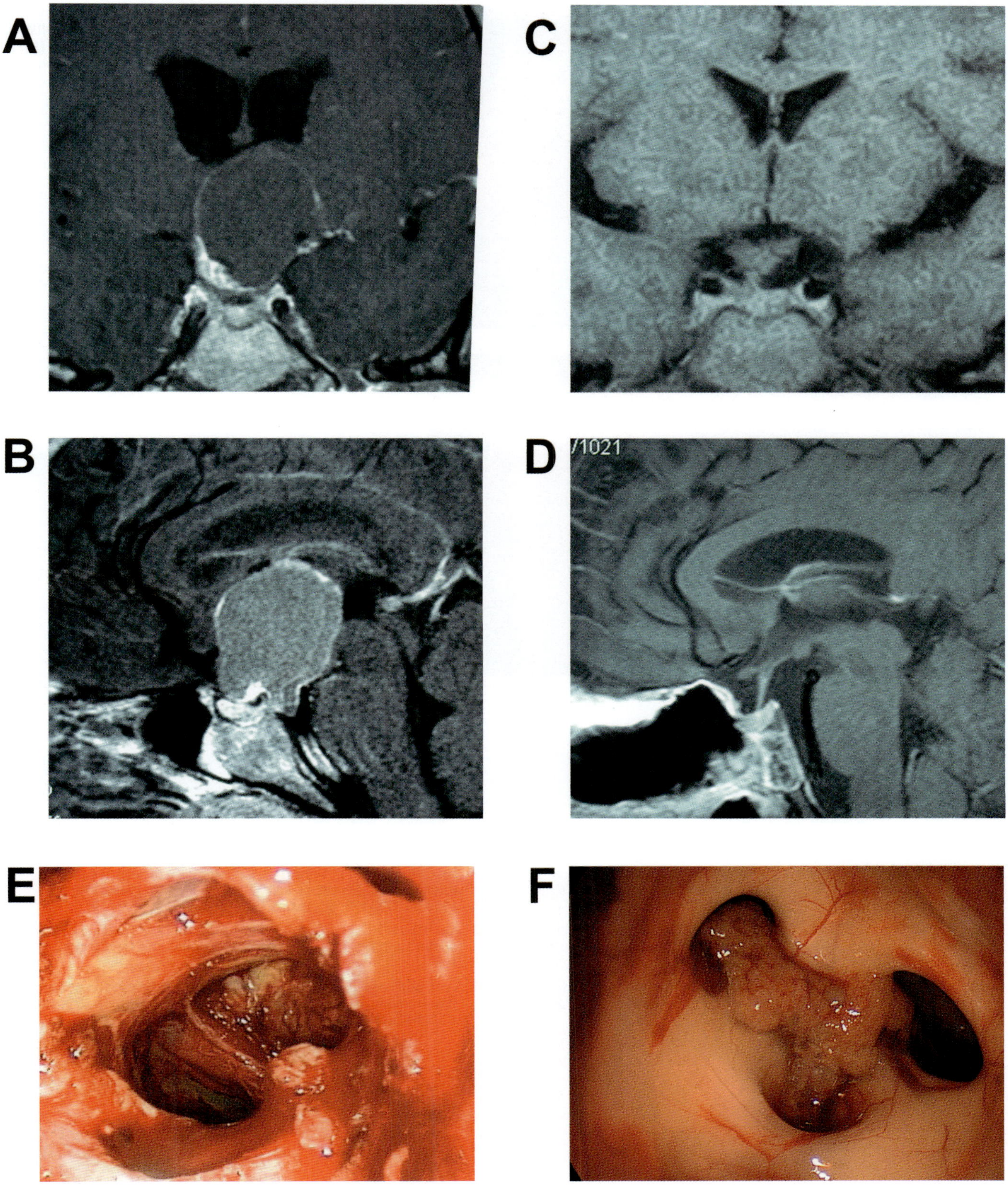

Fig. 20.5 Stalk preservation in large cystic craniopharyngioma. Preoperative coronal **(A)** and sagittal **(B)** contrast-enhanced MRI scans show a large cystic craniopharyngioma extending into the third ventricle. Postoperative coronal **(C)** and sagittal **(D)** contrast-enhanced MRI shows complete removal of the tumor with stalk preservation. **(E)** Intraoperative endoscopic view shows the stalk preserved after the surgery between the optic chiasm and pituitary gland. **(F)** Intraoperative endoscopic view of the roof off the third ventricle, foramina of Monro, choroid plexus, and fornices.

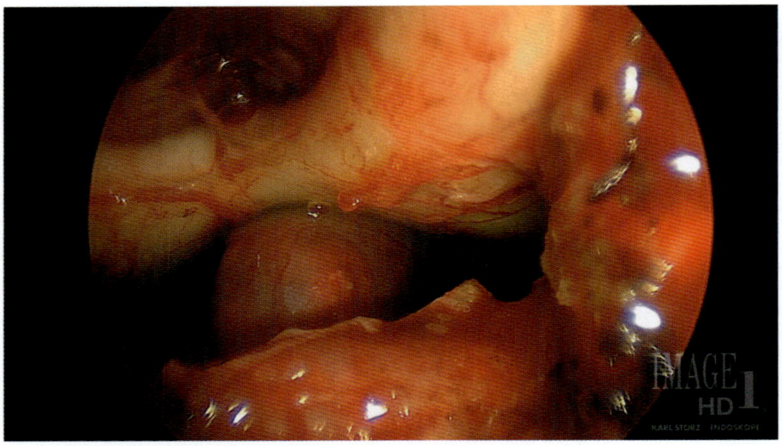

A

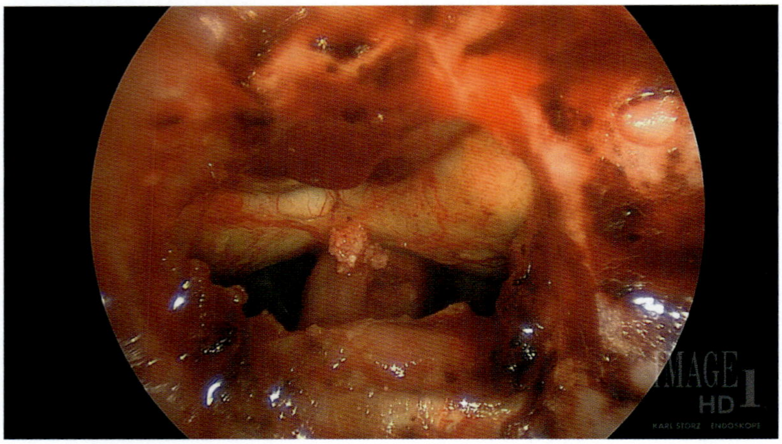

B

Fig. 20.6 Tumor biopsy. **(A)** A craniopharyngioma infiltrating into the stalk may not be removable without causing a postoperative panhypopituitary state. **(B)** In some situations, tumor biopsy followed by radiation may be preferable.

References

1. Kaptain GJ, Vincent DA, Sheehan JP, Laws ER Jr. Transsphenoidal approaches for the extracapsular resection of midline suprasellar and anterior cranial base lesions. Neurosurgery 2001;49:94–100, discussion 100–101
2. Frank G, Sciarretta V, Mazzatenta D, Farneti G, Modugno GC, Pasquini E. Transsphenoidal endoscopic approach in the treatment of Rathke's cleft cyst. Neurosurgery 2005;56:124–128, discussion 129
3. Laufer I, Anand VK, Schwartz TH. Endoscopic, endonasal extended transsphenoidal, transplanum transtuberculum approach for resection of suprasellar lesions. J Neurosurg 2007;106:400–406
4. de Divitiis E, Cavallo LM, Cappabianca P, Esposito F. Extended endoscopic endonasal transsphenoidal approach for the removal of suprasellar tumors: Part 2. Neurosurgery 2007;60:46–58, discussion 58–59
5. Kassam AB, Gardner PA, Snyderman CH, Carrau RL, Mintz AH, Prevedello DM. Expanded endonasal approach, a fully endoscopic transnasal approach for the resection of midline suprasellar craniopharyngiomas: a new classification based on the infundibulum. J Neurosurg 2008;108:715–728
6. Gardner PA, Kassam AB, Thomas A, et al. Endoscopic endonasal resection of anterior cranial base meningiomas. Neurosurgery 2008;63:36–52, discussion 52–54
7. Ross DA, Norman D, Wilson CB. Radiologic characteristics and results of surgical management of Rathke's cysts in 43 patients. Neurosurgery 1992;30:173–178, discussion 178–179
8. Jho HD, Ha HG. Endoscopic endonasal skull base surgery: Part 1—The midline anterior fossa skull base. Minim Invasive Neurosurg 2004;47:1–8
9. Leng LZ, Brown S, Anand VK, Schwartz TH. "Gasket-seal" watertight closure in minimal-access endoscopic cranial base surgery. Neurosurgery 2008;62(5, Suppl 2):E342–E343, discussion E343

21 The Endonasal Transplanum-Transtuberculum Endoscopic Approach in Pituitary Adenomas

Giorgio Frank, Diego Mazzatenta, Vittorio Sciarretta, Matteo Zoli, Giovanni Farneti, and Ernesto Pasquini

Tips and Pearls

- The endonasal transplanum-transtuberculum endoscopic approach (ETTEA) is an alternative to the transcranial approach for selected suprasellar tumors not otherwise suitable for the standard transsphenoidal procedure.
- In pituitary adenomas, the main indications are ectopic adenomas of the pituitary stalk, adenomas having a transdiaphragmatic growth to the periinfundibular area, and midline adenomas extending to the subfrontal region.
- Apart from cerebrospinal fluid (CSF) leaks, which are inherent to this type of intervention, the morbidity is higher than in the transsphenoidal procedure. This is the reason why caution and balance are required in adopting it.

Introduction

In 1987, Weiss,[1] using a sublabial microscopic approach, first described the transplanum-transtuberculum approach. Its application using the microsurgical technique was confirmed and popularized by other authors.[2–8] The advent of the endoscopic technique helped in reducing the difficulties related to a narrow and deep surgical field and helped to overcome the reduced peripheral vision normally associated with the microscope.[9] This made its use more frequent and applicable to a variety of pathologies (craniopharyngiomas, meningiomas, and adenomas).[10–13] In theory, the use of the endonasal transplanum-transtuberculum endoscopic approach (ETTEA) in comparison with the standard transsphenoidal approach increases the extent of tumor removal and reduces morbidity with respect to the intracranial approach. In fact, the surgical management of pituitary adenomas rarely requires a transcranial approach (less than 10% in the series of Buchfelder and Kreutzer[14] in 2008) and only a few, very select cases are suitable for an ETTEA. The surgical treatment of choice for pituitary adenomas still remains the transsphenoidal approach because it is safe, well tolerated, and effective.[12] The transsphenoidal approach facilitates an endocapsular selective adenomectomy, which means selective tumor removal with preservation of the pituitary gland.

The ETTEA induces the pituitary surgeon to take two actions that are contrary to customary practice: the intentional penetration of the subarachnoid space, and an extracapsular dissection of the tumor. The former makes an intraoperative cerebrospinal fluid (CSF) leak unavoidable, and increases the risks of postoperative CSF rhinorrhea and meningitis. However, increased experience in CSF leak repair, using modern techniques that are quite effective (mainly, multilayer plastic repair or a pedicled vascularized flap[15,16]) has made this condition easier to control, making intraoperative CSF leak an acceptable risk. The postoperative CSF leak rate has dropped to less than 6%.[17] An extracapsular dissection of the tumor enables a more radical tumor removal, at the expense of including normal pituitary gland tissue in the excision. Conversely, it is well known that, in pituitary surgery, a partial removal with functional preservation is often preferable to a radical removal with pituitary insufficiency.

The decision to change the management of a pituitary adenoma from a standard transsphenoidal approach to an extended one is not easy, and should be restricted to a few selected cases. Some of these cases would previously have been considered for a transcranial approach.[14] It is well accepted that the endonasal extended approach compared with a transcranial approach has the advantage of being a minimally invasive approach, giving direct access to the lesion with no risk of brain manipulation and neurovascular dissection.

The characteristics that make a pituitary adenoma amenable to the ETTEA, as an alternative to the transcranial approach, are the anatomical factors and the midline position of the tumor.[11] The anatomical factors favoring an endonasal approach are (1) a well-pneumatized sphenoid sinus; (2) an adequate intercarotid distance; (3) absence of associated vascular anomalies, such as aneurysms; and (4) the absence of vascular encasement by the tumor (**Fig. 21.1**).

At present, we are convinced that the ETTEA is the procedure of choice for ectopic adrenocorticotropic hormone (ACTH) microadenomas of the pituitary stalk.[8]

In macroadenomas, such a decision may be facilitated by the presence of pituitary insufficiency and visual disturbances because, under these circumstances, the role of selective adenomectomy is less important with respect to optochiasmatic decompression. We believe that an ETTEA should be

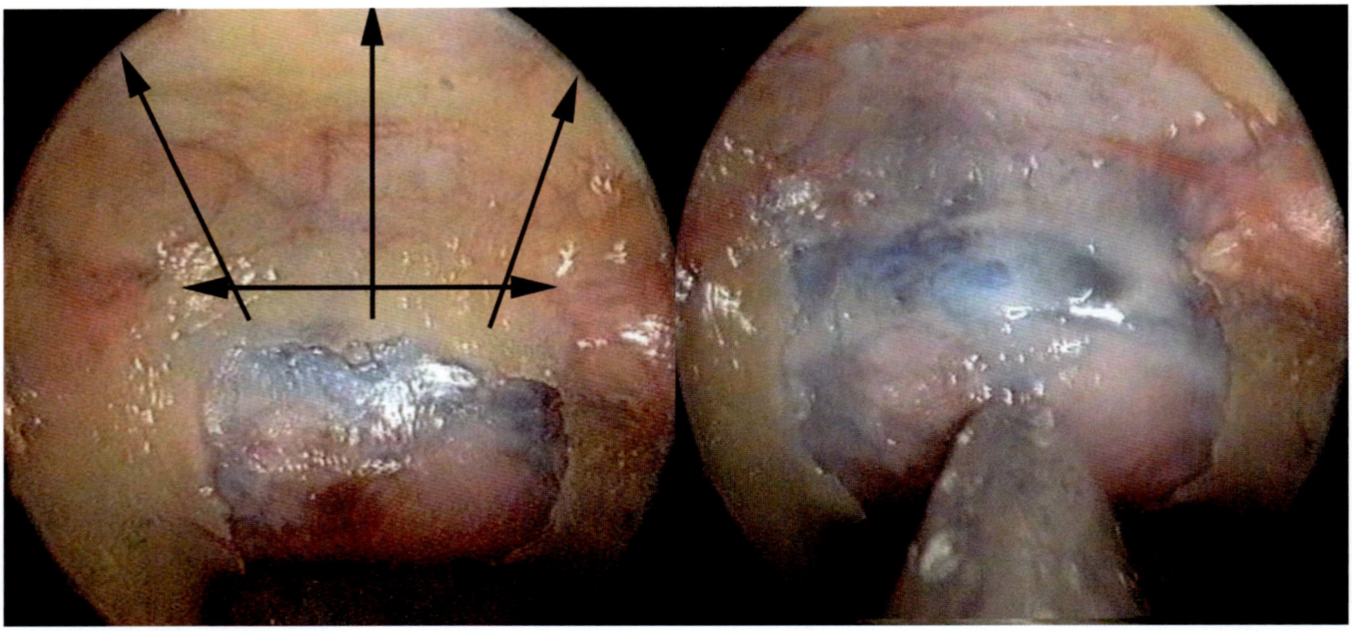

A B

Fig. 21.1 (A,B) Anatomic dissection in an injected specimen. After removal of the sellar bone, the next step is the removal of the bone from the planum following the direction indicated by the arrows in **A.** The extension of bone removal is related to sphenoidal pneumatization, tumor size, and intercarotid distance.

considered in adenomas with a midline subfrontal extension, in invasive adenomas growing through the diaphragma sella, and in fibrous tumors.

■ Technical Note

We have previously described our technique of ETTEA in several publications.[10,18] At present we would emphasize some interesting aspects of our procedure. We place the patient in a semi-sitting position, which we believe offers the advantage of a clearer operative field due to the reduced bleeding and gravity-induced drainage of blood and irrigation fluid away from the operative field. A disadvantage is the increased outflow of CSF and the increased risk of postoperative pneumocephalus. During the crucial phase of the procedure, we place the endoscope in a mechanical holder. This gives the surgeons the ability to carry out a bimanual dissection of the tumor. To increase the maneuverability of the instruments

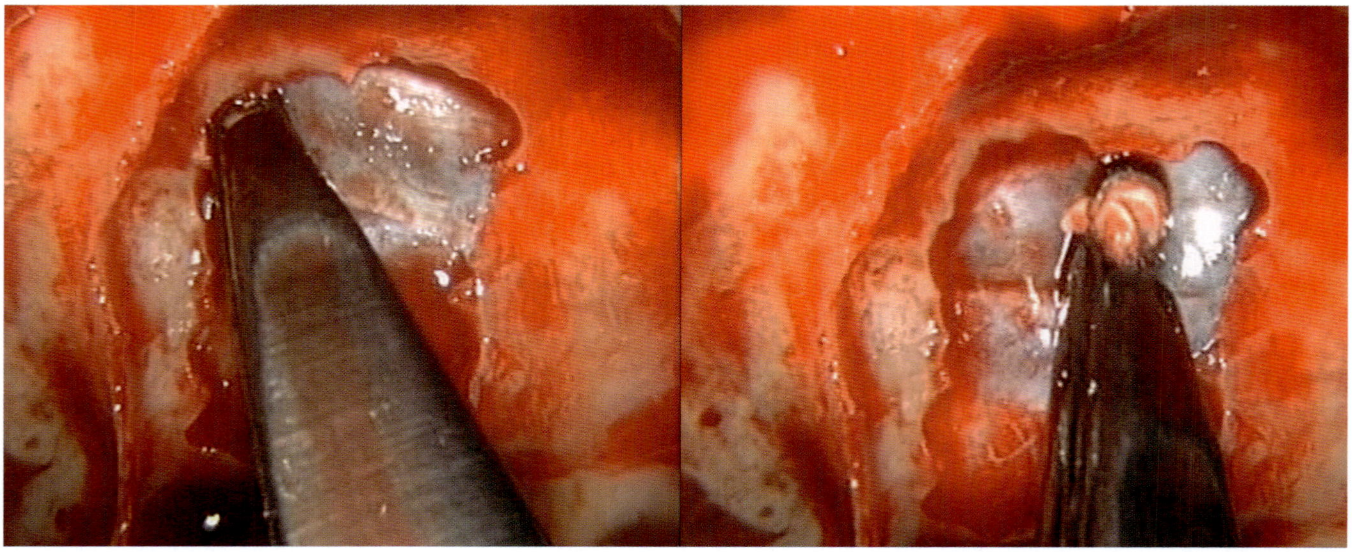

A B

Fig. 21.2 (A,B) Removal of the bone from the planum sphenoidalis is possible using a drill or cutting instrument, such as Kerrison's rongeurs. When the bone is thin, we prefer to use a cutting instrument to reduce the risk of damage from the heat generated by a high-speed diamond drill.

through the narrow surgical channel, we perform a unilateral middle turbinectomy at the beginning and laterally displace the contralateral middle turbinate. In doing so, we avoid also damage to the mucoperiosteum of the middle turbinate, which is needed in the multilayer closure. A wide anterior sphenoidotomy is then performed, and, depending on the size of the sphenoidal sinus, a uni- or bilateral posterior ethmoidectomy sometimes may be necessary to gain adequate control of the floor of the anterior cranial base. Bone removal is tailored to the lesion. It begins in the sellar region and extends to the tuberculum and the planum sphenoidale (**Fig. 21.1**).

We normally prefer to remove bone using Kerrison rongeurs, with the intention of avoiding tissue damage from the heat generated by a high-speed diamond drill (**Fig. 21.2**). An absolute limit to the lateral extension of the bone opening is the medial aspect of the opticocarotid recesses (**Figs. 21.1** and **21.2**); at these points, bone removal should be stopped to avoid optic nerve or carotid artery injury. The dural opening is also tailored to the lesion, keeping in mind that a wider and unnecessary opening increases the difficulty of the final watertight closure. The dural opening is in a horizontal H-shape fashion, with the two horizontal limbs of the H being on the sellar dura and on the frontal dura respectively, connected by a short vertical midline cut. The vertical incision is made after the superior intercavernous sinus (SICS) has been coagulated or clipped (**Figs. 21.3** and **21.4**). In this way, the subdural space is entered safely. The arachnoid plane should be preserved and sharply dissected from the dome of the tumor. The dome or "capsule" of the tumor is composed of the stretched dura of the diaphragma sella[4,19] (**Fig. 21.5**).

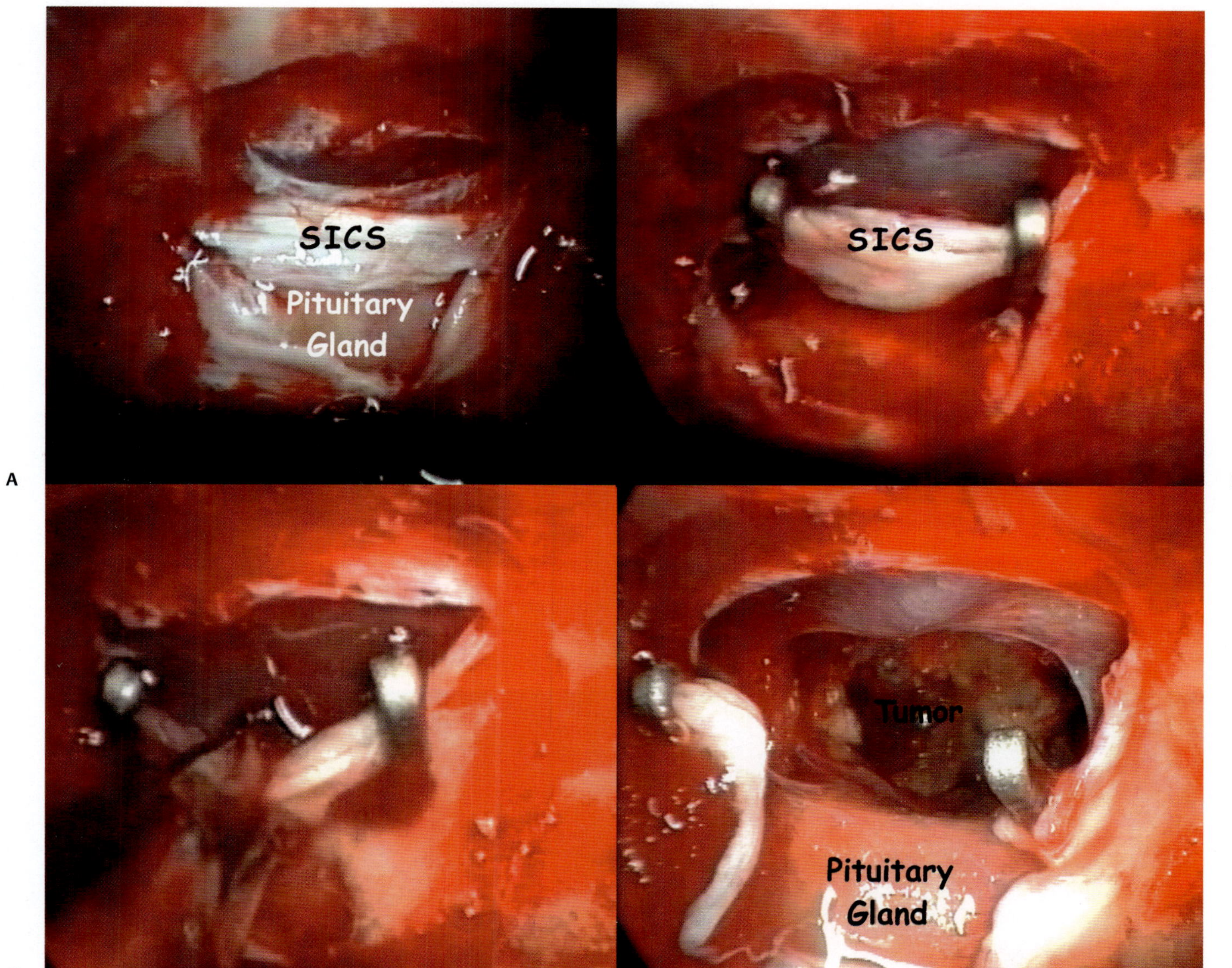

Fig. 21.3 The dural opening is in a horizontal H-shape fashion, with the two horizontal limbs of the H being on the sellar dura and on the frontal dura, respectively **(A,B)**, connected by a short vertical midline cut **(C,D)**. The vertical incision is made after the superior intercavernous sinus (SICS) has been coagulated or clipped **(B)**.

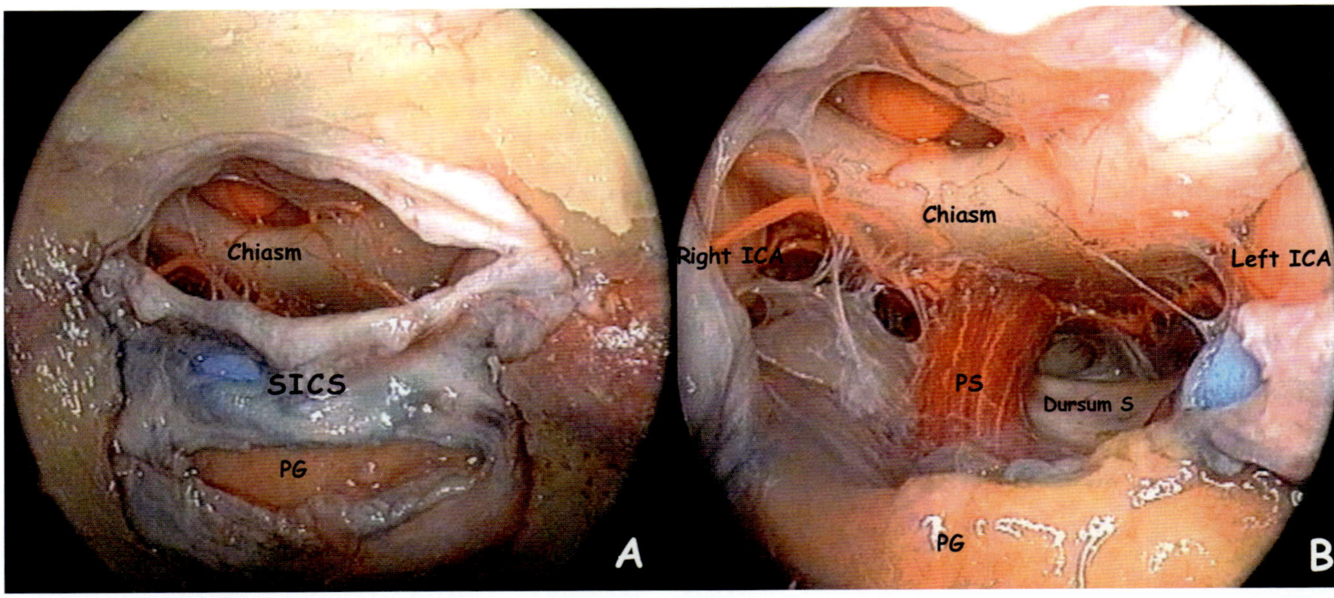

Fig. 21.4 **(A,B)** Anatomic dissection in an injected specimen. The supradiaphragmatic space is open after the dural opening with two horizontal incisions, one above and the other below the SICS **(A)**, and a vertical cutting of the SICS. The pituitary stalk (PS) is on the midline surrounded by an arachnoidal plane, which is important to follow during the dissection. The chiasm and the optic nerve are in the upper position. The upper internal carotid artery (ICA) segments are the lateral limits of this narrow space. PG: pituitary gland; S: sella.

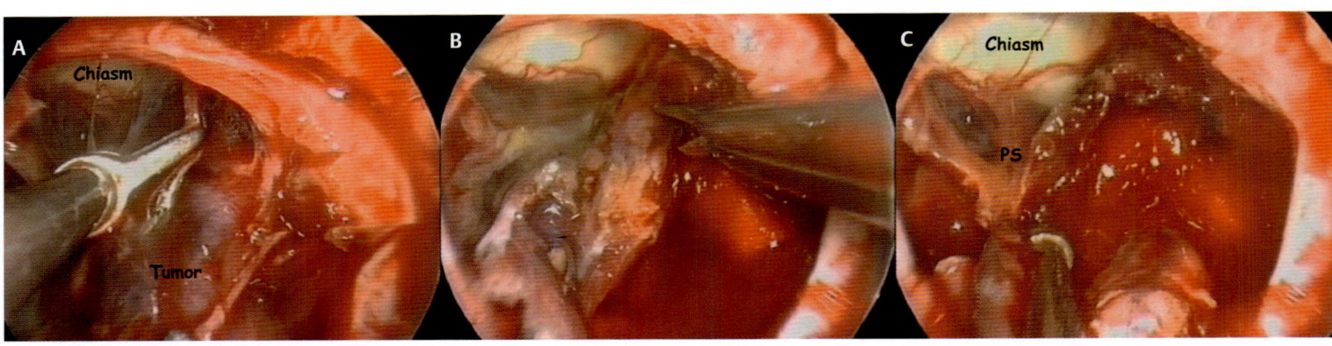

Fig. 21.5 A recurrent adenoma after a craniotomy approach. The tumor is adherent to the diaphragm. Subarachnoid and extracapsular dissection of the tumor is unavoidable. Meticulous coagulation of the vessels **(A)** following a sharp **(B)** and blunt **(C)** dissection is mandatory to obtain a radical removal of the tumor and to reduce the risk of intra- and postoperative hemorrhage. These types of tumors have a high risk of postoperative (3 to 4 hours) brain hemorrhage resulting from supradiaphragmatic/intradural residual tumors. PS: pituitary stalk.

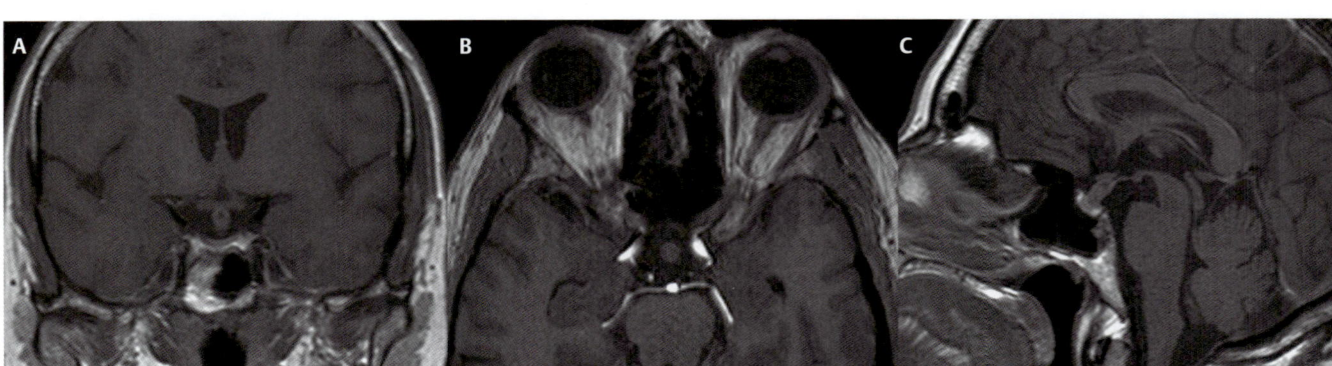

Fig. 21.6 Preoperative magnetic resonance imaging (MRI) in coronal **(A)**, axial **(B)**, and sagittal **(C)** views in a patient with ectopic adrenocorticotropic hormone (ACTH) microadenomas of the pituitary stalk. The pituitary stalk is enlarged by the tumor between the chiasm to the pituitary gland.

There are two reasons for preserving the arachnoidal plane: (1) the vessels are subarachnoidal, and working in the extraarachnoid space avoids vascular injury; (2) the arachnoidal plane, even if not completely preserved, helps during the reconstruction by acting as a barrier to the intradural displacement of the graft. When the target of the procedure is the pituitary stalk, it is necessary to pursue dural sectioning through the diaphragma sella after the sectioning of the SIS until the hiatus of the pituitary stalk is reached. In this way, the pituitary stalk is exposed at the epicenter of the operative field[8] (**Figs. 21.6, 21.7,** and **21.8**).

We normally reconstruct a dural defect using a multilayer technique. The first layer of fascia lata is inserted intracranially and intradurally, and it must be at least 30% larger than the dura defect. A second layer of fascia lata is applied intracranially and extradurally between the dura and the bone. This graft has to be tailored to the bone defect. If bone or cartilage is available, it is possible to apply one of them in the same position of the second layer so as to avoid the anterior displacement of the graft. The third layer is applied extradurally in an overlay position. We normally prefer a mucoperiosteum of the middle turbinate, but, if it is not available, a

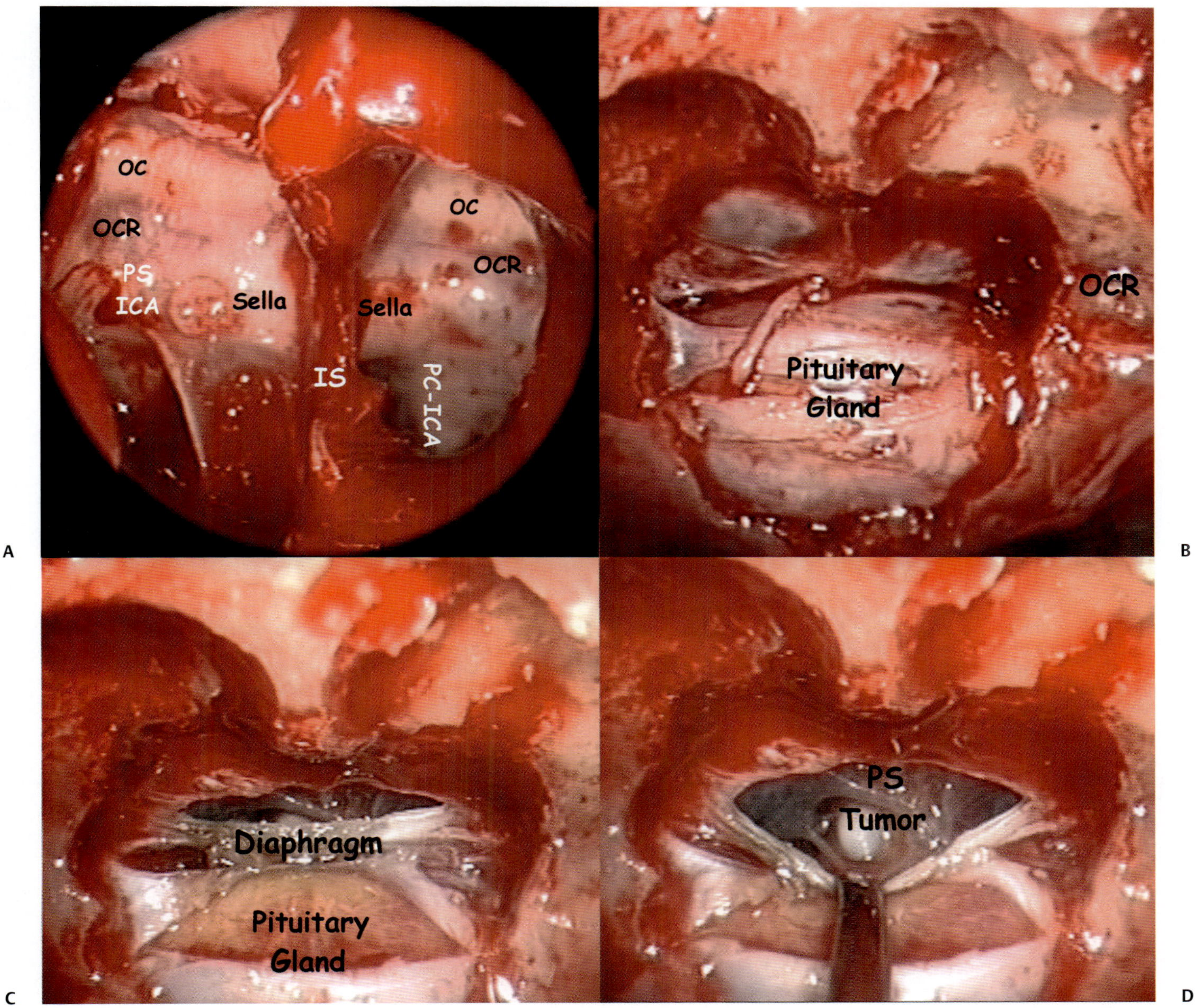

Fig. 21.7 Same patient as in Fig. 21.6 with ectopic ACTH microadenoma of the pituitary stalk. **(A)** A wide bilateral sphenoidotomy is performed with removal of the entire anterior wall of the sphenoid sinus and the upper part of the intersinusal septa (IS). The landmarks, well visible in the well-pneumatized sphenoid sinus, are the optic canal (OC), the optic carotid recess (OCR), and the parasellar and paraclival bulging of the internal carotid artery (PS-ICA; PC-ICA). After horizontal incisions, one below and the second above the SICS **(B,C),** it is possible to expose the pituitary stalk frontally and localize the microadenoma inside this structure **(D).**

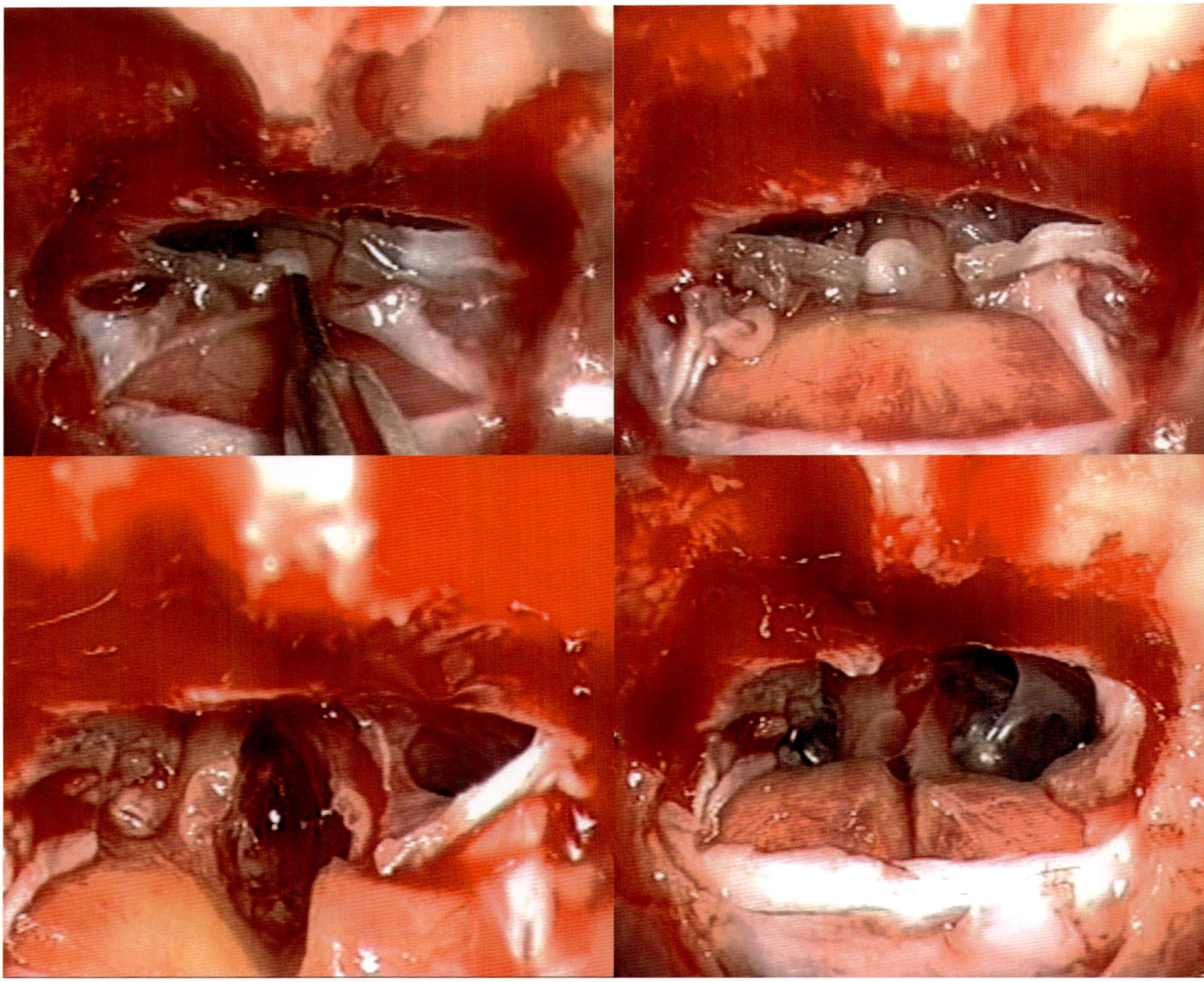

A B C D

Fig. 21.8 Same patient as in Figs. 21.6 and 21.7 with ectopic ACTH microadenoma of the pituitary stalk. After coagulation of the SICS, a vertical incision of the diaphragm is performed **(A)** to obtain the complete and frontal exposition of the pituitary stalk **(B).** The vertical incision is continued on the pituitary stalk and partially on the pituitary gland to easily and radically remove the ectopic tumor **(C).** When possible, we try to preserve the pituitary stalk to maintain pituitary functionality **(D).** Unfortunately, anatomic integrity does not always means functional preservation; however, it reduces surgical demolition, enables an easy duraplastic repair, and reduces the risk of postoperative CSF leak.

mucoperiosteum from the septum or fascia lata is useful as well (**Fig. 21.9**). Only Gelfoam is used to buttress the graft. We avoid the use of a foreign body in the repair. Lumbar drainage is used if there is preexisting CSF hypertension or if the floor of the third ventricle was opened during the procedure.

Results and Complications

Despite the fact that extended approaches have been described in the literature for nearly a quarter of a century, their application has been limited to a few pathologies such as craniopharyngiomas, meningiomas, and a few adenomas. This confirms the fact that an extended approach is indicated only in very few selected cases of pituitary adenomas. Furthermore, reports are focused on the technical details of the procedures, mixing all types of extended approaches, namely the transplanum-transtuberculum approach, and the various approaches to the cavernous sinus and the clivus. At present only sporadic cases of pituitary adenomas have been treated using the ETTEA 20. Furthermore in these few cases, endocrinological and visual results are not well detailed. The most frequent complication was CSF leak ranging up to 38.5%.[20]

A B C D

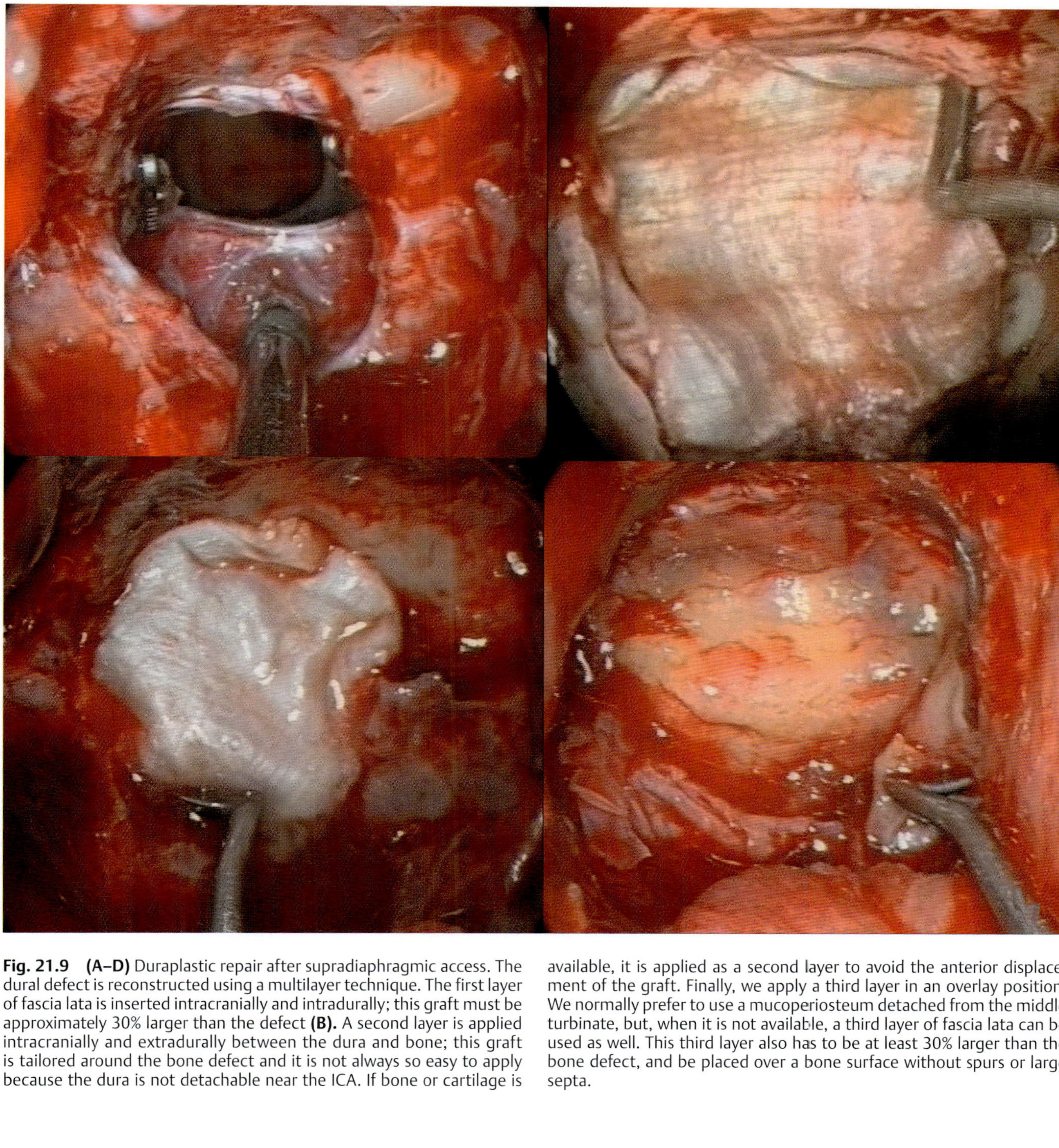

Fig. 21.9 (A–D) Duraplastic repair after supradiaphragmic access. The dural defect is reconstructed using a multilayer technique. The first layer of fascia lata is inserted intracranially and intradurally; this graft must be approximately 30% larger than the defect **(B).** A second layer is applied intracranially and extradurally between the dura and bone; this graft is tailored around the bone defect and it is not always so easy to apply because the dura is not detachable near the ICA. If bone or cartilage is available, it is applied as a second layer to avoid the anterior displacement of the graft. Finally, we apply a third layer in an overlay position. We normally prefer to use a mucoperiosteum detached from the middle turbinate, but, when it is not available, a third layer of fascia lata can be used as well. This third layer also has to be at least 30% larger than the bone defect, and be placed over a bone surface without spurs or large septa.

From these preliminary reports, it emerges that it is impossible to furnish credible data on the expected results and complications. Unfortunately, even if we review the various microscopic[2,5–8,17,19] and endoscopic-assisted[3] series, the problem remains.

Two studies from the literature merit special mention. One is the excellent study of Mason and colleagues[8] dealing with the transtuberculum approach for ectopic ACTH adenomas of the pituitary stalk; 10 patients were treated, and remission of the hypercortisol state with a low complication rate (one bitemporal hemianopia and one permanent panhypopituitarism) was obtained. The second is the study of Fatemi and colleagues,[3] in which the complication rates of the standard transsphenoidal approach and the extended approach were compared, demonstrating the increase in mortality and morbidity in the extended approach.

■ Conclusion

Preliminary results with the ETTEA in pituitary adenomas are insufficient to make a convincing argument in favor of the safety and effectiveness of the procedure. At present, we believe that the most convincing indication for its use is represented by the rare cases of ectopic pituitary stalk adenomas.

For other circumstances in which the ETTEA may be suggested (adenomas with midline subfrontal extension, invasive adenomas growing through the diaphragma sella, and fibrous adenomas), the indication is grounded in the still unproven conviction that it gives similar results using a less invasive approach than a craniotomy.

Certainly, in pituitary adenomas, the selection of the ETTEA should be carefully evaluated, and the procedure should be performed by well-trained endoscopic surgeons well versed in the procedure and having the skills to deal with possible complications.

References

1. Weiss MH. The transnasal transsphenoidal approach. In: Apuzzo MLJ, ed. Surgery of the Third Ventricle. Baltimore: Williams & Wilkins; 1987:476–494
2. Couldwell WT, Weiss MH, Rabb C, Liu JK, Apfelbaum RI, Fukushima T. Variations on the standard transsphenoidal approach to the sellar region, with emphasis on the extended approaches and parasellar approaches: surgical experience in 105 cases. Neurosurgery 2004;55: 539-547, discussion 547–550
3. Fatemi N, Dusick JR, de Paiva Neto MA, Kelly DF. The endonasal microscopic approach for pituitary adenomas and other parasellar tumors: a 10-year experience. Neurosurgery 2008;63(4, Suppl 2):244–256, discussion 256
4. Hashimoto N, Handa H, Yamagami T. Transsphenoidal extracapsular approach to pituitary tumors. J Neurosurg 1986;64:16–20
5. Kato T, Sawamura Y, Abe H, Nagashima M. Transsphenoidal-transtuberculum sellae approach for supradiaphragmatic tumours: technical note. Acta Neurochir (Wien) 1998;140:715–718, discussion 719
6. Kouri JG, Chen MY, Watson JC, Oldfield EH. Resection of suprasellar tumors by using a modified transsphenoidal approach. Report of four cases. J Neurosurg 2000;92:1028–1035
7. Maira G, Anile C, Rossi GF, Colosimo C. Surgical treatment of craniopharyngiomas: an evaluation of the transsphenoidal and pterional approaches. Neurosurgery 1995;36:715–724
8. Mason RB, Nieman LK, Doppman JL, Oldfield EH. Selective excision of adenomas originating in or extending into the pituitary stalk with preservation of pituitary function. J Neurosurg 1997;87:343–351
9. Jho HD, Carrau RL. Endoscopic endonasal transsphenoidal surgery: experience with 50 patients. J Neurosurg 1997;87:44–51
10. Cappabianca P, Frank G, Pasquini E, de Divitiis O, Calbucci F. Extended approach to the suprasellar region and planum sphenoidale. In: de Divitiis E, Cappabianca P, eds. Endoscopic Endonasal Transsphenoidal Surgery. New York: Springer; 2003:176–182
11. de Divitiis E, Cavallo LM, Cappabianca P, Esposito F. Extended endoscopic endonasal transsphenoidal approach for the removal of suprasellar tumors: Part 2. Neurosurgery 2007;60:46–58, discussion 58–59
12. Frank G, Pasquini E, Doglietto F, et al. The endoscopic extended transsphenoidal approach for craniopharyngiomas. Neurosurgery 2006; 59(1, Suppl 1):ONS75–ONS83, discussion ONS75–ONS83
13. Jho HD, Ha HG. Endoscopic endonasal skull base surgery: Part 1—the midline anterior fossa skull base. Minim Invasive Neurosurg 2004; 47:1–8
14. Buchfelder M, Kreutzer J. Transcranial surgery for pituitary adenomas. Pituitary 2008;11:375–384
15. Castelnuovo P, Locatelli D, Mauri S, De Bernardi F. Anterior cranial base CSF leaks. In: de Divitiis E, Cappabianca P, eds. Endoscopic Endonasal Transsphenoidal Surgery. New York: Springer; 2003:137–158
16. Hadad G, Bassagasteguy L, Carrau RL, et al. A novel reconstructive technique after endoscopic expanded endonasal approaches: vascular pedicle nasoseptal flap. Laryngoscope 2006;116:1882–1886
17. Zhao B, Wei YK, Li GL, et al. Extended transsphenoidal approach for pituitary adenomas invading the anterior cranial base, cavernous sinus, and clivus: a single-center experience with 126 consecutive cases. J Neurosurg 2010;112:108–117
18. Frank G, Pasquini E, Farneti G, et al. The endoscopic versus the traditional approach in pituitary surgery. Neuroendocrinology 2006;83:240–248
19. Kaptain GJ, Vincent DA, Sheehan JP, Laws ER Jr. Transsphenoidal approaches for the extracapsular resection of midline suprasellar and anterior cranial base lesions. Neurosurgery 2001;49:94–100, discussion 100–101
20. Ceylan S, Koc K, Anik I. Extended endoscopic approaches for midline skull-base lesions. Neurosurg Rev 2009;32:309–319, discussion 318–319

VII Tips and Pearls in the Sellar and Parasellar Approach

22 Microsurgical and Endoscopic Anatomy of the Parasellar Region

Carolina Martins, Alexandre Yasuda, Alvaro Campero, Luiz Felipe de Alencastro, Kohei Inoue, and Albert L. Rhoton, Jr.

Tips and Pearls

- The cavernous sinuses are located in the parasellar areas, formed by the union of the lateral part of the sphenoid body and the petrous apex of the temporal bone.
- The cavernous sinuses are bordered by the petrous apex and dorsum sellae posteriorly and the superior orbital fissure anteriorly, and extend from the level of the foramen rotundum inferiorly up to the level of the clinoids.
- Each cavernous sinus has four walls.
- The roof is divided into anterior (clinoidal) and posterior (oculomotor) triangles. It is most commonly used during anterior and posterior clinoidectomies or transcavernous approaches.
- The medial wall has two parts: sellar (superior) and sphenoidal (inferior). This wall may be breached by tumors arising on the sella or surgically used to approach cavernous sinus contents during endonasal or transmaxillary transsphenoidal approaches.
- The lateral wall is most commonly approached during middle fossa peeling. It is divided into three triangles—supratrochlear, infratrochlear, and anteromedial—which provide specific gates of entrance into the sinus.

Introduction

The parasellar area is part of the middle fossa, between the sellae and the temporal fossa. The parasellar area is considered to be the smallest area of the skull base with the highest concentration of important neural and vascular structures, as it houses the cavernous sinus.

The cavernous sinuses are bordered by the petrous apex and dorsum sellae posteriorly and by the superior orbital fissure anteriorly. They extend from the level of the foramen rotundum inferiorly up to the level of the clinoids. Each cavernous sinus has four walls. The roof faces the basal cisterns. The posterior wall faces the upper part of the posterior fossa. The medial wall, which separates the cavernous sinus from the contents of sella and sphenoid sinus, is formed by a thin dural layer, and this anatomical fact enables sellar tumors to extend toward the cavernous sinus. The lateral wall faces the medial temporal lobe. It has an inclination from medial to lateral, and is continuous with the floor of the temporal fossae.

Because of its acute-angled front and the shape of its back, the cavernous sinus has been compared with a boat.[1] It can also be viewed as a tent, in which fixed structures are covered by a cloth to create a compartment. In the cavernous sinus, these fixed structures belong to the skull base, and the cloth above them is the dura.

Knowledge of this special architecture is paramount in performing surgery in the parasellar area. The need to better understand the cavernous sinus has been a relentless effort, which started through a series of important anatomical contributions,[2–4] paving the way to the present understanding of the area.[5–8]

Bone Structures Along the Parasellar Area

The parasellar area is formed by a small contribution of the temporal bone and a major part of the sphenoid (**Fig. 22.1**). The temporal bone contributes to the parasellar area with its petrous apex, medial to the trigeminal impression. The petrous apex faces the lingula of the sphenoid bone and forms the posterior lip of the cranial opening of the carotid canal. In the articulated skull, both the lingula and the petrous apex are linked by the petrolingual ligament, which separates the petrous from the first vertical portion of the cavernous carotid. The sphenoid bone, the major bone structure responsible for supporting the cavernous sinuses, presents to the parasellar area the anterior clinoid process and the lateral part of the sphenoid body, along which the greater sphenoidal wing attaches.

The lesser sphenoid wings attach to each other along the sphenoid planum. Their posterior edges, the sphenoidal ridges, end medially as the anterior clinoid processes. Medial to the anterior clinoids are the intracranial openings of the optic canals, and, between them, the chiasmatic sulcus. The tuberculum sellae separates the chiasmatic sulcus and sphenoid planum from the sella turcica. On the most lateral part of this area the medial clinoid process may be present. In some instances, this process is linked to the anterior clinoid, forming the carotico-clinoidal foramen, through which the carotid artery passes. Across the sella, the tuberculum faces

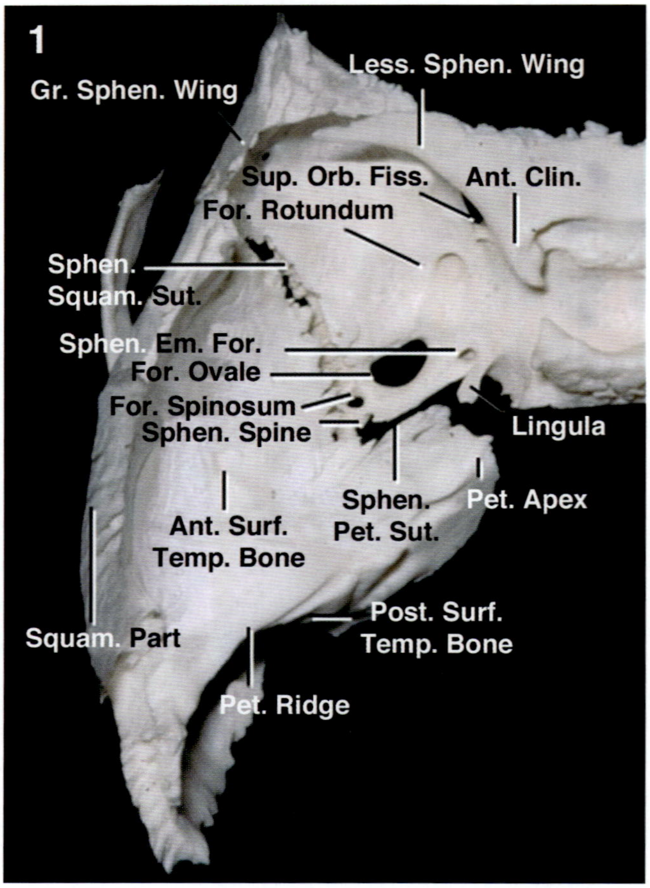

Fig. 22.1 Bone structures of the parasellar area. Ant.: anterior; Clin.: clinoid, clinoidal; Em.: emissary; Fiss.: fissure; For.: foramen; Gr.: greater; Less.: lesser; Orb.: orbital; Pet.: petrous, petrosal; Post.: posterior; Sphen.: sphenoidal; Squam.: squamosal; Sup.: superior; Sut.: suture; Temp.: temporal.

the dorsum sellae. On each side of dorsum, are the posterior clinoid processes.

The lateral part of the body of the sphenoid forms the inferior part of the medial wall of the cavernous sinus, which extends from the petrous apex to the superior orbital fissure. The upper part of the medial wall, up to the clinoids, is directly related to the contents of the sella. The portion of the sphenoid body that is related to the medial wall presents the carotid sulcus. The carotid sulcus runs along the lateral surface of the body of the sphenoid from its posterior part, near the lingula, where this sulcus is deeper, toward the superior orbital fissure, where the carotid sulcus fades along the optic strut. The carotid sulcus is the impression left at the body of the sphenoid by the carotid artery (**Fig. 22.2**).

To understand the structure of the cavernous sinus is fundamental to understanding the anterior clinoid and its attachments. Each anterior clinoid is attached to the sphenoid by three points (**Fig. 22.3**). Laterally, the anterior clinoid is continuous with the sphenoid ridge. Medially, the anterior clinoid attaches to the sphenoid by its anterior and posterior roots. The anterior root passes medially over the optic canal and along the sphenoid planum. This bone often is defective

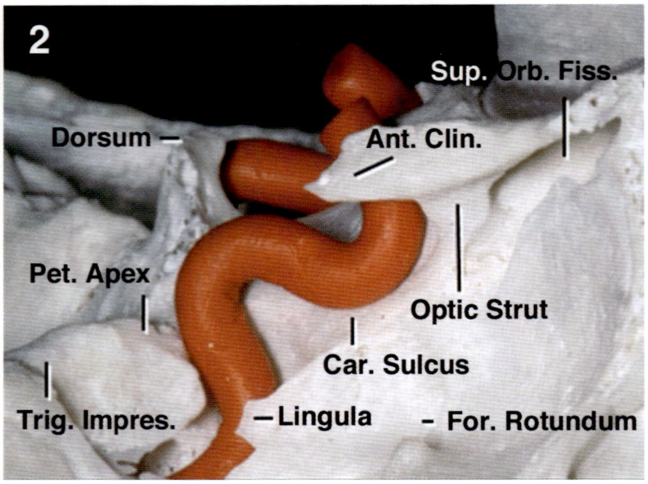

Fig. 22.2 Lateral view along the parasellar area. The internal carotid artery is shown in red. The lateral portion of the sphenoid body presents the carotid sulcus, the impression left at the body of the sphenoid by the carotid artery. Ant.: anterior; Car.: carotid; Clin.: clinoid; Fiss.: fissure; For.: foramen; Impres.: impression; Orb.: orbital; Pet.: petrous; Sup.: superior; Surf.: surface; Trig.: trigeminal.

and very thin, and the dura is the only element protecting the optic nerve in this area. The posterior root, also called the optic strut, is usually stout. It links the anterior clinoid to the sphenoid body, separating the optic canal from the superior orbital fissure. As the roof and floor of the optic canal are clinoidal attachments, the removal of the anterior clinoid decompresses the optic nerve.

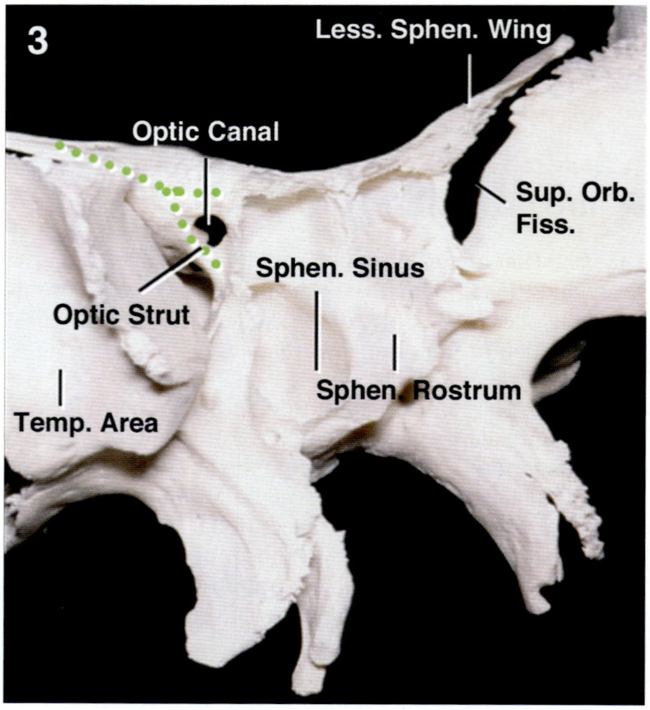

Fig. 22.3 Anterior oblique view of the sphenoid bone helps in understanding the anterior clinoid attachments. Fiss.: fissure; Less.: lesser; Orb.: orbital; Sphen.: sphenoidal; Sup.: superior; Temp.: temporal.

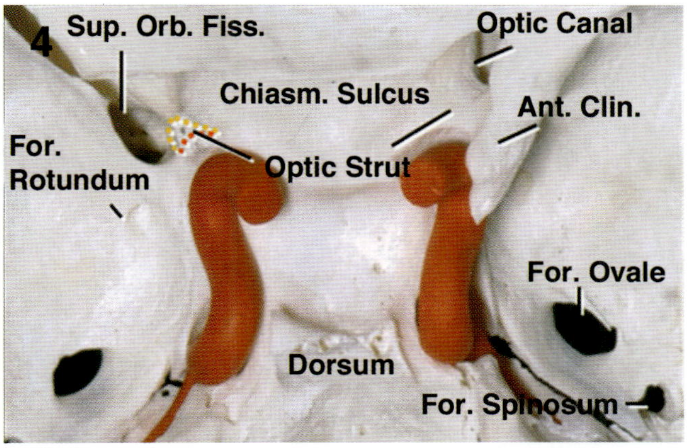

Fig. 22.4 Posterosuperior view into the parasellar area. The anterior clinoid process has been removed on the left, exposing the optic strut. The optic strut has two neural-facing surfaces, related to structures passing along the superior orbital fissure and optic canal (*yellow dotted lines*) and a vascular-facing surface, which relates to the carotid artery (*red dotted line*). Ant.: anterior; Chiasm.: chiasmatic; Clin.: clinoid; Fiss.: fissure; For.: foramen; Orb.: orbital; Sup.: superior.

The optic strut has three surfaces. The surface facing superiorly is the floor of the optic canal, the surface facing laterally forms, with the sphenoidal body, the medial border of the superior orbital fissure and is located at the anterior end of the cavernous sinus. The posterior-facing surface of the optic strut is concave and adapts to the anterior bend of the clinoidal portion of the carotid artery (**Fig. 22.4**). When removing the anterior clinoid—a common step in dealing with the cavernous sinus—the surgeon must recall that the optic strut has two neural-facing surfaces, related to the structures passing along the optic canal and superior orbital fissure, and a third, vascular-related surface, which faces the carotid.

Knowledge about the anterior clinoid is also important in understanding the roof of the cavernous sinus. The real roof of the sinus is located below the level of the anterior clinoid. The clinoid and its dural covering are extra protections for the anterior part of the roof, and can be compared to the attic of a house. At the level of the anterior clinoid, the carotid artery passes along the dural coverings of the parasellar area to reach the subarachnoid space. The part of the artery at the level of the anterior clinoid is not fully cavernous nor completely subarachnoidal, but is enclosed in this clinoidal intermediate space or attic and is named the clinoidal carotid.[5]

Mastering the anatomy of the anterior clinoid and clinoidal segment of the carotid is also paramount when dealing with the lateral wall of the sphenoid sinus, through an exocranial, endoscopic route.

On the exocranial side, the bony depression into the medial end of the optic strut is the opticocarotid recess (**Fig. 22.5**). The broad round prominence below the opticocarotid recess overlies the structures passing through the superior orbital fissure. Above the recess, on the superolateral part of the sinus wall, the optic nerve and ophthalmic artery are enclosed in the dura of the optic canal. The superior and inferior edges of the opticocarotid recess mark the position of the upper and lower carotid dural rings, and the arterial segment located between the two is the clinoidal segment (**Fig. 22.6**).

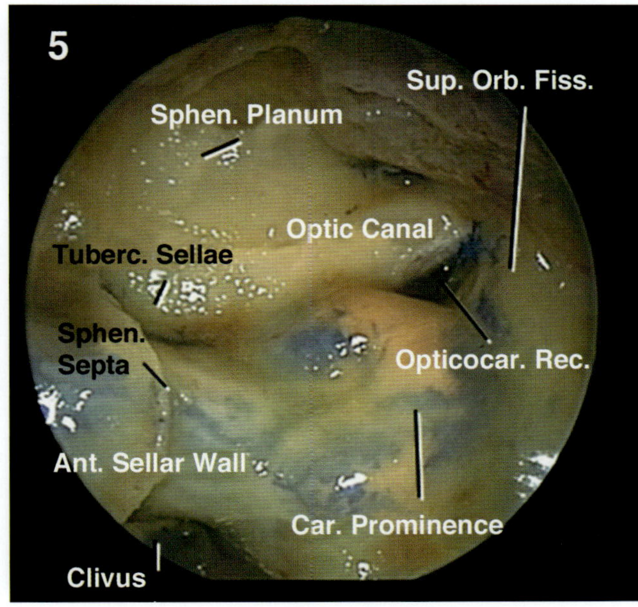

Fig. 22.5 Endoscopic dissection through the sphenoid sinus. The sphenoid planum and tuberculum sellae form the roof of the sphenoid sinus. The clivus, pneumatized up to the dorsum in this specimen, forms the posterior wall. The sella is located on the transition between the roof and posterior wall of the sphenoid sinus. The carotid sulcus produces a prominence within the sphenoid sinus, which is maximal in the most pronounced pneumatized sinuses. The carotid prominence can be divided into three segments: retrosellar, infrasellar, and presellar. Ant.: anterior; Car.: carotid; Fiss.: fissure; Opticocar.: opticocarotid; Orb.: orbital; Rec.: recess; Sphen.: sphenoidal; Sup.: superior; Tuberc.: tuberculum.

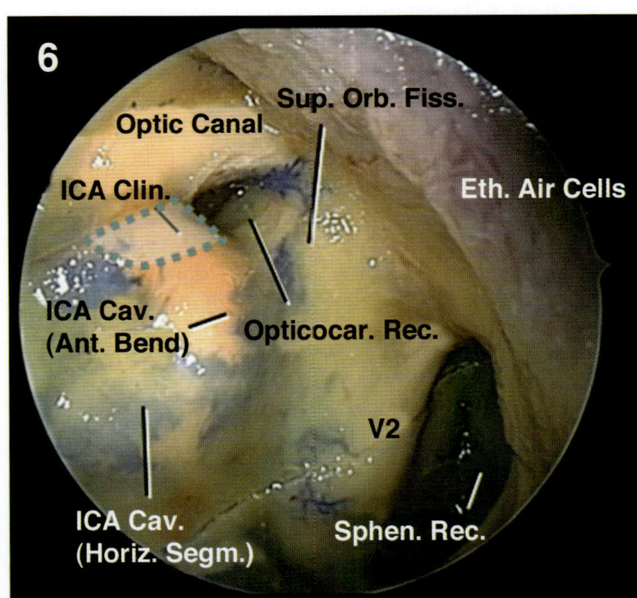

Fig. 22.6 Superolateral wall of the sphenoid sinus (*left side*); the clinoidal segment is highlighted by the dotted line. Ant.: anterior; Cav.: cavernous; Clin.: clinoid, clinoidal; Eth.: ethmoid, ethmoidal; Fiss.: fissure; Horiz.: horizontal; ICA: internal carotid artery; Opticocar.: opticocarotid; Orb.: orbital; Rec.: recess; Segm.: segment; Sphen.: sphenoidal; Sup.: superior; V2: seconc trigeminal nerve.

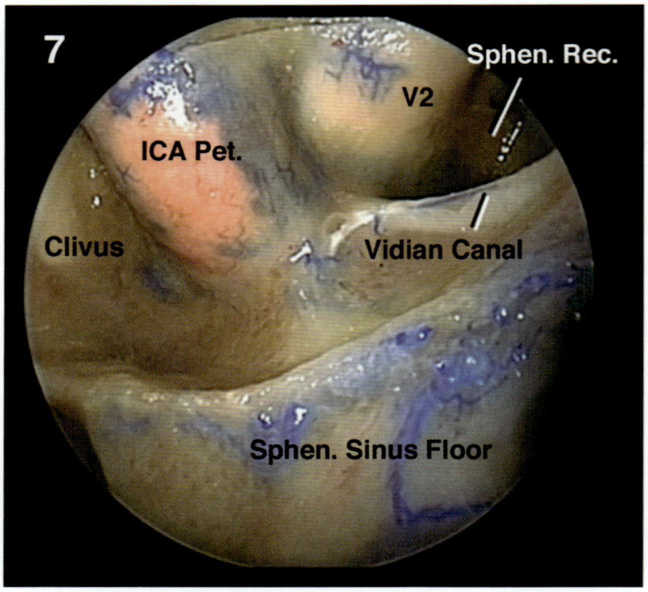

Fig. 22.7 Inferolateral wall and floor of the sphenoid sinus. As the cavernous sinus ends inferiorly at the level of the maxillary division (V2), the sphenoidal recess extends laterally below the sinus and lateral to the petrous part of the carotid artery. This segment of the carotid artery is signaled by the position of the vidian canal, which can be seen coursing along the floor of the sphenoid sinus. The vidian canal transmits the vidian nerve and the vidian artery. The vidian nerve is formed by the combination of the deep carotid nerve and the greater petrosal nerve and courses from the anterior wall of the foramen lacerum to the pterygopalatine ganglion into the pterygopalatine fossa. ICA: internal carotid artery; Pet.: petrous, petrosal; Rec.: recess; Sphen.: sphenoidal.

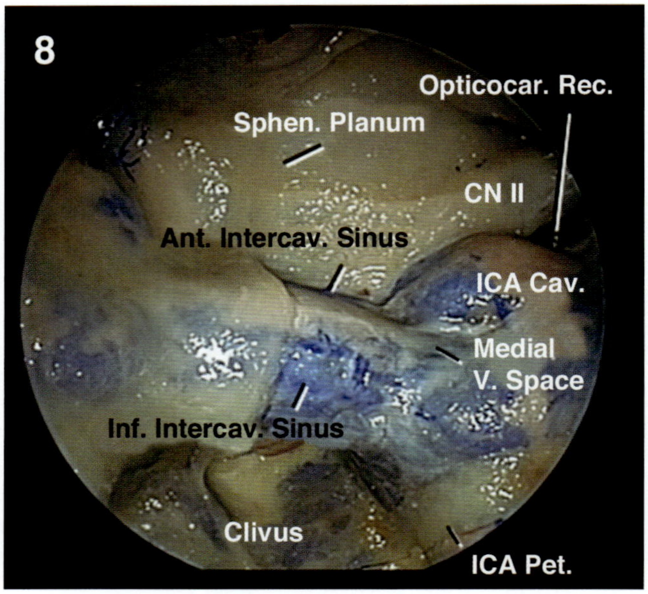

Fig. 22.8 The bone has been removed over the left half of the sellae and lateral wall of the sphenoid sinus. The retrosellar segment of the carotid prominence is seen on the posterolateral part of the sinuses in which the pneumatization extended laterally in the area of the dorsum. The retrosellar carotid prominence comprises the transition part between the distal petrous and the proximal cavernous carotid and is bound in place laterally by the petrolingual ligament. Several venous connections link the cavernous sinuses across midline, including the anterior and inferior intercavernous sinuses. These transsellar connections between the cavernous sinuses may exist at any point from the anterior to the posterior wall of the sella, including the diaphragma, or all connections between the two sides may be absent. The anterior intercavernous sinus, crossing the upper anterior margin of the sella, joins the cavernous sinus immediately behind the site at which the upper and lower rings fuse. The largest and most constant intercavernous connection is the basilar sinus, passing posterior to the dorsum and upper clivus and connecting the posterior aspect of both cavernous sinuses. The three main venous spaces within the sinus are identified by their relation to the carotid artery; they are the medial, anteroinferior, and posterosuperior compartments. Ant.: anterior; Cav.: cavernous; CN: cranial nerve; ICA: internal carotid artery; Inf.: inferior; Intercav.: intercavernous; Opticocar.: opticocarotid; Pet.: petrous; Rec.: recess; Sphen.: sphenoidal; V.: vein, venous.

A segment of the maxillary division of the trigeminal nerve, just peripheral to the ganglion, protrudes into the lateral wall, below the sella. The average length of the maxillary division bulging into the sinus is 10.9 mm.[3] The trigeminal ganglion and the first and third trigeminal divisions are usually separated from the sinus wall by the position of the carotid artery; however, when the sphenoid sinus is fully pneumatized into the greater sphenoid wing, creating the sphenoid sinus recess, the maxillary division becomes more clearly defined and the position of the superior orbital fissure and the mandibular division may be more clearly identified (**Figs. 22.6** and **22.7**).

Cavernous Sinus Contents

The dural envelope of the cavernous sinus is the site of a venous confluence that receives the terminal end of multiple veins draining the orbit, the sylvian fissure, and the middle and anterior fossae, and it has free communications with the basilar, superior and inferior petrosal and the intercavernous sinuses (**Fig. 22.8**). The three main venous spaces within the sinus are identified by their relation to the carotid artery; they are the medial, anteroinferior, and posterosuperior compartments.

Besides the medial venous plexus, the most medial structure inside the cavernous sinus is the carotid artery, coursing in intimate relationship with the abducens nerve (**Figs. 22.8, 22.9, 22.10, 22.11, 22.12,** and **22.13**). The terminal part of the petrous carotid exits the carotid canal and passes under the trigeminal nerve and the petrolingual ligament, where it turns upward to enter the posterior part of the cavernous sinus. The artery becomes enclosed in the dural envelope of the cavernous sinus only when it exits the region of the foramen lacerum and turns upward, after traveling below the petrolingual ligament to reach the carotid sulcus on the lateral surface of the sphenoid body.

The third and fourth nerves enter the posterior part of the roof, in close relation with the meningohypophyseal branch, and reach the lateral wall of the cavernous sinus, to pass, with the first trigeminal division, along the superior orbital

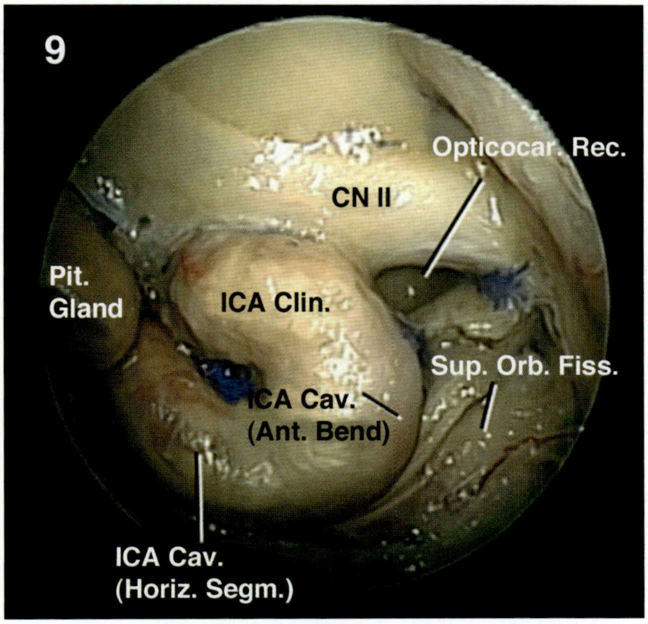

Fig. 22.9 The dura and venous structures have been removed, exposing the relationship of the carotid and pituitary gland. The infrasellar segment of the carotid prominence is located below the sellar floor and comprises the horizontal portion of the cavernous carotid. The presellar segment is located beside the anterior sinus wall and is the most frequently identified prominence related to the carotid inside the sphenoid sinus. It comprises the anterior carotid bend and the clinoidal segment of the carotid artery. The bone separating the artery and the sphenoid sinus is thinnest along the presellar part just below the tuberculum sellae. Ant.: anterior; Cav.: cavernous; Clin.: clinoid; CN: cranial nerve; Fiss.: fissure; Horiz.: horizontal; ICA: internal carotid artery; Opticocar.: opticocarotid; Orb.: orbital; Pit.: pituitary; Rec.: recess; Segm.: segment; Sup.: superior.

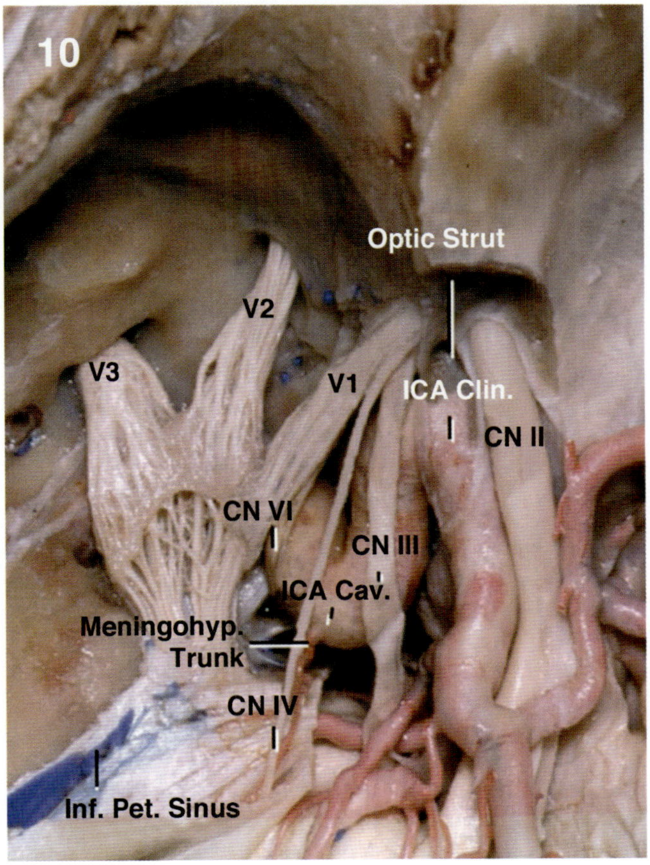

Fig. 22.10 The left cavernous sinus has been dissected to show its components. Cav.: cavernous; Clin.: clinoid; CN: cranial nerve; ICA: internal carotid artery; Inf.: inferior; Meningohyp.: meningohypophyseal; Pet.: petrosal; V1: first division; V2: second division; V3: third division of trigeminal nerve.

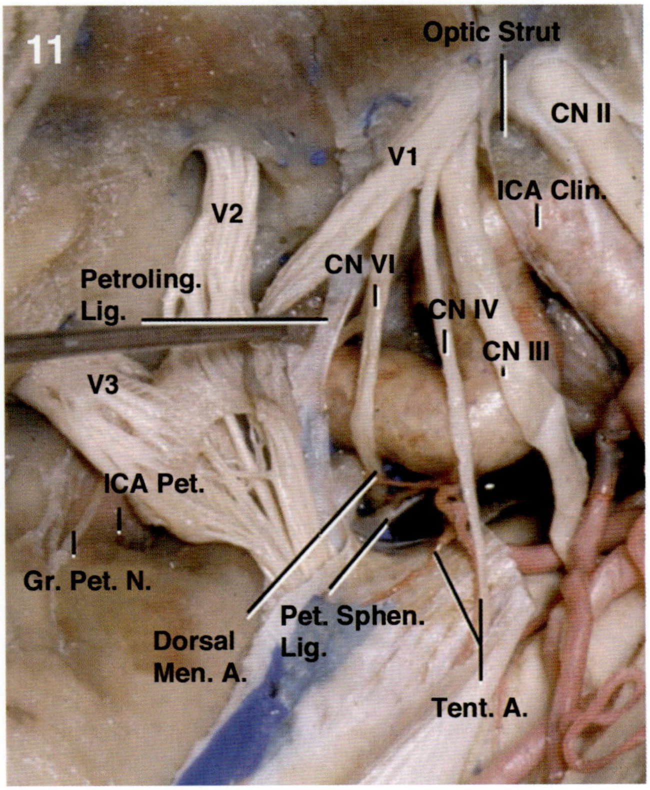

Fig. 22.11 The opthalmic division of the trigeminal nerve (V1) is displaced laterally, to view the petrolingual ligament and the point at which the sympathetic branches along the carotid nerve reach the abducens nerve. A.: artery; Clin.: clinoid, clinoidal; CN: cranial nerve; Gr.: greater; ICA: internal carotid artery; Lig.: ligament; Men.: meningeal; N.: nerve; Pet.: petrous, petrosal; Petroling.: petrolingual; Sphen.: spheno, sphenoid, sphenoidal; Tent.: tentorial; V1: first division; V2: second division; V3: third division of trigeminal nerve.

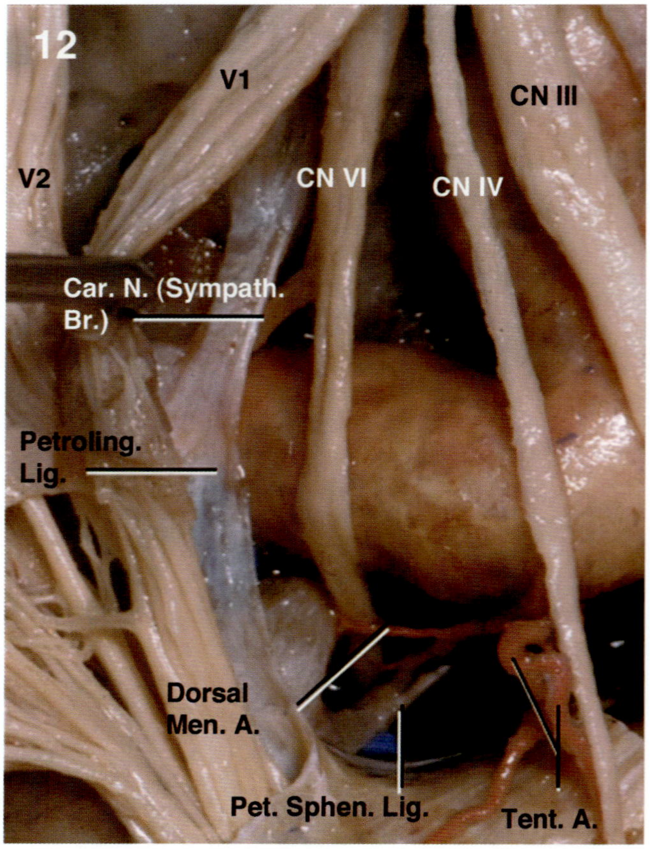

Fig. 22.12 Enlarged view of Fig. 22.11. A.: artery; Br.: branch; Car.: carotid; CN: cranial nerve; Lig.: ligament; Men.: meningeal; N.: nerve; Pet.: petrous, petrosal; Petroling.: petrolingual; Sphen.: spheno, sphenoid, sphenoidal; Sympath.: sympathetic; Tent.: tentorial; V1: first division; V2: second division; V3: third division of trigeminal nerve.

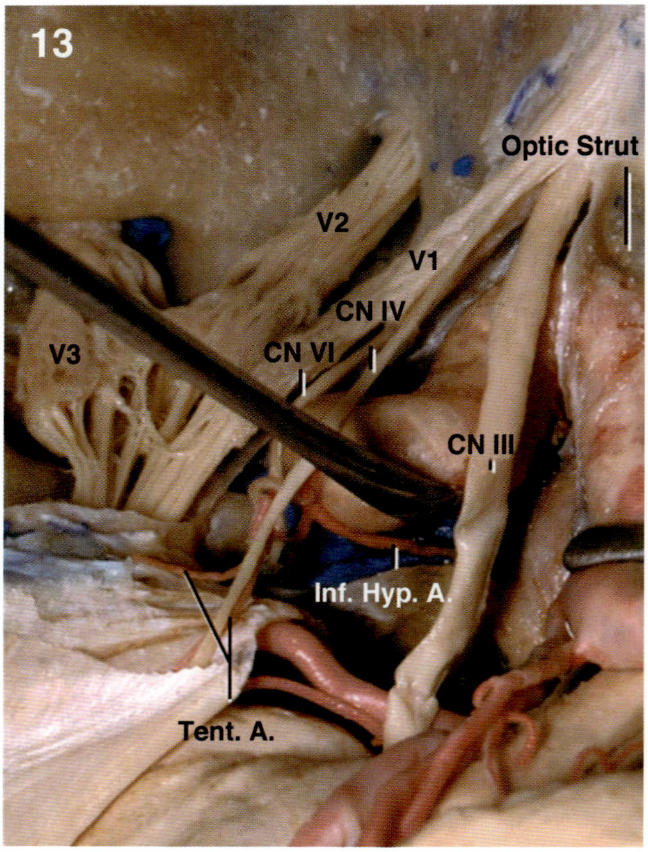

Fig. 22.13 The posterior bend of the cavernous carotid is displaced laterally to display the course of the inferior hypophyseal artery. A.: artery; CN: cranial nerve; Hyp.: hypophyseal; Inf.: inferior; Tent.: tentorial; V1: first division; V2: second division; V3: third division of trigeminal nerve.

fissure. The abducens nerve can be well seen when the first trigeminal division is displaced laterally (**Fig. 22.12**). The abducens nerve passes through the lower margin of the posterior wall of cavernous sinus, under the petrosphenoid ligament (Gubler's ligament). It courses inside the cavernous sinus and receives branches of the carotid nerve.

The carotid nerve, a branch of the sympathetic ganglia, branches into two parts near the genu of the petrous carotid artery: a larger anterior-superior and a smaller posterior-inferior trunk (**Figs. 22.14, 22.15, 22.16,** and **22.17**). The posterior branch sends rootlets that accompany the cerebral arteries and the trochlear and trigeminal nerves. The anterior branch gives origin to the deep petrosal nerve, which joins the greater petrosal nerve to form the vidian nerve (**Fig. 22.7**) and send smaller branches to the abducens and trigeminal nerves. The greater petrosal nerve detaches from the facial nerve at the level of the geniculate ganglion, passes through the facial hiatus, running under the dura in an anteromedial direction, parallel to and above the horizontal segment of the petrous carotid artery. From the abducens nerve, the sympathetic branches reach the ophthalmic division and enter the orbit.[9]

The cavernous carotid gives off several arterial branches. The meningohypophyseal trunk is a constant branch of the cavernous carotid (**Fig. 22.11**). In its complete form it gives rise to the dorsal meningeal, inferior hypophyseal, and tentorial arteries (**Figs. 22.12** and **22.13**). These arteries, besides supplying the meningeal layers of the parasellar area, also offer arterial supply to neural structures,[10] as is the case with the dorsal meningeal artery and the segment of the abducens nerve coursing inside Dorello's canal and the tentorial branches, which supply the trochlear nerve along the tentorial edge. The inferolateral trunk, which arises from the lateral portion of the horizontal segment of cavernous carotid, is another example of a neuromeningeal branch (**Figs. 22.17** and **22.18**). The divisions of the inferolateral trunk can be seen through the triangles of the parasellar area, and distribute to the oculomotor, trochlear, abducens, and ophthalmic nerves at the level of the superior orbital fissure, the maxillary division at the foramen rotundum, and the trigeminal ganglion and motor root, around which this branch anastomoses with branches of the middle and accessory meningeal arteries (**Fig. 22.19**). Sometimes the inferolateral branch may give rise to the tentorial arteries, in which case it assumes an

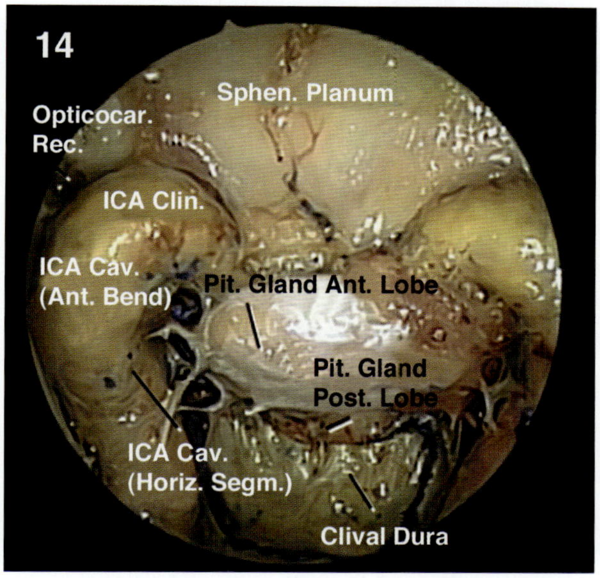

Fig. 22.14 Endoscopic dissection through the sphenoid sinus, in another specimen. The bone, dural, and venous structures over the sellar walls, cavernous carotid, and clivus have been removed. The anterior and posterior lobes of the pituitary gland are exposed. Ant.: anterior; Cav.: cavernous; Clin.: clinoid, clinoidal; Horiz.: horizontal; Opticocar.: opticocarotid; Pit.: pituitary; Post.: posterior; Rec.: recess; Segm.: segment; Sphen.: sphenoidal.

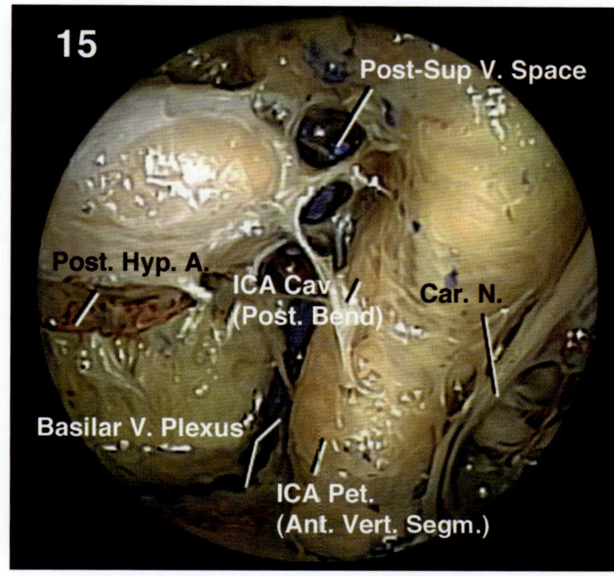

Fig. 22.15 The view is carried toward the left cavernous sinus area. The inferior hypophyseal artery arises from the posterior bend of the cavernous carotid, courses medially, supplying the dural floor of the posterior part of the sella, and reaches the posterior pituitary capsule and lobe and anastomoses with the its mate from contralateral side. The posterosuperior venous space of the cavernous sinus is located between the carotid and the posterior half of the roof of the sinus. The basilar sinus opens into the posterosuperior venous space. A.: artery; Ant.: anterior; Car.: carotid; Cav.: cavernous; Hyp.: hypophyseal; N.: nerve; Post.: posterior; Sup.: superior; V.: vein; Vert.: vertical.

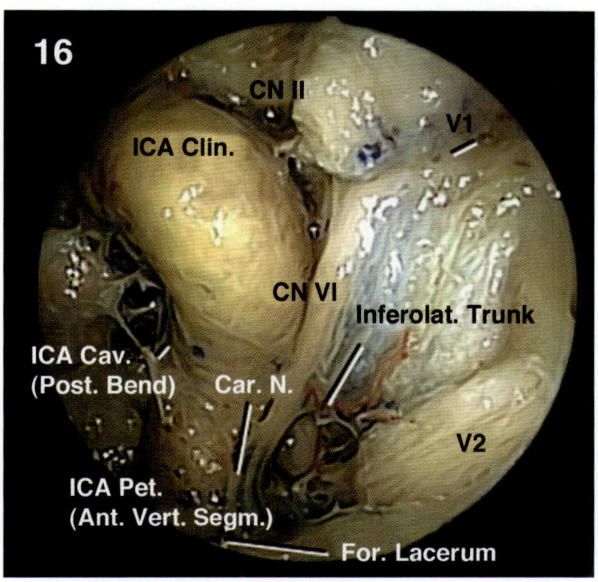

Fig. 22.16 The lateral wall of the sphenoid sinus has been dissected. The carotid nerve, a branch of the sympathetic ganglia, branches into two parts at the foramen lacerum area, near the genu of the petrous carotid artery: a larger anterior-superior and a smaller posterior-inferior trunk. The posterior branch sends rootlets that accompany the cerebral arteries and the trochlear and trigeminal nerves. The anterior branch gives origin to the deep petrosal nerve, which joins the greater petrosal nerve to form the vidian nerve (**see Fig. 22.7**) and send smaller branches to the abducens and trigeminal nerves. The inferolateral trunk, also called the artery of the inferior cavernous sinus, arises from the midportion of the horizontal segment of the cavernous carotid and passes medial to the first trigeminal division, superficial to the abducens nerve. Car.: carotid; Cav.: cavernous; CN: cranial nerve; For.: foramen; Inferolat.: inferolateral; V.: vein.

even larger role in the supply of the transdural segment of the nerves coursing along the parasellar area (**Fig. 22.20**). The capsular arteries arise from the medial side of the horizontal portion of the cavernous carotid, and pass along the medial wall of the cavernous sinus and join the inferior hypophyseal artery in the supply of the dura over the floor of the sella (**Fig. 22.21**).

Dural Arrangement in the Parasellar Area

It is the dural covering over the bone and the neural and vascular structures that define the cavernous sinus walls and compartments. The dura has a meningeal layer, which faces the brain and forms the diaphragma sellae and an endosteal layer, which is the periosteum of the sphenoid bone and extends along the roof and the posterior and lateral walls of the cavernous sinus.

It is along the lateral wall of the cavernous sinus that the distinction between the dural layers of the sinus is most easily demonstrated. On the lateral wall, elevating the meningeal layer as in a middle fossa surgical peeling, one exposes the

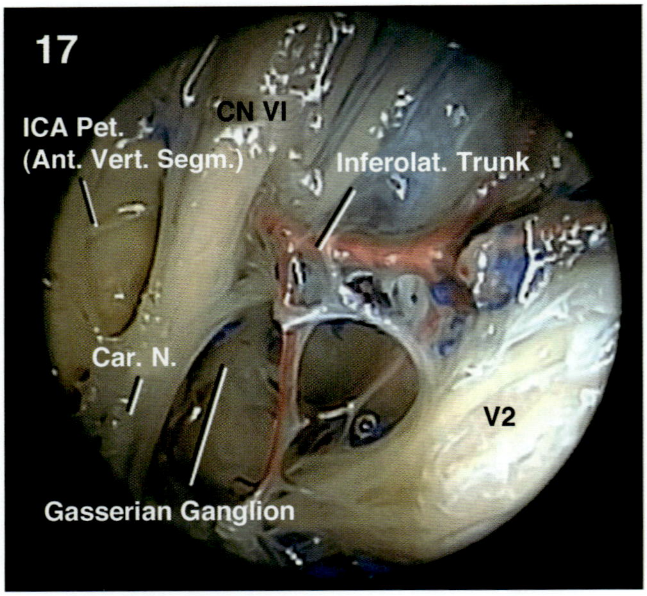

Fig. 22.17 Enlarged view of the area lateral to foramen lacerum. The inferolateral trunk provides supply to cranial nerves III, VI, V, and VI in their course along the parasellar area and to the dura covering the lateral wall of the cavernous sinus. The gasserian ganglion can be seen on the most posterior part of this area. The lower edge of the cavernous sinus, where the medial and lateral walls meet, is located just below the ophthalmic division; proceeding posteriorly, this inferior border is located medial to the junction of the upper and medial third of the gasserian ganglion. Ant.: anterior; Car.: carotid; CN: cranial nerve; ICA: internal carotid artery; Inferolat.: inferolateral; N.: nerve; Pet.: petrous; V2: second division of trigeminal nerve; Vert.: vertical.

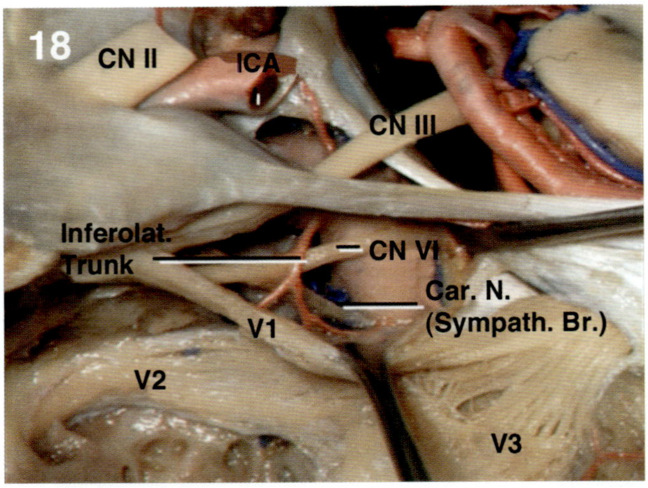

Fig. 22.18 Lateral view of the left cavernous sinus. V1 is displaced inferiorly exposing the inferolateral trunk. Br.: branch; CN: cranial nerve; ICA: internal carotid artery; Inferolat.: inferolateral; Sympath.: sympathetic; V1: first division; V2: second division; V3: third division of trigeminal nerve.

outer endosteal layer that covers the nerves and venous spaces (**Figs. 22.22** and **22.23**). Sometimes it is possible to see through this layer and recognize the structures running close to the lateral wall, but without fully entering into the sinus. In this situation, the surgeon must understand the importance of the triangular arrangements inside and around the cavernous sinus.

The cavernous sinus triangles are the spaces between the nerves and can be selectively opened to access specific areas of the cavernous sinus or surrounding structures (**Fig. 22.24**). Removing the endosteal layer and the venous plexus in the middle fossa and parasellar area exposes the supratrochlear, infratrochlear (or Parkinson's) anterolateral, posterolateral, and posteromedial triangles. As the inferior border of the cavernous sinus is located at the level of the maxillary division and foramen rotundum, the anterolateral, posterolateral, and posteromedial triangles are considered middle fossa

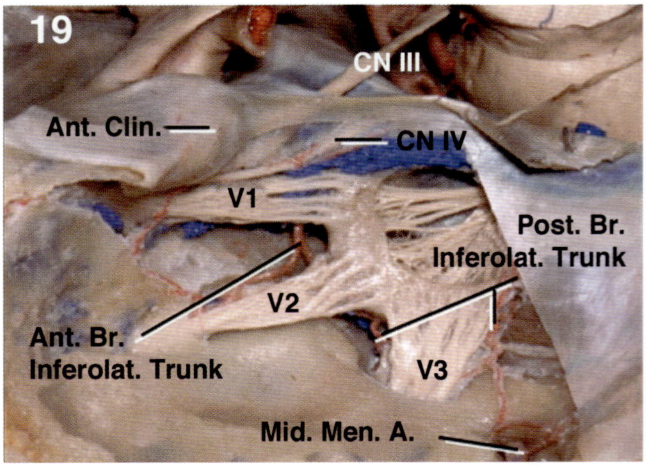

Fig. 22.19 Another dissected cavernous sinus. The branches of the inferolateral trunk can be seen along the parasellar and middle fossa triangles. A.: artery; Ant.: anterior; Br.: branch; Clin.: clinoid; CN: cranial nerve; Inferolat.: inferolateral; Men.: meningeal; Post.: posterior; V.: vein.

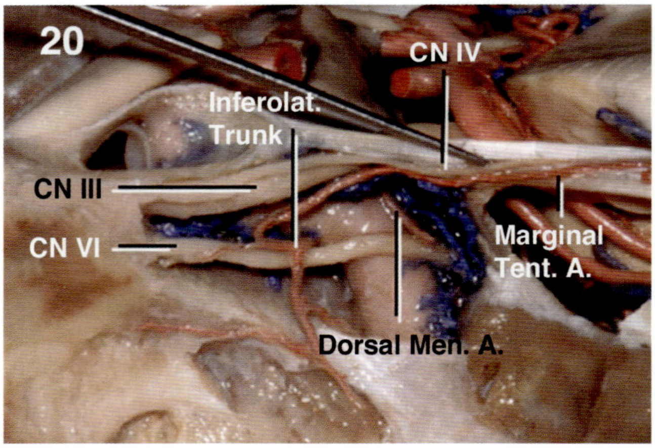

Fig. 22.20 Left cavernous sinus. The trigeminal nerve has been removed, exposing the inferolateral trunk and its branches. In this specimen, the marginal tentorial artery arises from the superior branch of the inferolateral trunk. A.: artery; CN: cranial nerve; Inferolat.: inferolateral; Men.: meningeal; Mid.: middle; Tent.: tentorial; V1: first division; V2: second division; V3: third division of trigeminal nerve.

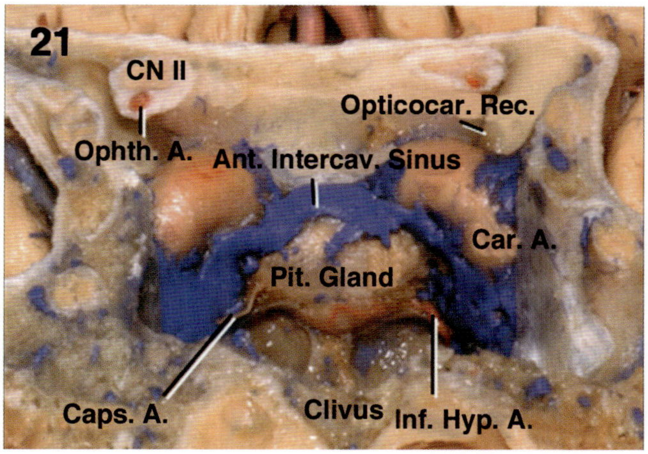

Fig. 22.21 Coronal cut through the skull base. The posterior wall of the sphenoid sinus has been partially removed. A.: artery; Ant.: anterior; Caps.: capsular; Car.: carotid; CN: cranial nerve; Hyp.: hypophyseal; Inf.: inferior; Intercav.: intercavernous; Ophth.: ophthalmic; Opticocar.: opticocarotid; Pit.: pituitary; Rec.: recess.

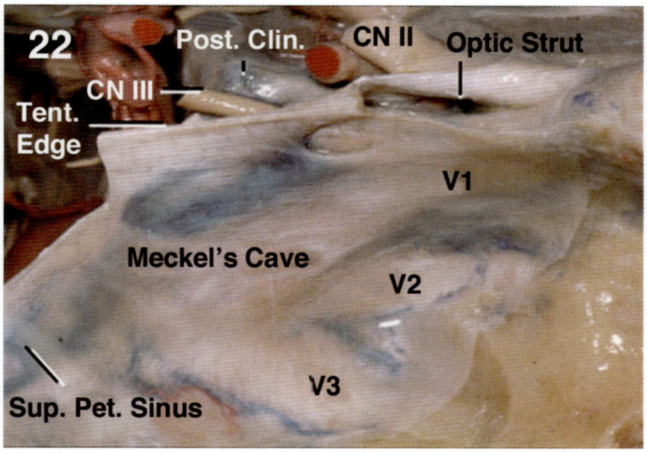

Fig. 22.22 Right lateral cavernous sinus wall. Clin.: clinoid; CN: cranial nerve; Pet.: petrous; Post.: posterior; Sup.: superior; Tent.: tentorial; V1: first division; V2: second division; V3: third division of trigeminal nerve.

triangles. The anterolateral triangle is located between the maxillary and mandibular divisions and contains the motor trigeminal root. The posterolateral triangle is bordered anteriorly by the mandibular division and medially by the greater petrosal nerve. The posteromedial or Kawase's triangle is located medial to the greater petrosal nerve and is related to the trigeminal ganglion and superior petrosal sinus.

The venous plexus contained in the middle fossa triangles open into the cavernous sinus through its inferior border and are called the pericavernous venous plexus. The openings of the pericavernous venous plexus can be observed at the point where the medial and lateral walls of the cavernous sinus meet, when dissecting the cavernous sinus from above (**Fig. 22.25**). These pericavernous plexuses can be considered to have a role similar to that of the ophthalmic veins and the superior petrosal sinuses.

The structural arrangement of the medial wall of the cavernous sinus differs from the lateral wall. The medial wall

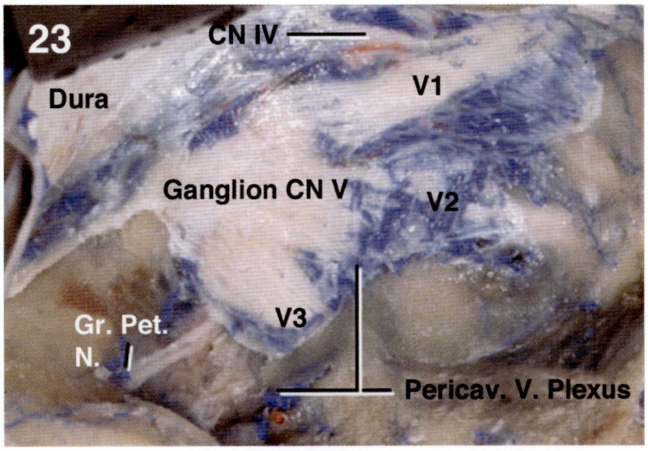

Fig. 22.23 The external dural layer of the right lateral wall of the cavernous sinus has been removed, while preserving the inner dural layer. The nerves coursing along the lateral wall can be seen by transparency. CN: cranial nerve; Gr.: greater; N.: nerve; Pericav.: pericavernous; Pet.: petrous; V.: vein, venous; V1: first division; V2: second division; V3: third division of trigeminal nerve.

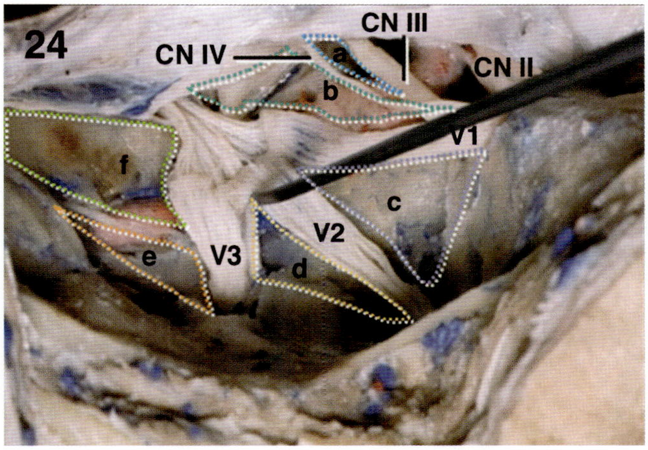

Fig. 22.24 The inner dural layer and the venous contents of the right cavernous sinus have been removed. The parasellar and middle fossa triangles are the spaces between the nerves and can be selectively opened to access specific areas of the cavernous sinus or surrounding structures. Removing the endosteal layer and the venous plexus in the middle fossa and parasellar area exposes the supratrochlear (a), infratrochlear (b) (or Parkinson's), anteromedial (c), anterolateral (d), posterolateral (e), and posteromedial (f) triangles. As the inferior border of the cavernous sinus is located at the level of the maxillary division and foramen rotundum, the anterolateral, posterolateral and posteromedial triangles are considered middle fossa triangles. The anterolateral triangle is located between the maxillary and mandibular divisions and contains the motor trigeminal root. The posterolateral triangle (e) is bordered anteriorly by the mandibular division, and medially by the greater petrosal nerve. The posteromedial or Kawase's triangle (f) is located medial to the greater petrosal nerve and is related to the trigeminal ganglion and superior petrosal sinus. CN: cranial nerve; V1: first division; V2: second division; V3: third division of trigeminal nerve.

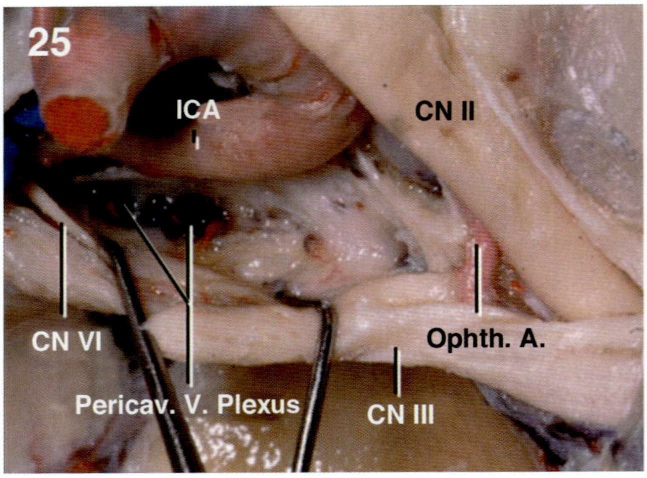

Fig. 22.25 Superior view into the right cavernous sinus. The venous plexus contained in the middle fossa triangles open into the cavernous sinus through its inferior border and are called pericavernous venous plexus. A.: artery; CN: cranial nerve; ICA: internal carotid artery; Ophth.: ophthalmic; Pericav.: pericavernous; V.: vein, venous.

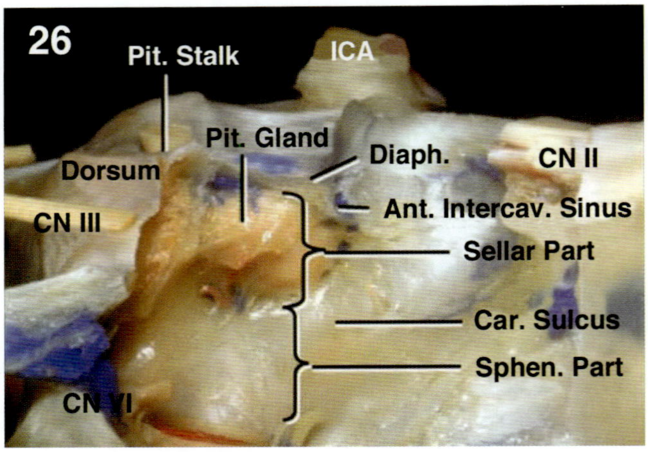

Fig. 22.26 Medial wall of the right cavernous sinus after removal of the cavernous carotid. Ant.: anterior; Car.: carotid; CN: cranial nerve; Diaph.: diaphragm; ICA: internal carotid artery; Intercav.: intercavernous; Pit.: pituitary; Sphen.: sphenoidal.

can be divided into superior and inferior parts.[7] The inferior part is related to the lateral part of the body of the sphenoid, whereas the superior part is directly related to the contents of sella (**Fig. 22.26**). Also in the dural arrangement, the medial wall seems to differ from the other cavernous sinus walls. Along the lower part, the medial wall is formed by the endosteal layer, which covers the body of the sphenoid. However, at the upper, sellar part, the medial wall is composed of the meningeal layer of the diaphragma sellae, which extends itself inferiorly and surrounds the hypophyseal capsule (**Fig. 22.27**). Knowledge of the anatomy of the medial sellar wall is important for understanding the cavernous sinus extension of pituitary tumors and transsphenoidally approaching the cavernous sinus either through an endonasal or transmaxillary route.

The roof of the cavernous sinus can be divided into anterior and posterior parts. The anterior part houses the clinoidal triangle, whereas the posterior part comprises the oculomotor triangle. The dura over the posterior roof of cavernous sinus is arranged in folds (**Fig. 22.28**). The anterior petroclinoid fold connects the petrous apex to the anterior clinoid and is the border between the roof and lateral wall. The posterior petroclinoid fold links the posterior clinoid and the

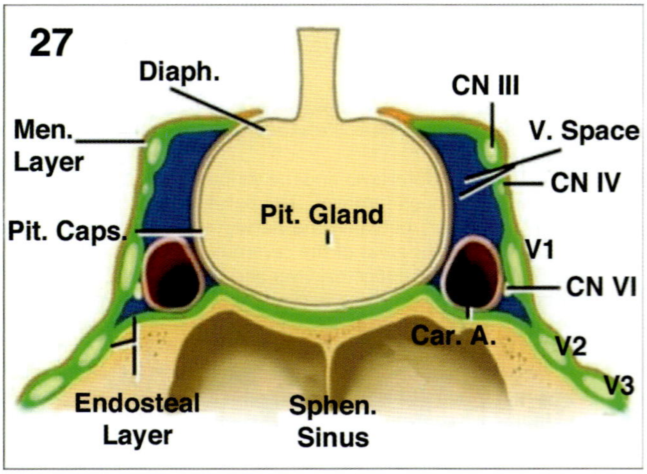

Fig. 22.27 Dural arrangement of the parasellar area. A.: artery; Caps.: capsule; Car.: carotid; CN: cranial nerve; Diaph.: diaphragm; Men.: meningeal; Pit.: pituitary; Sphen.: sphenoidal; V.: vein, venous; V1: first division; V2: second division; V3: third division of trigeminal nerve.

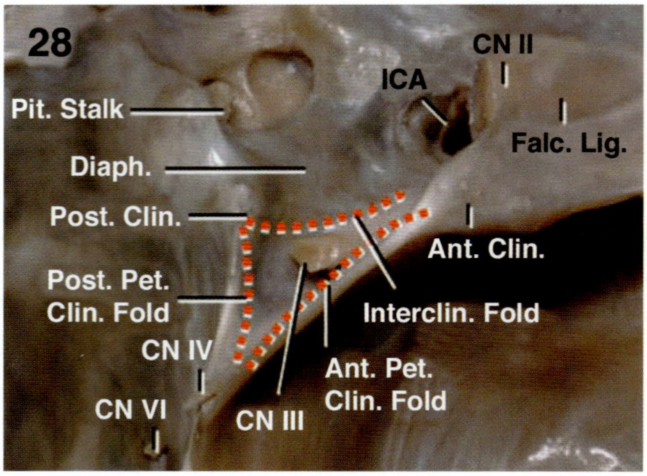

Fig. 22.28 Oblique view of the superior wall of the cavernous sinus. Ant.: anterior; Clin.: clinoid, clinoidal; CN: cranial nerve; Diaph.: diaphragm; Falc.: falciform; ICA: internal carotid artery; Interclin.: interclinoidal; Lig.: ligament; Pet.: petrous; Pit.: pituitary; Post.: posterior.

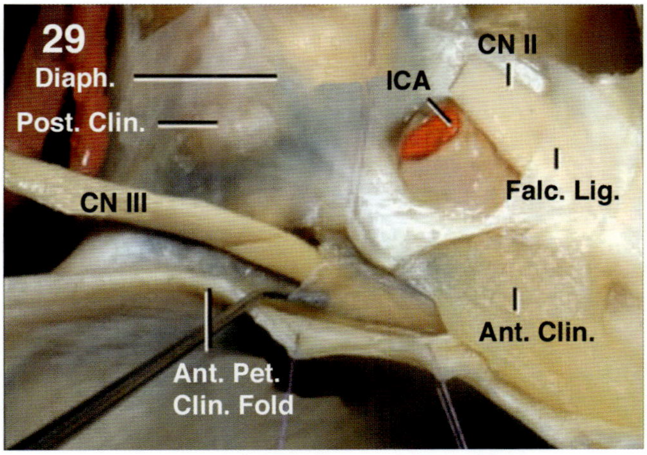

Fig. 22.29 The oculomotor triangle has been opened and the dissector inserted into the arachnoidal cuff of the oculomotor nerve, forming the walls of the oculomotor cistern. Ant.: anterior; Clin.: clinoid, clinoidal; CN: cranial nerve; Diaph.: diaphragm; Falc.: falciform; ICA: internal carotid artery; Lig.: ligament; Pet.: petro, petrous, petrosal.

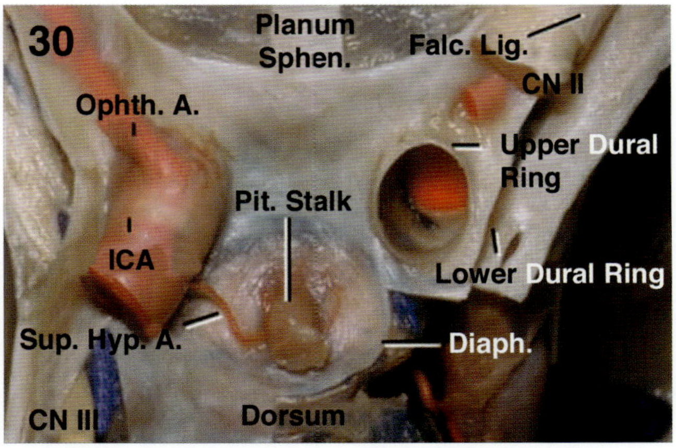

Fig. 22.30 Upper view of the parasellar area. The right carotid has been partially removed to highlight the dural arrangement of the clinoidal triangle. A.: artery; CN: cranial nerve; Diaph.: diaphragm; Falc.: falciform; Hyp.: hypophyseal; ICA: internal carotid artery; Lig.: ligament; Ophth.: ophthalmic; Pit.: pituitary; Sphen.: sphenoid; Sup.: superior.

petrous apex and is the border between the roof and the posterior wall. The interclinoid fold links the anterior and posterior clinoids. These three folds mark the borders of the oculomotor triangle, through which the oculomotor nerve and its arachnoidal cuff enter the roof to reach the lateral wall.

The arachnoidal cuff around the oculomotor nerve delimits a tiny cistern.[11] The oculomotor cistern follows the nerve from the porus up to the tip of the clinoid (**Fig. 22.29**). Although this cistern offers hydraulic protection to the nerve along the transition from its cisternal to its transdural parts, it also functions as a gate for tumoral extension into the cavernous sinus.[12] From a surgical point of view, this cistern provides a space to decompress or even mobilize this segment of the oculomotor nerve, favoring its preservation. In fact, arachnoidal cuffs and cisterns are also present along the course of other nerves passing along the cavernous sinus, and, as a set, they reinforce the meningeal wall of the sinus and might be used likewise.

On the anterior part of the sinus roof, the dura coursing over the anterior clinoid continues medially to form the falciform ligament over the optic nerve (**Figs. 22.30** and **22.31**). Below the nerve, the dura extends medially, forming the upper dural ring, over which the ophthalmic artery passes. It is just when removing the anterior clinoid that the lower dural ring, formed by the carotid oculomotor membrane, is exposed (**Fig. 22.32**). During an intracranial anterior clinoidectomy there may be minor bleeding, resulting from the opening of the diploic veins of the anterior clinoid. Usually, this kind of bleeding is easily controllable. True cavernous sinus bleeding occurs when opening the carotid oculomotor membrane. Opening the falciform ligament frees the optic nerve and provides easier access to the ophthalmic and superior hypophyseal branches of the supraclinoid carotid (**Figs. 22.33** and **22.34**). The posterior clinoidectomy is accomplished by working along the roof of the cavernous sinus, medial to

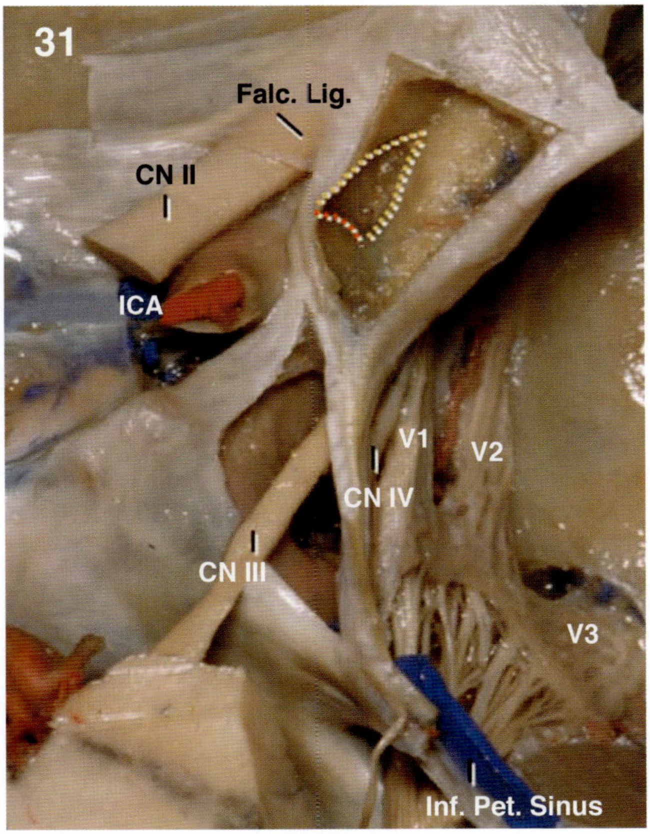

Fig. 22.31 Clinoidal and oculomotor triangles have been opened and the anterior clinoid removed up to the optic strut, exposing the carotido-oculomotor membrane. The optic strut has two neural-facing surfaces (*yellow dotted lines*) and one vascular-facing surface (*red dotted line*). CN: cranial nerve; Falc.: falciform; ICA: internal carotid artery; Inf.: inferior; Lig.: ligament; Pet.: petrosal; V1: first division; V2: second division; V3: third division of trigeminal nerve.

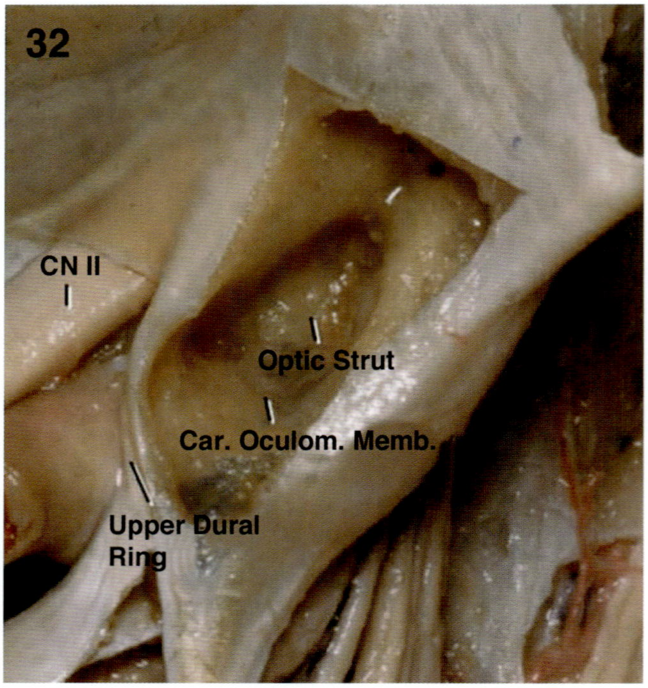

Fig. 22.32 The relationships of the optic strut are shown, as in Fig. 22.4. Car.: carotid; CN: cranial nerve; Memb.: membrane; Oculom.: oculomotor.

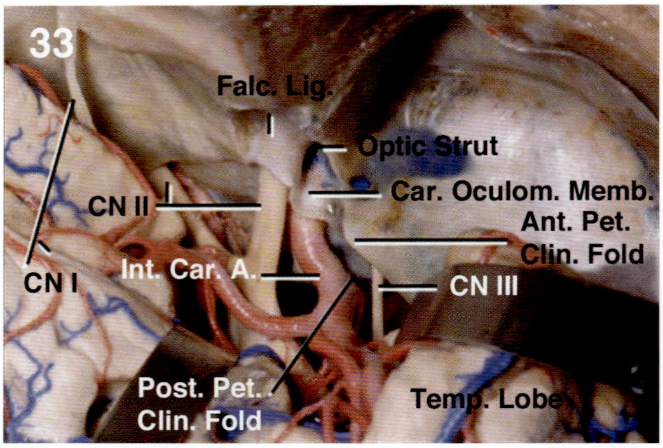

Fig. 22.33 Stepwise cadaveric dissection (*right side*), illustrating the surgical application of the anatomical concepts on the roof of cavernous (anterior and posterior parts). The dura over the anterior clinoid has been removed and the clinoid drilled as in an anterior clinoidectomy. By performing these maneuvers one is opening the upper compartment on the anterior roof of the cavernous sinus. It is possible to expose the falciform ligament over the optic nerve and the carotido-oculomotor membrane—the true cavernous sinus roof. Ant.: anterior; Car.: carotid; Clin.: clinoidal; CN: cranial nerve; Falc.: falciform; ICA: internal carotid artery; Lig.: ligament; Memb.: membrane; Oculom.: oculomotor; Pet.: petrous, petrosal; Post.: posterior; Temp.: temporal.

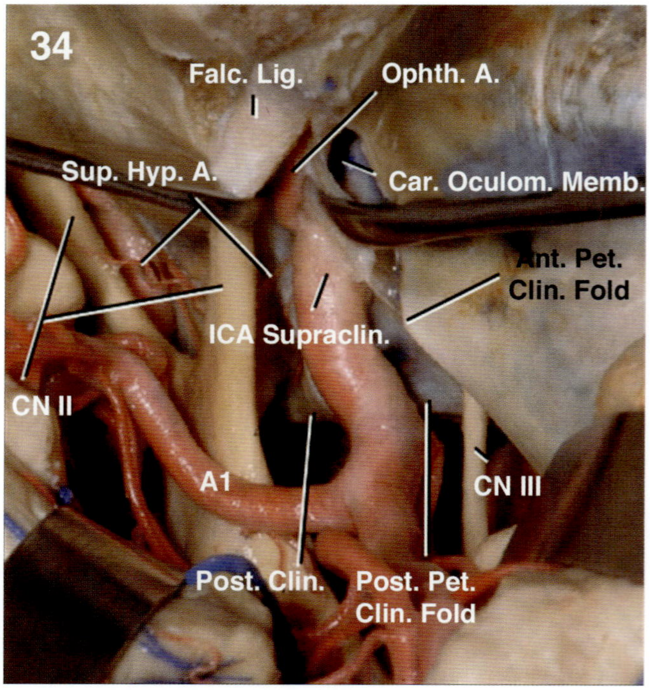

Fig. 22.34 Cutting through the lateral edge of the falciform ligament and upper dural ring, it is possible to free the optic nerve and expose the origin of the ophthalmic artery. A.: artery; A1: first segment of anterior cerebral artery; Ant.: anterior; Car.: carotid; Clin.: clinoid, clinoidal; CN: cranial nerve; Falc.: falciform; Hyp.: hypophyseal; ICA: internal carotid artery; Lig.: ligament; Memb.: membrane; Oculom.: oculomotor; Ophth.: ophthalmic; Pet.: petrosal; Post.: posterior; Sup.: superior; Supraclin.: supraclinoid.

the oculomotor nerve (**Figs. 22.35** and **22.36**). The removal of the posterior clinoid provides access to the upper part of the posterior fossa and is a fundamental part of the transcavernous approach to the basilar trunk and tip.[13]

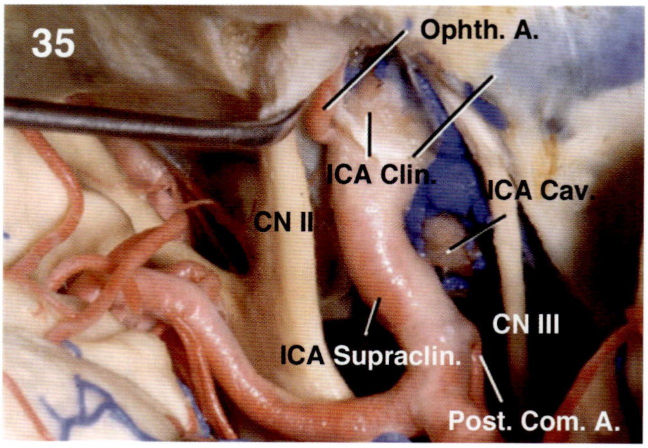

Fig. 22.35 It is only when cutting through the carotid oculomotor membrane that true cavernous sinus bleeding will be found. The posterior clinoidectomy is accomplished by working along the roof of the cavernous sinus, medial to the oculomotor nerve. A.: artery; Cav.: cavernous; Clin.: clinoid; CN: cranial nerve; Com.: communicating; ICA: internal carotid artery; Ophth.: ophthalmic; Post.: posterior; Supraclin.: supraclinoid.

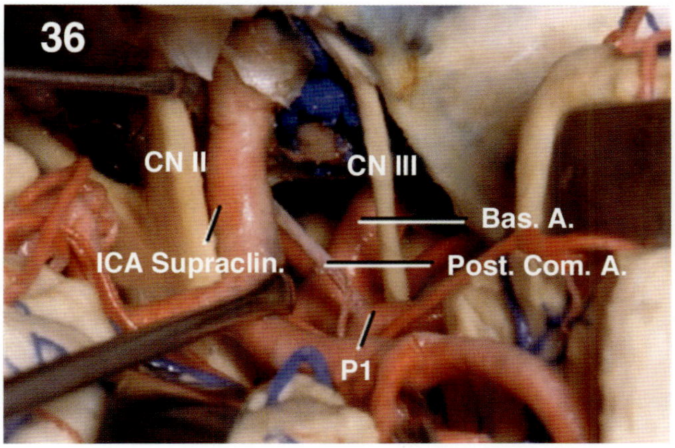

Fig. 22.36 The removal of the posterior clinoid provides access to the upper part of the posterior fossa and is a fundamental part of the transcavernous approach to the basilar trunk and tip. A.: artery; Bas.: basilar; CN: cranial nerve; Com.: Communicating; ICA: internal carotid artery; P1: first segment posterior communicating artery; Post.: Posterior; Supraclin.: supraclinoid.

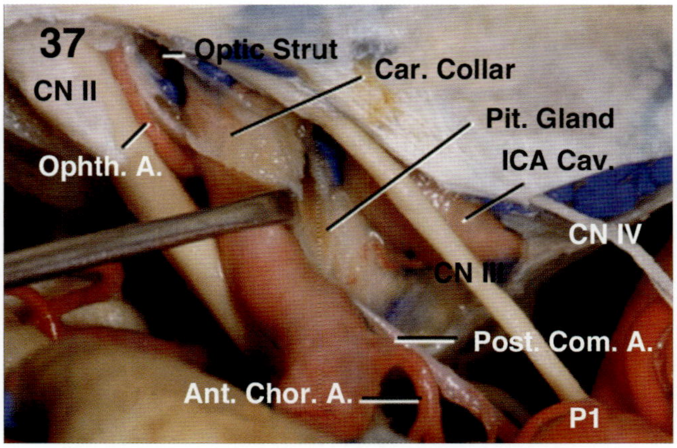

Fig. 22.37 The surgical application of the anatomical concepts of the cavernous sinus walls and triangles, including the middle fossa region triangles, can be applied to further extend this approach laterally. Cutting through the tent, exposing the infratrochlear triangle, and drilling the petrous apex through the Kawase triangle are a few examples. The transcavernous approach can also be extended medially, between the supraclinoid and horizontal portions of the cavernous carotid, through the medial wall and into the sella. A.: artery; Ant.: anterior; Car.: carotid; Cav.: cavernous; Chor.: choroidal; CN: cranial nerve; Com.: communicating; ICA: internal carotid artery; Ophth.: ophthalmic; P1: first segment posterior communicating artery; Pit.: pituitary; Post.: posterior.

The surgical application of the anatomical concepts of the cavernous sinus walls and triangles, including the triangles along the middle fossa region, can be applied to further extend this approaches laterally (**Fig. 22.36**) or to direct the approach medially, between the supraclinoid and horizontal portions of the cavernous carotid, through the medial wall and into the sella (**Fig. 22.37**).

Conclusion

A solid understanding of the osseous, dural, vascular, and neural structures and the anatomical concepts concerning the parasellar area and cavernous sinus is paramount in performing safe and successful surgery in this area.

References

1. Oliveira E, Tedeschi H, Siqueira M, Rhoton AL Jr. Microsurgical anatomy of the cavernous sinus. In: Salomon M, ed. Current Techniques in Neurosurgery, 2nd ed. New York: Churchill Livingstone, 1996:79–89
2. Harris FS, Rhoton AL Jr. Anatomy of the cavernous sinus. A microsurgical study. J Neurosurg 1976;45:169–180
3. Fujii K, Chambers SM, Rhoton AL Jr. Neurovascular relationships of the sphenoid sinus. A microsurgical study. J Neurosurg 1979;50:31–39
4. Inoue T, Rhoton AL Jr, Theele D, Barry ME. Surgical approaches to the cavernous sinus: a microsurgical study. Neurosurgery 1990;26:903–932
5. Seoane E, Rhoton AL Jr, de Oliveira EP. Microsurgical anatomy of the dural collar (carotid collar) and rings around the clinoid segment of the internal carotid artery. Neurosurgery 1998;42:869–884, discussion 884–886
6. Rhoton AL Jr. The cavernous sinus, the cavernous venous plexus, and the carotid collar. Neurosurgery 2002;51(4, Suppl):S375–S410
7. Yasuda A, Campero A, Martins C, Rhoton AL Jr, Ribas GC. The medial wall of the cavernous sinus: microsurgical anatomy. Neurosurgery 2004;55:179–189, discussion 189–190
8. Yasuda A, Campero A, Martins C, Rhoton AL Jr, de Oliveira E, Ribas GC. Microsurgical anatomy and approaches to the cavernous sinus. Neurosurgery 2005;56(1, Suppl):4–27, discussion 4–27
9. Johnston JA, Parkinson D. Intracranial sympathetic pathways associated with the sixth cranial nerve. J Neurosurg 1974;40:236–243
10. Martins C, Yasuda A, Campero A, Ulm AJ, Tanriover N, Rhoton AL Jr. Microsurgical anatomy of the dural arteries. Neurosurgery 2005;56 (2, Suppl):211–251, discussion 211–251
11. Martins C, Yasuda A, Campero A, Rhoton AL Jr. Microsurgical anatomy of the oculomotor cistern. Neurosurgery 2006;58(4, Suppl 2):ONS-220–ONS-227, discussion ONS-227–ONS-228
12. Dolenc VV. Cavernous sinus tumors. In: Yasargil MG, Dolenc VV, eds. Anatomy and Surgery of the Cavernous Sinus. Vienna: Springer Verlag; 1989:269–338
13. Seoane E, Tedeschi H, de Oliveira EP, Wen HT, Rhoton AL Jr. The pretemporal transcavernous approach to the interpeduncular and prepontine cisterns: microsurgical anatomy and technique application. Neurosurgery 2000;46:891–898, discussion 898–899

23 Surgical Indications for Pituitary Tumors

Marcello D. Bronstein

Tips and Pearls

Surgery for pituitary tumors is indicated:

- as first-line therapy for nonfunctioning pituitary adenomas (NFPA).
- as first-line therapy for Cushing's disease (both for micro. and macroadenomas).
- as first-line therapy for acromegaly: for microadenomas, enclosed macroadenomas, and macroadenomas with visual disturbances. Medical therapy is indicated as first-line treatment for invasive tumors. Additionally, debulking surgery, even noncurative, may improve the response to somatostatin analogues in primary resistant cases to these drugs.
- in special situations for prolactinomas, as medical therapy is the first option for this kind of pituitary tumor.

Introduction

Pituitary tumors are frequently occurring neoplasms, accounting for 10 to 15% of all intracranial neoplasias in surgical material and being found in up to 27% of nonselected autopsies.[1] They present with a broad spectrum of biologic presentation. Although almost invariably benign (adenomas), up to 20% of pituitary tumors exhibit invasive behavior. The exceedingly rare pituitary carcinomas do not diverge from adenomas by histologic features; distant metastasis is the sole diagnostic criterion.[2]

Pituitary tumors ate classified according to their morphologic and functional characteristics (**Table 23.1**). Such neoplasms are named secreting or "functioning" when they produce hormones in sufficient amounts to lead to clinical manifestations, including, from higher to lower prevalence, lactotrophic tumors (prolactinomas), somatotropinomas (acromegaly, gigantism), corticotropinomas (Cushing´s disease), and, rarely, tumors secreting the glucoproteic hormones thyroid-stimulating hormone (TSH) (thyrotropinomas: secondary hyperthyroidism), luteinizing hormone (LH), and follicle-stimulating hormone (FSH) (gonadotropinomas). Pituitary adenomas can also secrete two or more hormones, growth hormone (GH) and prolactin (PRL) co-secretion being the more prevalent of them. Pituitary neoplasms that do not produce circulating measurable amounts of intact hormones are called nonsecreting or nonfunctioning (NF) tumors.[3]

Table 23.1 Pituitary Adenomas Classification

Based on Morphology	Based on Function
Microadenomas	Secreting
Enclosed	Prolactin (PRL): prolactinomas
Invasive	Growth hormone (GH): acromegaly/ gigantism
Macroadenomas	Adrenocorticotropic hormone (ACTH): Cushing's disease
Enclosed	Follicle-stimulating hormone/luteinizing hormone (FSH/LH): gonadotrophic tumors
Invasive	Thyroid-stimulating hormone (TSH): central hyperthyroidism
Expanding	Mixed (mainly GH/PRL)
	Nonsecreting (clinically nonfunctioning)

Regarding their morphology, pituitary tumors are classified as microadenomas (less than 10 mm in diameter, generally enclosed, less frequently invasive) and macroadenomas (enclosed to sellar boundaries, expansive, or invasive (**Table 23.1**).[4] Microadenomas usually are diagnosed by the clinical picture or as a consequence of their hormonal hypersecretion or, when NF, by incidental findings from imaging performed for another indication, such as head trauma, or by autopsy finding. Macroadenomas are diagnosed by hormonal hypersecretion as well as hyposecretion, when present, or by neuro-ophthalmologic and neurologic manifestations. They can also be incidentally found.[1] Although there are no histologic differences, invasive tumors grow faster, leading to sellar erosion and infiltration of neighboring structures, such as the dura mater, bone, and sphenoid and cavernous sinuses. The morphology of pituitary tumors is assessed by imaging, and confirmed by surgery and pathology. Sometimes it is difficult to assess the degree of tumor invasiveness, as pituitary adenomas do not present a true capsule, just a "pseudocapsule" formed by pituitary cells and the reticulin network. Therefore, although invasiveness is more associated with macroadenomas, it can also be present in microadenomas.

The results of a surgical approach to pituitary adenomas depend not only on the surgeon's skill, but also on the tumor's features. A microadenoma or an enclosed macroadenoma has a much higher probability of cure than does a giant invasive tumor. Moreover, efficacious medical therapies, both for hormonal and tumor volume control, become the first-line treatment for pituitary tumors, especially prolactinomas and somatotropinomas, and mainly for those tumors that are not candidates for surgery. Nevertheless, surgical treatment, mainly by a microsurgical or endoscopic transsphenoidal approach, persists as a mainstream treatment for pituitary tumors. Its indications for each type of tumor are described in the following sections.

Secreting Pituitary Tumors

Prolactinomas

Prolactin-secreting adenomas are the most prevalent pituitary tumors.[5] An analysis of 50 surgical series by Gillam et al[6] encompassing 2137 microprolactinomas and 2226 macroprolactinomas found overall remission rates of 74.7% and 33.9%, respectively. Moreover, recurrence was observed in 18.2% of microadenomas and 22.8% of macroadenomas. Therefore, the overall surgical control for macroadenomas is far from ideal. On the other hand, prolactinomas respond very well to dopamine agonist (DA) drugs, such as bromocriptine and, especially, cabergoline; both PRL normalization and tumor shrinkage are observed in up to 80% of cases, including invasive ones, that are not candidates for surgery.[5] Additionally, a significant number of patients persist with normal serum PRL levels after DA drug withdrawal.[7] Nevertheless, medical treatment with DA also has disadvantages, mainly intolerance and resistance. Therefore, prolactinomas have the following surgical indications:

1. Failure of medical therapy (intolerance/resistance): 20% of cases
2. Patient´s personal choice (microprolactinomas)
3. Tumor enlargement on medical therapy: rare
4. Unstable pituitary apoplexy: 10% of cases
5. Cerebrospinal fluid (CSF) leakage during dopamine agonist therapy[8]: rare
6. Optic chiasm herniation on dopamine agonist therapy: rare
7. Previous pregnancy complicated by tumor expansion[9]
8. Symptomatic tumor enlargement during pregnancy that does not respond to reinstitution of dopamine agonist treatment[9]

Acromegaly

This disabling and rare disease, with a prevalence of 38 to 69 cases/million inhabitants, is almost invariably caused by a GH-secreting pituitary adenoma. About 10% of cases occur before adulthood, leading to gigantism. The life expectancy of acromegalic patients is reduced by about 10 years, and mortality, mainly due to cardiovascular complications, is three times higher than in the general population. Therefore, an aggressive approach to normalize GH/insulin-like growth factor 1 (IGF-1) is needed. Fortunately, many treatment modalities are currently availably for acromegaly (**Table 23.2**).[10]

Table 23.2 Treatment Modalities for Acromegaly

- Pituitary surgery
- Medical therapy
  - Somatostatin analogs
  - Dopamine agonists
  - GH-receptor antagonist
- Radiotherapy

Surgery, mainly by the transsphenoidal route, remains the first-line treatment for acromegaly. The main advantages are prompt results, the possibility of a definitive cure, resolution of the mass effects, and tumor debulking, which may improve further medical therapy. However, there are also disadvantages, such as the lack of availability of skilled surgeons, poor results in large/invasive tumors, the risk of complications (hypopituitarism, diabetes insipidus, CSF leakage), the 10% recurrence rate, and the comorbidities-dependent anesthesia and surgery risks. An analysis of four important surgical series encompassing all kinds of GH-secreting adenomas found, as expected, better results in microadenomas and enclosed macroadenomas, and overall surgical control in 57% of cases (**Table 23.3**). Therefore, acromegalic patients harboring large/invasive tumors may be primarily medically treated, mainly with the somatostatin analogues octreotide LAR and lanreotide autogel,[11] which are able to control GH/IGF-1 secretion in approximately 60% of cases but also lead to tumor shrinkage in up to 80% of patients. Furthermore, debulking surgery may improve the response to somatostatin analogues in resistant cases.[12] Also DA and the GH receptor antagonist pegvisomant have a place in the acromegaly treatment algorithm. Radiotherapy, in addition to the long latency period required to achieve disease control, presents a high incidence of complications (hypopituitarism, radionecrosis, secondary tumors, cerebrovascular disease, cognitive disturbances) and is currently reserved for only invasive/resistant cases.[13]

Cushing's Disease

Adrenocorticotropic hormone (ACTH)-secreting microadenomas are the main cause of Cushing's syndrome. Similarly to acromegaly, Cushing´s disease is associated with many comorbidities and increase mortality rate. Therefore, early and efficient therapy is highly desired.[14] Transsphenoidal pituitary surgery is the first-line treatment. According to the main published microsurgical series, it leads to disease control in 60 to 80% of cases (<15% for macroadenomas), with a

Table 23.3 Acromegaly: Surgical Results

Authors	Remission Criteria (in ng/mL)	Number of Patients	Microadenomas	Macroadenomas
Laws et al, 2000[18]	GH <2.5 GHGTT <1.0 Normal IGF-1	86	88%	65%
Freda et al, 1998[19]	GH <2.5 GHGTT <2.0 Normal IGF-1	115	88%	67% (noninvasive) 42% (invasive)
Shimon, et al, 2001[20]	GHGTT ≤2.0 Normal IGF-1	98	84%	64% (total) 20% (>20 mm)
Nomikos et al, 2005[21]	GH < 2.5 GHGTT <1.0 Normal IGF-1	688	85% (ni) 74% (i)	71% (ni) 8.3% (nigi) 19.3% (i) 0% (ig)

GH, growth hormone; GHGTT, growth hormone glucose tolerance test; I, invasive; IG, invasive giant; IGF-1, insulin-like growth factor 1; NI, noninvasive; NIGI, noninvasive giant.

recurrence rate of up to 20%.[14] The transsphenoidal endoscopic approach presents results comparable to the best microscopical approaches. The recurrence rates are apparently lower, but longer follow-up is needed to confirm this finding.[15] In addition, the endoscopic approach may be a good option for reoperation of patients with recurrent or persistent Cushing's disease.[16]

In cases of surgical failure, other therapies are available:

- Drug therapy: directed to the pituitary or the adrenals. Many drugs are available, but the success rate is relatively low, with a high incidence of side effects.[14]
- Radiotherapy: both conventional and stereotactic. With better results in children, radiotherapy presents the same problems described earlier for acromegaly.
- Bilateral adrenalectomy: although almost always curative, it requires lifelong glucocorticoid and mineralocorticoid replacement, and may lead to Nelson syndrome in a significant number of patients.

Clinically Nonsecreting (Nonfunctioning) Pituitary Adenomas (NFPA)

In these tumors, no hormone is secreted in excess, so the clinical features are related to the macroadenoma mass effect, and mainly include visual disturbances, headache, and hypopituitarism. Both micro- and macroadenomas can also be incidentally diagnosed. Therapy is indicated to relieve the tumor compression, when present, or to prevent future mass effects or the chance of pituitary apoplexy.[17] The surgical approach is the most effective treatment for NFPA. Radiotherapy is indicated to prevent tumor regrowth when tumor remnants are significant, but poses the problems already described. Drug therapy for NFPA is an emerging field, but still presenting poor overall results.[17]

References

1. Parent AD, Brown B, Smith EE. Incidental pituitary adenomas: a retrospective study. Surgery 1982;92:880–883
2. Kaltsas GA, Nomikos P, Kontogeorgos G, Buchfelder M, Grossman AB. Clinical review: diagnosis and management of pituitary carcinomas. J Clin Endocrinol Metab 2005;90:3089–3099
3. Osamura RY, Kajiya H, Takei M, et al. Pathology of the human pituitary adenomas. Histochem Cell Biol 2008;130:495–507
4. Hardy J. Transsphenoidal surgery of hypersecreting pituitary tumors. In: Kolhler G, Ross GT, eds. Diagnosis and Treatment of Pituitary Tumors. New York: Elsevier; 1973:179–194
5. Bronstein MD. Disorders of prolactin secretion and prolactinomas. In: DeGroot LJ, Jameson JL, eds. Endocrinology. Philadelphia: Elsevier/Saunders, 2006:485–510
6. Gillam MP, Molitch ME, Lombardi G, Colao A. Advances in the treatment of prolactinomas. Endocr Rev 2006;27:485–534
7. Bronstein MD. Potential for long-term remission of microprolactinoma after withdrawal of dopamine-agonist therapy. Nat Clin Pract Endocrinol Metab 2006;2:130–131
8. Bronstein MD, Musolino NR, Benabou S, Marino R Jr. Cerebrospinal fluid rhinorrhea occurring in long-term bromocriptine treatment for macroprolactinomas. Surg Neurol 1989;32:346–349
9. Bronstein MD. Prolactinomas and pregnancy. Pituitary 2005;8:31–38
10. Ben-Shlomo A, Melmed S. Acromegaly. Endocrinol Metab Clin North Am 2008;37:101–122, viii
11. Murray RD, Melmed S. A critical analysis of clinically available somatostatin analog formulations for therapy of acromegaly. J Clin Endocrinol Metab 2008;93:2957–2968
12. Jallad RS, Musolino NR, Kodaira S, Cescato VA, Bronstein MD. Does partial surgical tumour removal influence the response to octreotide-LAR in acromegalic patients previously resistant to the somatostatin analogue? Clin Endocrinol (Oxf) 2007;67:310–315
13. Jallad RS, Musolino NR, Salgado LR, Bronstein MD. Treatment of acromegaly: is there still a place for radiotherapy? Pituitary 2007;10:53–59
14. Pivonello R, De Martino MC, De Leo M, Lombardi G, Colao A. Cushing's Syndrome. Endocrinol Metab Clin North Am 2008;37:135–149, ix
15. Netea-Maier RT, van Lindert EJ, den Heijer M, et al. Transsphenoidal pituitary surgery via the endoscopic technique: results in 35 consecutive patients with Cushing's disease. Eur J Endocrinol 2006;154: 675–684

16. Wagenmakers MA, Netea-Maier RT, van Lindert EJ, Timmers HJ, Grotenhuis JA, Hermus AR. Repeated transsphenoidal pituitary surgery (TS) via the endoscopic technique: a good therapeutic option for recurrent or persistent Cushing's disease (CD). Clin Endocrinol (Oxf) 2009; 70:274–280

17. Dekkers OM, Pereira AM, Romijn JA. Treatment and follow-up of clinically nonfunctioning pituitary macroadenomas. J Clin Endocrinol Metab 2008;93:3717–3726

18. Laws ER, Vance ML, Thapar K. Pituitary surgery for the management of acromegaly. Horm Res. 2000;53 Suppl 3:71–75

19. Freda PU, Wardlaw SL, Post KD. Long-term endocrinological follow-up evaluation in 115 patients who underwent transsphenoidal surgery for acromegaly. Neurosurg. 1998; 89:353–358

20. Shimon I, Cohen ZR, Ram Z, Hadani M. Transsphenoidal surgery for acromegaly: endocrinological follow-up of 98 patients. Neurosurgery. 2001 Jun;48:1239–1243

21. Nomikos P, Buchfelder M, Fahlbusch R. The outcome of surgery in 668 patients with acromegaly using current criteria of biochemical "cure." Eur J Endocrinol. 2005;152:379–387

24 Do's and Don'ts in Pituitary Surgery

Dharambir S. Sethi and Beng Ti Ang

Tips and Pearls

- The endoscopic transnasal approach for pituitary tumors is a multidisciplinary team approach and should be done by neurosurgeons in conjunction with otolaryngologists.
- A careful preoperative endocrinologic and radiologic evaluation is paramount for assessing the surgical indications and for the success of the surgical procedure.
- Instrumentation plays an important role in performing safe and successful endoscopic sellar surgery.
- We currently use the transnasal modified approach with the removal of the most posterior aspect of the nasal septum.
- After nasal decongestion, the surgery itself is started on the side on which the sphenoid ostium is better visualized.
- The sphenoid ostium is widened inferiorly and medially down to the floor of the sphenoid sinus. Care is taken to avoid the septal branch of the sphenopalatine artery by not going too far inferolaterally.
- By direct visualization and tactile feedback, the thinnest part of the sellar floor is identified and gently fractured at the point of least resistance.
- The boundaries for the removal of the sellar floor are the planum sphenoidale superiorly, the clivus inferiorly, and the carotid prominence laterally.
- Care must be taken when removing the sellar floor over the intercavernous sinus to avoid tearing this vein, which can bleed profusely. In the event that this occurs, the intercavernous sinus may be cauterized with bipolar diathermy.
- Start to remove the tumor from the sellar floor, then work on the lateral extent next, and finally remove the suprasellar component if any. The diaphragma may descend rapidly in this region, giving the impression that the tumor has been completely removed, when in fact pockets of semisolid tumor or pockets where the tumor was adherent to the diaphragma may be left behind.

Introduction

Pituitary surgery has been traditionally performed by neurosurgeons using a sublabial, transseptal, transsphenoidal approach and the operating microscope.[1] The microscope provides excellent magnification, binocular vision, and a good depth of field essential for tumor removal. Transsphenoidal surgery has proven to be a safe and effective first-line therapy for most patients with sellar and suprasellar lesions. It is considered the "gold standard" and is effectively used by many pituitary surgeons around the world. More recently, since the description of endonasal resection of pituitary adenomas in three patients by Jankowski (an otolaryngologist) et al,[2] there has been a surge of interest in endonasal pituitary surgery. In the past decade, endonasal surgery for pituitary tumors has gained acceptance worldwide.[3–6]

Working as a combined rhinology-neurosurgery team, we performed our first endoscopic pituitary surgery in October 1994. This has been a longstanding partnership; close to 500 pituitary tumors have been operated upon using direct endonasal techniques.

Our initial approach was transseptal.[7] Though the results were encouraging, the transseptal approach had its limitations. One of the main limitations was having to work through a narrow tunnel created by elevating bilateral mucoperichondrial flaps on the nasal septum. Whereas the visualization was not compromised, instrumentation was often difficult, particularly when the situation required two surgeons to be working together while removing the tumor.

To overcome these limitations, we modified our approach to a direct endonasal transsphenoidal approach, avoiding a septoplasty and its inherent complications. This approach enables two surgeons to work through a common transnasal corridor using both hands and at times having four instruments in the operative field.[8,9]

This chapter provides some useful clinical pearls and pointers for practitioners venturing into endonasal pituitary surgery.[10-15]

Working As a Multidisciplinary Team

Since the introduction of endoscopic sinus surgery almost 25 years ago, otolaryngologists have become trained and experienced in endonasal sinus surgery and endonasal approaches to the sphenoid sinus. This accumulated experience of endoscopic-trained otolaryngologists may be utilized by neurosurgeons in providing endonasal access to the sphenoid sinus and the floor of the sella. The otolaryngologist's main roles during surgery are to provide relatively bloodless and unimpeded access to the sphenoid sinus through a wide midline sphenoidotomy, and to assist the neurosurgeon in tumor removal.

Although it is possible for a single surgeon to perform this surgery, a team approach is preferred. Once the initial approach is complete, both the neurosurgeon and the otolaryngologist can work together for the remainder of the procedure. In some situations it is important for the two of them to work together, with the otolarynologist holding the endoscope and providing manual manipulation of the endoscope to optimize the visualization, particularly near the end of the procedure when the angled scopes are used and the field of view is constantly changing.

Indications for Surgery

Endoscopic transnasal-transsphenoidal surgery for pituitary tumors is indicated in both endocrine active and nonfunctioning pituitary adenomas. Indications for surgery include all nonsecreting and most secreting pituitary tumors except for prolactinomas, which are usually well controlled by medical therapy with dopamine antagonist.[16]

Pre- and Perioperative Evaluation

All patients scheduled for pituitary surgery must undergo radiologic evaluation, endocrine assessment, and visual field tests pre- and postoperatively. A preoperative nasal endoscopic examination by the otolaryngologist should also be a part of the routine preoperative assessment. We have, in our institution, developed a "pituitary surgery pathway" for patients undergoing this operation. This is to ensure strict perioperative management compliance by all specialists.

Imaging Studies

Although both computed tomography (CT) and magnetic resonance imaging (MRI) have been used for imaging of the pituitary gland, MRI has become the preferred modality. MRI scanning of the pituitary region involving fine cuts and sagittal and coronal reconstruction is the gold standard imaging method for pituitary disease.[17] Radiologic evaluation should also include CT scans of the nose, paranasal sinuses, and sella turcica. CT scans are useful in studying the bony anatomy; moreover, calcified lesions such as craniopharyngiomas may be more easily identified with CT. CT scans are also a useful alternative to the MRI in patients who are claustrophobic and unable to tolerate an MRI study. The extent of sphenoid pneumatization, sphenoid dominance, internal sinus septa, and their termination on the optic nerve or the internal carotid artery are important anatomical considerations in planning transsphenoidal approach.

Although a conventional MRI scan of the pituitary fossa provides information about the location, size, and boundaries of the lesion and its relationship to adjoining structures, the prediction of the consistency of macroadenomas is controversial.[18–20] Prediction of the consistency of pituitary tumors on diffusion-weighted (DW) MRI has recently been reported.[21]

Visual Field Testing

Progressive deterioration of visual fields is often the principal neurologic criterion on which surgical management decisions are based. Humphrey and Goldmann visual field evaluations are useful even if there appears to be no contact between the optic pathway and the pituitary mass, because field defects may reflect previous impingement, potential vascular shunting, or displacement of the chiasm following decompression.

Endocrine Evaluation

The perioperative endocrine management of a patient undergoing pituitary surgery may vary depending on the size of the pituitary lesion, the type of the lesion, the surgical approach (transsphenoidal, craniotomy), and the preoperative endocrine function.

Otolaryngology Assessment

A preoperative nasal endoscopic examination to exclude any active rhinosinusitis is undertaken by the otolaryngologist. Preoperative nasal endoscopy also provides useful information about the nasal anatomy, such as turbinate hypertrophy, concha bullosa, or a gross septal deviation that may necessitate a septoplasty for access to the sphenoid sinus. Preoperative treatment of nasal and paranasal sinus infections until there is complete return to normal is essential. Perioperative prophylactic antibiotics are routinely used.

Having the Right Setup

One of the most important prerequisites for endonasal pituitary surgery is having a good videocamera system, sinus surgery and neurosurgical instruments, a dedicated neuroanesthesiologist, and assisting nursing staff members who have been specially trained for this type of surgery. Intraoperative neuronavigation and intraoperative MRI (iMRI) are not an absolute necessity but are employed in various institutions as adjuncts to maximize resection and also in expanded endonasal approaches.

Operative Setup

The Digital Endoscopic Video Camera System (Karl Storz Endoscopy, Flanders, NJ) is placed at the cephalic end of the table to enable both surgeons to view the surgery on the video monitor. The neuroanesthetist is at the caudal end of the table. The scrub nurse and the instrument trolley are at the left cephalic end. Imaging studies are displayed for intraoperative reference. The otolaryngologist stands on the right side of the operating table and the neurosurgeon on the left side.

The digital video camera is attached to the eyepiece of the telescope, and the entire procedure is monitored on a 19-inch thin-film transfer (TFT) flat-screen monitor. Video documentation of the surgical procedure is routinely done on a digital video recorder. A powered sinus dissection device is used for the sphenoidotomy. We use the microdebrider developed by Medtronic (Jacksonville, FL). A 4-mm bit with a serrated outer shaft is used for mucosal dissection.

■ Surgical Technique

Patient Positioning and Preparation

The nasal cavity is decongested by placing two neuropatties soaked in 4% cocaine, in each side approximately 20 minutes prior to induction. The patient is placed under general anesthesia and administered antibiotics, glucocorticoids, and antihistamines. We routinely use cephazolin (2 g, intravenous), dexamethasone (10 mg, intravenous), and diphenylhydramine (50 mg, intravenous). Oral endotracheal intubation is used and a pharyngeal pack is placed in the pharynx. A Foley urinary catheter is routinely inserted to monitor urinary output intraoperatively and postoperatively. The patient's head is placed on a horseshoe pad slightly extended, and turned slightly to the right. The head is elevated by approximately 30 degrees above the heart to facilitate venous drainage. Antiseptic solution (such as Povidine) is applied to the nose and mouth, and the area draped with sterile towels and a Steri-Drape. The lower abdomen is prepared and draped to obtain adipose tissue if necessary.

Nasal Preparation

The neuropatties that had been placed in the nasal cavity earlier are removed and discarded. The nasal cavity is once again decongested with topical application of cocaine. Sterile neuropatties soaked in 4% cocaine are endoscopically placed in the sphenoethmoid recess bilaterally. Allowing approximately 10 minutes for decongestion, the neuropatties are removed and the sphenoethmoid recess is infiltrated bilaterally, with 1% lidocaine with 1:80,000 epinephrine. A 21-gauge spinal needle is used for infiltration of the anterior wall of the sphenoid, sphenopalatine foramen, and the posterior part of the nasal septum.

Nasal Endoscopy and Identification of Sphenoid Ostia

After the nose has been adequately decongested an endoscopic examination is performed using a 0- or 30-degree endoscope (Karl Storz Endoscopy). The sphenoid ostia are identified bilaterally. The ostium lies just above the sphenoethmoid recess, approximately 1.5 cm above the choana. The shape and size of the sphenoid ostia may vary, but its location is almost constant. In some circumstances, the ostium is covered by a supreme turbinate, which can be gently retracted laterally or resected if necessary. Rarely, in the situation where the sphenoid ostium cannot be identified, entry into the sphenoid sinus can be gained using a blunt instrument or suction tip to exert controlled pressure to the anterior wall at the point of least resistance.

Midline Sphenoidotomy

Surgery is started on the side on which the sphenoid ostium is better visualized. Most of the time, we start on the right side. The microdebrider (with a 4-mm bit with a serrated outer shaft) is used to debride the mucosa in the sphenoethmoid recess around the sphenoid ostium, taking care not to traumatize the mucosa on the superior turbinates. The serrated blade of the microdebrider is directed medially and the outer sheath laterally, protecting the mucosa of the superior turbinate. The sphenoid ostium is widened inferiorly and medially down to the floor of the sphenoid sinus. Care is taken to avoid the septal branch of the sphenopalatine artery by not going too inferolaterally. Brisk bleeding may result if the septal branch of the sphenopalatine artery is encountered. This may be controlled by cauterizing the vessel with bipolar diathermy. In the rare situation where bleeding cannot be controlled, it may be necessary to expose and ligate the sphenopalatine artery at the sphenopalatine foramen, which is located in the superior meatus just posterior to the middle turbinate. Most endoscopic sinus surgeons are familiar with the technique.

If the bone of the sphenoid rostrum is thick, a 2-mm up- or down-biting Kerrison's rongeurs may be used to extend the sphenoidomy. Sometimes firm but controlled tapping of a hammer against the osteotome or a drill may be necessary to remove the sphenoid rostrum.

Mucosa is debrided from the posterior part of the vomer and the sphenoid rostrum. The sphenoidotomy is extended to the contralateral side by dislocating the attachment of the vomer from the sphenoid rostrum. The sphenoid ostium on the contralateral side is identified, and the sphenoidotomy extended as far as the contralateral superior turbinate by removing the sphenoid rostrum. The sphenoid rostrum is removed with a strong septal forceps. A wide sphenoidotomy that extends superiorly to the roof of the sphenoid, inferiorly to the floor of the sphenoid sinus, and laterally to the superior turbinate on either side is fashioned.

Removal of the Posterior Nasal Septum

About 1 cm of the posterior part of the vomer is removed with a reverse-cutting forceps to facilitate the introduction of instruments from both nostrils. This step permits a panoramic view of the sphenoid sinus and enables the two surgeons to use both hands to introduce up to four separate instruments, two through each nostril. The access to the sphenoid sinus is complete. For a very wide access, necessary in some patients with large tumors requiring an extended approach, the entire posterior bony nasal septum may be removed to facilitate instrumentation.

From this point onward, the neurosurgeon and the otolaryngologist work as a team. The otolaryngologist manually manipulates the endoscope and assists the neurosurgeon in removal of tumor.

Identifying the Sphenoid Sinus Landmarks

The sphenoid sinus is next examined with 0-, 30-, and 70-degree, 4-mm endoscopes, and important anatomical landmarks within noted (**Fig. 24.1**). Of particular importance are the structures on the lateral wall. The carotid prominence, optic prominence, and opticocarotid recess can be well identified when the sphenoid sinus is well pneumatized. On the lateral recess of a well-pneumatized sphenoid sinus, the second branch of the trigeminal nerve (V2) and the vidian canal may be identified superolaterally and inferomedially, respectively.

On the posterior wall, the tuberculum sella, the anterior wall of the sella, and the clivus are identified. The location of the intersinus septa, if any, is noted. If these septa have to be removed, extreme caution is exercised, as they often

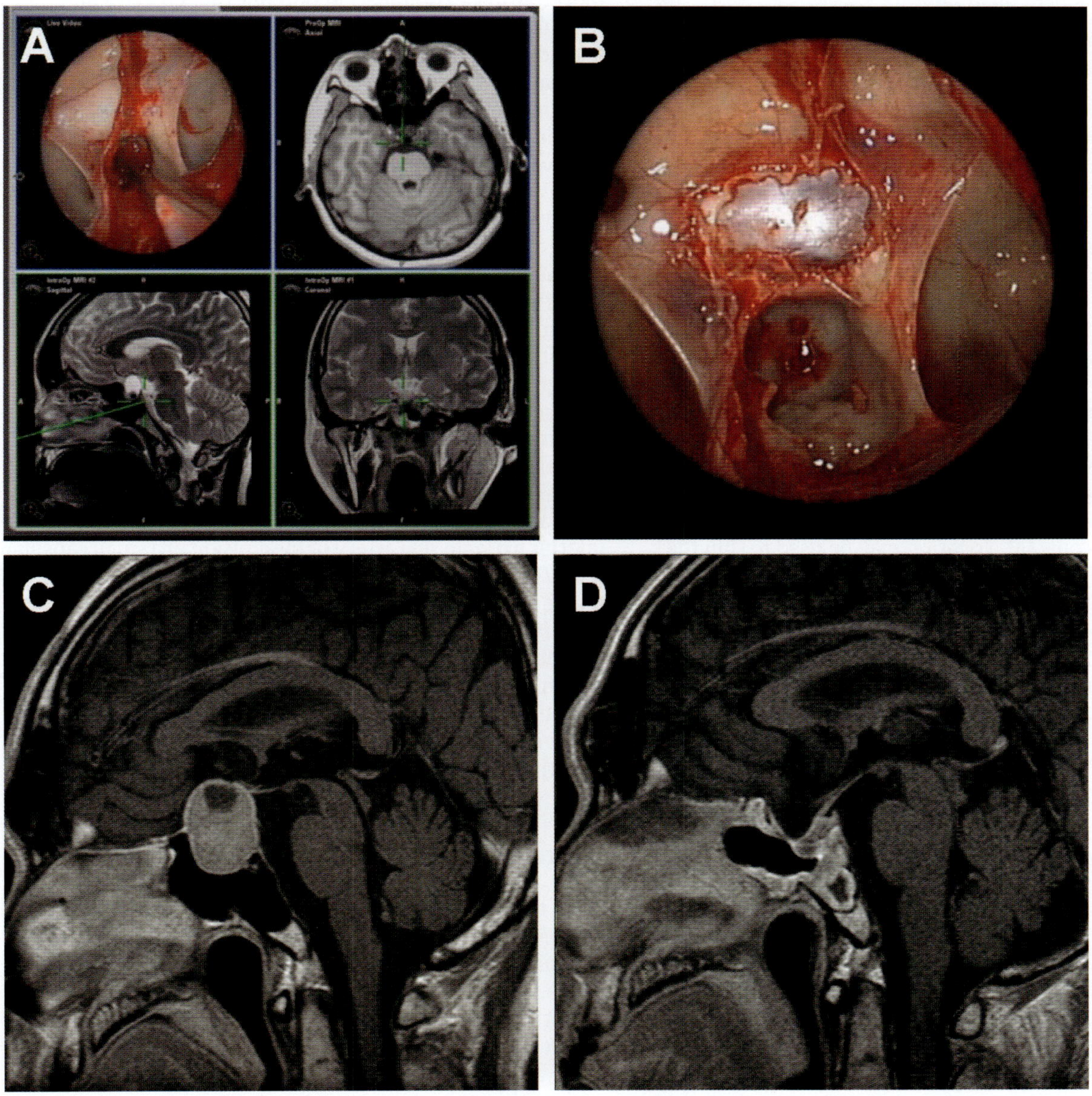

Fig. 24.1 **(A)** Endoscopic image showing the interior of the sphenoid sinus with a perspective of the bony sellar floor bulging into the sphenoid sinus and the presence of intersinus septa. Adjunctive neuronavigation is also demonstrated where the position of the tip of the probe is displayed in sagittal, coronal, and axial T2-weighted magnetic resonance images. **(B)** The bony sellar floor has been resected, and the sellar dura is exposed. The planum sphenoidale and optic nerve prominences can be visualized superior to the sellar, and the intersinus septa can be seen inserting onto the carotid prominences on either side of the clival recess. **(C,D)** Pre- and postoperative T1-weighted magnetic resonance images, respectively, detailing the extent of resection.

terminate on the carotid canal or the optic canal. It is safer to use Tru-Cut instruments to remove these septa. Injudicious avulsion of the septa with non–Tru-Cut instruments may cause fracture of the thin bone overlying the cavernous sinus or the optic nerve with resultant hematoma, intractable bleeding, or even blindness. Caution is also exercised in not stripping the sphenoid mucosa, as this may result in considerable bleeding.

Once a panoramic view of the entire sphenoid sinus and the surgical landmarks is obtained, the access to the sella turcica is complete.

The major landmarks for proper identification of the sellar floor are the planum sphenoidale above, the clivus below, and the carotid prominences bilaterally.

Fenestration of the Sellar Floor

Once the sellar floor has been identified, the mucosa over the sellar floor is cauterized with bipolar diathermy to expose the underlying bone. The extent of removal of the sellar floor varies depending on the size and location of the pathology. The thickness of the sellar floor may be assessed by gentle palpation with an instrument such as a ball probe. By direct visualization and tactile feedback, the thinnest part of the sellar floor is identified and gently fractured at the point of least resistance. A plane is developed between the dura and sellar floor with a right-angle hook. A 1-mm Kerrison punch or a curette may be used to delicately remove the sellar floor, exposing the dura. The boundaries of removal of the sellar floor are the planum sphenoidale superiorly, the clivus inferiorly, and the carotid prominence laterally.

If the anterior wall of the sella is thick, a high-speed diamond drill under constant irrigation may be used to thin the sellar floor to a point that the dura may be visualized imparting a bluish hue through the thinned sellar floor.

Care must be taken when removing the sellar floor over the intercavernous sinus to avoid tearing this vein, which can bleed profusely. In the event that this occurs, the intercavernous sinus may be cauterized with bipolar diathermy.

Incision of the Dura

Bipolar diathermy is used for hemostasis over the dura before incising it. The incision may be made using a sickle knife or a scalpel with a retractable blade or a 45-degree-angle alligator scissors. The type of incision made over the dura may vary depending on the surgeon's preference, the type and size of the tumor, and the exposure necessary to remove the tumor. Incisions may be vertical, horizontal, cruciate, and diagonal, or made in the shape of a flap reflected inferiorly. Care is taken not to extend the vertical segment of the incision too superiorly, so as not to encounter the subarachnoid space or the anterior intercavernous venous sinus. The lateral extent of the horizontal incision is limited by the cavernous sinus on both sides, and great caution must be exercised to avoid the carotid artery in the far lateral corners of the exposure. Incising the dura on the diagonal from corner to corner provides a wider opening than a cruciate incision. The upper leaf of dura may be further incised in the midline if exposure over the top of the gland is needed.

Removal of Tumor

The delivery of the tumor depends on the consistency of the tumor contents. A cystic tumor decompresses rapidly. Large gelatinous or semisolid tumors are usually under pressure and decompress on incising the tumor capsule. Tumor tissue is taken for a histologic examination. Once we have sufficient tumor tissue for a histologic examination, the tumor is removed using a combination of blunt ring curettes and pituitary forceps. The otolaryngologist and neurosurgeon work in tandem at this point. While one surgeon removes the tumor with a ring curette, the other provides continuous suction, enabling rapid removal. A systematic approach in removing the tumor is useful. Start to remove the tumor from the floor, then work on the lateral extent next, and finally remove the suprasellar component if any. Often the tumor decompresses rapidly in areas where it is cystic or gelatinous. The diaphragma may descend rapidly in this region, giving the impression that the tumor has been completely removed, when in fact pockets of semisolid tumor or pockets where the tumor was adherent to the diaphragma may be left behind. Therefore, it is useful to attempt to control the descent of the diaphragma by systematic removal of the tumor.

It is extremely important to be gentle while working on the lateral aspect of the sella, as the medial layer of the cavernous sinus can be extremely thin. Arterial bleeding has been reported due to carotid artery injury, but may also arise from a tear in the arterial branch of the carotid, such as the inferior hypophyseal artery or by avulsion of a small capsular artery from the carotid artery.[13] Blunt curettes should be used, as the arachnoid can be extremely thin and cerebrospinal fluid (CSF) leakage may result even with gentle manipulation. If the diaphragma descends unequally, there may be a pocket of tumor left behind. In this situation it is useful for one surgeon to gently retract the diaphragma away to enable visualization of and removal of the retained tumor by the other surgeon.

Endoscopic Inspection of Sellar Cavity

Once the tumor has been removed, a 4-mm angled endoscope, 30-, 45-, or 70-degree, is used to view the sellar cavity and suprasellar cistern to ensure that there is no residual tumor. Lateral visualization with angled endoscopes enables exploration of the medial wall of the cavernous sinus. The extent to which neurovascular structures in the cavernous sinus are encased by the pathology must be carefully assessed. Although encasement is not a contraindication to this approach, surgeons must decide if they are able to safely dissect the tumor off the carotid artery, and should consider the possibility of radiosurgery and fractionated radiation to control the growth of residual unresectable tumor. In some cases, what appears to be tumor encasement of a vessel on preoperative MRI scan turns out to represent a vessel coursing along the capsule of the tumor that can be separated by an excellent arachnoid plane.

Sellar Hemostasis

Once the tumor has been completely removed, minor oozing from the sella is controlled by packing the sella with neuropatties providing tamponade for about 5 minutes. Upon removal of the neuropatties, the sella is once again endoscopically examined, and any localized oozing is controlled with placement of Surgicel (Johnson & Johnson, New Brunswick, NJ) over the area. In the situation where oozing from the sella persists despite the above measures, it may controlled by application of thrombin-infused gelatin matrix[22] (FloSeal; Baxter International, Deerfield, IL).

Management of a Cerebrospinal Fluid Leak

In the event that a CSF leak is recognized intraoperatively, the defect is plugged with abdominal fat and sealed with fibrin matrix (Tisseel; Baxter International). In our practice, for the standard transsphenoidal approach to pituitary lesions, a lumbar drain is not routinely placed for intraoperative leaks.

Nasal Hemostasis

Once the surgery is concluded, nasal hemostasis is ensured. Any minor mucosal oozing or bleeding from the septal branch of the sphenopalatine artery (SPA) is controlled with bipolar diathermy. If the bleeding from the septal branch of the SPA is persistent, it may be necessary to expose the SPA at the sphenopalatine foramen and ligate the vessel by applying arterial clips.

Nasal Packs

To facilitate postoperative mucosal healing, ensure the bone of the sphenoid rostrum is not exposed and that it is adequately covered by mucosa. Nasal Merocels (Medtronic Xomed Surgical Products, Jacksonville, FL), 8 cm, are placed in the nasal cavity on either side and hydrated with saline to expand. They are removed after 24 hours.

Modifications to the Technique

The technique described above is used for most lesions confined to the sella turcica. However, modifications to the approach may be necessary in certain situations where there is considerable extension of the sellar lesion through the diaphragma sella into the suprasellar cistern. Removal of the tuberculum sella and part of the planum sphenoidale is required in such cases to visualize and remove the tumor from the suprasellar cistern.

For wider access to the sphenoid sinus and wider exposure of the planum sphenoidale, the approach may be combined with bilateral ethmoidectomies and removal of the entire posterior bony nasal septum. The wide exposure of the sphenoid and the skull base provides excellent access to the planum sphenoidale and tuberculum sella. With this exposure the removal of the sellar floor can be extended superiorly to remove the tuberculum sella and part of the planum sphenoidale. Incision of the dura provides excellent visualization of the suprasellar cistern, enabling more complete removal of sellar lesions that extend through the diaphragma sella into the suprasellar cistern. The approach may also be used for some purely suprasellar prechiasmal and postchiasmal lesions that rest above a normal-sized sella. This endoscopic-extended transsphenoidal approach to the suprasellar cistern has been reported by several authors.[23–25]

■ Postoperative Care

Once the surgery is complete, the patient is extubated and brought to the recovery room where the patient's vital signs are monitored. For the next 24 hours the patient is monitored in the neurosurgical intensive care unit, particularly for diabetes insipidus and for visual deterioration. A fasting morning cortisol level is obtained on the morning of the second postoperative day, and cortisol replacement is initiated only if the level is abnormally low. Nasal packing is removed on the first postoperative day. If no lumbar drain has been placed, patients ambulate on the second postoperative day and may be discharged on the third postoperative day or as soon as they are ambulating and eating well. During the postoperative period, the patient is monitored for any CSF leak, or symptoms and signs of meningitis or any hemorrhage. Antibiotics and analgesics are routinely prescribed. The patient is examined following the removal of the packs. Any blood clots in the nasal cavity are aspirated under endoscopic guidance.[26–28]

The first office visit is scheduled for a week following the surgery. After application of topical 4% cocaine, blood clots are endoscopically removed from the nasal cavity and sphenoid sinus. The sella is carefully examined for any bleeding or CSF leakage. The patient is seen by the otolaryngologist once a week for the first 3 weeks, followed by two more appointments at 3-week intervals. Healing usually take about 3 to 6 weeks. Further appointments are scheduled as necessary. Postoperative follow-up is also provided by the endocrinologist, ophthalmologist, and the neurosurgeon.

■ Conclusion

The endoscopic transsphenoidal approach is the most direct and least invasive method for reaching the sellar floor and is now widely accepted in most institutions around the world. However, it is emphasized that detailed knowledge of the surgical anatomy and endoscopic techniques is essential prior to undertaking this surgery. This surgery should always be performed with a neurosurgeon and only by surgeons with significant experience in both transsphenoidal and endoscopic surgery, preferably after considerable practice on cadaver specimens. With experience, the technique may be used for lesions extending to the suprasellar cistern or located purely in the suprasellar cistern with an intact sella.

This surgery not only is a partnership between the neurosurgeon and the otolaryngologist, but also should be a partnership among all specialists involved in the management of pituitary tumors.

References

1. Hardy J. Transsphenoidal hypophysectomy. J Neurosurg 1971;34:582–594
2. Jankowski R, Auque J, Simon C, Marchal JC, Hepner H, Wayoff M. Endoscopic pituitary tumor surgery. Laryngoscope 1992;102:198–202
3. Jho HD, Carrau RL. Endoscopic endonasal transsphenoidal surgery: experience with 50 patients. J Neurosurg 1997;87:44–51
4. Nasseri SS, Kasperbauer JL, Strome SE, McCaffrey TV, Atkinson JL, Meyer FB. Endoscopic transnasal pituitary surgery: report on 180 cases. Am J Rhinol 2001;15:281–287
5. Cappabianca P, Alfieri A, de Oivitiis F. Endoscopic endonasal transsphenoidal approach to the sella: towards functional endoscopic pituitary surgery (FEPS). Minim Invasive Neurosurg 1998;41:66–73
6. Sethi DS, Stanley RE, Pillay PK. Endoscopic anatomy of the sphenoid sinus and sella turcica. J Laryngol Otol 1995;109:951–955
7. Sethi DS, Pillay PK. Endoscopic surgery for pituitary tumors. Op Tech Otolaryngol Head Neck Surg 1996;7:264–268
8. Sethi DS, Leong JL. Endoscopic pituitary surgery. Otolaryngol Clin North Am 2006;39:563–583
9. Sethi DS, Kumar K. Endoscopic pituitary surgery. Op Tech Otolaryngol Head Neck Surg 2006;18:57–64
10. Fujii K, Chambers SM, Rhoton AL Jr. Neurovascular relationships of the sphenoid sinus. A microsurgical study. J Neurosurg 1979;50:31–39
11. Renn WH, Rhoton AL Jr. Microsurgical anatomy of the sellar region. J Neurosurg 1975;43:288–298
12. Jho HD, Ha HG. Endoscopic endonasal skull base surgery: Part 1—The midline anterior fossa skull base. Minim Invasive Neurosurg 2004;47:1–8
13. Rhoton AL Jr. Anatomy of the pituitary gland and sellar region. In: Thapar K, Kovacs K, Scheithauer BW, Lloyd RV, eds. Diagnosis and Management of Pituitary Tumors. Totowa, NJ: Humana Press; 2000:13–40
14. Laws ER Jr, Kern EB. Complications of trans-sphenoidal surgery. Clin Neurosurg 1976;23:401–416
15. Rhoton AL Jr, Hardy DG, Chambers SM. Microsurgical anatomy and dissection of the sphenoid bone, cavernous sinus and sellar region. Surg Neurol 1979;12:63–104
16. Molitch ME. Medical treatment of prolactinomas. Endocrinol Metab Clin North Am 1999;28:143–169, vii
17. Elster AD. Modern imaging of the pituitary. Radiology 1993;187:1–14
18. Naganuma H, Satoh E, Nukui H. Technical considerations of transsphenoidal removal of fibrous pituitary adenomas and evaluation of collagen content and subtype in the adenomas. Neurol Med Chir (Tokyo) 2002;42:202–212, discussion 213
19. Iuchi T, Saeki N, Tanaka M, Sunami K, Yamaura A. MRI prediction of fibrous pituitary adenomas. Acta Neurochir (Wien) 1998;140:779–786
20. Chakrabortty S, Oi S, Yamaguchi M, Tamaki N, Matsumoto S. Growth hormone-producing pituitary adenomas: MR characteristics and pre- and postoperative evaluation. Neurol Med Chir (Tokyo) 1993;33:81–85
21. Pierallini A, Caramia F, Falcone C, et al. Pituitary macroadenomas: preoperative evaluation of consistency with diffusion-weighted MR imaging initial experience. Radiology 2006;239:223–231
22. Ellegala DB, Maartens NF, Laws ER Jr. Use of FloSeal hemostatic sealant in transsphenoidal pituitary surgery: technical note. Neurosurgery 2002;51:513–515, discussion 515–516
23. Schwartz TH, Anand VK. The endoscopic endonasal transsphenoidal approach to the suprasellar cistern. Clin Neurosurg 2007;54:226–235
24. de Divitiis E, Cavallo LM, Cappabianca P, Esposito F. Extended endoscopic endonasal transsphenoidal approach for the removal of suprasellar tumors: Part 2. Neurosurgery 2007;60:46–58, discussion 58–59
25. Laufer I, Anand VK, Schwartz TH. Endoscopic, endonasal extended transsphenoidal, transplanum transtuberculum approach for resection of suprasellar lesions. J Neurosurg 2007;106:400–406
26. Black PM, Zervas NT, Candia GL. Incidence and management of complications of transsphenoidal operation for pituitary adenomas. Neurosurgery 1987;20:920–924
27. Wilson CB, Dempsey LC. Transsphenoidal microsurgical removal of 250 pituitary adenomas. J Neurosurg 1978;48:13–22
28. Cappabianca P, Cavallo LM, Valente V, et al. Sellar repair with fibrin sealant and collagen fleece after endoscopic endonasal transsphenoidal surgery. Surg Neurol 2004;62:227–233, discussion 233

25 Endoscopic Transnasal Pituitary Surgery

Aldo Cassol Stamm, Eduardo Vellutini, Daniel Timperley, and Leonardo Balsalobre

Tips and Pearls

- A wide sphenoidotomy improves visualization and orientation, and enables two surgeons to operate simultaneously without the crowding of instruments.
- Preservation of the sphenoid mucosa reduces bleeding from the exposed bone and provides a simple reconstructive option.
- Wide sellar bony resection enables visualization into the sella and the use of the two-surgeon technique, enabling capsular dissection rather than blind scraping techniques.
- A large, quadrangular dural opening also facilitates access and visualization.
- The 45-degree endoscope is useful to confirm tumor removal, especially laterally.
- In macroadenomas, the arachnoid of the diaphragma is the border of the resection and should be cleared of disease.
- Capsular dissection facilitates complete tumor removal with preservation of normal glandular tissue.

Introduction

Endoscopic pituitary surgery (EPS) is a well-established technique for the treatment of sellar tumors, especially pituitary adenomas. It offers some advantages compared with microscopic approaches, such as a superior close-up view of the relevant anatomy, an enlarged working angle, and increased panoramic vision inside the surgical area.[1-4]

Several studies, including a large systematic review, show that EPS decreases the operating time, the use of lumbar drains, the risk of postoperative diabetes insipidus, the length of hospital stay, patient discomfort, and rhinologic complications.[1-6]

The pituitary gland is well accessed through the nasal cavity and sphenoid sinus, and since the last century several approaches have been described.

This chapter discusses techniques that can improve the results in pituitary surgery, with more radical removal, optic chiasm decompression, and better endocrinologic results.

Pituitary surgery can be divided into nasal, sellar, and reconstructive stages. The nasal stage provides access to the sphenoid sinus via various approaches and is discussed in more depth in Chapter 14. The sellar stage is the main focus of this chapter, and the reconstructive options are discussed briefly.

Nasal Stage

Adequate exposure of the sphenoid sinus is essential. In addition to maximizing the lateral extent of the sphenoidotomy, lowering the opening to the floor of the sinus is important to provide access to the inferior aspect of the sella. The panoramic view possible with the endoscope enables visualization of anatomic landmarks, which aids surgical orientation (**Fig. 25.1**). A wide opening into the sphenoid also enhances the ability of two surgeons to operate simultaneously without the crowding of instruments, enabling sharp capsular dissection and improving the ability to control bleeding. Small openings restrict both visualization and the number of instruments that can be used simultaneously, resulting in reliance on curettage and blind scraping techniques with limited ability to manage bleeding.[7] The various approaches are discussed in Chapter 14.

Sellar Stage

The sellar stage of the procedure begins with the identification of landmarks through the wide sphenoidotomy created during the nasal stage. A panoramic view should be obtained, enabling bilateral identification of the opticocarotid recesses, internal carotid arteries, and optic nerves in one view of the endoscope. The sella, clivus, and planum are identified in the midline (**Fig. 25.1**).

The intersinus septum and accessory septa are removed. Particular care is taken where a septum is attached over the carotid artery to avoid an uncontrolled fracture, which may result in arterial injury. The sphenoid mucosa is displaced laterally, rather than stripping the lining of the sinus. Bleeding from exposed bone is reduced, and the mucosa can be used to supplement sella reconstruction.

The bone of the sella is thinned using a diamond drill, or if thin, gently fractured. A Kerrison rongeur is then used to remove the bone in an extradural manner. Bone removal continues until the "four blues" are identified: the cavernous sinuses on each side and the superior and inferior intercavernous sinuses. A rectangular dural opening is then made just inside these vascular boundaries (**Fig. 25.2**).

After exposure of the tumor, tumor fragments are sent for pathologic examination. Excision is performed using micro-

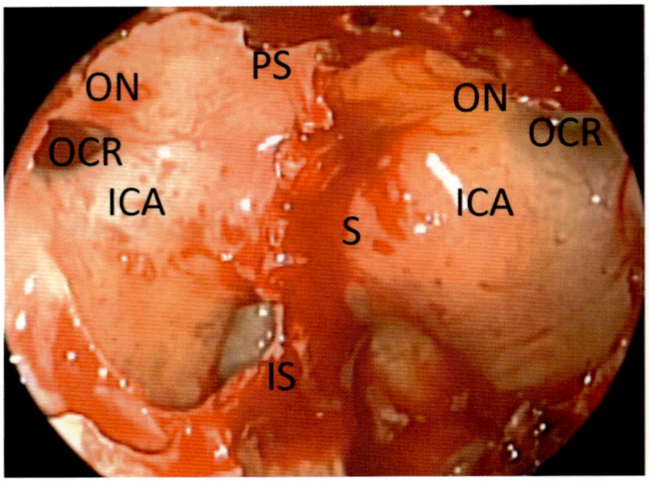

A

Fig. 25.1 **(A)** Endoscopic view of the sphenoid sinuses. A wide view of the anatomic structures facilitates surgical orientation. **(B)** Cadaver dissection demonstrating the position of the venous sinuses. C: clivus; ICA: internal carotid arteries; IIS: inferior intercavernous sinus; IS: intersinus septum; OCR: opticocarotid recess; ON: optic nerve; PS: planum sphenoidale; S: sella turcica; SIS; superior intercavernous sinus.

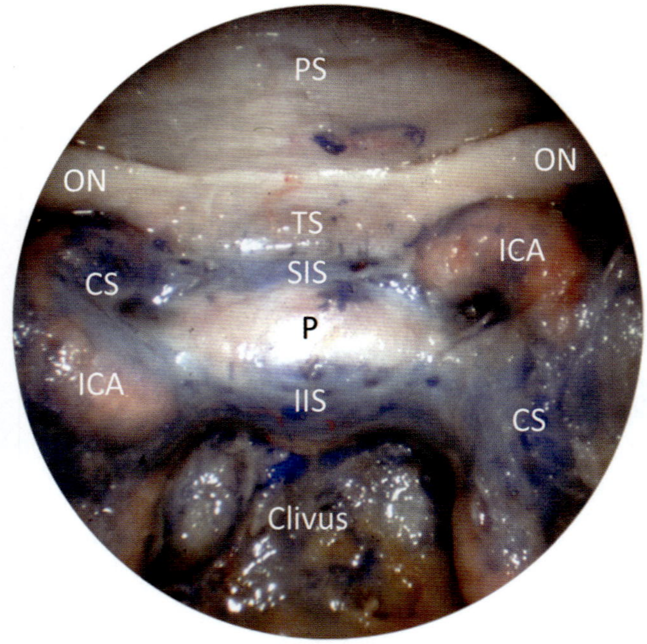

B

surgical techniques to separate the tumor from the normal gland and sellar walls. Capsular dissection of the tumor is favored as opposed to curettage and scraping techniques. Dissection in the plane between the tumor and normal structures facilitates complete tumor removal with maximal preservation of normal tissues, particularly residual pituitary gland. For larger tumors, initial debulking is required so that the tumor collapses and dissection of the capsule is possible (**Fig. 25.2**). In macroadenomas, tumor resection is not complete until the arachnoid membrane of the diaphragma is identified and separated from the lesion (**Fig. 25.2**). Although dissection is most safely performed using a 0-degree endoscope, a 45-degree endoscope is useful to check the completeness of the resection, particularly laterally around the carotids and cavernous sinus. Venous bleeding from the cavernous or intercavernous sinuses is controlled with hemostatic materials, compression, and patience.

Once resection is complete, reconstruction of the sella floor is performed. If there is a significant cerebrospinal fluid (CSF) leak, fat and fascia lata are used in an underlay fashion and the nasoseptal flap is placed over the repair. When the arachnoid is exposed but there is no significant CSF leak, the

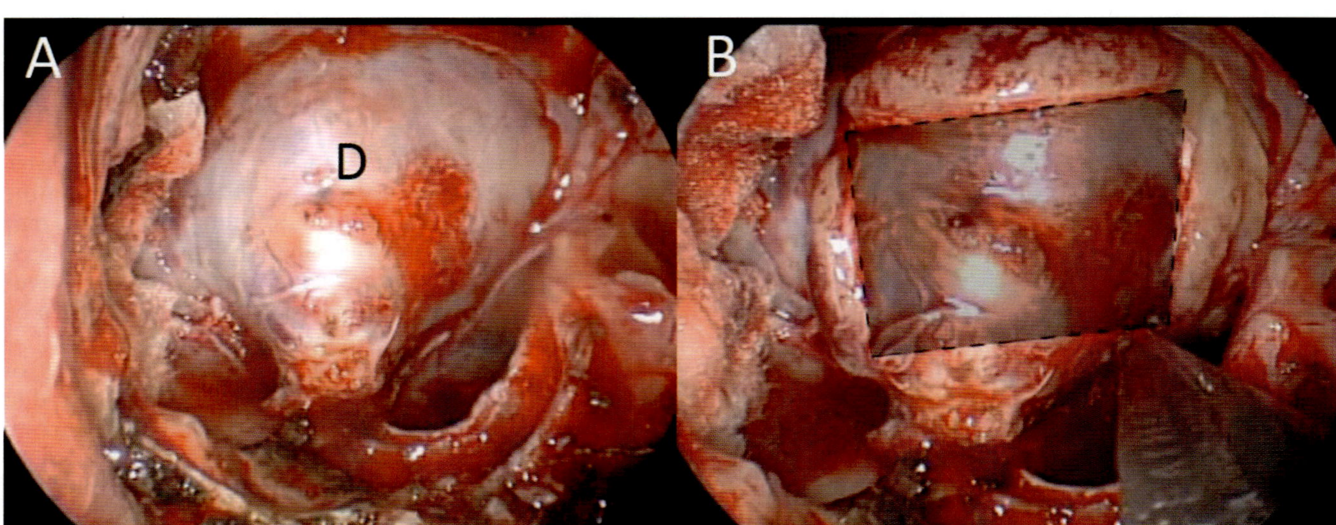

Fig. 25.2 Resection of pituitary macroadenoma. **(A)** A wide bony opening is made to ensure adequate access for the endoscope and the instruments. **(B)** A quadrangular dural incision is made, defined by the cavernous and intercavernous sinuses.

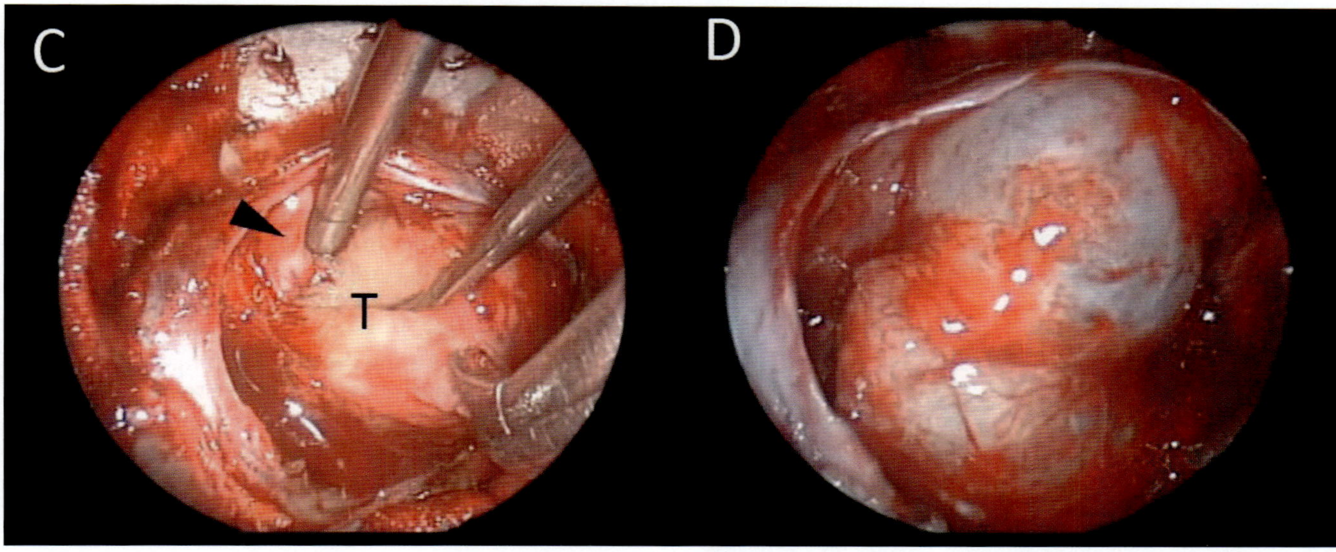

Fig. 25.2 (*Continued*) **(C)** Four-handed capsular dissection. Following initial tumor debulking, traction on the tumor capsule reveals the plane between the tumor and normal tissue, which can then be dissected (*arrowhead*). Dissection in this plane maximizes tumor removal while preserving normal structures. **(D)** At the end of the procedure, a final check is made with the 45-degree endoscope. The resection is incomplete unless the arachnoid has been cleared of tumor. A: arachnoid; D: dura of sella; T: tumor.

flap is used alone. In intrasellar microadenomas without exposed arachnoid, the sphenoid mucosa is used to cover the defect and the flap replaced in its original location.

Expanded Access

Expanded approaches are necessary where tumor extends outside the sellar and access is inadequate via the sellar approach alone. Inferior access is achieved via the transclival approach, superior access by the suprasellar/transplanum approach, and lateral access by the transpterygoid approach.

Transclival

The transclival approach provides access inferior to the sella turcica (**Fig. 25.3**). The nasal stage of the procedure is similar to the sellar approach, except that the sphenoid face must be lowered even further, possibly with removal of the sphenoid floor, depending on the extent of the lesion. Resection of the

A

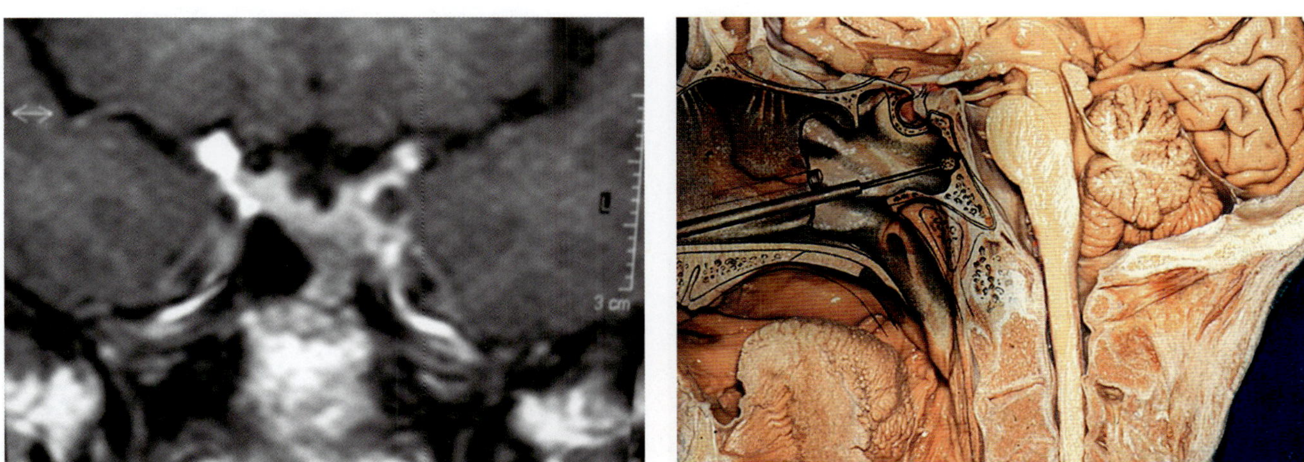

B

Fig. 25.3 Transclival approach. **(A)** Magnetic resonance imaging (MRI) scan of a 50-year-old man with acromegaly. Tumor is seen extending into the clivus. **(B)** A schematic drawing of a clival resection via a bi-nostril approach. The anterior face of the sphenoid is lowered, and the floor resected as required to gain access. Care is taken to avoid injury to the basilar plexus lying between the dural layers on the posterior aspect of the upper clivus.

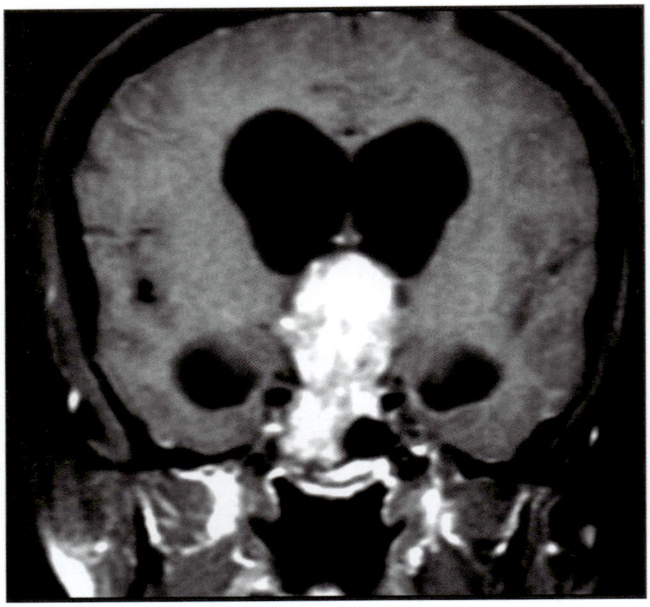

Fig. 25.4 An MRI of a 54-year-old man with a nonfunctioning pituitary macroadenoma who presented with increased intracranial pressure, headache, and visual loss. A transplanum approach is required to access the superior extension.

upper clivus and sphenoid floor is performed with the drill. Care must be taken laterally to avoid the clival carotid arteries, and posteriorly due to the possibility of bleeding from the basilar plexus. If there is tumor infiltration, the basilar plexus is usually obstructed. Bleeding from the basilar plexus is treated similarly to other venous sinuses, with pressure, hemostatic agents, and patience.[8]

Transplanum

The transplanum approach is the anterosuperior extension of the sellar approach (**Fig. 25.4**). It is used where there is significant tumor extension above the sella or where sella access is limited by medial protrusion of the internal carotid arteries. A posterior ethmoidectomy is required to access the planum as far anteriorly as the posterior ethmoid arteries. The boundaries of the planum removal are the posterior ethmoid arteries anteriorly and the optic nerves laterally, resulting in a trapezoidal opening with the narrow end situated posteriorly (**Fig. 25.5**). The bone over the sella and the planum are thinned using the drill and removed with Kerrison rongeurs. Removal of the tuberculum sellae joins the two approaches. The dura of the planum is opened with a trapezoidal dural incision. This dural opening is joined to the sella opening by coagulating and then dividing the superior intercavernous sinus in the midline.[9]

Transpterygoid

This is the lateral extension of the sellar approach, used for removal of adenomas that invade the cavernous sinus (**Fig. 25.6**). The approach is detailed in Chapter 14. When planning this approach, it should be remembered that the sphenopalatine artery is often compromised, so a contralateral septal flap is planned. Dissection within the cavernous sinus is challenging, and is performed using gentle movements of a nontraumatic suction device. Tumor consistency and vascularity may be limiting factors for an aggressive surgical approach. Hemostasis is achieved with pressure, Surgicel (or similar), and time. Even in cases where there is no CSF leak, use of a vascularized flap over the exposed internal carotid is recommended.

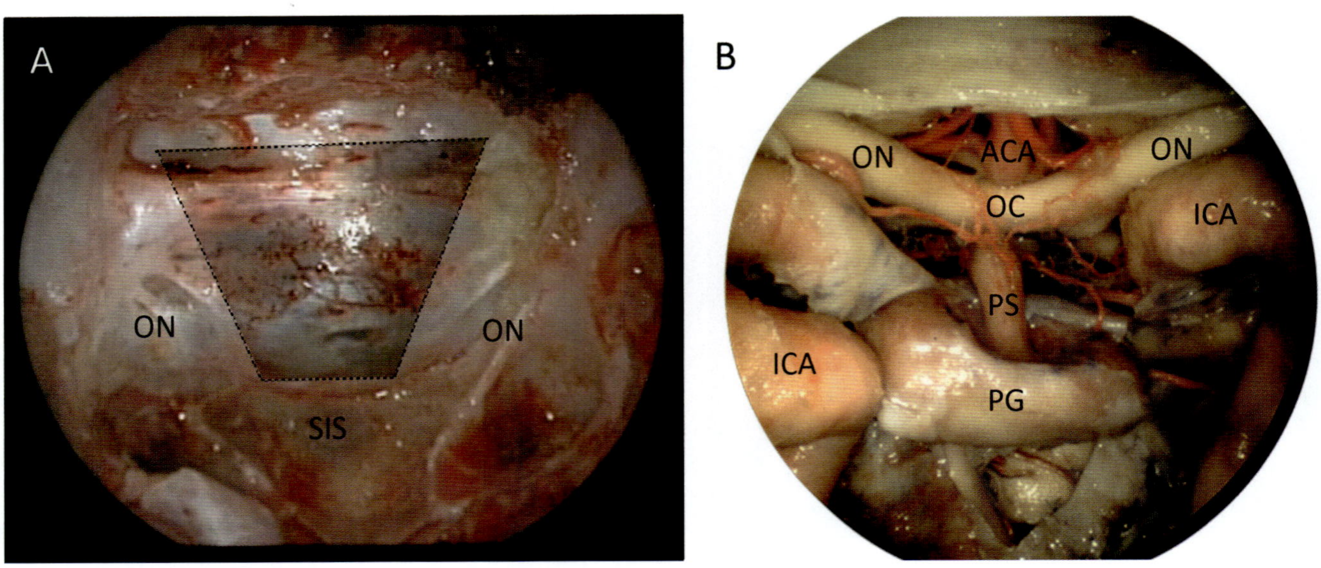

Fig. 25.5 Transplanum approach. **(A)** The trapezoidal dural incision is marked. ON: position of optic nerves; SIS: superior intercavernous sinus. **(B)** Structures accessed by the transplanum approach. ACA: anterior cerebral complex; ICA: internal carotid artery; OC: optic chiasm; ON: optic nerve; PG: pituitary gland; PS: pituitary stalk.

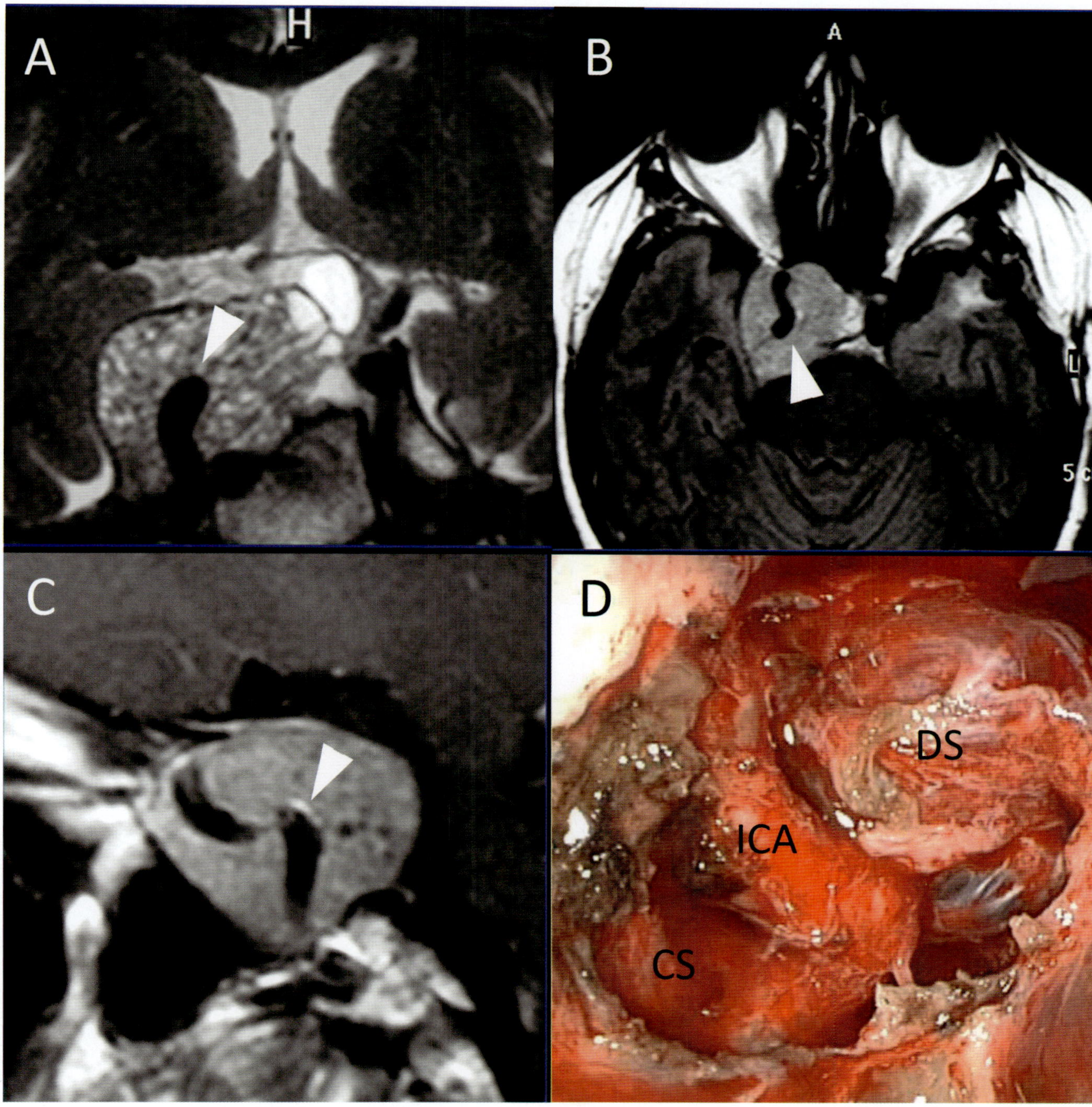

Fig. 25.6 A 41-year-old woman with recurrent Cushing's disease following two previous procedures. A large tumor extends into the left cavernous sinus, encasing the internal carotid artery (*arrowheads*). A transpterygoid approach is required in this case. **(A)** Coronal view. **(B)** Axial view. **(C)** Sagittal view. **(D)** Intraoperative view following transpterygoid approach. The ICA is in the center of the operating field with good access to the cavernous sinus. CS: cavernous sinus; DS: diaphragma sella; ICA: internal carotid artery.

Conclusion

Endoscopic pituitary surgery provides significant advantages over traditional microsurgery. Adequate access is essential to allow panoramic views and unimpeded access for multiple instruments in a two-surgeon approach, particularly where expanded approaches are required. Teamwork is vital in endoscopic skull base surgery, and pituitary surgery represents an excellent opportunity to develop the working relationship between the neurosurgeon and the otorhinolaryngologist, as well as others in the multidisciplinary team.

References

1. Cappabianca P, Alfieri A, de Divitiis E. Endoscopic endonasal transsphenoidal approach to the sella: towards functional endoscopic pituitary surgery (FEPS). Minim Invasive Neurosurg 1998;41:66–73
2. Har-El G. Endoscopic transnasal transsphenoidal pituitary surgery—comparison with the traditional sublabial transseptal approach. Otolaryngol Clin North Am 2005;38:723–735
3. Jho HD. Endoscopic transsphenoidal surgery. J Neurooncol 2001;54:187–195
4. Jarrahy R, Berci G, Shahinian HK. Assessment of the efficacy of endoscopy in pituitary adenoma resection. Arch Otolaryngol Head Neck Surg 2000;126:1487–1490
5. Badie B, Brooks N, Souweidane MM. Endoscopic and minimally invasive microsurgical approaches for treating brain tumor patients. J Neurooncol 2004;69:209–219
6. Rotenberg B, Tam S, Ryu WHA, Duggal N. Microscopic versus endoscopic pituitary surgery: a systematic review. Laryngoscope 2010;120:1292–1297
7. Stamm AC, Vellutini E, Harvey RJ, Nogeira JF Jr, Herman DR. Endoscopic transnasal craniotomy and the resection of craniopharyngioma. Laryngoscope 2008;118:1142–1148
8. Stamm AC, Pignatari SS, Vellutini E. Transnasal endoscopic surgical approaches to the clivus. Otolaryngol Clin North Am 2006;39:639–656, xi
9. Stamm AM. Transnasal endoscopy-assisted skull base surgery. Ann Otol Rhinol Laryngol Suppl 2006;196:45–53

26 Hydroscopy: Application to Pituitary Surgery

W. Derek Leight and Brent A. Senior

Tips and Pearls

- Hydroscopy is a novel technique for examining the sella turcica after minimally invasive pituitary surgery, employing gentle fluid distention of the sella while performing endoscopy.
- It frequently results in removal of additional, unseen tumor, and has been shown to result in a lower revision surgery rate.
- It is associated with a lower risk of cerebrospinal fluid (CSF) leak.
- It is a safe and effective technique and a useful adjunct to pituitary tumor removal that should be in the armamentarium of endoscopic skull base surgeons.

Introduction

Endoscopic transsphenoidal pituitary surgery as we know it today has been enabled by a series of advances in our understanding of physiology, medicine, and technology, in addition to advances in other fields, including endocrinology, microbiology, general surgery, urology, orthopedics, neurosurgery, and otolaryngology. Paradigm shifts in one field of medicine or surgery often come from borrowing and adapting techniques from other fields. In this fashion, endoscopic techniques have been transferred from one field to another, adapting to the specific requirements of each field. Neurosurgery, although a relative latecomer to endoscopic surgery, recently adapted traditional endoscopic techniques from the fields of urology, orthopedic surgery, and otolaryngology. This has produced a novel technique that is gaining worldwide acceptance: hydroscopy. Hydroscopy refers to the process of endoscopically visualizing the sella turcica using saline for low-pressure fluid distention. This technique has led to improvements in surgical techniques and outcomes for endoscopic transsphenoidal pituitary surgery.[1,2]

History

The history of hydroscopy begins with the development of the cystoscope. While Bozzini developed the "Lichtleiter" in the early 1800s, modern endoscopy began with Nitze's development of a functional cystoscope in 1878.[3] This cystoscope was the first to utilize a lens and an electric light source at the tip of the instrument (**Fig. 26.1**). Cystoscopes were adapted to other disciplines, which led to the advancement of endoscopic techniques in many branches of medicine. Early cystoscopes used only air insufflation, which was very difficult in males and required patients to be in the uncomfortable genupectoral position to allow air to be vacuumed into the bladder by the downward pull of the abdomen. Application of a second cylinder for fluid instillation by Couriard and Evermann and advances in electronics and lighting led to fluid distention cystoscopy, which provided better visualization, easier exams in males, cooling for the light element, improved safety, and allowed the patient to be in the more comfortable lithotomy position.[3,4]

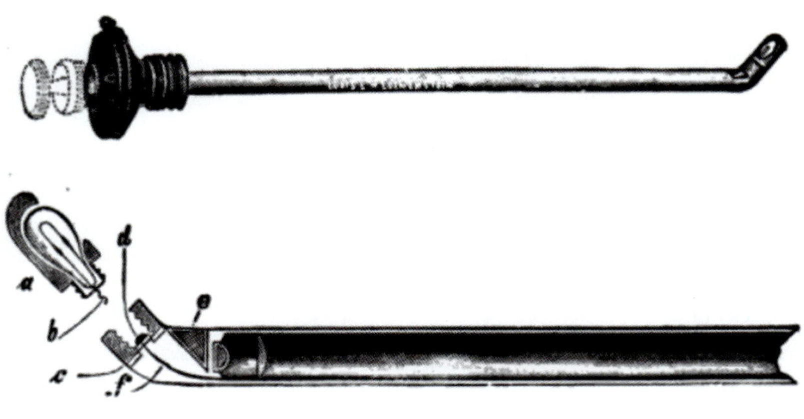

Fig. 26.1 Nitze's cystoscope featured the first lens system and the first feasible light source at the tip of the endoscope, which paved the way for fluid distention cystoscopy. (From Luys G. A Treatise on Cystoscopy and Urethroscopy. St. Louis: Mosby, 1918. [This book is in the public domain.])

Although fluid distention eventually became standard in cystoscopy, most other branches of medicine adopted the method of air insufflation. In 1912, when Severin Nordentoft published his results of knee examinations using the trochar endoscope, arthroscopy using fluid distention was born.[5] Japanese professor Kenji Takagi, unaware of Nordentoft's findings, developed the first widely used arthroscopic instruments. Takagi's protégé, Masaki Watanabe, developed the standard technique and instrumentation for arthroscopy using fluid distention, removed the first knee lesion arthroscopically in 1955, and eventually became known as the father of modern arthroscopy.[6,7]

Early neuroendoscopy centered on endoscopy of the ventricles and cerebrospinal fluid (CSF)-containing spaces. The first neuroendoscopic procedure was performed by urologist Victor L'Espinasse in 1910. He used a cystoscope to ablate the choroid plexus in two infants with hydrocephalus.[8] Neuroendoscopic procedures such as choroid plexectomy and endoscopic ventriculostomy were performed by Dandy and others; however, the field did not catch on due to the technical difficulty, lack of adequate instrumentation, high mortality rates, and the development of the ventricular shunt and the operating microscope. By the 1970s, advances in endoscope and camera technology permitted the reintroduction of neuroendoscopic techniques.[9] By 1992, Jankowski reported the first pure endoscopic transsphenoidal pituitary resection. In 1997, Jho and Carrau published the first large series of results using the pure endoscopic endonasal transsphenoidal approach. This approach became the basis for endoscopic skull base surgery.[10] In 2005, Senior et al,[1] combining the techniques of fluid distention endoscopy, nasal endoscopy, and neuroendoscopy, published the first description of hydroscopy of the sella turcica during endoscopic endonasal transsphenoidal pituitary surgery.

Rationale

The sella turcica is not a rigid space (**Fig. 26.2**). The bony tuberculum sella and dorsum sella tent up the diaphragma superiorly and the cavernous sinuses laterally. It is very distensible superiorly and relatively distensible laterally. After excision of a pituitary tumor, the potential space is filled in as the diaphragma collapses and the pituitary is decompressed. The result is that the lateral and superior corners of the sella become extremely difficult to thoroughly evaluate. Often, pockets of solid tumor may be left behind after an initial aspiration of a gelatinous portion of tumor. Other groups have advocated addressing this problem by having one surgeon retract the diaphragma superiorly and examine the cavity with angled endoscopes, while the other removes residual tumor with curettes and suction.[11] In our experience, this technique has produced suboptimal visualization and been technically difficult, requiring two surgeons to have three or four instruments inside the sella at once. Other groups have tried using suction curettes as retractors in the sella; however, in our experience, this increases the risk of CSF leak by tearing the diaphragma, and it still provides only a focal view of the sella.

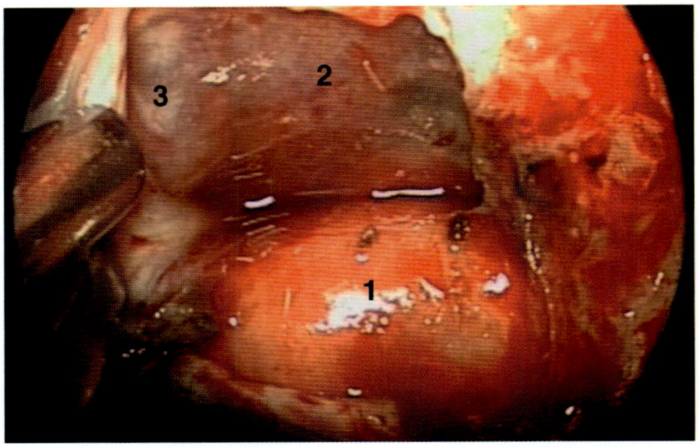

Fig. 26.2 This expanded view illustrates that the sella is a potential space, not a cerebrospinal fluid (CSF)-containing space. The tuberculum sella and planum sphenoidale have been removed. The pituitary (1), planar dura (2), diaphragma and C6 carotid segment (3) are visualized. (Courtesy of Dr. Adam M. Zanation.)

In examining ways to distend the sella without using extra instrumentation, we looked to the history of endoscopy and the techniques of cystoscopy and arthroscopy. Arthroscopy, in particular, provides excellent visualization of small, partially distensible spaces (**Fig. 26.3**). It also facilitates identification of abnormal tissue, particularly partially attached or torn tissue, as it floats around the saline medium. Another advantage of using fluid is the ability to remove blood from the field without having to use suction, which frees up an-

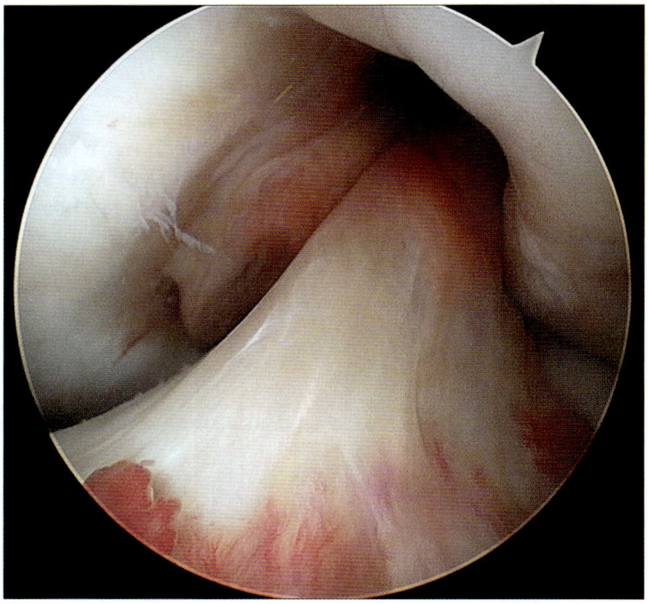

Fig. 26.3 Fluid distention arthroscopy of the knee provides excellent visualization of narrow, partially distensible spaces, and facilitates discrimination of pathologic tissue. This technique was the inspiration for hydroscopy of the sella.

other hand for other instrumentation. Additionally, because saline is nearly identical in density to CSF, it will not expand under pressure into the brain cavity. This is a major theoretical advantage over using air, due to the risk of tension pneumocephalus.

Patient Selection

Nearly all patients undergoing endoscopic endonasal pituitary surgery at our institution have hydroscopy performed during the procedure. Patients with secreting adenomas will undergo thorough hydroscopic examination of the sella to ensure complete tumor removal. Patients with Rathke's cleft cysts generally do not require hydroscopy. However, if a CSF leak is suspected, it can be a useful adjunct.

Preoperative Evaluation

At our institution, all patients found to have pituitary tumors undergo a thorough evaluation by multiple specialties, including endocrinology, otolaryngology, neurosurgery, and ophthalmology. Patients are presented at a multidisciplinary pituitary conference where a treatment plan is formulated. Surgical intervention for hormonally inactive tumors is reserved for compressive symptoms, rapid growth, apoplexy, or severe headache. Intervention for prolactinomas is reserved for failed medical management. Patients with growth hormone secreting tumors, with or without acromegaly, and adrenocorticotropic hormone (ACTH)-secreting tumors are offered surgery upon diagnosis. All patients undergo preoperative nasal endoscopy, paranasal sinus computed tomography (CT) scan, and magnetic resonance imaging (MRI). The vast majority of cases are performed using stereotactic CT guidance using fused MRI and CT images for better visualization of tumor, as well as important neurovascular structures. When possible, patients receive preoperative visual acuity and visual field exam by an ophthalmologist.

Surgical Technique

Our operative technique for pituitary surgery has been described elsewhere.[2] Briefly, the patient is turned 90 degrees counterclockwise from the anesthetist and placed in the beach-chair position. A fused CT/MRI file is registered to a stereotactic guidance system. This provides valuable neurovascular anatomical detail not available from CT alone. The abdomen is sterilely prepared for a fat graft if necessary. A zero-degree, 4-mm Hopkins rod is used initially. The ClearESS suction/irrigation system (PhotoMedex, Montgomery, PA) is applied to the Hopkins rod, which will later be used for hydroscopy. This increases the diameter of the scope to 5.5 mm (**Fig. 26.4**). The ClearESS irrigation system utilizes a standard pressure bag applied around a bag of saline to force sterile saline through the irrigation channel. The operation is done in the standing position, as this better accommodates the two-surgeon, four-handed technique. The approach is performed using a paraseptal corridor. The middle turbinate is lateralized. The superior turbinate is partially resected. If a large defect or high-flow CSF leak is anticipated, a nasoseptal flap is performed prior to sphenoidotomy. Next, the sphenoid ostium is identified and enlarged with curettes. A wide sphenoidotomy is then performed with Kerrison rongeurs. Next, the posterior septectomy is performed and the intersinus septum is taken down. A wide sphenoidotomy is performed on the contralateral side. This is usually completed by changing nostrils and lateralizing the opposite middle turbinate. Binarial access is then obtained. Unless there is an obvious contraindication, the endoscope is placed in the right nostril. Next, the mucosa on the face of the sella is cauterized with the bipolar cautery and the face of the sella is then thinned with a high-speed drill, usually with a 4-mm rough-cut diamond burr. If the face of the sella has been thinned out by tumor, a small chisel or curette can be used to fracture the bone. Kerrison rongeurs are then used to remove the sellar bone. Next, the dura is cauterized and incised, and the tumor is removed with a variety of neurosurgical suctions, curettes, and forceps.

After the tumor is grossly resected, hydroscopy is performed. The endoscope is carefully inserted into the sella, where the diaphragma, depending on the size of tumor removed, is

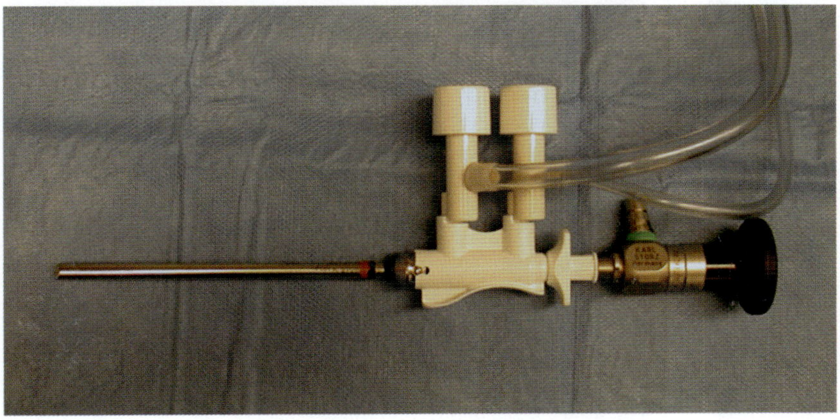

Fig. 26.4 ClearESS endoscopic suction/irrigation system (PhotoMedex, Montgomery, PA).

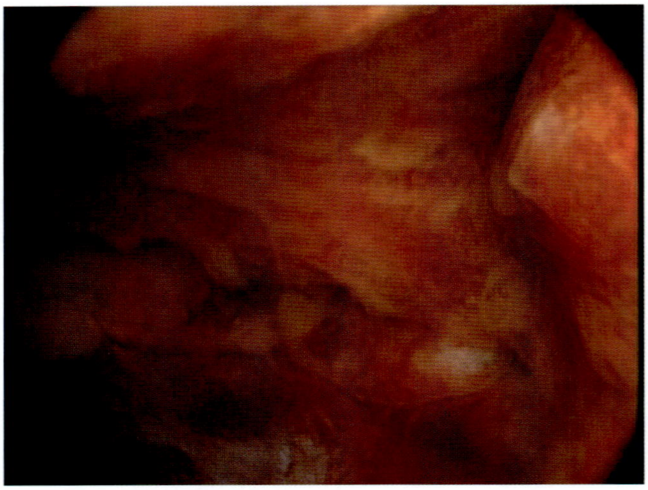

Fig. 26.5 Expanded view of the sella during hydroscopy.

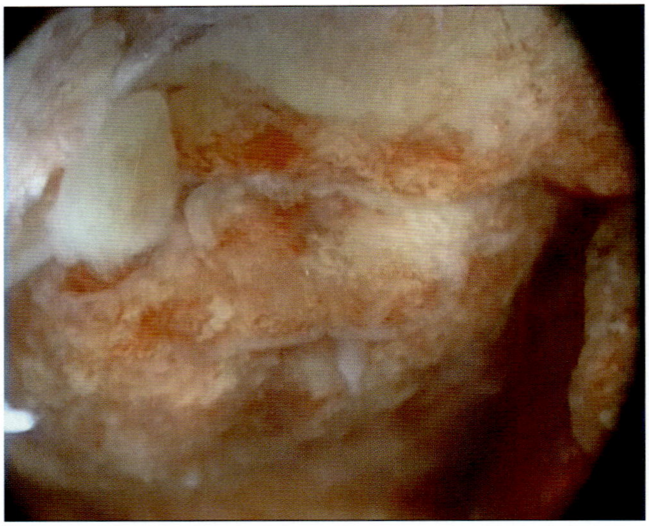

Fig. 26.6 Hydroscopic view of a residual piece of pituitary tumor on the diaphragma sella discovered during hydroscopy.

usually nearly fully collapsed. The irrigation channel is then opened, and the sella is gently pressurized with sterile, room-temperature normal saline. As the sella expands, the focus on the camera must be adjusted to account for the light diffraction properties of water (**Fig. 26.5**). The suction port on the ClearESS is not used, as this creates turbulent saline flow, which decreases visualization. Generally, the overall amount of saline used in hydroscopy does not fill the nasal cavities and nasopharynx; thus, it usually does not spill out onto the field, and suction is not immediately necessary. A clear image of the expanded sella is then obtained. Bleeding is minimized by the low-pressure saline, and blood in the field is immediately diluted and washed away, producing a clear field of vision in the sella and also a clear view of the soft tissue structures without a layer of blood. At this point, usually only one surgeon is necessary, as the operating surgeon can hold the scope in one hand to examine the sella and has the other hand free to use instrumentation, such as curettes or forceps. As the sella is under a low-pressure laminar flow system, loosely attached tissue waves freely in the saline medium, making it readily identifiable. In this manner, residual tumor is often identified during hydroscopy (**Fig. 26.6**). Tumor may be removed with curettes (**Fig. 26.7**) or washed out of the sella and removed via suction from the nasal cavity at the conclusion of the procedure. To examine the corners of the sella, a 45-degree sheath for the ClearESS system is available (**Fig. 26.8**). If an expanded approach is taken, suprasellar structures can be readily seen.

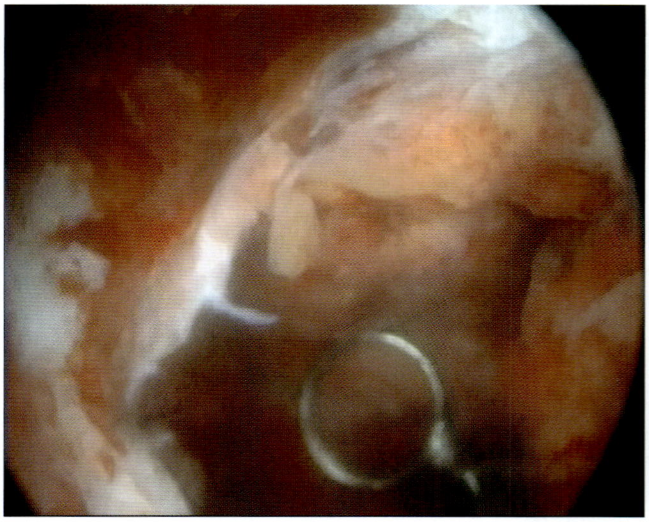

Fig. 26.7 Ring curette entering the sella during hydroscopy to remove residual tumor discovered during hydroscopy.

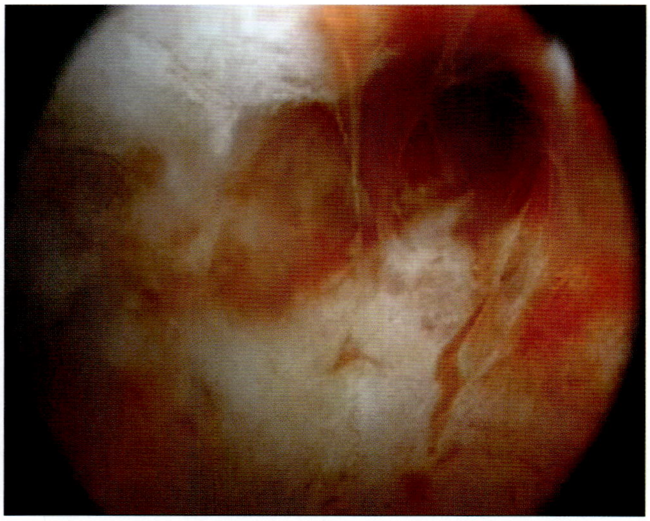

Fig. 26.8 Expanded view of the left posterior superior sella provided by hydroscopy.

Results

Hydroscopy has been performed on over 200 patients thus far. Our initial intuitive experience demonstrated that performing hydroscopy led to a substantial improvement in tumor removal. We found that hydroscopy often resulted in the discovery and subsequent removal of additional tumors. Whether or not these tumors would have been identifiable using nonhydroscopic techniques was initially difficult to determine. However, when we examined our series of over 190 surgeries, we found that hydroscopy lowered the probability of needing a repeat surgery significantly. Additionally, we found that hydroscopy was associated with a significantly lower rate of postoperative CSF leak.[2] We found no association with diabetes insipidus. By placing an arterial line in the sella during hydroscopy, we determined that the pressure required to inflate the sella in most cases was only 2 or 3 mm Hg.

Conclusion

Hydroscopic examination of the sella turcica during minimally invasive pituitary surgery is safe and effective. It substantially improves visualization of the sella and surrounding structures. It improves surgical outcomes by reducing the need for revision surgery. It is associated with a decreased risk of postoperative CSF leak, likely due to the surgeon's ability to visualize the diaphragma without retraction. There are currently no known detrimental side effects to employing this technique. Hydroscopy is a valuable tool in the armamentarium of the endoscopic skull base surgeon.

References

1. Senior BA, Dubin MG, Sonnenburg RE, Melroy CT, Ewend MG. Increased role of the otolaryngologist in endoscopic pituitary surgery: endoscopic hydroscopy of the sella. Am J Rhinol 2005;19:181–184
2. Senior BA, Ebert CS, Bednarski KK, et al. Minimally invasive pituitary surgery. Laryngoscope 2008;118:1842–1855
3. Mouton WG, Bessell JR, Maddern GJ. Looking back to the advent of modern endoscopy: 150th birthday of Maximilian Nitze. World J Surg 1998;22:1256–1258
4. Nicholson P. Problems encountered by early endoscopists. Urology 1982;19:114–119
5. Kieser CW, Jackson RW. Severin Nordentoft: the first arthroscopist. Arthroscopy 2001;17:532–535
6. Bigony L. Arthroscopic surgery: a historical perspective. Orthop Nurs 2008;27:349–354, quiz 355–356
7. Jackson RW. Quo venis quo vadis: the evolution of arthroscopy. Arthroscopy 1999;15:680–685
8. Walker ML. History of ventriculostomy. Neurosurg Clin N Am 2001; 12:101–110, viii
9. Li KW, Nelson C, Suk I, Jallo GI. Neuroendoscopy: past, present, and future. Neurosurg Focus 2005;19:E1
10. Doglietto F, Prevedello DM, Jane JA Jr, Han J, Laws ER Jr. Brief history of endoscopic transsphenoidal surgery—from Philipp Bozzini to the First World Congress of Endoscopic Skull Base Surgery. Neurosurg Focus 2005;19:E3
11. Sethi DS, Leong JL. Endoscopic pituitary surgery. Otolaryngol Clin North Am 2006;39:563–583, x

27 Endoscopic Cavernous Sinus Surgery

Giorgio Frank, Diego Mazzatenta, Vittorio Sciarretta, Matteo Zoli, Giovanni Farneti, and Ernesto Pasquini

Tips and Pearls

- Adenomas and chordomas, especially those of soft consistency having an extradural location, are ideally suited for endoscopic cavernous sinus surgery.
- The approach should be selected in accordance with the growth of the tumor in the cavernous sinus (CS) compartments; the midline transsphenoidal approach is sufficient when the tumor grows in the medial and posterosuperior compartments of the CS.
- The ethmoido-pterygo-sphenoidal (EPS) approach is preferred if the tumor also involves the anteroinferior or lateral compartments of the CS.
- Endoscopic CS surgery should be done by surgeons well trained with the endoscopic technique and in centers where endovascular support is available and where it is possible to switch to open surgery, if necessary.

Introduction

A single gold standard in cavernous sinus (CS) surgery does not exist, because the technique must be adapted to the features of the particular tumor. Anterior extracranial approaches and transcranial approaches are complementary, and both techniques facilitate obtaining the best surgical result with the minimal morbidity. Both have to be in the armamentarium of the skull base surgeon operating on CS tumors. Anterior extracranial approaches present three advantages over the transcranial approaches: (1) They are extracerebral, avoiding any brain manipulation. 2) They enable penetrating the CS through the medial wall, which is devoid of any nerves. Conversely, in transcranial approaches, the CS is penetrated, crossing the lateral wall through narrow windows between the cranial nerves. (3) Working within the CS in anterior extracerebral approaches, there are areas, such as the medial and the posterosuperior compartments, that do not run the risk of nerve damage, and there are others area, such as the anteroinferior and the lateral compartments, that have a well-defined point where there is a risk of nerve damage. The abducens nerve (cranial nerve VI) runs the main risk of damage because it runs free in the CS space; the others nerves are embedded and protected between the two layers composing the lateral wall of the CS (**Fig. 27.1**).

The main disadvantage of anterior extracerebral approaches is the difficulty of controlling the carotid artery and protecting it from injury. Jho and Carrau[1] in 1997 reported the first series of pituitary adenomas treated using an endonasal endoscopic technique. Since that time, we have recognized the possibility of extending this technique to use it in surgery of the parasellar region. One year later we started our experience with endoscopic endonasal surgery of the CS, and our preliminary results were reported to the Fifth European Skull Base Society Congress in 2001.[2] We prefer the endoscopic technique because it overcomes the limitations of the microsurgical technique,[3] such as the necessity to utilize wider surgical channels with limited peripheral vision, and the necessity to utilize metallic retractors.

We recommend the endoscopic approach only to surgeons who are well trained with this technique and only in centers where endovascular support is available, and where it is possible to switch to open surgery, if needed.

Selection Criteria

The selection criteria for an endoscopic CS surgery are mainly the biological behavior of the tumor and its location. Tumors involving the vessels and nerves, such as meningiomas and carcinomas, are not good candidates for this approach (**Fig. 27.2**). Conversely, tumors not involving the vessels and the nerves, such as adenomas and chordomas or chondrosarcomas, are amenable to this type of surgery. The consistency of the tumor may be a further criterion for selecting the endoscopic approach, with soft tumors being more suitable for this type of surgery. Only tumors that are totally extradural or have limited intradural extension are suitable for endonasal endoscopic approach. But if the tumor has a large intradural extension, we use the transcranial approach.

Technical Note

A detailed description of our endonasal approach to the CS is available elsewhere.[4–7] In this chapter we focus on the tips and pearls that can result in a successful operation.

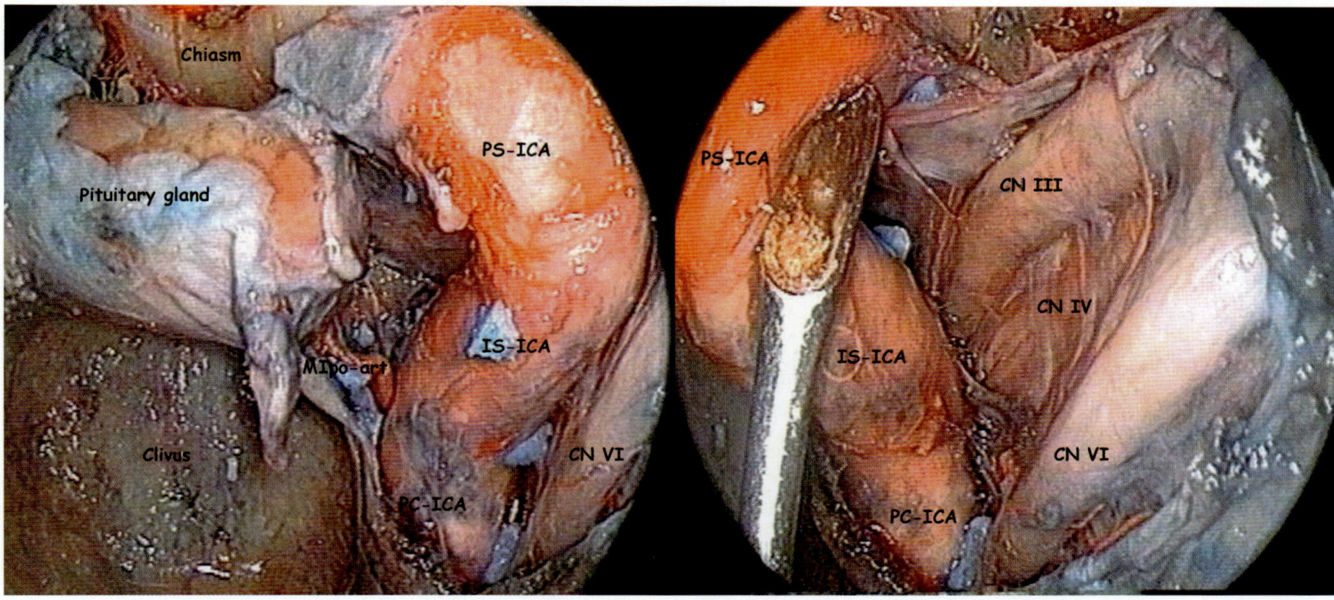

A B

Fig. 27.1 Left cavernous sinus (CS) anatomical dissection in a venous and artery injected specimen. **(A)** The medial and posterosuperior compartments. The parasellar (PS-ICA) and infrasellar (IS-ICA) portion of the internal carotid artery delimit this area laterally. The posteroinferior border of the medial compartment is the meningohypophyseal artery. No nerve crosses this area. The anteroinferior compartment is in front of the paraclival internal carotid artery (PC-ICA). Medially and inferiorly to the lower portion of the PC-ICA is the vidian artery (not visible in these images). Cranial nerve VI runs free into the lateral portion of the CS attached to the lateral wall of PC-ICA, in the medial to lateral and inferior to superior directions. **(B)** After the medial displacement of the PS-ICA and IS-ICA, the lateral compartment and posterosuperior compartment of CS are well viewed. All nerves (with the exception of cranial nerve VI) run embedded between the two layers of the lateral wall of CS: the endosteal layer medially and the meningeal layer laterally.

We recommend placing the patient in the semi-sitting position, which reduces the bleeding and enables the spontaneous outflow of blood, making the operatory field clearer and facilitating visual control of the surgical bed. The main risk of the semi-sitting position is an air embolism, but we have never observed an air embolism during the endoscopic endonasal procedure, even if we routinely apply a device necessary to detect a similar complication.

The mechanical holder maintains the position of the endoscope during the crucial phase of the procedure; it enables

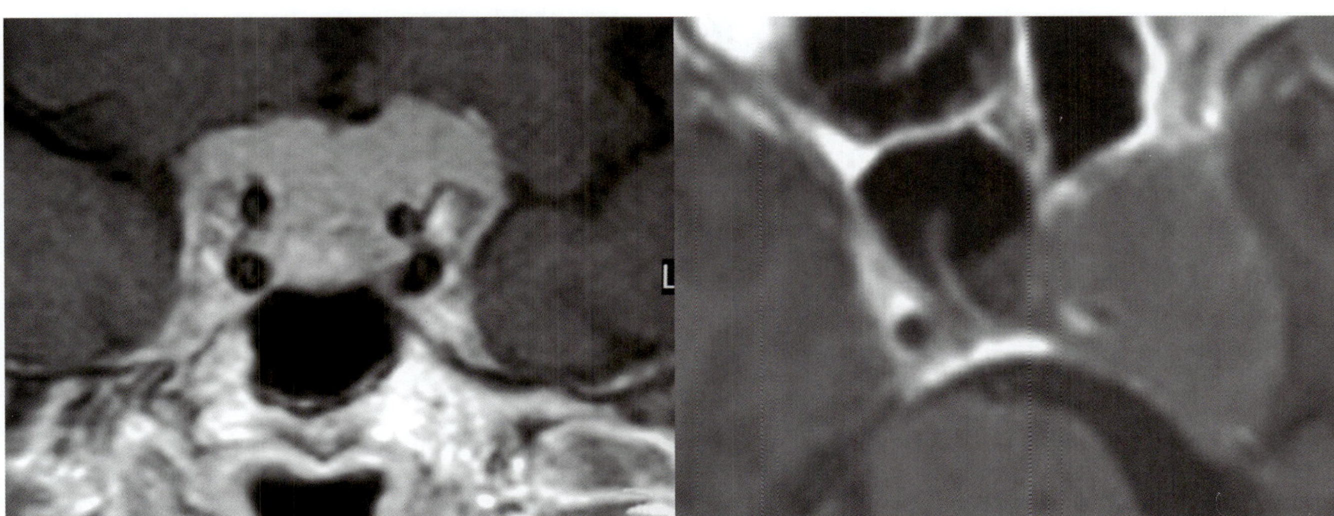

A B

Fig. 27.2 Two cases of meningioma involving the CS. **(A)** First case: A coronal view demonstrates that both CSs are infiltrated and the ICAs are totally encased by meningioma. **(B)** Second case: An axial view demonstrates the right parasellar segment of the ICA being strangled by meningioma with a small lumen.

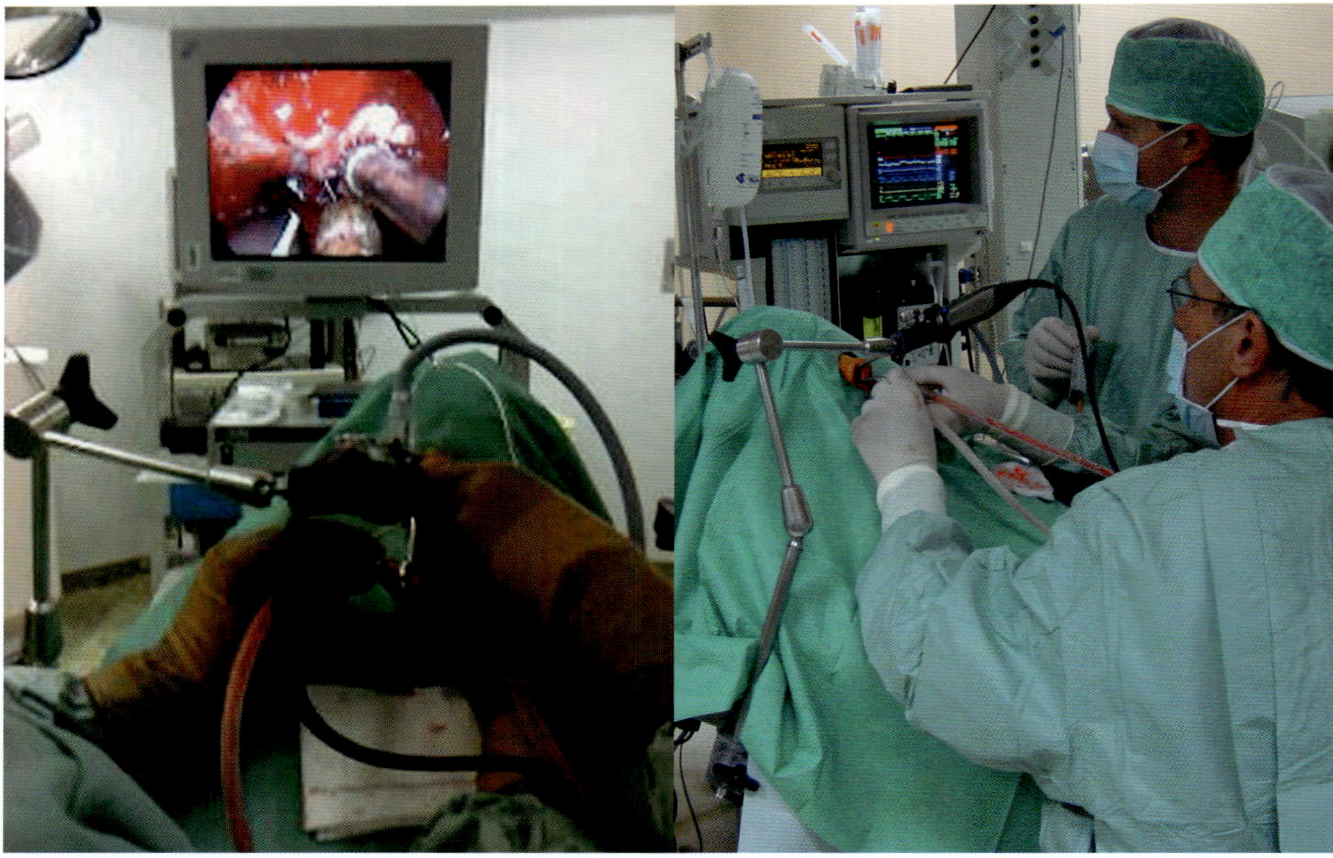

A B

Fig. 27.3 The mechanical holder and the endoscope. **(A)** Three instruments plus the endoscope are introduced simultaneously. **(B)** The adenomectomy phase. The neurosurgeon works bimanually and the other surgeon assists with another instrument or performs small adjustments to the endoscope to improve the vision.

both surgeons to work bimanually, permitting safe and precise adjustments of the position of the optics, which is necessary to avoid instrument crowding and to provide the best vision of the surgical field (**Fig. 27.3**).

Surgical Approaches

Midline Transsphenoidal Endoscopic Approach

The midline transsphenoidal endoscopic approach (MTEA) is suitable for performing an endoscopic CS surgery when the tumor involves only the medial or the posterosuperior compartments of the CS.[4,5] This approach differs from the standard approach because it is necessary to remove also the bone covering the anterior surface of the CS extending in the craniocaudal direction from the optocarotid recess to the paraclival carotid prominence and extending laterally to the border of the bulk of the tumor (**Fig. 27.4**). The dural opening begins in the sella and is extended toward the involved cavernous sinus. Normally it is possible to penetrate into the medial and posterosuperior compartments of the CS following the direction of tumor growth (**Fig. 27.5**). To improve the view into the medial compartment, it may be useful to cut the medial wall starting from its anteromedial border. The 30-degree endoscope may further increase the visual control of these compartments. The use of the Doppler helps to identify the course of the internal carotid artery (ICA) within the CS and facilitates a safe tumoral resection.

Ethmoido-Pterygo-Sphenoidal Endoscopic Approach

The ethmoido-pterygo-sphenoidal endoscopic approach (EPSEA)[1,4–7] is the procedure of choice when the tumor also involves the anteroinferior and the lateral compartments of the CS (**Fig. 27.6**).

The key point of this approach is represented by the drill-out of the superomedial portion of the pterygoid process (**Fig. 27.7A,B**). To better expose this structure, it is necessary to perform a wide medial meatotomy, which facilitates the exposure of the sphenopalatine foramen and the sphenopalatine artery, and, behind these structures, the pterygoid process. In this way a frontal exposure of the bone of the lateral sphenoid process in front to the CS is obtained (**Fig.

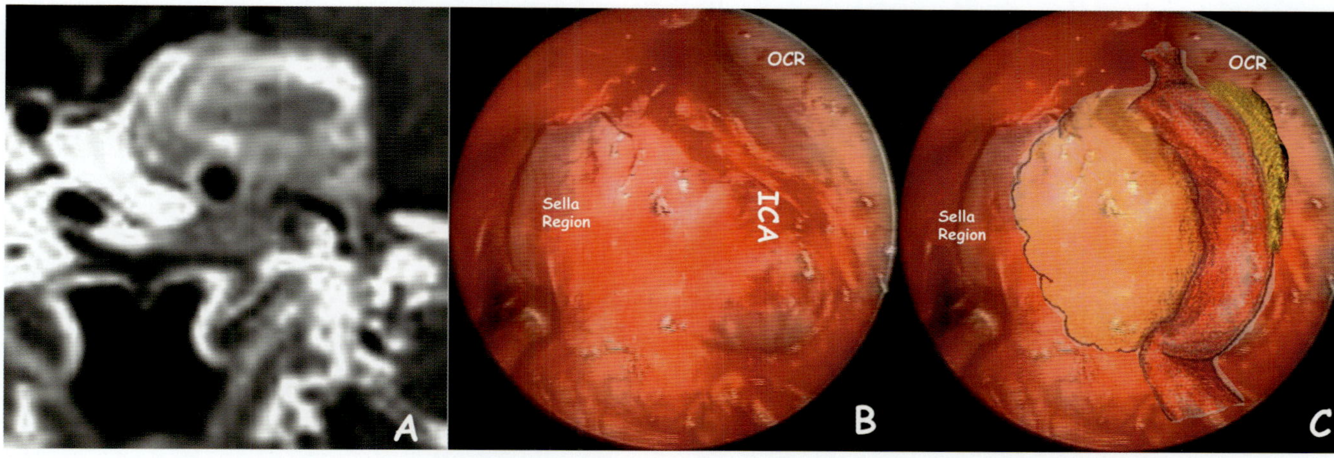

Fig. 27.4 A patient with recurrent nonfunctioning (NF) macroadenoma who was previously operated on via a transsphenoidal microsurgical approach. (A) Magnetic resonance imaging (MRI) shows the tumor growing in the left CS with total encasement of the ICA. In the sella region the fat utilized for the sella reconstruction during the previously operation is well viewed. **(B)** The bulging of the tumor in the sella and parasella area after the removal of the bone in front of the CS. **(C)** The relationship between the bulging tumor and the ICA. The only two landmarks are seen: the midline indicated by the suction tube, and the optic carotid recess (OCR).

27.7C,D). The bone to be removed to expose the sinus is a quadrilateral-shaped area. The borders are represented anterosuperiorly by the orbital apex, posterosuperiorly by the optocarotic recess, anteroinferiorly by the prominence of the second trigeminal branch, and posteroinferiorly by the prominence of the paraclival carotid artery. The opening of the periosteum in front of the lateral and anteroinferior compartment of the CS requires recognizing the displacement of the carotid artery on the MRI. Furthermore, neuronavigation with CT angiography and the Doppler helps to verify our

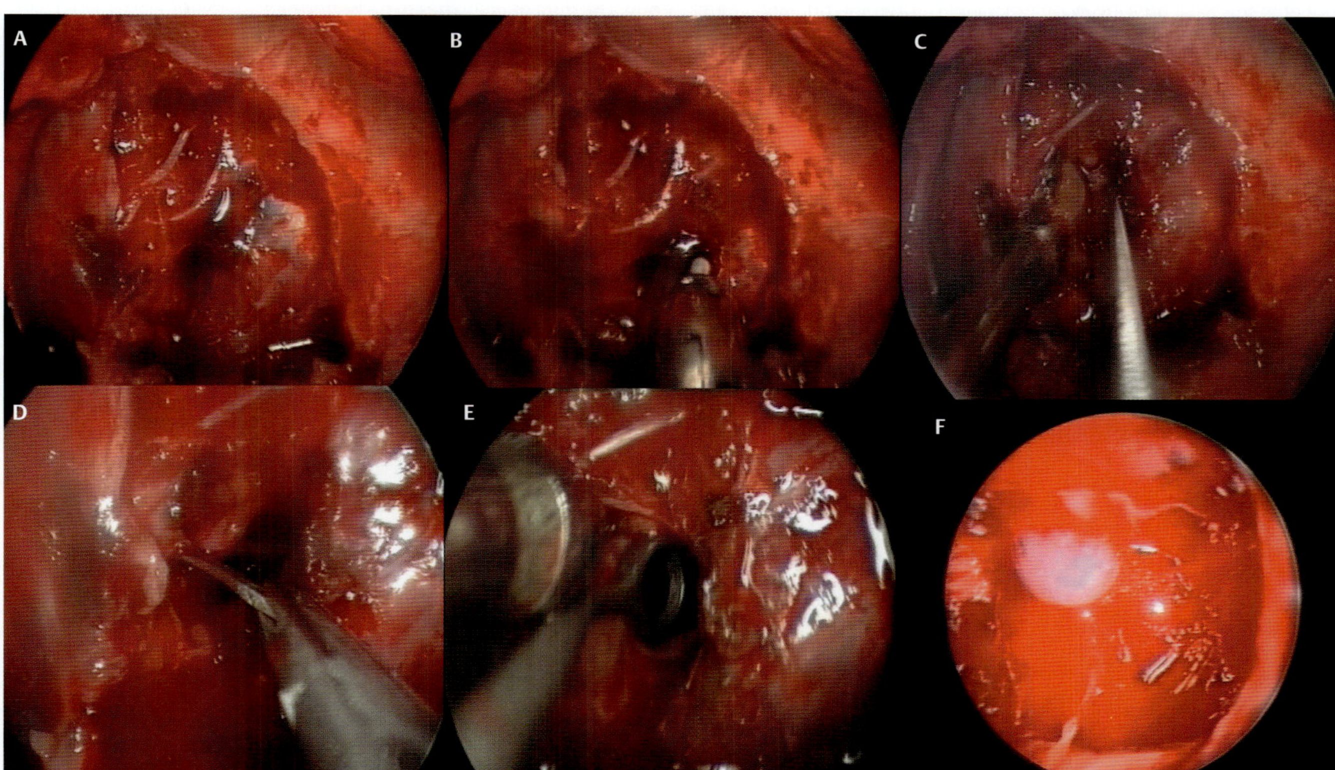

Fig. 27.5 Same patient as in Fig. 27.4. **(A)** The surgical step after the dura opening. **(B)** The intraoperative Doppler helps to localize the ICA course into the CS. After the ICA localization with a knife **(C)** and scissors **(D),** the left medial wall of the CS is opened and enlarged. **(E)** The ring curette enables the surgeon to remove the tumor piece by piece through the anterior loop of the ICA. **(F)** The exploration of the CS through the anterior loop of the ICA with the 30-degree endoscope. No macroscopic residual of the tumor is visible.

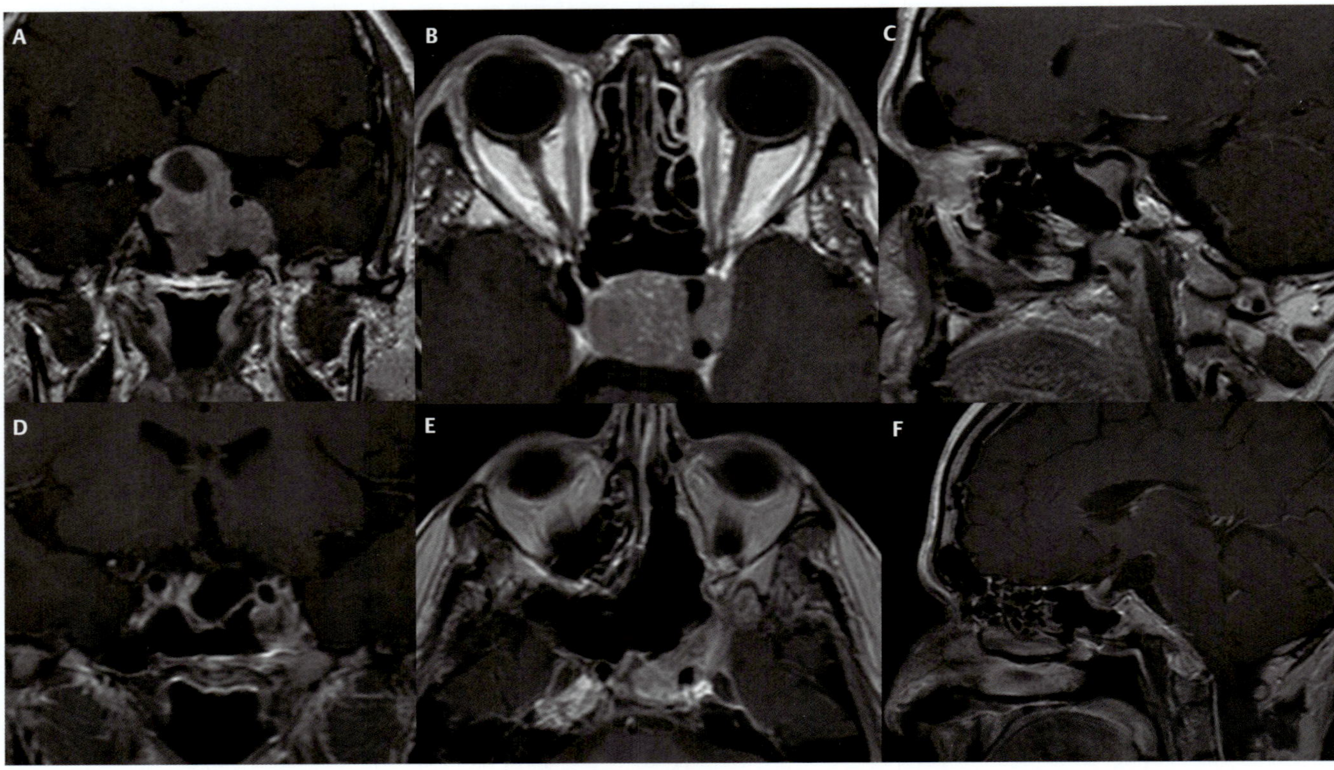

Fig. 27.6 **(A–C)** A patient with an NF macroadenoma with a cystic component in the sellar area involving the medial, anteroinferior, and lateral compartments of the CS. The sagittal view **(C)** demonstrates the intracavernous tract of the ICA. The tumor dislocates the ICA posterosuperiorly. The dura opening has to be performed inferolaterally to avoid damaging the ICA. **(D–F)** Postoperative MRI scans.

anatomical orientation, suggesting the safest point (farthest from the carotid artery) at which to start the incision (**Figs. 27.8** and **27.9**). The incision of the periosteum should be made extremely cautiously until the carotid and the sixth nerve are identified; then, the opening of the periosteum can be safely tailored to the tumor (**Figs. 27.10** and **27.11**).

In an uneventful procedure, the intervention is concluded by obtaining hemostasis, and, if no CSF leak occurred, plastic repair is not performed. Anterior nasal packing using Merocel is done only in the EPSEA, and the packing is removed after 48 hours.

Conclusion

Our technique for performing endoscopic CS surgery was briefly reported, focusing on the selection criteria and on some fundamental technical issues. Keeping in mind these suggestions, this technique appears to be safe and effective.[5,6] Nonetheless, it can be considered a complementary approach to the craniotomic route rather than an alternative. We think that this technique should be present in the armamentarium of surgeons dealing with CS tumors.

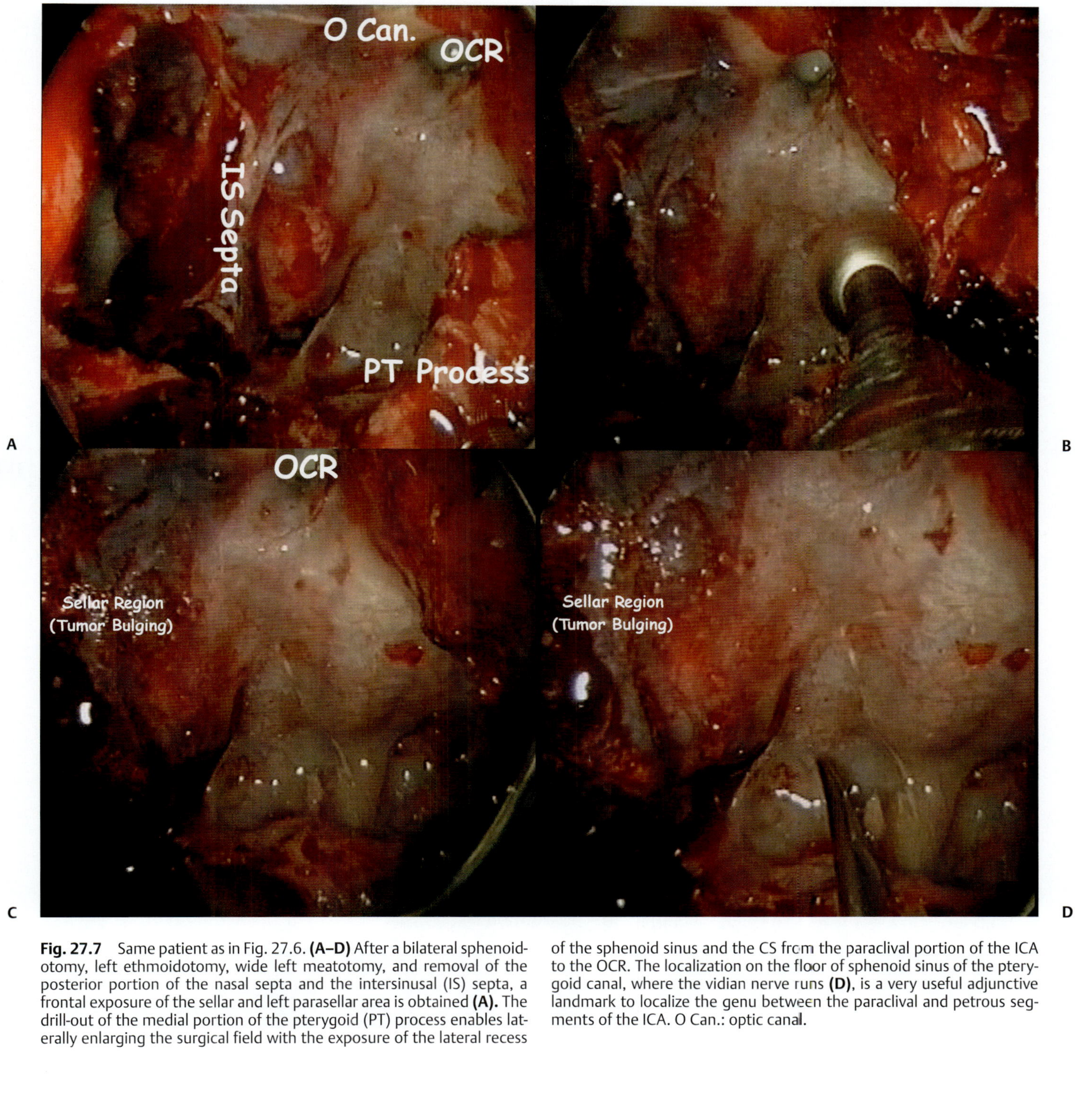

Fig. 27.7 Same patient as in Fig. 27.6. **(A–D)** After a bilateral sphenoidotomy, left ethmoidotomy, wide left meatotomy, and removal of the posterior portion of the nasal septa and the intersinusal (IS) septa, a frontal exposure of the sellar and left parasellar area is obtained **(A).** The drill-out of the medial portion of the pterygoid (PT) process enables laterally enlarging the surgical field with the exposure of the lateral recess of the sphenoid sinus and the CS from the paraclival portion of the ICA to the OCR. The localization on the floor of sphenoid sinus of the pterygoid canal, where the vidian nerve runs **(D)**, is a very useful adjunctive landmark to localize the genu between the paraclival and petrous segments of the ICA. O Can.: optic canal.

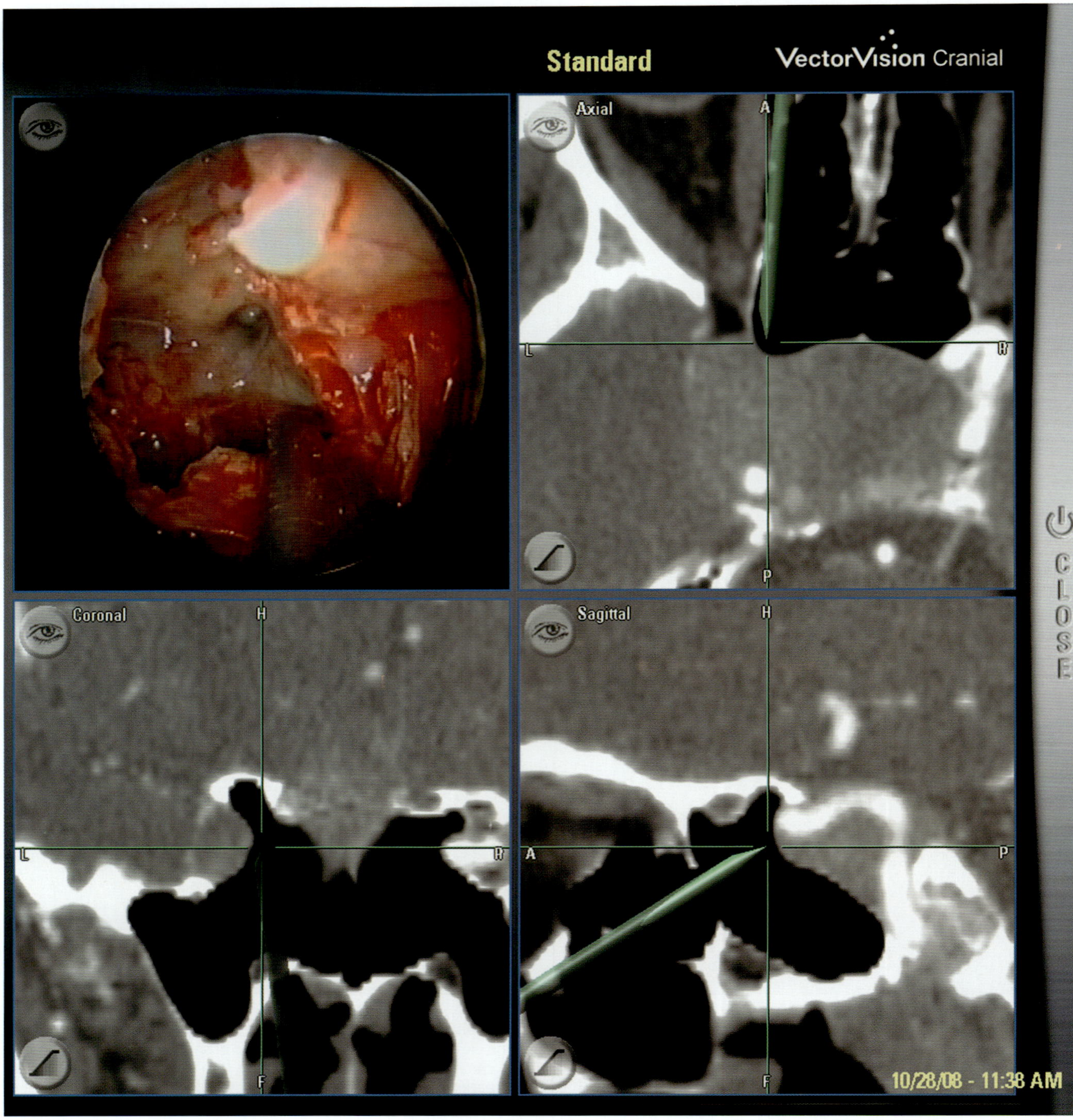

A B C D

Fig. 27.8 The neuronavigation system is a very useful device to facilitate recognizing the ICA position during the bone removal and dura opening. After the tumoral removal, the accuracy of the neuronavigation evaluation diminishes for the possible displacement of the soft tissue and the ICA.

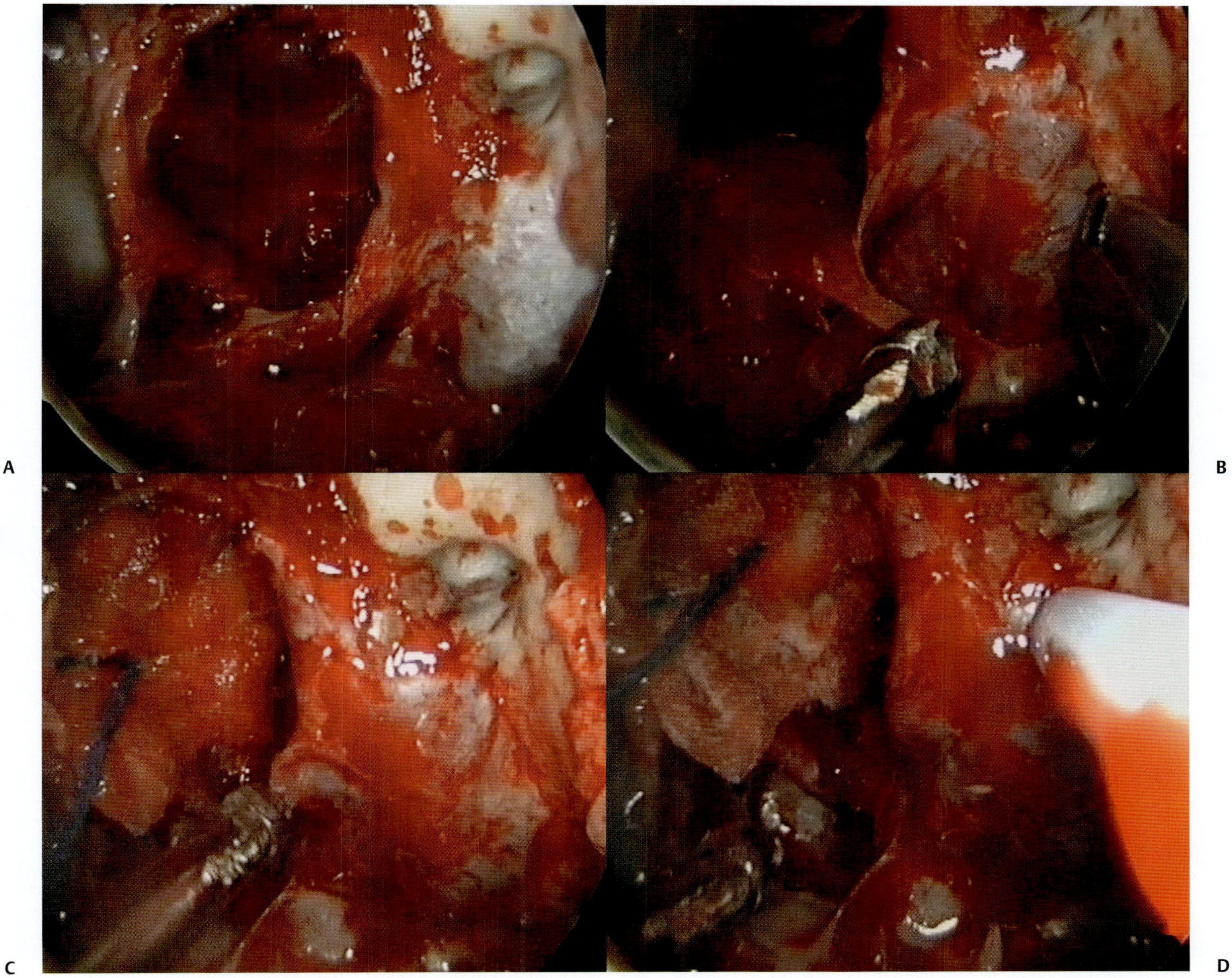

Fig. 27.9 Same patient as in Fig. 27.6. The first step of the adenomectomy is to remove the tumor from the sella cavity **(A)** as in the midline access. **(B,C)** Then the bone in front of the CS has to be removed from the sella to the lateral wall of the sphenoid sinus in front of the ICA, which is bulging below the OCR. **(D)** Another useful device to localize the ICA before the dura opening is the Doppler.

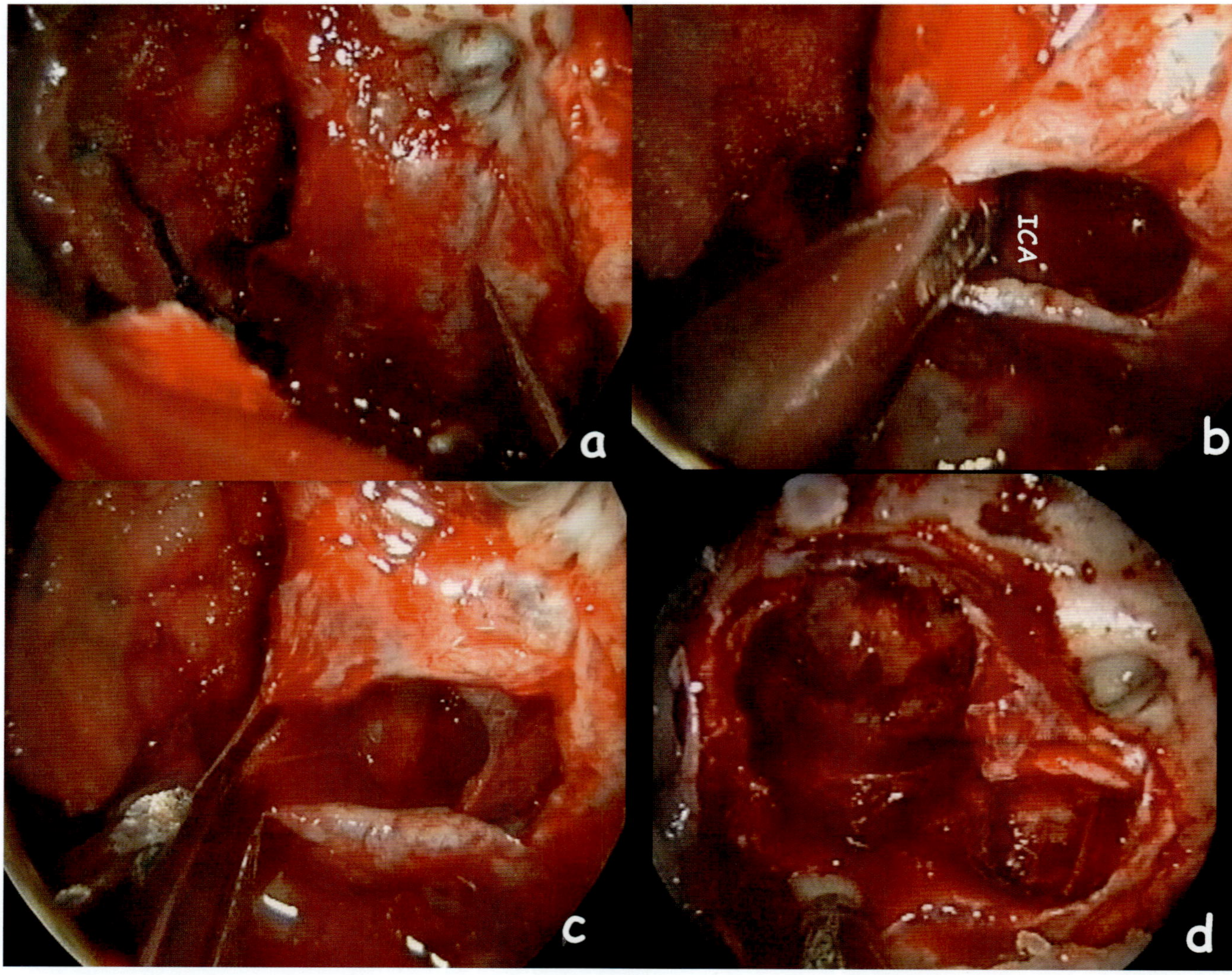

Fig. 27.10 Same patient as in Fig. 27.6. **(A–D)** The opening of the periosteum in front to the lateral and anteroinferior compartment of the CS requires recognizing the displacement of the carotid artery on MRI, confirmed by the neuronavigation system and Doppler. Then it is possible to open the periosteum with a thin knife **(A).** The incision in the periosteum should be made extremely cautiously until the carotid and the sixth nerve are identified; then the opening of the periosteum can be safely tailored to the tumor **(C). (D)** The final view of the surgical field after the adenomectomy from the sellar and parasellar region.

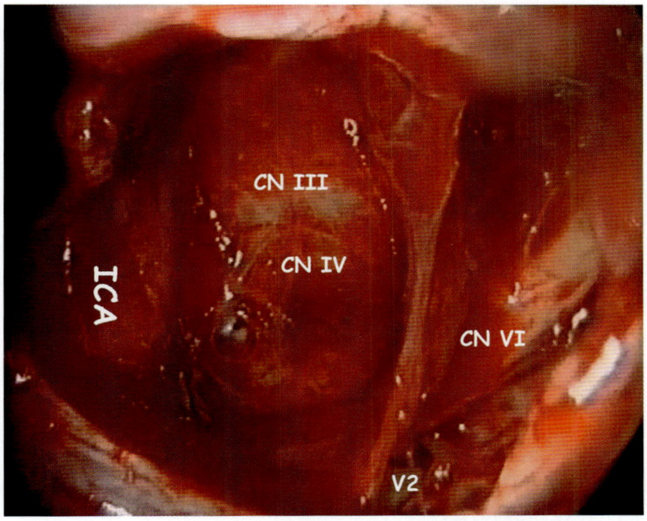

Fig. 27.11 Same patient as in Fig. 27.6. The final endocavitary exploration with the 30-degree endoscope. No residual tumor is visible. Well viewed is cranial nerve VI running free, and the other cranial nerves run into the lateral wall of the CS between the endosteal and the meningeal layer.

References

1. Jho HD, Carrau RL. Endoscopic endonasal transsphenoidal surgery: experience with 50 patients. J Neurosurg 1997;87:44–51
2. Frank G, Pasquini E, Calbucci F. Endoscopic approach to the CS via an ethmoido-pterygo-sphenoidal route. Presented at the 5th European Skull Base Society Congress, Copenhagen, Denmark, June 15–17, 2001 (additional abstract, p. 96)
3. Doglietto F, Lauretti L, Frank G, et al. Microscopic and endoscopic extracranial approaches to the cavernous sinus: anatomic study. Neurosurgery 2009;64(5, Suppl 2):413–421, discussion 421–422
4. Frank G, Pasquini E. Approach to the cavernous sinus. In: de Divitiis E, Cappabianca P, eds. Endoscopic Endonasal Transsphenoidal Surgery. New York: Springer; 2003:159–175
5. Frank G, Pasquini E. Endoscopic endonasal cavernous sinus surgery, with special reference to pituitary adenomas. Front Horm Res 2006;34:64–82
6. Frank G, Sciarretta V, Calbucci F, Farneti G, Mazzatenta D, Pasquini E. The endoscopic transnasal transsphenoidal approach for the treatment of cranial base chordomas and chondrosarcomas. Neurosurgery 2006;59(1, Suppl 1):ONS50–ONS57, discussion ONS50–ONS57
7. Pasquini E, Sciarretta V, Farneti G, Mazzatenta D, Modugno GC, Frank G. Endoscopic treatment of encephaloceles of the lateral wall of the sphenoid sinus. Minim Invasive Neurosurg 2004;47:209–213

28 Transsellar/Transdorsal Approach via a Pituitary Transposition to the Interpeduncular Cistern

Daniel M. Prevedello, Amin B. Kassam, Juan C. Fernandez-Miranda, Paul A. Gardner, Ricardo L. Carrau, and Carl H. Snyderman

Tips and Pearls

- Endoscopic endonasal management of lesions located in the interpeduncular fossa requires a multidisciplinary team.
- Common indications for an endoscopic endonasal pituitary transposition to access the interpeduncular fossa are craniopharyngiomas, meningiomas, chordomas, and other retroinfundibular lesions such as granular cell tumors, germinomas, and teratomas, among others.
- Advantages of an endoscopic ventral access transposing the pituitary gland for the management of lesions located in the interpeduncular fossa are no need for brain retraction, no manipulation of the third or optic nerves, and no need to manipulate the posterior communicating artery and its perforators.
- Contraindications to this approach include patient comorbidities, lack of availability of a multidisciplinary team, and lack of specialized equipment/instruments.
- A careful preoperative evaluation should include a physical examination, imaging studies, and pituitary panel function.
- Surgical technique includes a bilateral nasal approach by two surgeons working with a four-hand technique and dynamic real-time camera movements that facilitate continuous visualization and bimanual dissection.
- As a first step, a nasoseptal flap (if available) is designed and dissected for the reconstruction of the subsequent skull base defect. Its dimensions should be anticipated according to the planned dural defect.
- A sinonasal corridor is opened by the removal of the posterior septum, rostrum of the sphenoid sinus, face of the sella, planum sphenoidale, tuberculum sellae, and the middle third of the clivus.
- Opening of the sella is followed by the ligation and transection of the superior intercavernous sinus, to open the dura of the chiasmatic groove.
- Wide exposure of the pituitary gland is followed by lysis of the pituitary ligaments that attach its capsule to the dura. The aperture of the diaphragm is opened and the gland is transposed superiorly over the chiasm.
- Drilling of the dorsum sellae follows the ligation, cauterization, or thrombosis of the posterior intercavernous sinus. The posterior clinoids are removed and the retroclival dura is opened. Control of the basilar plexus requires intraluminal packing with hemostatic material.
- Visualization and resection of a lesion located in the interpeduncular fossa usually requires a cephalad view provided by a 45- or 70-degree angled lens endoscope.
- Reconstruction of the skull base and dural defect is completed with the vascularized nasoseptal flap.

Introduction

Few locations in the human body are guarded by as many vital structures as the interpeduncular fossa. Its anatomical boundaries consist of the optic apparatus and the third ventricle superiorly, the mamillary bodies and mesencephalon posteriorly with the basilar artery and posterior cerebral arteries, and the posterior communicating artery with its perforators along with the oculomotor nerve bracketing the region laterally.[1–3] The entire region is bordered anteriorly by the sella and its contents, including the pituitary gland and infundibulum.[3–6] Therefore, access to this region is a challenge irrespective of the surgical approach.

Conventional anterolateral skull base approaches to the interpeduncular fossa have been described. However, they all require manipulation of the lateral contents of the interpeduncular cistern, and in particular of the oculomotor nerve and posterior communicating artery.[2,7–13] Despite significant and extensive dissection, the final working space is often a small corridor between the optic nerves and tracts, cranial nerve III, and the branches of the posterior communicating artery. Ipsilateral visualization of the region directly located under the optic nerve and tract is particularly challenging.

Advances in endoscopic endonasal techniques have made possible the resection of skull base pathologies (expanded EEA endoscopic endonasal approaches).[4,14–17] This work is performed by a skull base team consisting of two surgeons working with four hands through both of the patient's nostrils. A dynamic and real-time movement of the endoscope facilitates the visualization and bimanual dissection. Endoscope holders are not recommended, as the continuous movement of the camera provides magnification as well as depth perception.[17]

Following a pituitary transposition, the EEA approach provides a direct route to the interpeduncular area without manipulation of cranial nerves. We believe that the pituitary gland is more tolerant of mobilization than any of the other structures within the interpeduncular cistern. In the event of postoperative dysfunction, it can be managed with endocrine replacement. All other surrounding structures, particularly the cranial nerves, are very sensitive, and their manipulation can produce iatrogenic deficits.[18]

Indications and Advantages

The indication for this procedure is directly related to the location and site of origin of the pathology. Any lesion behind the pituitary infundibulum requiring resection or decompression constitutes an indication for this approach. Tumors that are commonly located in this area are meningiomas, craniopharyngiomas, chordomas, chondrosarcomas, germinomas, teratomas, and granular cell tumors.

To better understand the advantages of the endoscopic endonasal pituitary gland transposition to reach the interpeduncular fossa, it is important to understand the limitations of the other approaches.

During a standard pterional approach, the structures limiting adequate exposure of the interpeduncular cistern are the optic nerves and the chiasm that limit access, mainly superiorly.[1,19] An orbitozygomatic osteotomy augments the angle of exposure; however, the approach is still limited by the position of the optic apparatus.[12] Sugita et al[20] noted these issues and described the need to retract the optic tract and mamillary bodies to reach superior aspects of the interpeduncular cistern.

The carotid-oculomotor recess can be expanded by drilling the anterior and posterior clinoid processes, unroofing the optic nerve, and opening the cavernous sinus, with mobilization of the internal carotid artery (ICA) and cranial nerve III.[1,8,21] Nevertheless, these variations generate greater morbidity by virtue of the need to mobilize neurovascular structures.[1] Most, if not all, patients who undergo this procedure suffer a transient third nerve palsy.[1,8,18,21]

An alternative access to tumors that fill the interpeduncular cistern and extend into the third ventricle involves opening the lamina terminalis through a more anterior subfrontal or interhemispheric approach.[22] However, this approach is equally limited in accessing the inferior portion of the interpeduncular cistern, and cannot be used when the floor of the third nerve is not eroded by tumor.[22,23]

Other approaches through the temporal fossa such as the transsylvian translimen insular approach and transchoroidal approach are other options to access the interpeduncular cistern.[12] However, these approaches carry the potential for significant temporal lobe dysfunction.[24]

The anterior transpetrosal approach proposed by Harsh and Sekhar[25] and the petrosectomy proposed by Kawase et al[7] provide access to the prepontine cistern, but, as with other approaches, they are limited in exposing the retrosellar area.[1]

The posterior transpetrosal approach described by Hakuba et al[2] in 1985 provides an improved caudal-cranial angle, thereby improving the access to the rostral portion of this region. However, adequate visualization of the interpeduncular cistern is obtained only by aggressive drilling of the petrous bone, which threatens hearing and balance functions.[26] Additionally, the approach still takes a lateral to medial trajectory; therefore, a corridor between the optics and the oculomotor nerve is still required. Furthermore, visualization under the ipsilateral optic tract can prove to be difficult.[2,26,27]

The extended transsphenoidal route has been used by some to approach suprasellar pathologies located in the suprasellar space adjacent to the tuberculum sellae and planum sphenoidale.[3,28–36] However, the microscopic transsphenoidal approach is limited in its parasellar exposure, particularly for lesions that extend far superiorly, laterally, or posteriorly into the perimesencephalic cisterns.[3,28,30,31,33,36–38] Kouri et al[39] pointed out that the presence of a lesion behind the stalk is one of the major limitations of the extended transsphenoidal approach. Others have suggested the use of an endoscope to improve visualization during transsphenoidal-microsurgical approaches. However, the limited working space within the speculum prevents effective maneuverability of instruments, and thus also prevents an adequate dissection.[3,14,28,30–33,36–38]

The main advantage of the pituitary transposition is to obtain adequate access and visualization to the retroinfundibular region, generating a midline approach to a midline lesion in a caudal to cranial orientation, thus avoiding manipulation of brain or cranial nerves. A total hypophysectomy should be considered when accessing lesions that have already compromised gland function, as is often the case with craniopharyngiomas.[6]

Contraindications

Care should be taken when considering a pituitary transposition in children or young adults because there is a risk of pituitary dysfunction and infertility.[40] All risks and benefits should be taken into consideration and they should be part of the informed-consent discussion with the patient and family before proceeding. Similarly, elderly patients and patients with comorbidities should be thoroughly evaluated preoperatively because they are prone to systemic complications.

We believe that the lack of multidisciplinary team cooperation is a contraindication for the procedure. The main team should include at a minimum a neurosurgeon, an otolaryngologist, and an endocrinologist, all of whom should have adequate experience. Similarly, the lack of specialized equipment, instruments (endoscope, bipolar, endo-scissors, etc.) or adequate infrastructure (intensive care unit, monitors, etc.) is also considered a contraindication for the procedure. Image-guidance systems are highly recommended.

Diagnostic Workup

Physical examination should include a neurologic assessment with special focus on cranial nerve function. A neuro-ophthalmologic examination including a formal visual field test is recommended because many lesions in the suprasellar and retroinfundibular space compromise vision.

A preoperative endocrine evaluation is critical to determine the baseline function of the pituitary gland. Furthermore, confirmation of panhypopituitarism opens the possibility for total gland resection and avoiding unnecessary surgical dissection.

Imaging

Magnetic resonance imaging (MRI) with contrast is performed on all patients to elucidate the relationship among the skull base, brain, pituitary gland, and optic nerves. A computed tomography angiography (CTA) is also performed to better establish the relationship of the tumor with the intracranial vessels, particularly the basilar artery, posterior cerebral arteries, and posterior communicating arteries. Furthermore, the CT provides better visualization of the bone, which helps in planning the approach. MRI and CTA are often fused in the image guidance system to combine all the above-mentioned characteristics.

Surgery

Instrumentation

Adequate instrumentation is paramount for the endoscopic approach to the interpeduncular fossa. Necessary equipment includes high-quality endoscopes (0-, 45-, and 70-degree), preferably high-definition (HD); video equipment (camera and monitor); long endoscopic bipolar forceps; long and precise high-speed drills (hybrid 1-, 2-, 3-, and 4-mm); long dissection instruments; and hemostatic materials such as microfibrillar cellulose and foam/paste of collagen matrix mixed with thrombin.

Operative Setup

Patients are positioned supine on the operating table with their head fixed in a Mayfield head holder, attached to the image guidance system, with the head in a neutral position and the neck slightly rotated to the right side and tilted to the left. The nose is prepared with pledgets soaked with 0.05% oxymetazoline, followed by the external application of povidone iodine solution.

Preparation

The procedure begins with the removal of the right middle turbinate. A nasoseptal flap is elevated from the widest nasal cavity (discussed below; see Repair). A posterior septectomy is performed after disarticulating the rostrum from the sphenoid bone, creating a bilateral binostril exposure to allow freedom of movement.[41] The left middle turbinate is generally lateralized and not resected.

The natural sphenoid ostium on the left side is widened to form one single cavity communicating the sphenoid sinuses with the posterior aspect of both nasal compartments. The lateral margins of the anterior sphenoidotomies are extended to the level of the medial pterygoid plates, and wide bilateral sphenoidotomies are performed.

Then, the sphenoidotomy is widened to include the lateral recess of the sphenoid extending lateral to the carotid canal, and the exposure is extended rostrally to expose the posterior cells of the ethmoid sinus to define the junction between the planum sphenoidale and the tuberculum sellae. Intrasphenoidal septations are carefully reduced with a drill, because they often lead to the vertical segment of the cavernous internal carotid artery (ICA).[42] Finally, the floor of the sphenoid is drilled back to the level of the clivus, providing adequate space for the endoscope. This creates a caudal-to-rostral trajectory into the subchiasmatic space.

Bone removal over the sellar face is initially extended laterally over the medial portions of each cavernous sinus and rostrocaudally exposing both the superior (SIS) and inferior intercavernous sinus (IIS). The tuberculum is thinned using a high-speed drill and then removed.

Approach

The dura mater over the tuberculum, the SIS, and the entire pituitary fossa is now exposed and can be opened in a cruciate fashion. During the opening, the dura overlying the sella is opened carefully along the midline to avoid transgressing the thinner underlying soft tissue layer that forms the pituitary capsule. Once this plane is established, it is followed superiorly underneath the SIS. The SIS is ligated, clipped, or preferably coagulated with a bipolar electrocautery and then transected, communicating the suprasellar and sellar dural openings.

The sellar opening is completely widened laterally and inferiorly in a cruciate manner, facilitating visualization of the entire anterior face of the gland (**Fig. 28.1**). As the dissection progresses laterally, one can appreciate that the dense dura of the sellar floor bifurcates in the direction of the cavernous

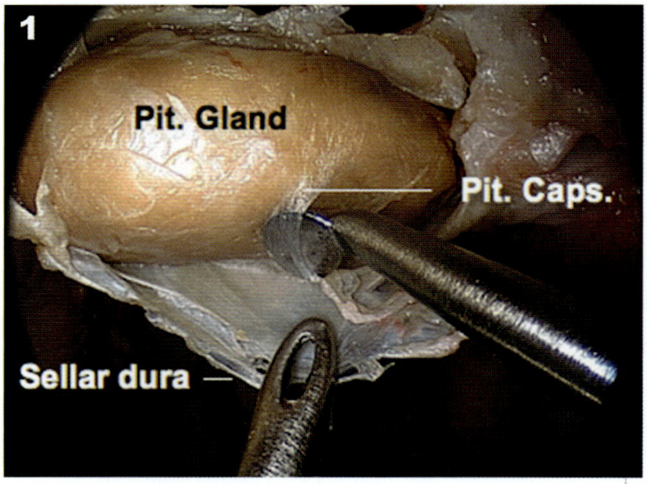

Fig. 28.1 The key for a successful pituitary transposition is preservation of the pituitary capsule, a distinct layer that must be preserved when opening sellar dura. Caps.: capsule; Pit.: pituitary.

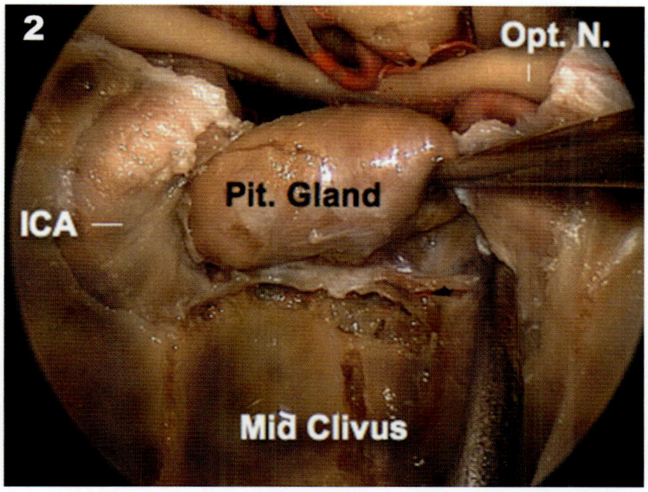

Fig. 28.2 The gland is being dissected from the floor of the sella toward the right medial cavernous sinus wall. ICA: internal carotid artery; N.: nerve; Opt.: optic; Pit.: pituitary.

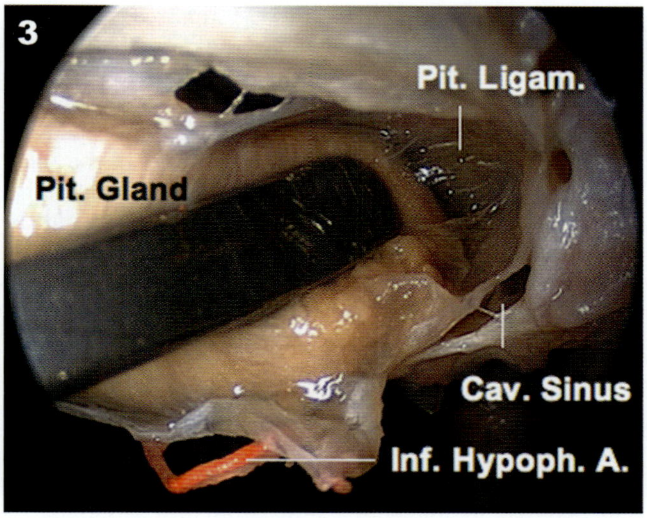

Fig. 28.3 Separation of the gland from the medial cavernous wall requires dissection of the pituitary ligaments, soft tissue attachments running between the pituitary capsule, and the wall of the cavernous sinus. A.: artery; Cav.: cavernous; Hypoph.: hypophyseal; Inf.: inferior; Ligam.: ligament; Pit.: pituitary.

sinus (**Fig. 28.2**). This fact is well appreciated when openings near the inferolateral corners of the sellar dura result in vigorous venous bleeding from projections of the cavernous sinus in between the two layers of dura. Consequently, the lateral aspect of the IIS has to be clipped occasionally.

The pituitary gland is then released from the soft tissue attachments along the plane in between the dura that forms the medial cavernous sinus wall and the pituitary capsule itself. This separation is performed in a sequence of blunt and sharp dissection. There are numerous fibrous projections connecting the pituitary capsule to the lateral sellar dura or medial cavernous sinus wall. We refer to these as the pituitary ligaments (**Fig. 28.3**). These ligaments must be systematically transected along the lateral contour of the gland along with the inferior hypophyseal and the McConnell's arteries, if present, to completely free the gland (**Fig. 28.4**).

The projection of dura that covers the sella is densely attached to the superior aspect of the capsule of the pituitary gland, and it has to be divided and finally incised in a midline direction, opening the central aperture exposing the stalk. Once the pituitary aperture is completely opened and the stalk freed, the gland can be mobilized superiorly without any resistance (**Fig. 28.5**). Once the transposition is complete, the infundibulum abuts the ventral surface of the optic

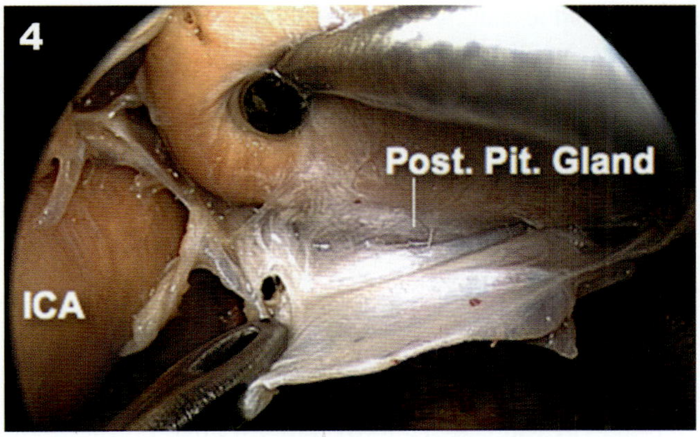

Fig. 28.4 Complete dissection of the gland from the dura at the level of the sellar floor exposes the posterior pituitary gland. ICA: internal carotid artery; Pit.: pituitary; Post.: posterior.

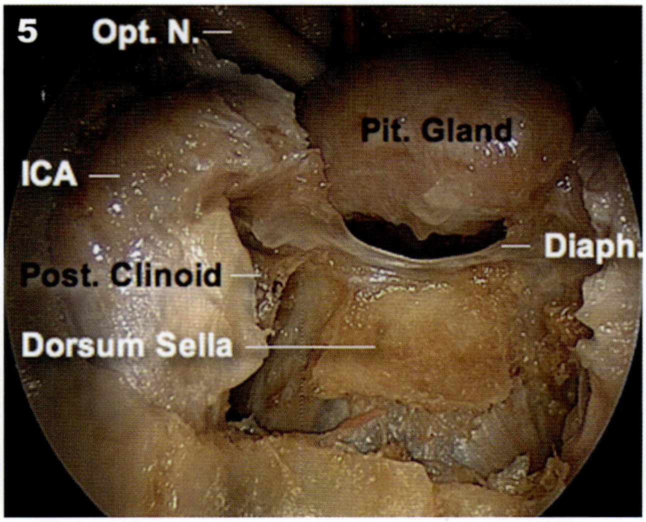

Fig. 28.5 Once the gland has been completely dissected from the surrounding dura, the pituitary aperture or diaphragm should be transected along with the superior intercavernous sinus. This allows the transposition of the gland into the suprasellar space, between the optic nerves. This maneuver exposes the dorsum sella and posterior clinoids that can now be safely removed. An osteotomy between the dorsum sella and the posterior clinoids is advised to avoid excessive traction while removing the clinoid, which can be risky for the third nerve and carotid artery. Diaph.: diaphragm; ICA : internal carotid artery; N.: nerve; Opt.: optic; Pit.: pituitary; Post.: posterior.

chiasm and the pituitary gland fills the suprasellar space and the prechiasmatic cistern. The gland is covered with fibrin glue to prevent desiccation and hold its position in the suprasellar space.

Once the pituitary gland is transposed, the entire posterior wall of the sella is visualized. The dura mater of the sellar floor is coagulated and dissected posteriorly and superiorly, exposing the dorsum sellae. This posterior dura contains the posterior intercavernous plexus.[13,43] This represents a very vascular region, and copious venous bleeding is often encountered during incision of this dura. This venous bleeding is controlled systematically using packing with hemostatic agents.

The upper third of the clivus is drilled flat along with the dorsum sellae. The posterior clinoids are also drilled and divided until they can be mobilized medially. It is imperative not to try to mobilize the posterior clinoid prior to creating a medial fracture line with a 1- or 2-mm drill bit, otherwise the posterior carotid canal could move with the posterior clinoid, creating a laceration of the internal carotid artery in the cavernous segment.

Once the exposure is completed, the dura is opened, providing access to the prepontine and interpeduncular cisterns, providing for direct access to the structures behind Liliequist's membrane. The intradural dissection proceeds with strict adherence to the neurosurgical principles. These cisterns contain critical arterial perforating vessels from the posterior circulation along with the third and sixth cranial nerves inferiorly. Identification of these structures as well as the posterior communicating artery laterally is recommended prior to proceeding with the dissection (**Fig. 28.6**).

Resection of retroinfundibular lesions proceeds with caution, often under the view of 45- or 70-degree endoscopes. The technique varies depending on the pathology of the case. The use of two suctions applying traction and countertraction during the resection is the often-employed technique to debulk the tumors. Very calcified lesions are more challenging and may require the use of ultrasonic aspirators. If the tumor extends into the anterior recess of the third ventricle, it can then be followed through the interpeduncular fossa and infundibular recess above the level of the mamillary bodies (**Fig. 28.6**) and behind the optic chiasm until the third ventricle is opened. Under direct visualization of critical neurovascular structures, the arachnoid bands covering the tumor capsule are sharply dissected, taking care to preserve the small perforators and the hypothalamic walls. It should be noted that sharp dissection is the only technique used in this region.

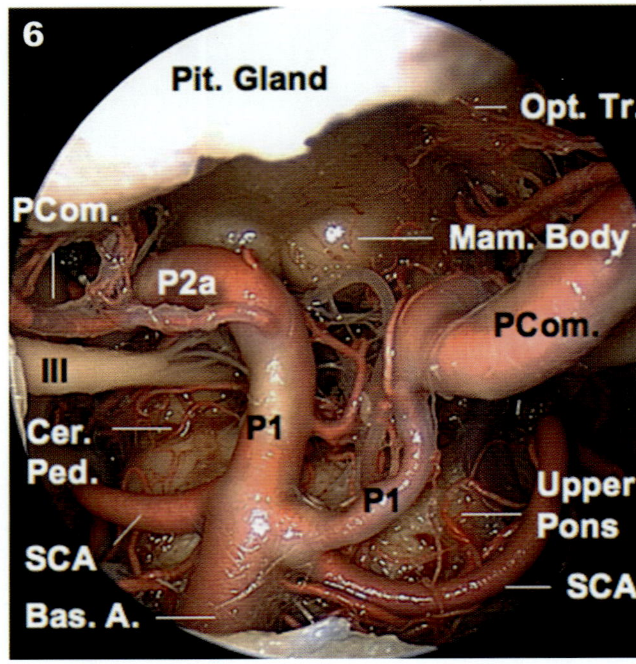

Fig. 28.6 Removal of the upper clivus (dorsum sella and posterior clinoids) provides an excellent view of the interpeduncular cistern and its contents, including basilar bifurcation, superior cerebellar arteries, posterior cerebral arteries and their branches, optic tracts, third nerves, mammillary bodies, and hypothalamic region. A.: artery; Bas.: basilar; Cer.: cerebral; Mam.: mammillary; Opt.: optic; PCom.: posterior communicating artery; Ped.: peduncle; Pit.: pituitary; SCA: superior cerebellar artery; Tr.: tract.

Repair

The defect is reconstructed with a subdural inlay graft between the brain and the dura mater. We favor the use of collagen matrix (Duragen; Integra Life Sciences, Plainsboro, NJ) as it has good tissue-handling properties, and we use it to reconstruct the arachnoid layer. Subsequently, a vascularized pedicle flap based on the posterior nasal septal artery is used for reconstruction.[44] The flap is harvested during the exposure phase of the procedure, and it is positioned in the nasopharynx. Following resection, the nasoseptal flap hinged on the posterior nasal septal artery is then positioned over the dural edges of the defect. Care should be taken to ensure that the flap makes direct and complete contact with the bony edges to promote rapid healing and a water-seal. Also, the flap should be oversized, as it has approximately a 20% contraction over time. A very thin layer of dural sealant is then used to coat the edges of the flap in a "picture frame" fashion. Sealant should not be allowed to migrate between the flap and underlying bone, as this will preclude direct contact and healing. Sponge packing or a balloon of a Foley catheter is then positioned to further buttress the flap and to mitigate the possibility of separation or migration of the flap edges. If a balloon is deemed advantageous, we use a 14-French Foley catheter that is passed from the left nostril across the residual portion of the nasal septum to the right nasal cavity, and the distal portion is placed into the upper nasopharynx across the midline and filled with saline.[15] The patient must be examined immediately postoperatively to ensure that the balloon is not compressing the optic nerves or brain. Occasionally, a lumbar spinal drain is inserted at the end of the procedure (obesity, subarachnoid hemorrhage, high flow leak).

Complications

In our initial series of pituitary transpositions, we were able to preserve the gland function in all six non-craniopharyngioma patients. In patients with craniopharyngiomas, we were able to preserve gland function in 75%.[40] Seven of eight patients (87.5%) with normal preoperative pituitary function maintained it postoperatively.

A pituitary transposition with extensive arachnoid dissection of the interpeduncular cistern, and occasional opening of the third ventricle, results in a high-flow cerebrospinal fluid (CSF) leak. Two of seven patients who had a reconstruction of the skull base utilizing a nasal septum flap developed CSF leak postoperatively. Conversely, all three patients who did not have a vascularized flap for reconstruction had a CSF leak in the postoperative period. Thus, the use of a vascularized flap significantly diminished the possibility of postoperative CSF leak in these situations ($p < .038$).[40]

Postoperative Care

Pituitary function is assessed the morning following surgery, checking the serum cortisol level. Our protocol also follows fluid balance and sodium to identify the development of diabetes insipidus. Even if the preservation of the pituitary gland function is confirmed postoperatively, it is rechecked 8 to 12 weeks later with a complete pituitary panel.

A CT of the brain is performed the same day of surgery to rule out any hemorrhagic events. A postoperative MRI is performed during the initial 24 hours postoperatively to assess the surgical resection and to rule out complications.

After removal of the packing (5 to 7 days after surgery), the operative corridor is carefully suctioned under endoscopic control. The patient is instructed to irrigate with 0.9% saline solution three to four times a day.

Patients are instructed to avoid straining physical activities, nose blowing, and sneezing with a closed mouth for a period of 6 weeks. All patients are also recommended to take stool softeners. Follow-up visits take place at least every 2 weeks or even more frequently if there is any concern. At each visit the cavity is debrided of crusts, granulation tissue, clots, and secretions. If a CSF leak is detected, the patient is taken back to the operating room as soon as possible, as a delay results in an increased risk of infection and meningitis.

A second MRI is obtained 3 months after surgery to serve as a baseline for future comparisons and surveillance.

Conclusion

The endoscopic endonasal approach with pituitary transposition is an effective way to expose the retroinfundibular region at the interpeduncular cistern. It has the advantage of being a midline approach to access midline lesions, avoiding all the lateral boundaries of the interpeduncular cistern, which are rich in vital neurovascular structures. In addition, transposition of the pituitary gland followed by removal of the dorsum sellae and the posterior clinoids facilitates direct subchiasmatic/retrochiasmatic access into the heart of any lesion located in the interpeduncular, prepontine cistern as well as the anterior recess of the third ventricle.

Reconstruction using a vascularized flap is essential to reduce the postoperative morbidity related to CSF leaks. We strongly recommend that the endoneurosurgeon only consider this approach after accumulating a reasonable amount of experience, as the risk of complications is significant.

References

1. Figueiredo EG, Zabramski JM, Deshmukh P, Crawford NR, Preul MC, Spetzler RF. Anatomical and quantitative description of the transcavernous approach to interpeduncular and prepontine cisterns. Technical note. J Neurosurg 2006;104:957–964
2. Hakuba A, Nishimura S, Inoue Y. Transpetrosal-transtentorial approach and its application in the therapy of retrochiasmatic craniopharyngiomas. Surg Neurol 1985;24:405–415
3. Kaptain GJ, Vincent DA, Sheehan JP, Laws ER Jr. Transsphenoidal approaches for the extracapsular resection of midline suprasellar and anterior cranial base lesions. Neurosurgery 2001;49:94–100, discussion 100–101
4. Kassam A, Snyderman CH, Mintz A, Gardner P, Carrau RL. Expanded endonasal approach: the rostrocaudal axis. Part II. Posterior clinoids to the foramen magnum. Neurosurg Focus 2005;19:E4
5. Maira G, Anile C, Albanese A, Cabezas D, Pardi F, Vignati A. The role of transsphenoidal surgery in the treatment of craniopharyngiomas. J Neurosurg 2004;100:445–451
6. Zuccaro G. Radical resection of craniopharyngioma. Childs Nerv Syst 2005;21:679–690
7. Kawase T, Toya S, Shiobara R, Mine T. Transpetrosal approach for aneurysms of the lower basilar artery. J Neurosurg 1985;63:857–861
8. Krisht AF. Transcavernous approach to diseases of the anterior upper third of the posterior fossa. Neurosurg Focus 2005;19:E2
9. Menovsky T, Grotenhuis JA, de Vries J, Bartels RH. Endoscope-assisted supraorbital craniotomy for lesions of the interpeduncular fossa. Neurosurgery 1999;44:106–110, discussion 110–112
10. Perneczky A, Fries G. Endoscope-assisted brain surgery: part 1—evolution, basic concept, and current technique. Neurosurgery 1998;42:219–224, discussion 224–225
11. Shirane R, Hayashi T, Tominaga T. Fronto-basal interhemispheric approach for craniopharyngiomas extending outside the suprasellar cistern. Childs Nerv Syst 2005;21:669–678
12. Ulm AJ, Tanriover N, Kawashima M, Campero A, Bova FJ, Rhoton A Jr. Microsurgical approaches to the perimesencephalic cisterns and related segments of the posterior cerebral artery: comparison using a novel application of image guidance. Neurosurgery 2004;54:1313–1327, discussion 1327–1328
13. Yasuda A, Campero A, Martins C, Rhoton AL Jr, de Oliveira E, Ribas GC. Microsurgical anatomy and approaches to the cavernous sinus. Neurosurgery 2005;56(1, Suppl):4–27 discussion 4–27
14. Frank G, Pasquini E, Doglietto F, et al. The endoscopic extended transsphenoidal approach for craniopharyngiomas. Neurosurgery 2006; 59(1, Suppl 1):ONS75–ONS83, discussion ONS75–ONS83
15. Kassam A, Carrau RL, Snyderman CH, Gardner P, Mintz A. Evolution of reconstructive techniques following endoscopic expanded endonasal approaches. Neurosurg Focus 2005;19:E8
16. Kassam A, Snyderman CH, Mintz A, Gardner P, Carrau RL. Expanded endonasal approach: the rostrocaudal axis. Part I. Crista galli to the sella turcica. Neurosurg Focus 2005;19:E3
17. Kassam AB, Gardner P, Snyderman C, Mintz A, Carrau R. Expanded endonasal approach: fully endoscopic, completely transnasal approach to

the middle third of the clivus, petrous bone, middle cranial fossa, and infratemporal fossa. Neurosurg Focus 2005;19:E6

18. Seoane E, Tedeschi H, de Oliveira E, Wen HT, Rhoton AL Jr. The pretemporal transcavernous approach to the interpeduncular and prepontine cisterns: microsurgical anatomy and technique application. Neurosurgery 2000;46:891–898, discussion 898–899
19. Sano H, Kato Y, Akashi K, et al. Operation on high-lying basilar bifurcation aneurysms. Surg Neurol 1997;48:458–464
20. Sugita K, Kobayashi S, Shintani A, Mutsuga N. Microneurosurgery for aneurysms of the basilar artery. J Neurosurg 1979;51:615–620
21. Krisht AF, Kadri PA. Surgical clipping of complex basilar apex aneurysms: a strategy for successful outcome using the pretemporal transzygomatic transcavernous approach. Neurosurgery 2005;56(2, Suppl): 261–273, discussion 261–273
22. Fahlbusch R, Honegger J, Paulus W, Huk W, Buchfelder M. Surgical treatment of craniopharyngiomas: experience with 168 patients. J Neurosurg 1999;90:237–250
23. Maira G, Anile C, Colosimo C, Cabezas D. Craniopharyngiomas of the third ventricle: trans-lamina terminalis approach. Neurosurgery 2000; 47:857–863, discussion 863–865
24. Nagata S, Sasaki T. The transsylvian trans-limen insular approach to the crural, ambient and interpeduncular cisterns. Acta Neurochir (Wien) 2005;147:863–869
25. Harsh GR IV, Sekhar LN. The subtemporal, transcavernous, anterior transpetrosal approach to the upper brain stem and clivus. J Neurosurg 1992;77:709–717
26. Tummala RP, Coscarella E, Morcos JJ. Transpetrosal approaches to the posterior fossa. Neurosurg Focus 2005;19:E6
27. Seifert V, Raabe A, Zimmermann M. Conservative (labyrinth-preserving) transpetrosal approach to the clivus and petroclival region—indications, complications, results and lessons learned. Acta Neurochir (Wien) 2003; 145:631–642, discussion 642
28. Couldwell WT, Weiss MH, Rabb C, Liu JK, Apfelbaum RI, Fukushima T. Variations on the standard transsphenoidal approach to the sellar region, with emphasis on the extended approaches and parasellar approaches: surgical experience in 105 cases. Neurosurgery 2004;55: 539–547, discussion 547–550
29. Doglietto F, Prevedello DM, Jane JA Jr, Han J, Laws ER Jr. Brief history of endoscopic transsphenoidal surgery—from Philipp Bozzini to the First World Congress of Endoscopic Skull Base Surgery. Neurosurg Focus 2005;19:E3
30. Dumont AS, Kanter AS, Jane JA Jr, Laws ER Jr. Extended transsphenoidal approach. Front Horm Res 2006;34:29–45
31. Dusick JR, Esposito F, Kelly DF, et al. The extended direct endonasal transsphenoidal approach for nonadenomatous suprasellar tumors. J Neurosurg 2005;102:832–841
32. Frank G, Pasquini E, Mazzatenta D. Extended transsphenoidal approach. J Neurosurg 2001;95:917–918
33. Kim J, Choe I, Bak K, Kim C, Kim N, Jang Y. Transsphenoidal supradiaphragmatic intradural approach: technical note. Minim Invasive Neurosurg 2000;43:33–37
34. Kitano M, Taneda M. Extended transsphenoidal approach with submucosal posterior ethmoidectomy for parasellar tumors. Technical note. J Neurosurg 2001;94:999–1004
35. Laws ER Jr. Transsphenoidal microsurgery in the management of craniopharyngioma. J Neurosurg 1980;52:661–666
36. Laws ER, Kanter AS, Jane JA Jr, Dumont AS. Extended transsphenoidal approach. J Neurosurg 2005;102:825–827, discussion 827–828
37. de Divitiis E. Endoscopic transsphenoidal surgery: stone-in-the-pond effect. Neurosurgery 2006;59:512–520, discussion 512–520
38. de Divitiis E, Cappabianca P. Microscopic and endoscopic transsphenoidal surgery. Neurosurgery 2002;51:1527–1529, author reply 1529–1530
39. Kouri JG, Chen MY, Watson JC, Oldfield EH. Resection of suprasellar tumors by using a modified transsphenoidal approach. Report of four cases. J Neurosurg 2000;92:1028–1035
40. Kassam AB, Prevedello DM, Thomas A, et al. Endoscopic endonasal pituitary transposition for a transdorsum sellae approach to the interpeduncular cistern. Neurosurgery 2008;62(3, Suppl 1):57–72, discussion 72–74
41. Kassam AB, Snyderman C, Gardner P, Carrau R, Spiro R. The expanded endonasal approach: a fully endoscopic transnasal approach and resection of the odontoid process: technical case report. Neurosurgery 2005;57(1, Suppl):E213, discussion E213
42. Fernandez-Miranda JC, Prevedello DM, Madhok R, et al. Sphenoid septations and their relationship with internal carotid arteries: anatomical and radiological study. Laryngoscope 2009;119:1893–1896
43. Théron J, Chevalier D, Delvert M, Laffont J. Diagnosis of small and micro pituitary adenomas by intercavernous sinus venography. A preliminary report. Neuroradiology 1979;18:23–30
44. Kassam AB, Thomas A, Carrau RL, et al. Endoscopic reconstruction of the cranial base using a pedicled nasoseptal flap. Neurosurgery 2008; 63(1, Suppl 1):ONS44–ONS52, discussion ONS52–ONS53

VIII Tips and Pearls in Endoscopic Transclival Surgery

29 Endoscopic Anatomy of the Clivus and Posterior Fossa

Luigi Maria Cavallo, Isabella Esposito, Matteo De Notaris, Felice Esposito, Manfred Tschabitscher, and Paolo Cappabianca

Tips and Pearls

Key points of the endonasal approaches to the midline posterior cranial fossa are as follows:

Cranial level

- Wide anterior sphenoidotomy
- Sellar floor and tuberculum sellae removal
- Pituitary gland elevation/transposition (superior/inferior hypophyseal arteries)
- Dorsum sellae and posterior clinoids removal (oculomotor nerve)

Middle level

- Mucosal dissection up to the vomero-sphenoid junction/vidian nerves
- Vomer resection
- Removal of the inferior sphenoid sinus wall (intrapetrous carotid artery)
- Clival bone removal (paraclival carotid arteries, abducent nerve)

Caudal level

- Mucosal dissection up to the vomero-sphenoid junction/vidian nerves
- Vomer resection
- Removal of the inferior sphenoid sinus wall (intrapetrous carotid artery)
- Mucosal and muscles dissection (parapharyngeal carotid artery)
- Exposure of the foramen magnum (hypoglossal nerve)
- C1 anterior arch removal (vertebral artery)
- Dens removal

Introduction

The idea driving the evolution of skull base surgery is the creation of surgical corridors molded on the three-dimensional orientation of the main neurovascular structures. The part of the ventral skull base extended from the retrosellar area to the upper cervical spine has been exposed through several anterior, anterolateral, and posterolateral routes,[1–5] performed with conventional or keyhole exposure,[6] or with microsurgical,[7] endoscope-assisted or pure endoscopic techniques.[8–11] Such variety of surgical strategies corresponds to the challenging complex anatomy of this region.

Because the lesions arising in the midline posterior skull base often displace the neurovascular structures dorsally and laterally, an anterior surgical window through the natural endonasal corridor is attractive and the endoscopic technique provides a dynamic close-up view of such deep areas and of the neurovascular structures bordering the surgical corridors itself.

The endoscopic endonasal approach enables access to the entire sphenoid, clivus, and craniovertebral junction; this route has been used for the management of either extradural or intradural lesions from the retrosellar area down to the craniovertebral junction.[10,12–22]

The main preconditions for using this technique are multidisciplinary cooperation,[23] thorough anatomic knowledge,[24,25] advanced surgical skills,[26,27] and familiarity with state-of-the-art imaging techniques, dedicated surgical instruments, and reconstruction strategies and materials.[28] Cadaver-laboratory endoscopic dissections represent the first step in improving the surgeon's orientation and self-confidence; such exercises are mandatory to understand the anatomy of the skull base and to acquire a three-dimensional orientation, which will be of value also when unlocking the posterior cranial fossa through lateral and posterior routes.

This chapter describes the endoscopic endonasal approach to the posterior cranial fossa and highlights the main anatomic relationships and potential problems of the technique. To simplify the anatomic description, we divide the posterior skull base into three levels (**Fig. 29.1**):

- Cranial: from the posterior interclinoid line to the floor of the sella turcica, which corresponds to the retrosellar area
- Middle: from the floor of the sella turcica to the line connecting the hypoglossal canals
- Caudal: at level of the craniovertebral junction

The measures reported in this chapter derive from several anatomic studies.[24] However, they are highly variable, as demonstrated by the wide standard deviations reported in the original papers. Furthermore, to improve the incisiveness of the anatomic description, we have omitted the analysis of many important anatomic variations; nevertheless, the surgeon must have thorough knowledge about these variations before applying this technique on patients.

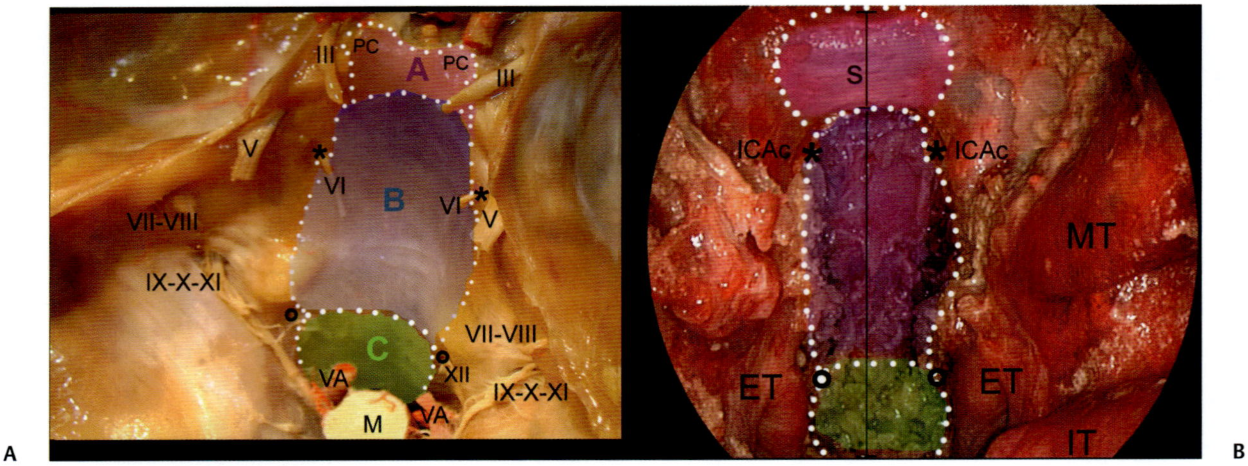

Fig. 29.1 Transcranial **(A)** and endoscopic endonasal **(B)** views of the midline posterior cranial base. The overlapped drawing shows the extension of the bone window during the endoscopic endonasal approach to the posterior skull base. The dotted lines border the surgical windows to expose the retrosellar area (*pink area,* A), retroclival area (*blue area,* B), and craniovertebral junction (*green area,* C). ET: eustachian tube; ICAc: paraclival segment of the internal carotid artery; IT: inferior turbinate; M: medulla; MT: middle turbinate; PC: posterior clinoid; S: sella; VA: vertebral artery; *: Dorello's point; circle: hypoglossal canal; black line: midline. *Nerves:* III: oculomotor nerve; V: trigeminal nerve; VI: abducens nerve; VII-VIII: acoustic-facial bundle; IX-X-XI: lower cranial nerves; XII: hypoglossal nerve.

Imaging Techniques

Recent advances in three-dimensional reconstruction techniques and measurement software have greatly improved the surgeon's ability to perform detailed preoperative planning.[29,30] State-of-the-art imaging technologies (Amira® Visage Imaging Inc., San Diego; Osirix®, Advanced Open-Source PACS Workstation DICOM viewer) permit the study of the individual anatomy, thus spurring the virtual reality of the imaging to be part of the preoperative workup.

High-resolution computed tomography scan with coronal and sagittal reconstruction and both soft tissues and bone algorithms addresses the paranasal sinuses, skull base foramina, and canals. In particular, the following points should be assessed in determining the feasibility of the approach:

- Pneumatization of the sphenoid sinus: in a conchal-type sphenoid sinus, the clival indentation below the sella is not visible; sphenoidal and rhinopharyngeal segments of the clivus are not clearly identified, which makes the exposure more difficult
- Bone dehiscence at the level of both parasellar and paraclival carotid prominences
- Vidian canal on axial and coronal images and its relation to the foramen lacerum
- Carotid canal
- Configuration of the posterior clinoids
- Configuration of the craniovertebral junction

Magnetic resonance imaging is complementary to computed tomography, but it is unable to delineate the fine osseous details required for endoscopic skull base surgery; the examination is performed in the axial, coronal, and sagittal planes with 3-mm sections. The comparison between a T2-weighted image, a T1-weighted image, and contrast-enhanced T1-weighted images enables assessment of either normal anatomy or pathology of the skull base. Inflammatory tissue and fluid in the paranasal sinuses can be separated from tumoral tissue with the T2-weighted image. Fat-saturation T1-weighted sequences reduce misinterpretation of signal from adipose tissue. They are mandatory to evaluate the parapharyngeal space adjacent to the skull base; the exit foramina of the cranial nerves, which contain fatty tissue; and recurrent skull base lesions. These sequences also improve the definition of clival pathology because it contains bone marrow. The internal carotid artery and the other vascular structures are better defined by magnetic resonance angiography and digital subtraction angiography; this latest is the best method to delineate the vascular supply of a specific anatomical area or lesion; however, it rarely has a diagnostic value and its main indication is preoperative tumor endovascular embolization.

Endoscopic Endonasal Approach

According to the guidelines highlighted by the creation of the endonasal corridor for an extended endoscopic endonasal approach to the skull base and namely to the clival area requires the following steps:

- Removal of one middle turbinate, usually the right one; the other middle turbinate is pushed laterally
- Middle meatal antrostomy preserving the uncinate process and extending inferiorly as necessary, on the side where the middle turbinate has been removed
- Creation of a pedicled nasoseptal flap on the septal branch of the right sphenopalatine artery, which is positioned into the maxillary sinus through the created antrostomy; this flap is used to reconstruct the surgical access in the multilayered reconstruction

- Detachment of the nasal septum from the sphenoid keel and removal of its posterior part (approximately 2 cm) to widen the working corridor
- Posterior or total bilateral ethmoidectomy, as necessary
- Wide anterior sphenoidotomy (taking care of the posterior nasal artery)
- Removal of the intrasphenoidal septa, with flattening the whole sphenoid wall to better host the nasoseptal flap for the reconstruction
- Identification of sphenoidal bony landmarks—sella, planum sphenoidale, medial and lateral opto-carotid recesses, and clival indentation—could help the surgeon's orientation

At this point two surgical corridors can be used, one above and the other below the inferior wall of the sphenoid sinus. The *superior corridor* leads to the sellar area and to the sphenoidal portion of the clivus. The *inferior corridor* leads to the rhinopharyngeal segment of the clivus, the foramen magnum, and craniovertebral junction.

As stated above, we divide the posterior cranial fossa in three levels (**Fig. 29.2**). This conceptual classification was inspired by the neurovascular structures bordering the surgical window, and for each level we will describe the exposure and the intradural exploration.

The main steps to expose the retrosellar area (cranial level of the posterior skull base) are as follows:

- Opening of the sella and the tuberculum sellae
- Removal of the medial opto-carotid recess and the sellar floor
- Identification of the superior and inferior hypophyseal arteries

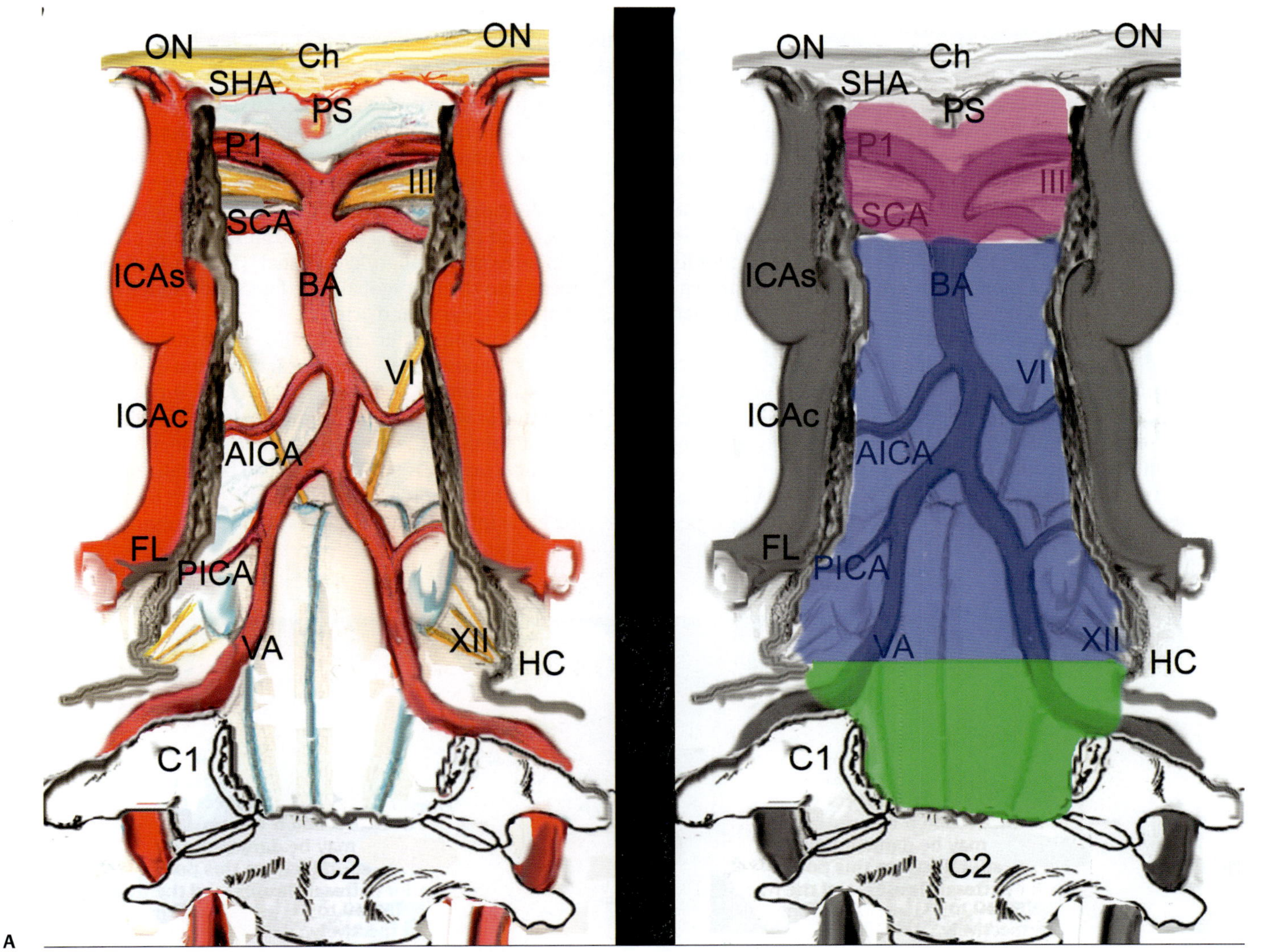

Fig. 29.2 Schematic drawings showing the intradural neurovascular structures exposed through the endonasal route **(A)** and the borders of the three surgical windows (retrosellar, retroclival, and craniovertebral junction) **(B)**. C1: atlas; C2: epistropheus; Ch: chiasm; FL: foramen lacerum; HC: hypoglossal canal; ICAc: paraclival segment of the internal carotid artery; ICAs: parasellar segment of the internal carotid artery; ON: optic nerve; P1: precommunicating segment of the posterior cerebral artery; PICA: posterior inferior cerebellar artery; PS: pituitary stalk; SCA: superior cerebellar artery; VA: vertebral artery; pink area: cranial level; blue area: middle level; green area: caudal level. *Nerves:* III: oculomotor nerve; VI: abducens nerve; XII: hypoglossal nerve.

- Mobilization of the gland[17]
- Drilling of the sellar floor and dorsum sellae
- Removal of the posterior clinoids

The parasellar segment of the internal carotid artery borders laterally the surgical corridor; "kissing carotid arteries" should be ruled out preoperatively and are a contraindication to the transdorsum exposure of the retrosellar area.

Depending on the superior extension of the area to be exposed, the gland can be mobilized on one side or reflected upward. The Pittsburgh group has applied an en-bloc transposition technique.[17] This technique requires complete disconnection of the gland from the pituitary fossa, which is obtained by cutting the ligaments that anchor the capsule to the medial wall of the cavernous. The neurohypophysis, which has a jelly-like appearance, is more firmly attached posteriorly and should be detached sharply. During this last maneuver, overpressure of the dissector should be avoided because a certain degree of dehiscence of the dorsum can be found. Furthermore, a persistent trigeminal artery may be located just posterior to the neurohypophysis; in fact, such a vessel can leave the cavernous sinus through either the dorsum or the dura lateral to it. During such maneuvers, the hypophyseal cistern should be preserved; in elderly patients it may become larger and extend laterally or to the neurohypophysis. These arachnoidal diverticula can be dissected and fixed out from the surgical corridor with a few drops of fibrin glue. The same technique can be used to fix the gland after its dislocation. The critical point of this step is avoiding stretching the pituitary stalk and the subsequent possible wallerian degeneration of the hypothalamic neurons.

In our dissection, selective dislocation of the central part of the gland could be obtained with a V-shaped cut; the lateral parts of the gland are left in place (**Fig. 29.3**). This strategy may reduce the length of this step and the stretching of the infundibulum.

These techniques need larger surgical series before being validated as standard procedures and are controversial, especially in the case of purely retrosellar lesions that do not alter the pituitary function.

Drilling of the sellar floor enhances the working area before starting the transdorsum approach and provides a certain degree of pituitary mobility, which could be enough when exposing of the prepontine cistern.

During the drilling of the dorsum sellae, the working area is funnel-shaped because the intercarotid distance at the anterior wall of the sella is approximately 20 mm[24] whereas the posterior interclinoidal distance is approximately 15 mm[24]; this places the neurovascular structures into the parasellar area at risk of injury.

Furthermore, the lateral surface of the sella should be inspected for the presence of sellar bridges, which are bands of bone running between the anterior and posterior clinoids and should be fractured carefully before removal of the posterior clinoids.

The removal of both sphenoidal and rhinopharyngeal segments of the clivus exposes the middle level of the posterior skull base, through the following steps (**Fig. 29.4**)[8]:

- Identification, in a medial to lateral direction, of the vomer-sphenoid junction, the anterior foramen of the palatovaginal canal, and the pterygoid canal. The vaginal process of the medial pterygoid plate has a groove on its inferior surface that articulates with the sphenoidal process of the palatine bone, thus forming the palatovaginal canal (or pharyngeal canal) (**Fig. 29.4A,B**), which opens into the pterygopalatine fossa and carries the pharyngeal nerve and artery.
- Removal of the vomer and drilling of the inferior wall of the sphenoid sinus. The lateral extension of bone removal is limited by the pterygoid canal. It runs through the inferior wall of the sphenoid sinus, toward the anterior genu of the petrous segment of the internal carotid artery (ICA).[31] This canal can be localized 0.5 cm laterally to the vomero-sphenoid junction.[32] By drilling the bone inferomedially to this canal, the surgical

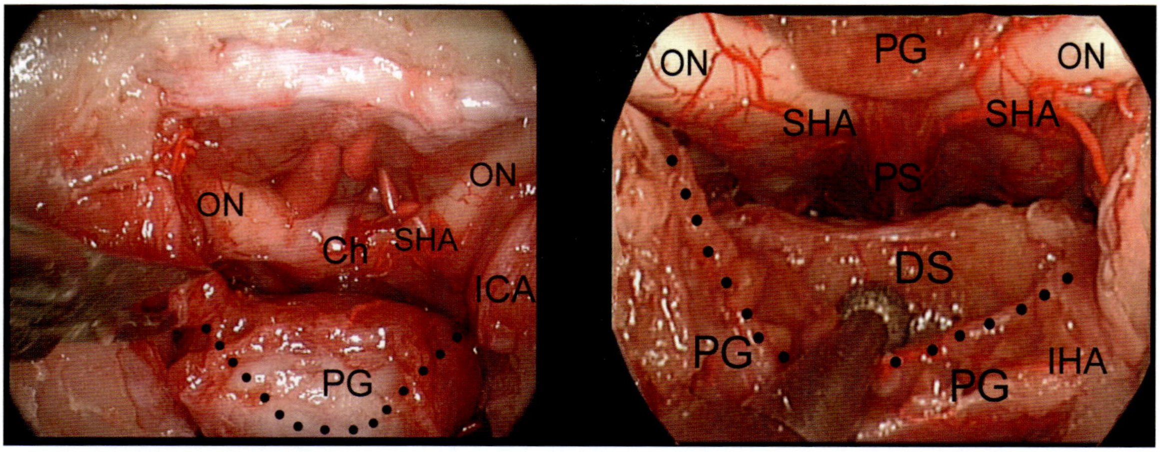

Fig. 29.3 (A,B) Exposure of the upper clivus (cranial level) realized through an upward transposition of the pituitary gland. Ch: chiasm; DS: dorsum sellae; ICA: internal carotid artery; IHA: inferior hypophyseal artery; ON: optic nerve; PG: pituitary gland; PS: pituitary stalk; SHA: superior hypophyseal artery; dotted line: borders of the transglandular transposition.

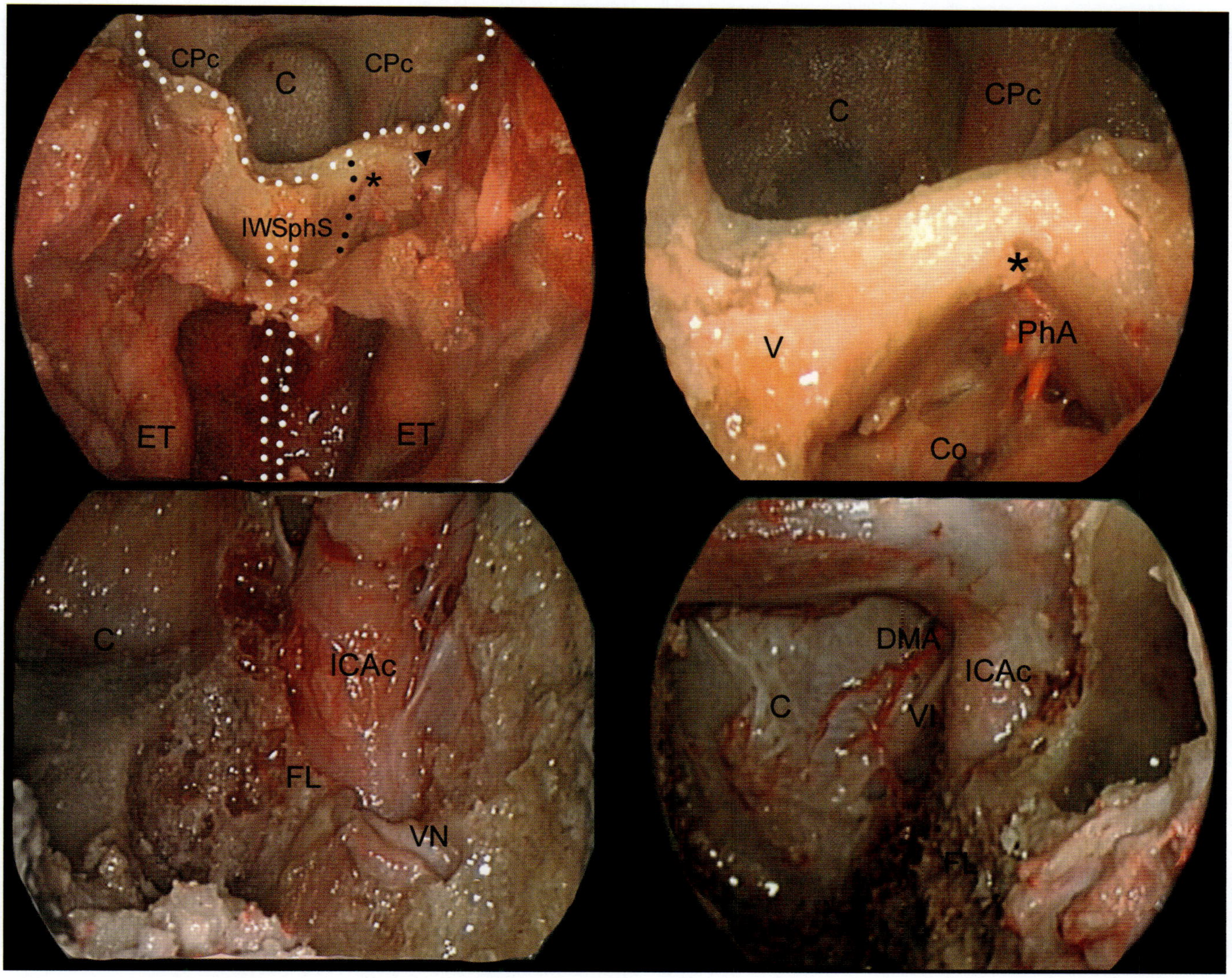

Fig. 29.4 (A–D) Exposure of the clivus (middle level). C: clivus; Co: choana; CPc: paraclival tract of the carotid protuberance; DMA: dorsal meningeal artery; ET: eustachian tube; FL: foramen lacerum; ICAc: paraclival segment of the internal carotid artery; IWSphS: inferior wall of the sphenoid sinus; PhA: pharyngeal artery; V: vomer; VN: vidian nerve; VI: abducens nerve; the white dotted lines border the anterior sphenoidotomy and vomer removal; the black dotted line borders the vomerosphenoid junction; *: palatovaginal canal; arrowhead: vidian canal.

corridor can be widened while reducing the risk of tearing the ICA (**Fig. 29.4C**).

- Dissection of the rhinopharyngeal mucosa and lateralization of the *longus capitis* and *longus colli* muscles
- Identification of the foramen magnum and hypoglossal canals
- Drilling of the clival bone

The lateral boundaries of the surgical corridor are represented on both sides by the following:

- Paraclival segment of the ICA and foramen lacerum
- Abducens nerve
- Medial pterygoid plate and eustachian tube
- Hypoglossal canal

Paraclival carotid arteries are separated by a distance of approximately 17 mm.[24] Cranial nerve VI crosses the basilar plexus when entering the cavernous sinus[33]; its dural porus, under the superior sphenopetrous ligament, at Dorello's point, is situated an average of 20 mm below the posterior clinoid process and 1 cm from the midline. The dorsal meningeal artery is in close relationship with the nerve at this level, thus representing a useful landmark to preserve the nerve itself (**Fig. 29.4D**).

The foramen lacerum is formed by the body of the sphenoid bone anteromedially, by the petrous apex posteriorly, and by the border of the great sphenoidal wing laterally. Medially it is plugged by fibrous tissue and cartilage, being a point of minor resistance, and special care should be taken when exposing the petrous apex. Below this landmark the surgical window enlarges.

The eustachian tube lies parallel and lateral to the petrous ICA, representing a valuable landmark to preserve it when approaching the infratemporal fossa or the jugular foramen through the rhinopharynx.[15]

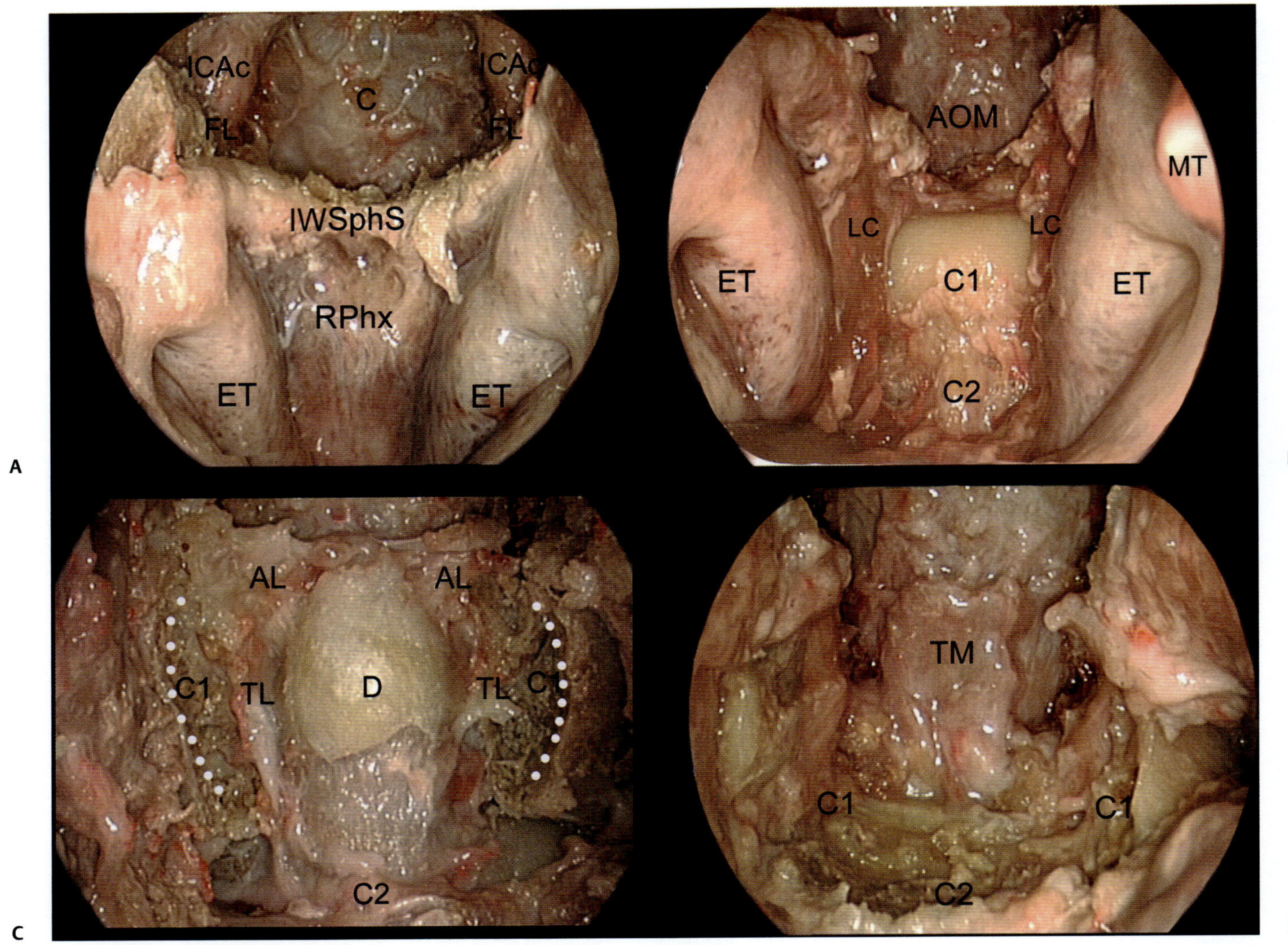

Fig. 29.5 (A–D) Exposure of the craniovertebral junction (caudal level). AL: alar ligament; AOM: atlo-occipital membrane; C: clivus; C1: atlas; C2: axis; D: dens; ET: eustachian tube; FL: foramen lacerum; ICAc: paraclival segment of the internal carotid artery; IWSphS: inferior wall of the sphenoid sinus; LC: longus colli muscle; MT: middle turbinate; RPhx: rhinopharynx; TL: transverse ligament; TM: tectorial membrane; dotted line: lateral borders of the removal of the anterior arch of C1.

The caudal level of the posterior skull base is exposed in correspondence to the craniovertebral junction through the following steps (**Fig. 29.5**)[34,35]:

- Flattening the vomer down to the hard palate
- When necessary, the soft palate can be pulled downward with a suture applied through the mouth
- C-shaped incision of the mucosa of the rhinopharynx
- Elevation of longus colli and longus capitis muscles from their medial attachment and their shifting to the side
- Identification of the caudal edge of the clivus and disinsertion of the atlanto-occipital membrane from C1
- Removal of the anterior edge of the foramen magnum and drilling of the medial third of the occipital condyles
- Identification of the anterior tubercle of the atlas
- Removal of the anterior arc of C1
- Cut of the apical and alar ligaments
- Drilling of the dens until it becomes eggshell-like, keeping the base intact
- Removal of the dens fracturing its base in a postero-anterior direction
- Sharp dissection of the transverse ligament and the tectorial membrane from the underlying dura

The C-shaped incision of the mucosa of the rhinopharynx protects the blood supply of the soft parts through the ascending and greater palatine and the ascending pharyngeal arteries. At the level of the craniovertebral junction, the dura is covered by the tectorial membrane, which extends downward from the middle clivus and represents the superior extension of the posterior longitudinal ligament of the spinal canal; this membrane and the longitudinal part of the cruciform ligament are incised with the dura.

The surgical window is bordered by the hypoglossal canal.[36] It is possible to wide the opening by removing the anterior third of the occipital condyles, without entering the hypoglossal canal, which is located above the junction of the anterior and middle third of each occipital condyle.[37] This bony canal is approximately 15 mm from the midline and 9 mm above the intradural entry of the vertebral artery.[24] During drilling of the occipital condyle, the change from cancellous to cortical bone indicates that the hypoglossal canal has been reached. Opening it will cause bleeding from the venous plexus surrounding the nerve.

Intradural Exploration

A T-shaped dura incision allows the dura to be retracted back to the edges of the bone window. The basilar venous sinus should be managed upon opening the dura.

After opening the dura mater, it is important to identify the different neurovascular structures; knowledge of the anticipated anatomical variations is an important contributor to the safety of the operation.

Cranial Level

The endonasal view of the cranial level can be expanded up to the floor of the third ventricle, interpeduncular fossa, and the mesial surface of the temporal lobe. The oculomotor nerve emerges from the midbrain on the medial surface of the cerebral peduncle, bordered by the posterior cerebral artery (PCA) above, and the superior cerebellar artery (SCA) below it (**Fig. 29.6A,B**). It runs along the lateral aspect of the anterior incisural space, inferomedial to the uncus, toward the roof of the cavernous sinus. The posterior communicating artery courses posteromedially below the floor of the third ventricle; from its superior and lateral aspect several perforators penetrate the floor of the third ventricle between the optic chiasm and the cerebral peduncle (**Fig. 29.6C**). Running the endoscope below the oculomotor nerve, the inferior surface and the free edge of the tentorium are visualized with the trochlear nerve running below the free edge of the

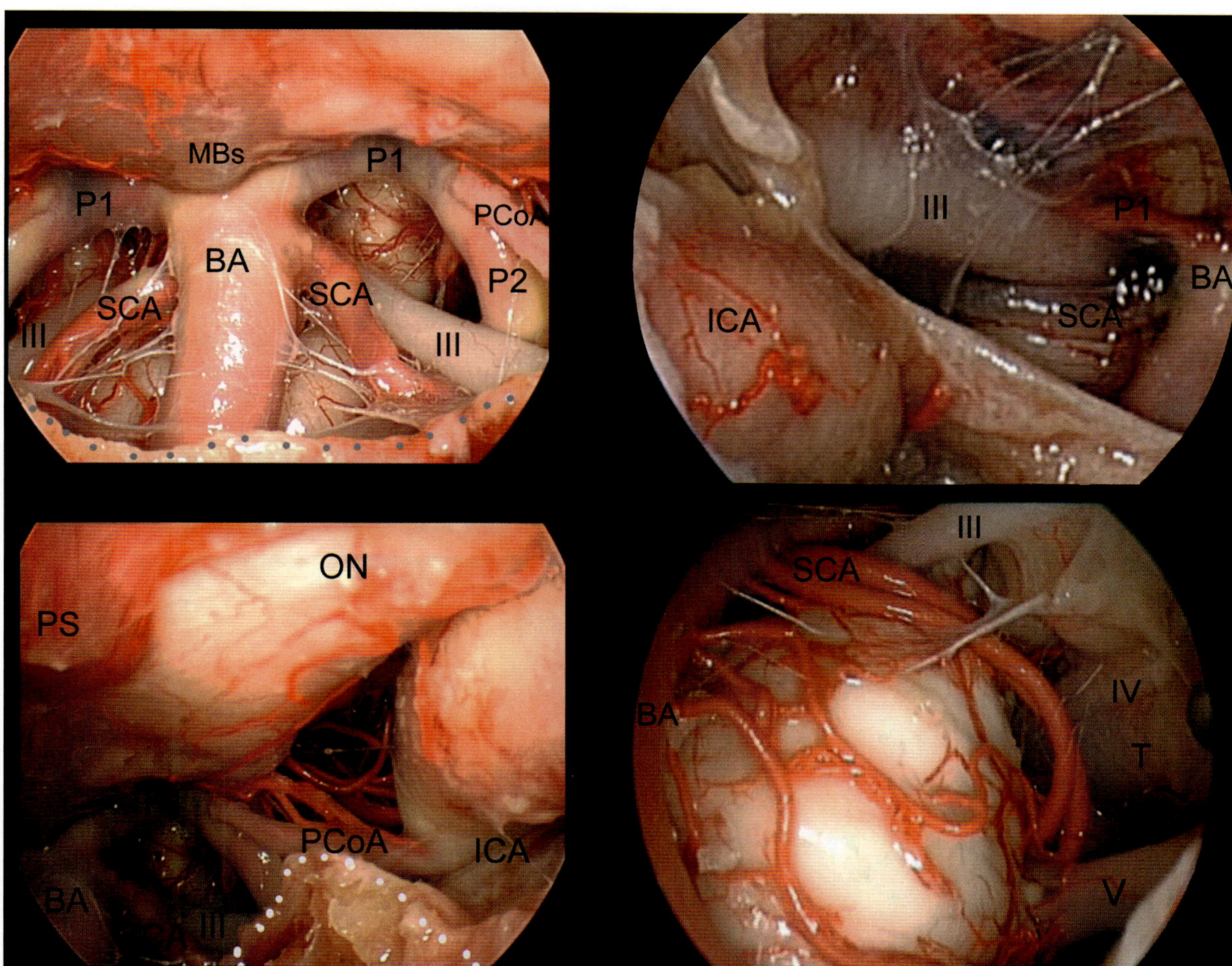

Fig. 29.6 (A–D) Cranial level: intradural exploration of the retrosellar space. BA: basilar artery; MBs: mammillary bodies; ON: optic nerve; P1: precommunicating segment of the posterior cerebral artery; P2: postcommunicating segment of the posterior cerebral artery; PCoA: posterior communicating artery; PS: pituitary stalk; SCA: superior cerebellar artery; T: tentorium. *Nerves:* III: oculomotor nerve; IV: trochlear nerve; V: trigeminal nerve.

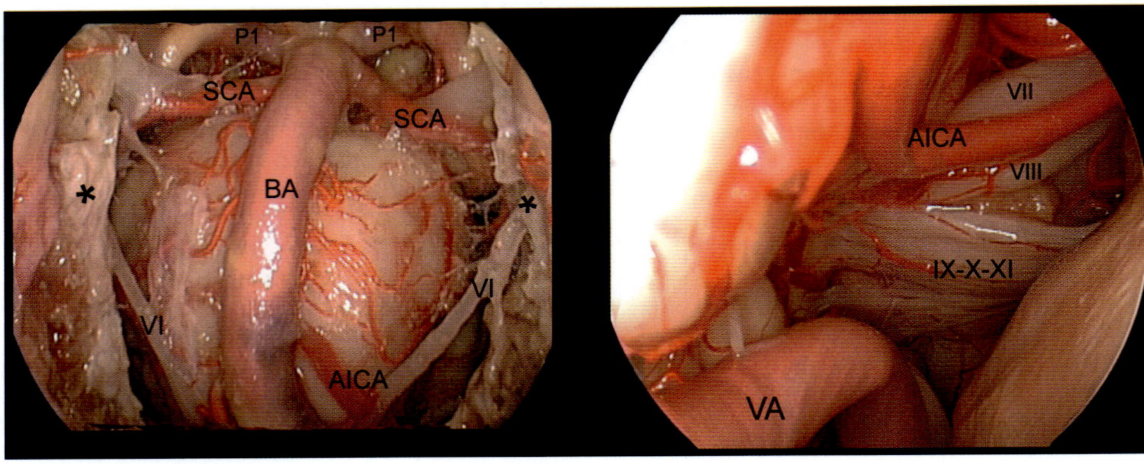

A B

Fig. 29.7 (A,B) Middle level: intradural exploration. AICA: anteroinferior cerebellar artery; BA: basilar artery; P1: precommunicating segment of the posterior cerebral artery; SCA: superior cerebellar artery; VA: vertebral artery; *: entry point of the abducens nerve. *Nerves:* VI: abducens nerve; VII-VIII: acoustic-facial bundle.

tentorium. The pontomesencephalic segment of the SCA leads to the entry zone of the trigeminal nerve (**Fig. 29.6D**).

Middle Level

The cisternal segment of the abducens nerve ends when it pierces the dura mater of the clivus (Dorello's point) (**Fig. 29.7**). On the midline, the entire ventral surface of the pons and the medulla oblongata and the basilar artery, arising from the two vertebral arteries, are visualized. Pointing the endoscope above the cisternal segment of the abducens nerve, upward, the entry zone of the trigeminal nerve can be exposed; the trigeminal porus lies approximately 5 mm above and lateral to the Dorello's point. Pointing laterally the endoscope, below the abducens nerve, the anteroinferior cerebellar artery (AICA) can be followed toward the acoustic-facial bundle; just below it lie the lower cranial nerves; the jugular foramen lies approximately 14 mm lateral to the Dorello's point. The posteroinferior cerebellar artery (PICA) or its branches can be found anterior to the lower cranial nerves.

Caudal Level

The vertebral artery and the origin of the PICA are identified (**Fig. 29.7**). The rootlets of the hypoglossal nerve may be stretched by these vessels, and sometimes they look so small and flimsy that they are mistaken for arachnoid bands. These rootlets converge toward the hypoglossal canal through one or more small dural pori (**Fig. 29.8A**). Extending bone removal

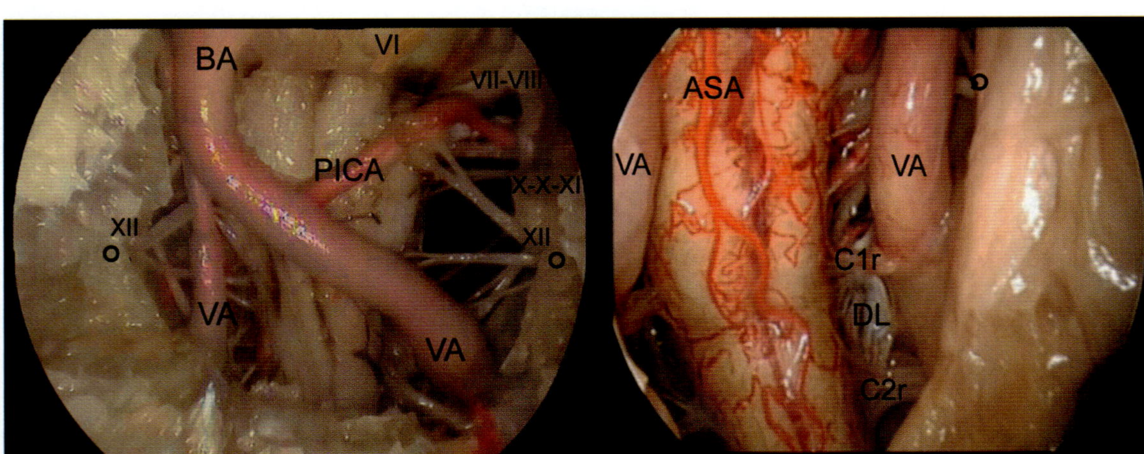

A B

Fig. 29.8 (A,B) Caudal level: intradural exploration. ASA: anterior spinal artery; BA: basilar artery; C1r: first cervical rootlets; C2r: second cervical rootlets; DL: dentate ligament; PICA: posteroinferior cerebellar artery; VA: vertebral artery; circle: hypoglossal canal. *Nerves:* VI: abducens nerve; VII-VIII: acoustic-facial bundle; XII: hypoglossal nerve.

below the hypoglossal canal and angling the endoscope laterally, the intradural segment of the vertebral artery can be followed toward its dural entry. The anterior spinal artery, the ventral and dorsal rootlets of C1 and C2, and the dentate ligament between them are identified (**Fig. 29.8B**).

■ Pedicled Flaps Used to Reconstruct the Posterior Skull Base

Several vessels offer the opportunity to reinforce the multilayered reconstruction[38] of the skull base with a pedicled flap:

- The posterior nasal artery can feed a mucosal nasoseptal flap.[39]
- The artery of the inferior turbinate can feed a mucoperichondrial flap.
- The descending palatine artery is the root of the posterior palatal flap, which may be of value for redo cases.[40]

The mucosal nasoseptal flap, initially described by Hadad et al[41] and popularized by the Pittsburgh group,[38] is created ipsilaterally to the middle turbinectomy and middle antrostomy and is obtained through the following steps:

1. Sagittal incision at the junction between the floor of the nasal cavity and the nasal septum (anterior to the soft palate, which can be palpated with the instrument)
2. Mucosal incision over the sphenoid rostrum, just below the level of the sphenoidal rostrum, in a lateral to medial direction
3. Sagittal septal incision approximately 1.5 cm below the roof of the nasal cavity, and connection of this incision with the first one
4. Anterior vertical septal incision joining the two sagittal incisions (posterior to the projection of the most anterior aspect of the inferior turbinate over the septum)
5. Dissection of the flap from the nasal septum with a sharp instrument in an anterior to posterior direction
6. Harvesting of the flap in the homolateral maxillary sinus

During the positioning of the flap, the stretching of the vascular pedicle should be avoided and the perichondral surface should be carefully identified and positioned over the bony defect. The flap and its vascular pedicle will shrink approximately 30%[39]; however, if needed, the reconstruction surface can be widened by applying free mucoperichondrium from the middle turbinate or other pedicled flaps. The inferior turbinate flap provides less vascularized tissue and has a limited arch of rotation.

The posterior palatal flap requires the creation of a palatal flap with preservation of its vascular pedicle, the descending palatine vessels, which are mobilized from the pterygopalatine canal; the flap is then transposed into the nasal cavity through the palatal defect. Care should be taken in preserving the nasal floor mucosa overlying the palatal defect, to reduce the risk of oronasal fistula.

References

1. Beals SP, Joganic EF, Hamilton MG, Spetzler RF. Posterior skull base transfacial approaches. Clin Plast Surg 1995;22:491–511
2. Welch WC, Kassam A. Endoscopically assisted transoral-transpharyngeal approach to the craniovertebral junction. Neurosurgery 2003;52:1511–1512
3. Bambakidis NC, Gonzalez LF, Amin-Hanjani S, et al. Combined skull base approaches to the posterior fossa. Technical note. Neurosurg Focus 2005;19:E8
4. Kassam AB, Patel A, Welch W, et al. The carotid-vertebral space: an "extended" lateral window to the ventromedial cranial base and lower craniocervical junction. Ear Nose Throat J 2005;84:312–315
5. De Monte F, Dannenbaum M, Hanna E. Clival tumors. In: Hanna E, De Monte F, eds. Comprehensive Management of Skull Base Tumors. New York: Informa Healthcare USA; 2009:277–292
6. Lan Q, Gong Z, Quian Z, et al. Microsurgical treatment of posterior cranial fossa tumors via keyhole approaches. In: Kato TKY, ed. Minimally Invasive Neurosurgery and Multidisciplinary Neurotraumatology. Tokyo: Springer-Verlag; 2006:202–211
7. Al-Mefty O, Ayoubi S, Kadri PA. The petrosal approach for the resection of retrochiasmatic craniopharyngiomas. Neurosurgery 2008;62(5, Suppl 2):ONS331–ONS335, discussion ONS335–ONS336
8. Cavallo LM, Messina A, Cappabianca P, et al. Endoscopic endonasal surgery of the midline skull base: anatomical study and clinical considerations. Neurosurg Focus 2005;19:E2
9. Schwartz TH, Fraser JF, Brown S, Tabaee A, Kacker A, Anand VK. Endoscopic cranial base surgery: classification of operative approaches. Neurosurgery 2008;62:991–1002, discussion 1002–1005
10. Stippler M, Gardner PA, Snyderman CH, Carrau RL, Prevedello DM, Kassam AB. Endoscopic endonasal approach for clival chordomas. Neurosurgery 2009;64:268–277, discussion 277–278
11. Cappabianca P, Cavallo LM, Esposito F, De Divitiis O, Messina A, De Divitiis E. Extended endoscopic endonasal approach to the midline skull base: the evolving role of transsphenoidal surgery. Adv Tech Stand Neurosurg 2008;33:151–199
12. Jho HD, Ha HG. Endoscopic endonasal skull base surgery: Part 3—The clivus and posterior fossa. Minim Invasive Neurosurg 2004;47:16–23
13. Kassam AB, Snyderman C, Gardner P, Carrau R, Spiro R. The expanded endonasal approach: a fully endoscopic transnasal approach and resection of the odontoid process: technical case report. Neurosurgery 2005;57(1, Suppl):E213, discussion E213
14. Frank G, Sciarretta V, Calbucci F, Farneti G, Mazzatenta D, Pasquini E. The endoscopic transnasal transsphenoidal approach for the treatment of cranial base chordomas and chondrosarcomas. Neurosurgery 2006;59(1, Suppl 1):ONS50–ONS57, discussion ONS50–ONS57
15. Zanation AM, Snyderman CH, Carrau RL, Gardner PA, Prevedello DM, Kassam AB. Endoscopic endonasal surgery for petrous apex lesions. Laryngoscope 2009;119:19–25
16. Al-Mefty O, Kadri PA, Hasan DM, Isolan GR, Pravdenkova S. Anterior clivectomy: surgical technique and clinical applications. J Neurosurg 2008;109:783–793
17. Kassam AB, Prevedello DM, Thomas A, et al. Endoscopic endonasal pituitary transposition for a transdorsum sellae approach to the interpeduncular cistern. Neurosurgery 2008;62(3, Suppl 1):57–72, discussion 72–74
18. Carrabba G, Dehdashti AR, Gentili F. Surgery for clival lesions: open resection versus the expanded endoscopic endonasal approach. Neurosurg Focus 2008;25:E7
19. Magrini S, Pasquini E, Mazzatenta D, Mascari C, Galassi E, Frank G. Endoscopic endonasal odontoidectomy in a patient affected by Down syndrome: technical case report. Neurosurgery 2008;63:E373–E374, discussion E374
20. Dehdashti AR, Karabatsou K, Ganna A, Witterick I, Gentili F. Expanded endoscopic endonasal approach for treatment of clival chordomas: early results in 12 patients. Neurosurgery 2008;63:299–307, discussion 307–309
21. Stamm A, Pignatari SSN. Transnasal endoscopic surgical approach to the posterior fossa. In: Anand V, Schwartz T, eds. Practical Endoscopic Skull-Base Surgery. San Diego: Plural Publishing; 2007:155–161

22. Stamm AC, Pignatari SS, Vellutini E. Transnasal endoscopic surgical approaches to the clivus. Otolaryngol Clin North Am 2006;39:639–656, xi

23. Cappabianca P, Alfieri A, de Divitiis E. Endoscopic endonasal transsphenoidal approach to the sella: towards functional endoscopic pituitary surgery (FEPS). Minim Invasive Neurosurg 1998;41:66–73

24. Lang J. Skull Base and Related Structures: Atlas of Clinical Anatomy. Stuttgart: Schattauer Verlag; 1995

25. Seeger W. Endoscopic and Microsurgical Anatomy of the Upper Basal Cisterns. Vienna: Springer-Verlag; 2008

26. Fortes FS, Sennes LU, Carrau RL, et al. Endoscopic anatomy of the pterygopalatine fossa and the transpterygoid approach: development of a surgical instruction model. Laryngoscope 2008;118:44–49

27. Snyderman C, Kassam A, Carrau R, Mintz A, Gardner P, Prevedello DM. Acquisition of surgical skills for endonasal skull base surgery: a training program. Laryngoscope 2007;117:699–705

28. Cappabianca P, Decq P, Schroeder HW. Future of endoscopy in neurosurgery. Surg Neurol 2007;67:496–498

29. Cavallo LM, Dal Fabbro M, Jalalod'din H, et al. Endoscopic endonasal transsphenoidal surgery. Before scrubbing in: tips and tricks. Surg Neurol 2007;67:342–347

30. Gardner PA, Kassam AB, Rothfus WE, Snyderman CH, Carrau RL. Preoperative and intraoperative imaging for endoscopic endonasal approaches to the skull base. Otolaryngol Clin North Am 2008;41:215–230, vii

31. Kassam AB, Vescan AD, Carrau RL, et al. Expanded endonasal approach: vidian canal as a landmark to the petrous internal carotid artery. J Neurosurg 2008;108:177–183

32. Endoscopic endonasal transclival approach and retrosigmoid approach to the clival and petroclival regions. de Notaris M, Cavallo LM, Prats-Galino A, Esposito I, Benet A, Poblete J, Valente V, Gonzalez JB, Ferrer E, Cappabianca P. Neurosurgery. 2009 Dec;65(6 Suppl):42–50; discussion 50-2.

33. Iaconetta G, Fusco M, Cavallo LM, Cappabianca P, Samii M, Tschabitscher M. The abducens nerve: microanatomic and endoscopic study. Neurosurgery 2007;61(3, Suppl):7–14, discussion 14

34. Alfieri A, Jho HD, Tschabitscher M. Endoscopic endonasal approach to the ventral cranio-cervical junction: anatomical study. Acta Neurochir (Wien) 2002;144:219–225, discussion 225

35. Messina A, Bruno MC, Decq P, et al. Pure endoscopic endonasal odontoidectomy: anatomical study. Neurosurg Rev 2007;30:189–194, discussion 194

36. Karasu A, Cansever T, Batay F, Sabanci PA, Al-Mefty O. The microsurgical anatomy of the hypoglossal canal. Surg Radiol Anat 2009;31: 363–367

37. Cavallo LM, Cappabianca P, Messina A, et al. The extended endoscopic endonasal approach to the clivus and cranio-vertebral junction: anatomical study. Childs Nerv Syst 2007;23:665–671

38. Cavallo LM, Messina A, Esposito F, et al. Skull base reconstruction in the extended endoscopic transsphenoidal approach for suprasellar lesions. J Neurosurg 2007;107:713–720

39. Kassam AB, Thomas A, Carrau RL, et al. Endoscopic reconstruction of the cranial base using a pedicled nasoseptal flap. Neurosurgery 2008; 63(1, Suppl 1):ONS44–ONS52, discussion ONS52–ONS53

40. Oliver CL, Hackman TG, Carrau RL, et al. Palatal flap modifications allow pedicled reconstruction of the skull base. Laryngoscope 2008; 118:2102–2106

41. Hadad G, Bassagasteguy L, Carrau RL, et al. A novel reconstructive technique after endoscopic expanded endonasal approaches: vascular pedicle nasoseptal flap. Laryngoscope 2006;116:1882–1886

30 Endoscopic Transnasal Craniectomy: Approaches to the Clivus and Posterior Fossa

Aldo Cassol Stamm, Shirley S.N. Pignatari, Eduardo Vellutini, Diego Hermann, and Daniel Timperley

Tips and Pearls

- Endoscopic management of lesions of the posterior cranial fossa requires a multidisciplinary team approach.
- The current indications for the endoscopic transnasal craniectomy approach to the posterior cranial fossa are clival chordomas, chondrosarcomas, cholesterol granulomas, and mucoceles.
- The advantages of endoscopic transnasal craniectomy in the management of these lesions are the ability to avoid cerebral retraction and to decrease the incidence of injury to the lower cranial nerves.
- Contraindications for this approach include patient comorbidities, unfavorable anatomy, lack of availability of multidisciplinary team cooperation and interaction, and lack of specialized equipment/instruments.
- A careful preoperative evaluation should always be performed in these patients, and must include both physical examination and imaging studies.
- The first step of the surgery is the creation of a nasal septum flap (if available) for the reconstruction of the large skull base defect. This flap should be designed for the planned dural defect.
- The drilling of the clival bone is difficult, and carries significant risk to the patient. Always check for the internal carotid arteries. The midline is generally a safe spot to start drilling.
- Bleeding in the basilar plexus cannot be cauterized safely but is usually controlled with packing using hemostatic material.
- The opening of the internal layer of the dura at the level of the middle and superior clivus must be accomplished with great care to avoid injury to the underlying basilar artery.
- Straight and angled endoscopes should be used to appreciate the anatomy of the region as well as to look for any residual disease. Care should be taken with the tip of these instruments.
- At the end of the procedure, the dural defect is sealed with fat and fascia lata, and covered with the flap. The packing is positioned and stays for as long as necessary.

Introduction

Before the endoscopic era, the management of lesions in these regions required extensive craniotomies resulting in significant morbidity to patients.[1,2] However, even with several endoscopic proposed approaches, effective and safe treatment of lesions involving these regions is still a challenge.[3–7] The problems of infection, cerebrospinal fluid leakage, difficulty controlling intradural bleeding, lack of experience, and appropriate surgical instruments still exist.[8] The combination of a team approach, with neurosurgery, otolaryngology, intensive care, anesthesiology, pathology, endocrinology, and paramedical staff, including specialist nursing, good patient selection, a thorough understanding of the anatomy, and appropriate expertise and equipment, facilitates extending the transnasal craniectomy approach to the clivus and posterior fossa.[9]

Indications and Advantages

The endoscopic transnasal craniectomy approach to the posterior cranial fossa is used for lesions involving the clivus or retroclival region. The most common lesions for which this approach is indicated are clival chordomas and chondrosarcomas, followed by cholesterol granulomas and mucoceles (**Table 30.1**).

The advantages of this approach include the ability to avoid any cerebral retraction and to decrease the incidence of injury to the lower cranial nerves. In addition, the approach is direct, and does not require any external incisions.

Contraindications

Contraindications include patient comorbidities that might preclude them from prolonged general anesthesia; unfavorable anatomy, such as small sphenoid sinus or diminished space between the internal carotid arteries, which makes drilling the clival bone more difficult and risky; lack of multidisciplinary team cooperation and interaction; and lack of specialized equipment/instruments.

Diagnostic Workup

The physical examination includes neurologic assessment with a special focus on cranial nerve function. Endoscopic assessment of the nasal cavity is recommended to visualize

Table 30.1 Patients with Clival Lesions (Chordomas and Chondrosarcomas) Treated at Hospital Professor Edmundo Vasconcelas, a Tertiary Referral Hospital

Case	Gender	Age	Symptoms/Signs	Anatomic Extension	Tumor Type
1	F	12	VI nerve palsy	SS, clivus	Chordoma
2	F	53	NO, occipital pain	SS, clivus	Chordoma
3	F	46	VL; V nerve palsy	SS, clivus, CS bilateral, PA bilateral	Chordoma
4	M	18	VI nerve palsy, cervical pain	SS, clivus, PF	Chordoma (chondroid)
5	M	36	III and VI nerve palsies	SS, clivus, CS left	Chordoma
6	M	74	VI nerve palsy, headache	SS, clivus, PF	Chordoma
7	F	45	III and VI nerve palsies, ND	SS, clivus, CS bilateral	Chordoma
8	M	43	III and VI nerve palsies; VL	SS, clivus, CS bilateral, PF	Chordoma
9	M	24	VI and VII nerve palsies	Clivus, CS right, PA right	Chordoma
10	F	26	VII nerve palsy, HL	Clivus, PA right	Chondrosarcoma
11	F	22	Headache	Clivus, PF	Chordoma
12	F	45	Right hemiparesis	Clivus, PF	Chordoma
13	F	63	VI nerve palsy	Clivus	Chordoma
14	M	56	VI nerve palsy, dysphasia	SS, clivus, PF, PP, CS bilateral	Chordoma
15	F	53	VL; III, V, and bilateral VI nerve palsies	SS, clivus, PP, CS bilat	Chordoma
16	M	29	VI nerve palsy	SS, clivus, PF	Chordoma
17	F	64	VI nerve palsy	SS, clivus	Chordoma
18	M	33	VI, X, and XI nerve palsies	SS, clivus, PF	Chordoma (chondroid)
19	F	6	Brainstem syndrome, dyspnea	SS, clivus, PF	Chordoma
20	M	59	Headache, vertigo	Petrous apex	Chordoma (chondroid)
21	F	78	III and VI nerve palsies, headache	SS, clivus	Chordoma
22	M	15	Headache	SS, clivus, PF	Chordoma
23	M	28	Headache	SS, clivus	Chordoma

Abbreviations: CS: cavernous sinus; HL: hearing loss; ND: neurologic defect; NO: nasal obstruction; PA: petrous apex; PF: posterior fossa; PP: parapharyngeal space; SS: sphenoid sinus; VL: visual loss.
Source: Data courtesy of A. Stamm.

any nasal lesions and document septal integrity, deviations, and other anatomical findings. An ophthalmologic examination is suggested if the optic nerve or orbital integrity is compromised, including a visual field examination (**Fig. 30.1**).

Imaging

Coronal, axial, and parasagittal computed tomography (CT) images of the paranasal sinuses and skull base are essential in the preoperative assessment for surgery. It is also necessary to evaluate the size of the sphenoid sinus, the position of the internal carotid artery, especially its paraclival portion, and the thickness of the clivus in the sagittal plane.

Magnetic resonance imaging (MRI) is important to demonstrate the morphology of the soft tissues. Additionally, MRI should be evaluated for involvement of the carotid artery, vertebrobasilar system, and dural sinuses (**Fig. 30.2**).

Magnetic resonance angiography (MRA) or CT angiography (CTA) can also be helpful to look at the relationship between the basilar and internal carotid arteries and the pathology. Particular attention should be given to the cavernous sinus, the inferior end of the superior intercavernous sinuses, and the basilar venous plexus.

Angiography can also be important to verify the functional integrity of the circle of Willis and the extent of any carotid artery compromise, and to differentiate an aneurysm from a tumor (**Fig. 30.3**).

Surgery

Instrumentation

Adequate instrumentation is paramount for the endoscopic approach to the clivus and posterior fossa. The necessary

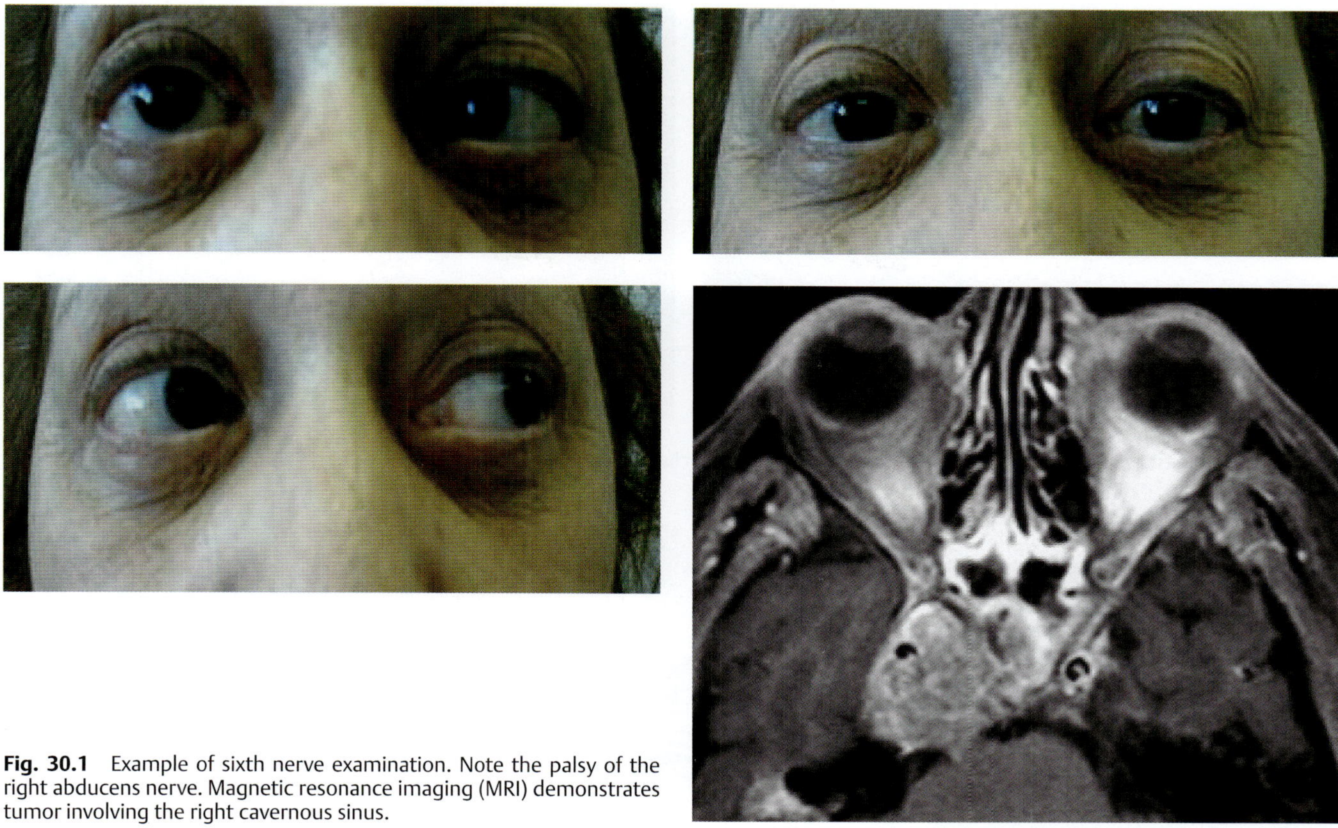

Fig. 30.1 Example of sixth nerve examination. Note the palsy of the right abducens nerve. Magnetic resonance imaging (MRI) demonstrates tumor involving the right cavernous sinus.

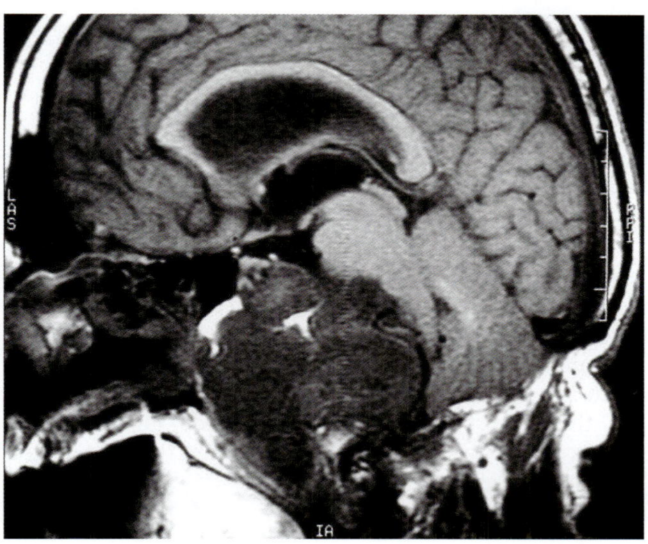

Fig. 30.2 Sagittal reconstruction of MRI showing large mass involving the clival area, compressing the posterior fossa structures with resultant hydrocephalus.

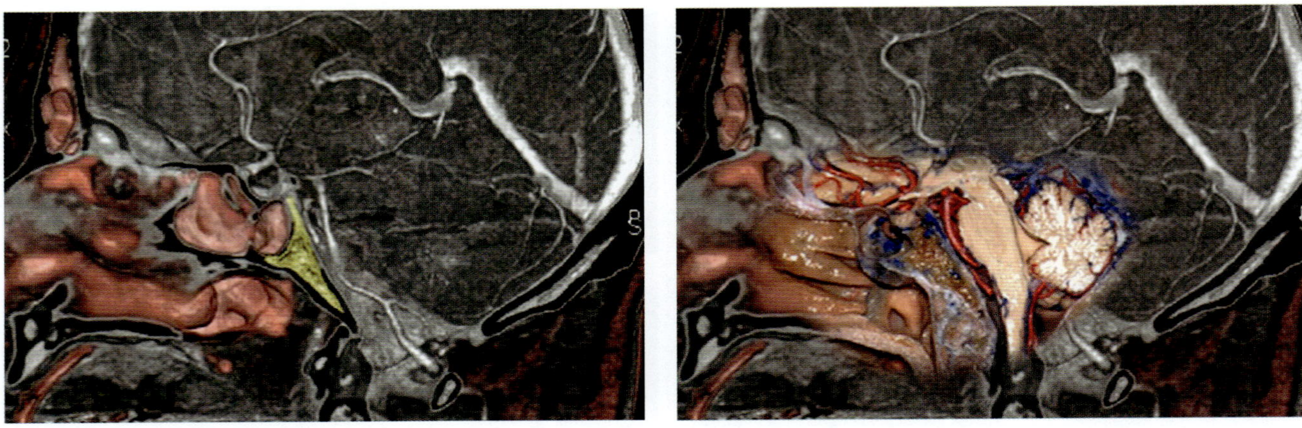

A B

Fig. 30.3 Midsagittal view through the nasal cavity and clivus. **(A)** The clival bone is shown in yellow, and the sinonasal and oral mucosa are shown in pink. **(B)** The soft tissue structures.

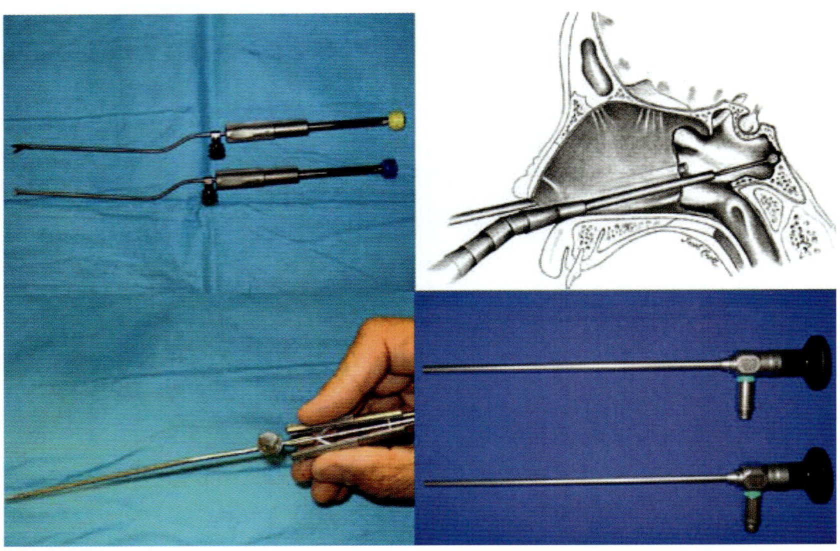

Fig. 30.4 Specialized skull base equipment. The instruments are longer than those designed for surgery within the paranasal sinuses, and designed to be held as shown. The pistol-style grips used in standard sinus instruments result in movement of the tip of the instrument when it is opened or closed, a significant problem in delicate intracranial dissection. The upper endoscope is 5 mm in diameter (Karl Storz Endoscopy), providing a wider field of view and improved illumination for skull base surgery.

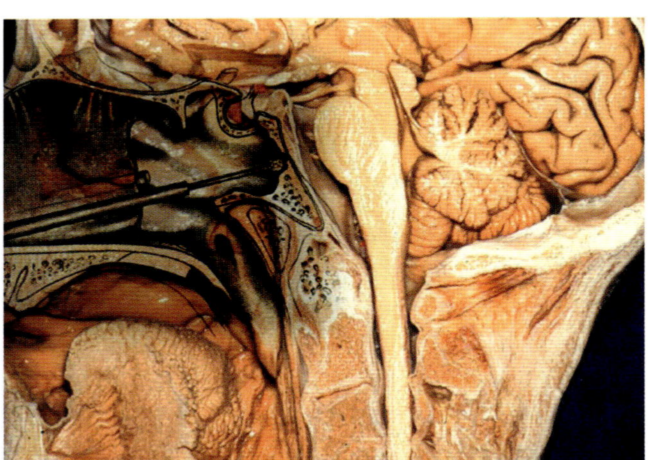

Fig. 30.5 Drawing of an anatomical sagittal specimen, showing the long drill and instruments used to reach the clival bone.

equipment includes high-quality endoscopes (0- and 45-degree); video equipment (camera and monitor); long endoscopic bipolar forceps, preferably suction bipolar; long and delicate drills; long dissection instruments; and hemostatic materials. In conjunction with Karl Storz Endoscopy (Flanders, NJ), the authors developed a 5-mm, wide-angle, 0-degree endoscope for these procedures to increase the field of view and illumination (**Figs. 30.4** and **30.5**).

Operative Setup

The surgery is performed with the patient under hypotensive general anesthesia. The patient is placed in a supine position on the operating table, with the head elevated 30 degrees, the neck slightly flexed, and the head extended and turned toward the surgeon. High-concentration adrenaline-soaked cottonoids (1:1000) are placed in the nasal cavity for

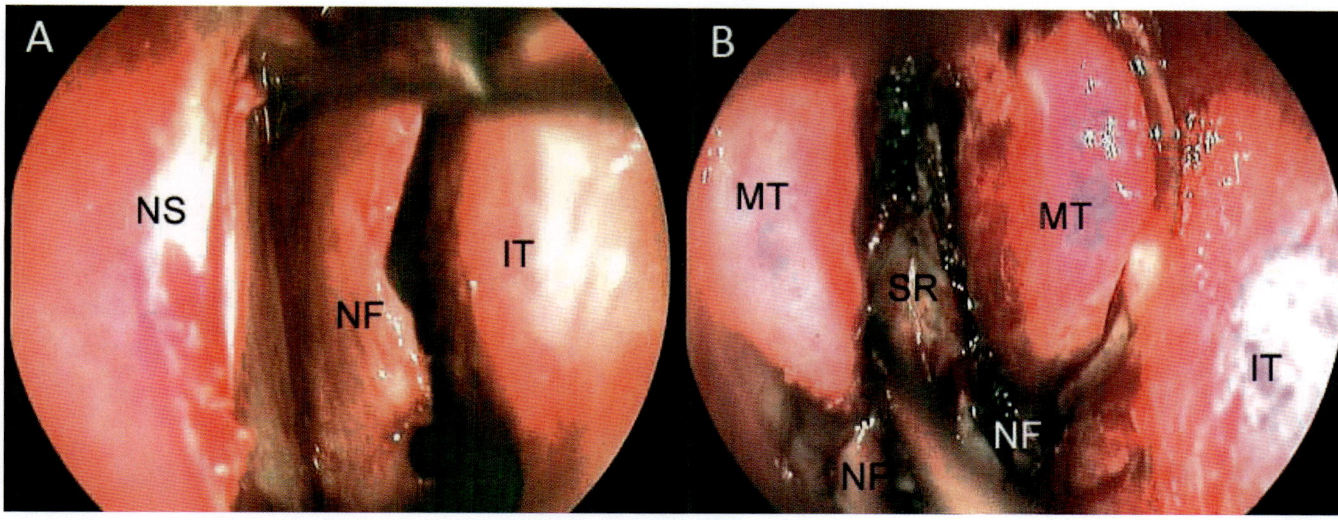

Fig. 30.6 Creation of nasal septal flaps. **(A)** Raising the flap. The vertical incision has been made at the level of the head of the inferior turbinate. The flap is being elevated in a subperichondrial plane. **(B)** Bilateral nasoseptal flaps have been elevated and placed in the nasopharynx. A partial septectomy has been performed, providing a view of both sides of the nose and the sphenoid rostrum. IT: inferior turbinate; MT: middle turbinate; NF: nasal flap; NS: nasal septum; SR: sphenoid rostrum.

10 minutes before the surgical procedure begins. The septum is infiltrated with lidocaine with adrenaline 1:100,000.

Preparation

A nasal septal flap, pedicled at the sphenopalatine bundle, is created on one side. This flap can be as long and as wide as necessary to cover the skull base defect. The creation of the flap starts with incisions at the choanal arch that are brought forward as anteriorly as necessary for the planned dural defect. In some cases the flap can be harvested from the nasal floor or even from the inferior turbinate. Multiple modifications regarding length and width are possible, and the flap should be created based on the size and shape of the planned defect (**Fig. 30.6**).[10] A maxillary antrostomy can be created on the same side to store the nasal septal flap and keep it safe during the procedure.

The sphenoid rostrum and anterior wall of the sphenoid sinus are exposed. The mucosal flap is lifted until both natural sphenoid ostia are in view. Prior to the opening of the sphenoid sinus, a complete ethmoidectomy is performed bilaterally to improve the surgical access.

A wide opening of the anterior sphenoid sinus wall is created with a micro-Kerrison punch, and a drill is used to lower the sphenoid rostrum. A wide exposure at this point is the key to the subsequent surgical procedure. The sinus mucosa that lines the clival area is reflected carefully, exposing the clival bone. Care is taken to ensure complete hemostasis at this point in the procedure. The field should be completely dry before proceeding to the next stage of the procedure (**Fig. 30.7**).

Approach

The clival bone is fully exposed, and its removal is initiated with a diamond burr drill and continued carefully with a micro-Kerrison punch if necessary. The limits of the clival bone removal are the floor of the sella superiorly, the foramen magnum inferiorly, and the internal carotid arteries and occipital condyles laterally.

To create an intradural exposure, the external layer of the dura is first incised with a No. 11 blade. Bleeding in the basilar

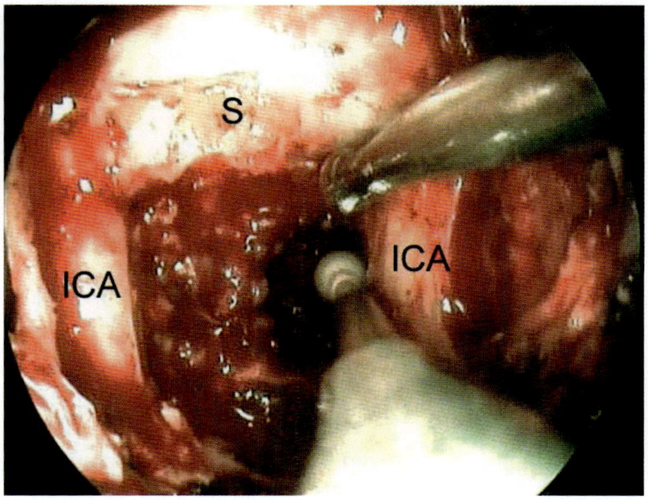

Fig. 30.7 Exposure at the start of drilling the clival bone. The distance between the internal carotid arteries is an important factor in determining surgical access to this area. ICA: internal carotid artery; S: sella.

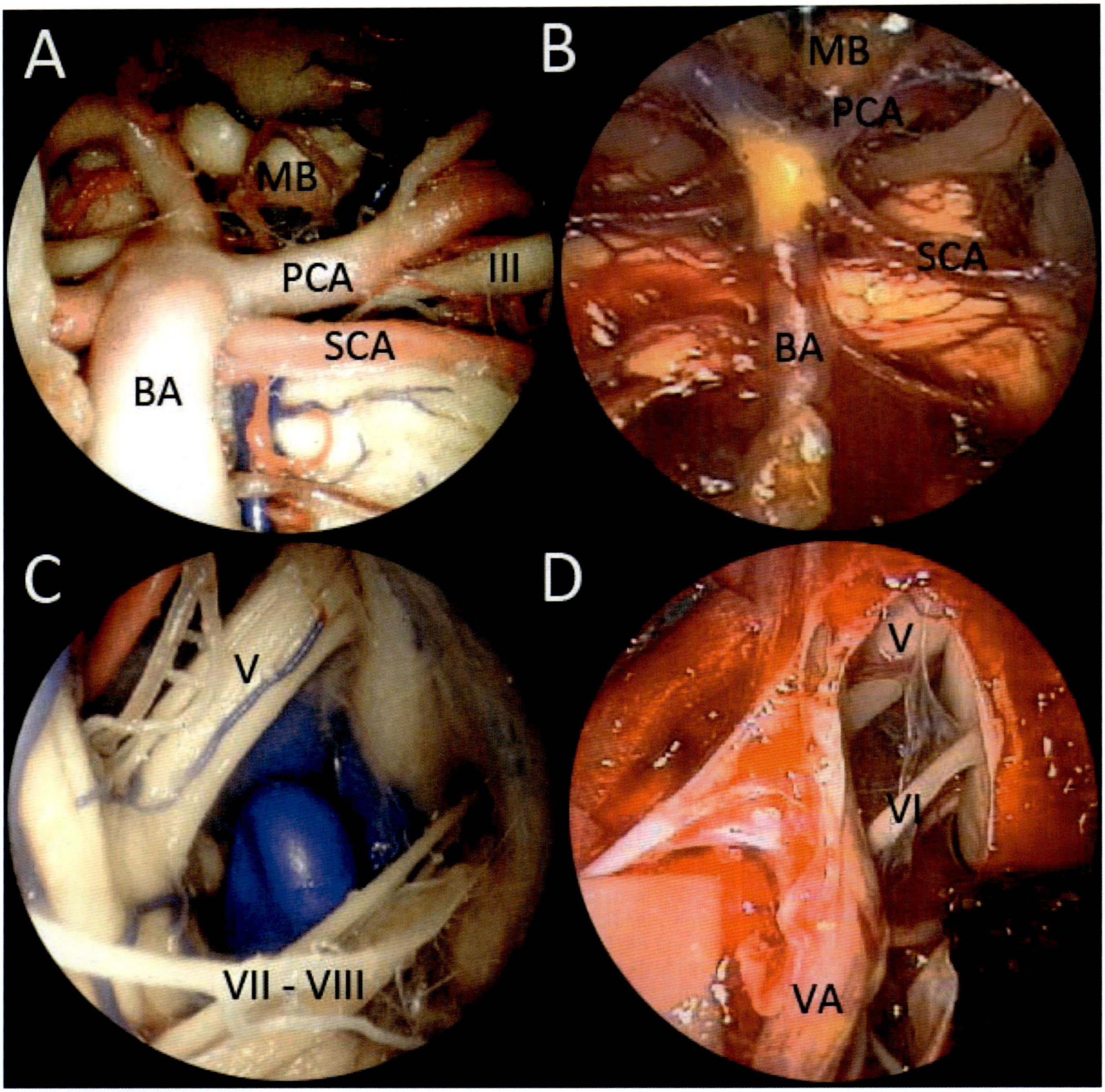

Fig. 30.8 Endoscopic anatomy following clival resection. **(A)** Anatomical specimen demonstrating midline structures. **(B)** Corresponding intraoperative view. **(C)** Anatomical specimen demonstrating left cerebellopontine angle (CPA) using a 45-degree endoscope. **(D)** Corresponding intraoperative view of the left CPA. In this view, the right vertebral artery (VA) can be seen and obscures the view of the left VA. BA: basilar artery; MB: mamillary body; SCA: superior cerebellar artery; VA: right vertebral artery; III, V, VI, VII, VIII: cranial nerves III to VIII.

plexus cannot be cauterized safely but is usually controlled with packing using hemostatic material, such as Surgicel, among others. Large lesions often encroach on and obliterate much of the plexus, but if the lesion is not large or if the plexus is not completely compressed, profuse and intense bleeding can occur. Judicious packing, time, patience, and experience are required to control it.[10]

The opening of the internal layer of the dura at the level of the middle and superior clivus must be accomplished with great care to avoid injury to the underlying basilar artery. Once the dura is opened, minor bleeding is stopped by bipolar coagulation, and it is finally possible to introduce the 0-degree endoscope carefully into the intradural space.

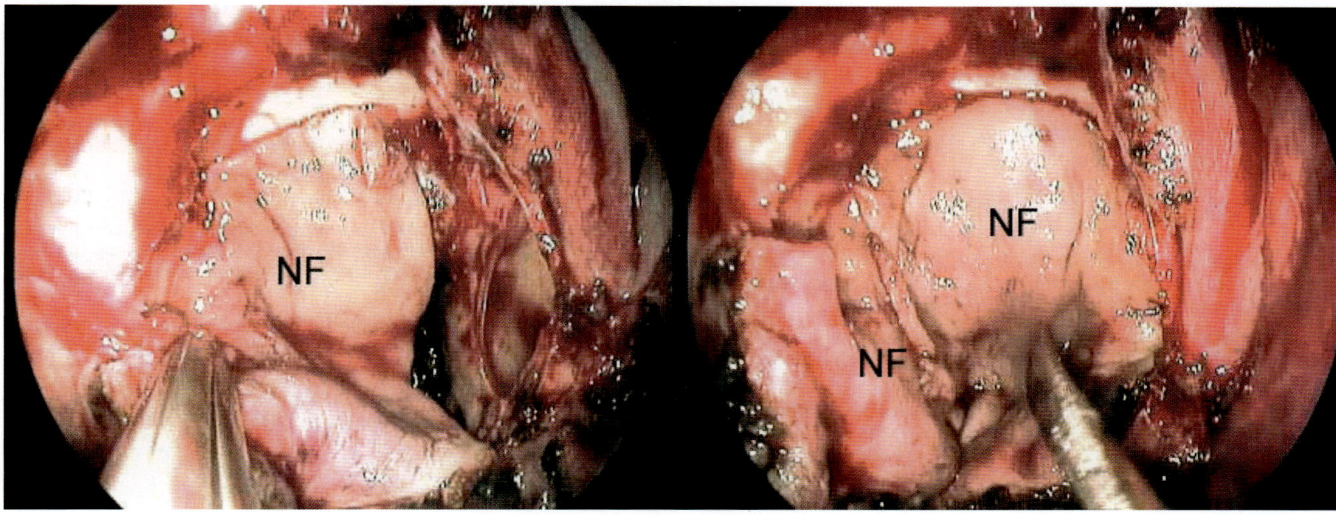

Fig. 30.9 Repair with nasoseptal flaps. In this case, bilateral flaps were used to completely close the defect. NF: nasal flap.

Once the anatomy is appreciated, identify the major vessels of the posterior fossa (basilar artery and branches, anterior inferior cerebellar artery [AICA], vertebral arteries, superior cerebellar and posterior cerebral arteries); the intradural course of cranial nerves III, IV, V, and VI; the brainstem; and the mamillary bodies. The cerebellopontine angle, cranial nerves VII through XII, and retrosellar regions are best visualized with the 45-degree endoscope (**Fig. 30.8**).

Meticulous dissection is required to remove the lesion. Frequent irrigation and suction with neurosurgical tip-protected low suction is used to maintain good vision. Once removal is completed, the surgeon can proceed to repair of the surgical site.

Repair

Dural repair in the region of the clivus is difficult. If the defect is large, it can be occluded with abdominal fat first and then covered with grafts of fascia lata or synthetic material such as Duragen® (Integra Life Sciences Corp.; Plainsboro, NJ) or Duraform® (Codman; Raynham, MA). These grafts are covered by the sphenopalatine-based pedicled nasal septal flap(s). The flap(s) is(are) secured with fibrin glue and pieces of Gelfoam or Spongostan. Should the defect be larger than the previously harvested flap, the closure of the defect is augmented by the addition of a free mucosal graft. Antibiotic ointment is placed over the Gelfoam, and a Foley catheter balloon is inflated to support the repair and to avoid displacement of the nasal packing into the nasopharynx. The balloon must be positioned under direct vision and inflated with no more than 10 cc of saline solution. It is left for about 5 days. The nasal cavity is packed using gauze with antibiotic ointment for about 10 days. Broad-spectrum antibiotics are used for 10 days or as long as necessary (**Fig. 30.9**).[8,9]

Complications

The fast and precise identification of the complications involved with this surgery are paramount for correct management of the patient. The management of these complications is discussed in other chapters. The complications include cerebrospinal fluid (CSF) leakage, nasal bleeding, bleeding from internal carotid artery, intracranial bleeding, venous bleeding, cranial nerve injuries, infections, orbital hematoma due to the nasal approach, nasal synechia, and nasal infection.

Postoperative Care

After the removal of the packing, the operative cavity is carefully suctioned, and any residual bony fragments are removed under endoscopic view. The patient is instructed to perform frequent nasal irrigations with 0.9% saline solution. After any dural repairs it is recommended to avoid physical activities, nose blowing, and sneezing with a closed mouth for a period of approximately 30 days. Stool softeners are recommended for all patients. Long-term restrictions should also be recommended to patients. Follow-up takes place at least every 2 weeks, or more often if there are any concerns. At each visit the operated nasal cavity is cleaned of crusts, granulation tissue, clots, and secretions. Imaging is performed only after the cavity has satisfactorily healed.

Conclusion

The transnasal craniectomy is an alternative way to treat these patients, and in expert hands, this technique can obtain good results. Comfort and expertise with endoscopic techniques to control intracranial bleeding, reconstruct skull base defects, and manage intradural structures are all prerequisites for the operative team. These skills combined with a detailed knowledge of endoscopic anatomy of the region, and its distortion from disease, serve as a foundation for addressing this complex pathology.

References

1. Mullan S, Naunton R, Hekmat-Panah J, Vailati G. The use of an anterior approach to ventrally placed tumors in the foramen magnum and vertebral column. J Neurosurg 1966;24:536–543
2. Sano K, Jinbo M, Saito I. [Vertebro-basilar aneurysms, with special reference to the transpharyngeal approach to basilar artery aneurysm]. No To Shinkei 1966;18:1197–1203
3. Crockard HA. The transoral approach to the base of the brain and upper cervical cord. Ann R Coll Surg Engl 1985;67:321–325
4. Draf W, Weber R, Keerl R. Endonasale chirurgie von tumoren der nasennebenhohlen und rhinobasis. Medizin im Bild 1995;2:13–17
5. Harsh GR IV, Joseph MP, Swearingen B, Ojemann RG. Anterior midline approaches to the central skull base. Clin Neurosurg 1996;43:15–43
6. Alfieri A, Jho HD. Endoscopic endonasal cavernous sinus surgery: an anatomic study. Neurosurgery 2001;48:827–836, discussion 836–837
7. Jho HD. The expanding role of endoscopy in skull-base surgery. Indications and instruments. Clin Neurosurg 2001;48:287–305
8. Stamm AC, Pignatari SSN. Transnasal endoscopic-assisted surgery of the skull base. In: Cummings CW, Flint PW, Harker LA, eds. Otolaryngology Head Neck Surgery, 4th ed. Philadelphia: Elsevier Mosby; 2005: 3855–3876
9. Beals SP, Joganic EF, Holcombe TC, Spetzler RF. Secondary craniofacial problems following skull base surgery. Clin Plast Surg 1997;24:565–581
10. Kaylie DM, Wittkopf JE, Coppit G, Warren FM III, Netterville JL, Jackson CG. Revision lateral skull base surgery. Otol Neurotol 2006;27:225–233

IX Tips and Pearls in Endoscopic Transmaxillary/Transpterygoid/Infratemporal Approaches

31 Endoscopic Transethmoid-Pterygoid-Sphenoid Approach

Davide Locatelli, Ilaria Acchiardi, Matteo Vitali, Frank Rikki Canevari, and Paolo Castelnuovo

Tips and Pearls

- The "diving" technique is a technique we have used since 1997 for the complete resection of tumors; it facilitates stopping oozing blood, cleaning the tumoral cavity, and demonstrating cerebrospinal fluid (CSF) fistulas and cavernous sinus perforations.
- Neuronavigation is needed, together with a thorough understanding of anatomical markers, verified by a preoperative neuroradiologic study, to avoid dangerous disorientation in the surgery.
- Intraoperative Doppler sonography is essential to locate the intracavernous carotid because visualization may be poor at the beginning of the operation due to tumoral compression.
- Bleeding control: cavernous sinus bleeding may be significant if the tumor has incompletely filled the sinus. We suggest a preoperative evaluation to avoid unnecessary risks. Check the complete obstruction of the sinus by the tumor, locate the carotid position inside the sinus, be prepared to control venous bleeding by gentle cottonoid compression, and use the diving technique with saline irrigation and hemostatic agents.
- Arterial bleeding is very rare, but we are prepared to control this bleeding by direct cottonoid compression, micropolar coagulation, hemostatic agents, endovascular coiling after initial bleeding control, immediate and delayed angiography any time bleeding is suspected, and most of all extensive experience in this type of surgery before being confronted with such a risk.

Introduction

The transethmoid-pterygoid-sphenoid (TPS) approach provides surgical access to lateral regions of the anterior and middle cranial base and to the infratemporal fossa. It is an extended application of the endoscopic transethmoid approach.

Indications and Advantages

A TPS approach is indicated for all pathologies with lateral extension to the course of the internal carotid artery at the base of the skull, such as cerebrospinal fluid (CSF) fistulas of Sternberg's canal,[1,2] pituitary macroadenomas, cranial pharyngiomas, chordomas and chondrosarcomas, meningiomas, tumors of the sellar cavity (metastases), angiofibromas, and retrobulbar, dermoid, and epidermoid tumors.[3]

Contraindications

There are no absolute contraindications to using a TPS approach, although, in view of the importance of anatomical landmarks in the various stages of surgery, any alteration in normal anatomy is a risk factor, such as the recurrence of lesions after previous surgical procedures.

Another risk factor is alteration in vessel walls. For this reason, patients who have undergone previous radiotherapy or patients with lesions involving the tunica adventitia of vessels should be carefully assessed prior to surgery.

Surgical Planning

Surgical planning entails gadolinium-enhanced magnetic resonance imaging (MRI) of the lesion, maxillofacial computed tomography (CT), and three-dimensional (3D) CT angiography. If necessary, a carotid occlusion test is done (**Figs. 31.1, 31.2, 31.3,** and **31.4**).

Surgical Approach

The transethmoid-pterygoid-sphenoid approach involves four main surgical steps:

1. The ethmoid step
2. The pterygoid step
3. The pterygoid-sphenoid step
4. The intracavernous step

The Ethmoid Step

This step involves anterior-posterior ethmoidectomy, sphenoidectomy, and partial removal of the middle and superior turbinates. The anatomical structures and the surgical phases are well known and are the same as those involved in

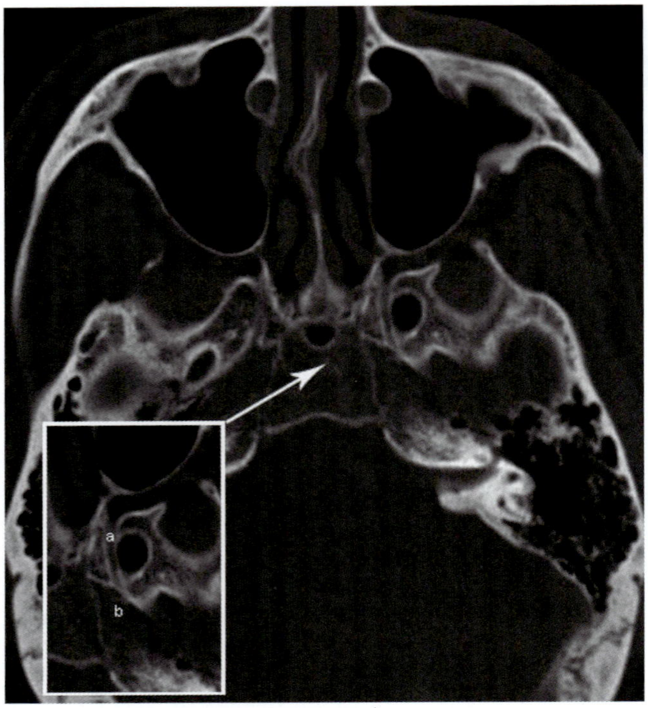

Fig. 31.1 Axial computed tomography (CT) of the skull base showing the vidian canal (a) and the internal carotid artery (b).

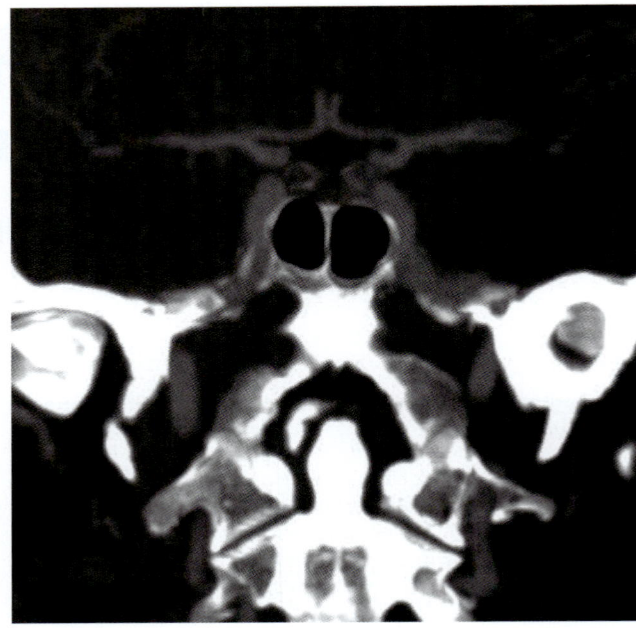

Fig. 31.2 Angio-CT with visualization of the paraclival carotid artery bilaterally.

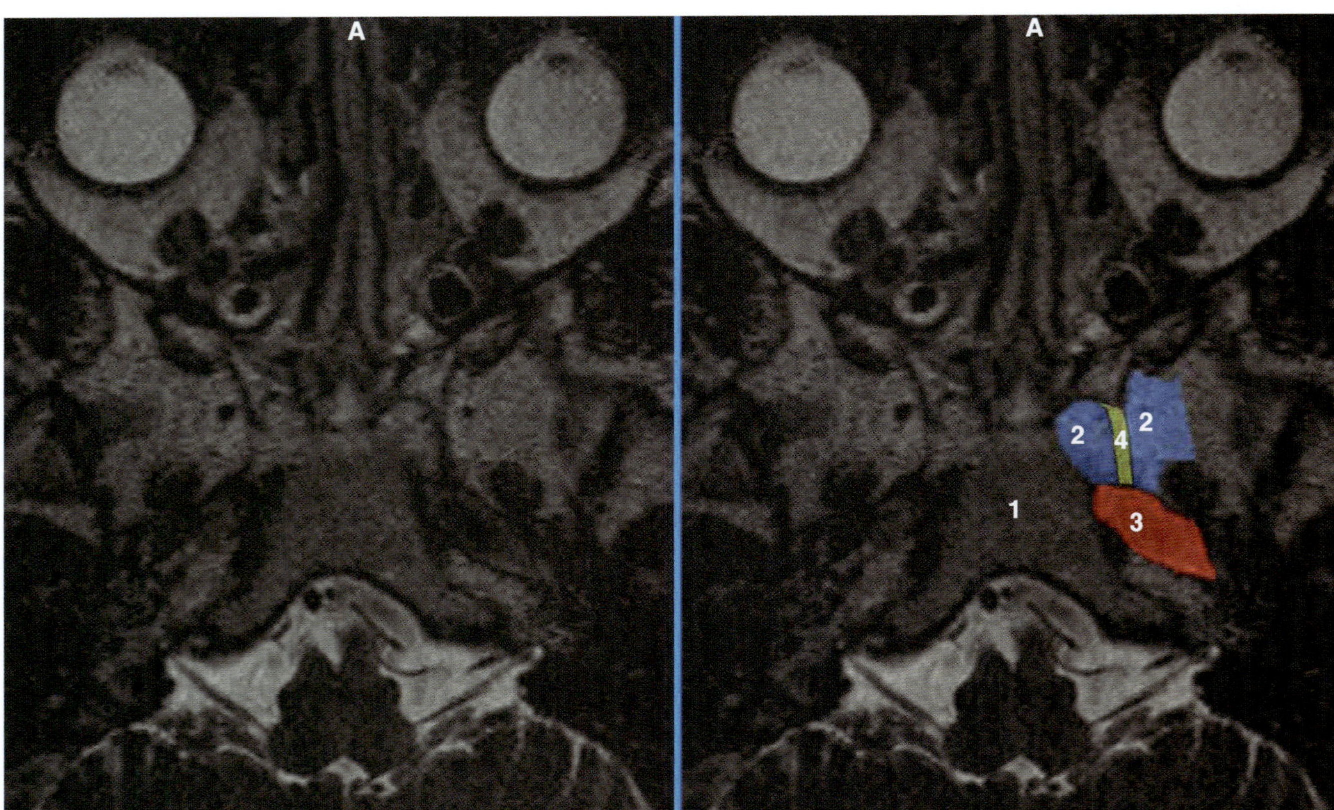

Fig. 31.3 Axial T2-weighted magnetic resonance imaging (MRI) sequence at the level of the vidian canal: 1, clivus; 2, pterygoid; 3, horizontal tract of the internal carotid artery (ICA); 4, vidian canal.

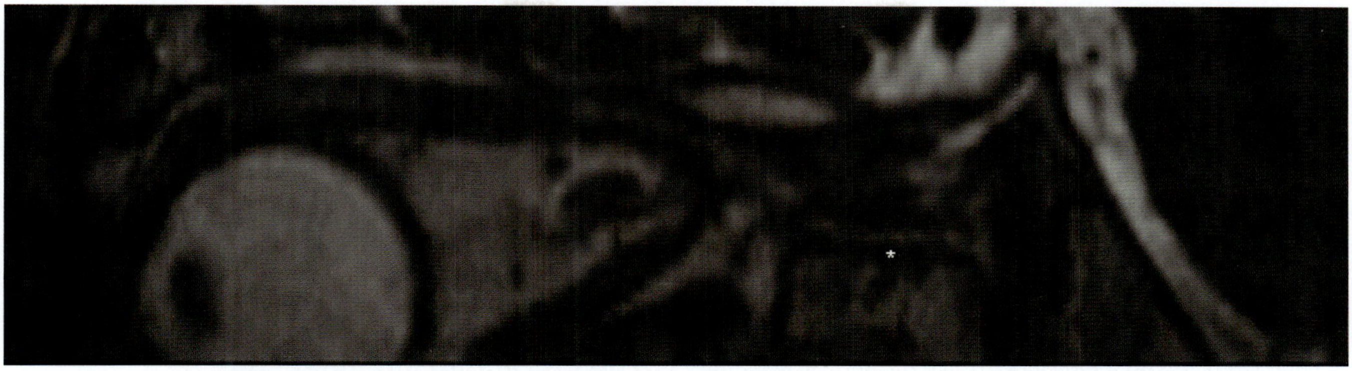

Fig. 31.4 Multiplanar reconstruction (MPR) of the T2-weighted MRI sequence showing the vidian canal and the internal carotid artery.

sinonasal phlogistic diseases, albeit with some specific technical details. First, the anterior ethmoid region is explored, and the inferior tip of the uncinate is identified and removed with a backward-cutting punch, using the inferior middle margin of the ethmoid bulla as a landmark. Once partial inferior uncinectomy has been performed and the infundibulum opened, the natural ostium of the maxillary sinus can be explored. The uncinate process can be completely removed with angled forceps and a microdebrider. The inferior medial margin of the bulla is exposed, opened, and removed in a mediolateral direction as far as the lamina papyracea. Once the bulla has been removed, the natural ostium of the maxillary sinus is widened posteriorly. Following anterior ethmoidectomy, the second portion of the middle turbinate is opened from the inferomedial margin to the lamina papyracea, providing access to the posterior ethmoid. The next step consists of partially resecting the middle turbinate with cutting forceps starting from the sagittal portion. The superior insertion of the middle turbinate and the lateral edges, with the branches of the sphenopalatine artery, are preserved.

The sagittal portion of the superior turbinate is identified and removed in an anterior-to-posterior direction up to its posterior insertion into the anterior sphenoid wall, preserving the superior portion of the basal lamella. The natural ostium of the sphenoid sinus opens medial to the tip of the superior or supreme turbinate and is then widened using a circular cutting punch. Once the sphenoid has been explored, the sphenoidectomy is extended laterally until the orbital apex is identified (**Fig. 31.5**). Technical expertise in this stage lies in identifying the lamina papyracea and orbital apex, which defines the upper boundary of the TPS approach.[4–6]

The Pterygoid Step

This step involves the identification and management of vascular structures that cross over during the approach. Thorough knowledge of this anatomy is crucial even for the endoscopic treatment of phlogistic diseases. The sphenopalatine artery is the first vessel encountered; it emerges from the pterygopalatine fossa into the nasal cavity through the sphenopalatine foramen, which is made up of the orbital and sphenoidal processes of the palatine bone, and above by the sphenoid bone, located posterior to the tip of the middle turbinate.

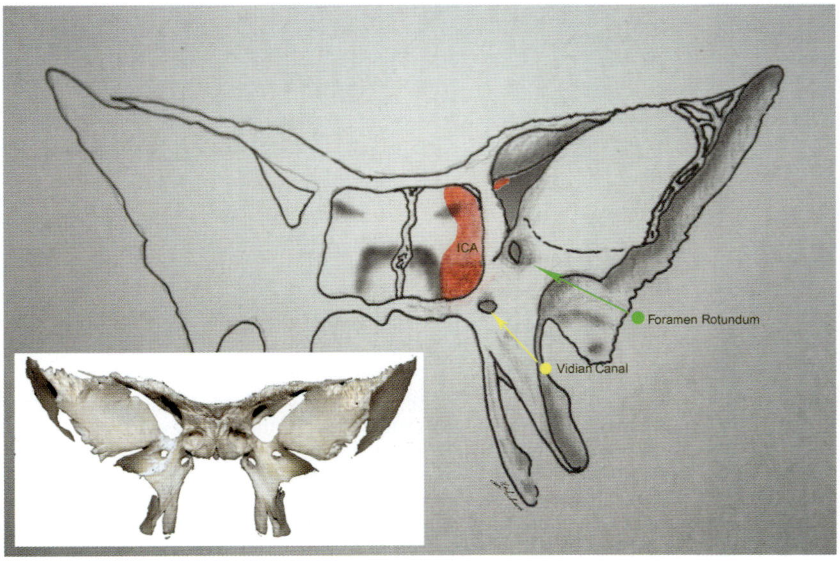

Fig. 31.5 Schematic drawing of the sphenoid bone and of the landmarks correlated with the picture of the sphenoid (*inset*).

Once the middle antrostomy has been enlarged posteriorly, the periosteum of the palatine bone is exposed. Dissecting backward in the subperiosteal plane, a bony crest is exposed that serves as a landmark for the palatine artery.

The artery is cauterized using bipolar forceps or clipped with vascular microclips and then cut. The pterygopalatine fossa and the sphenopalatine foramen are opened using a diamond burr drill. The posterior wall of the maxillary sinus is then removed with an angled cutting punch following the subperiosteal plane. A bone window is opened in the posterior wall of the maxillary sinus, and the portion of the sphenopalatine artery in the pterygopalatine fossa can be cauterized. It is preferable not to open the periosteal plane immediately and not to expose the contents of the fossa, but to make a subperiosteal dissection in a mediolateral, supero-inferior direction starting from the basi-sphenoid. As dissection proceeds laterally, the vidian canal can be seen, into which the vidian nerve and artery run. The opening of the pterygoid follows the vidian canal in the floor of the sphenoid sinus in an anteroposterior direction to the lateral wall of the sphenoid sinus, where the vidian artery emerges from the internal carotid artery in the first tract of the paraclival segment. The path of the vidian artery is a fundamental surgical landmark for identifying the internal carotid artery, and especially for the passage between the horizontal petrous tract and the vertical paraclival tract. Once the vidian artery has been identified, it can be electrocauterized with bipolar forceps and, if necessary, clamped with vascular microclips (**Figs. 31.6** and **31.7**).

The Pterygoid-Sphenoid Step

This step involves the removal of the basi-sphenoid and the pterygoid process of the sphenoid. This surgical step requires considerable experience in endoscopic skull base surgery due to the complexity of the anatomical structures. However, knowledge of this phase is crucial in managing diseases of

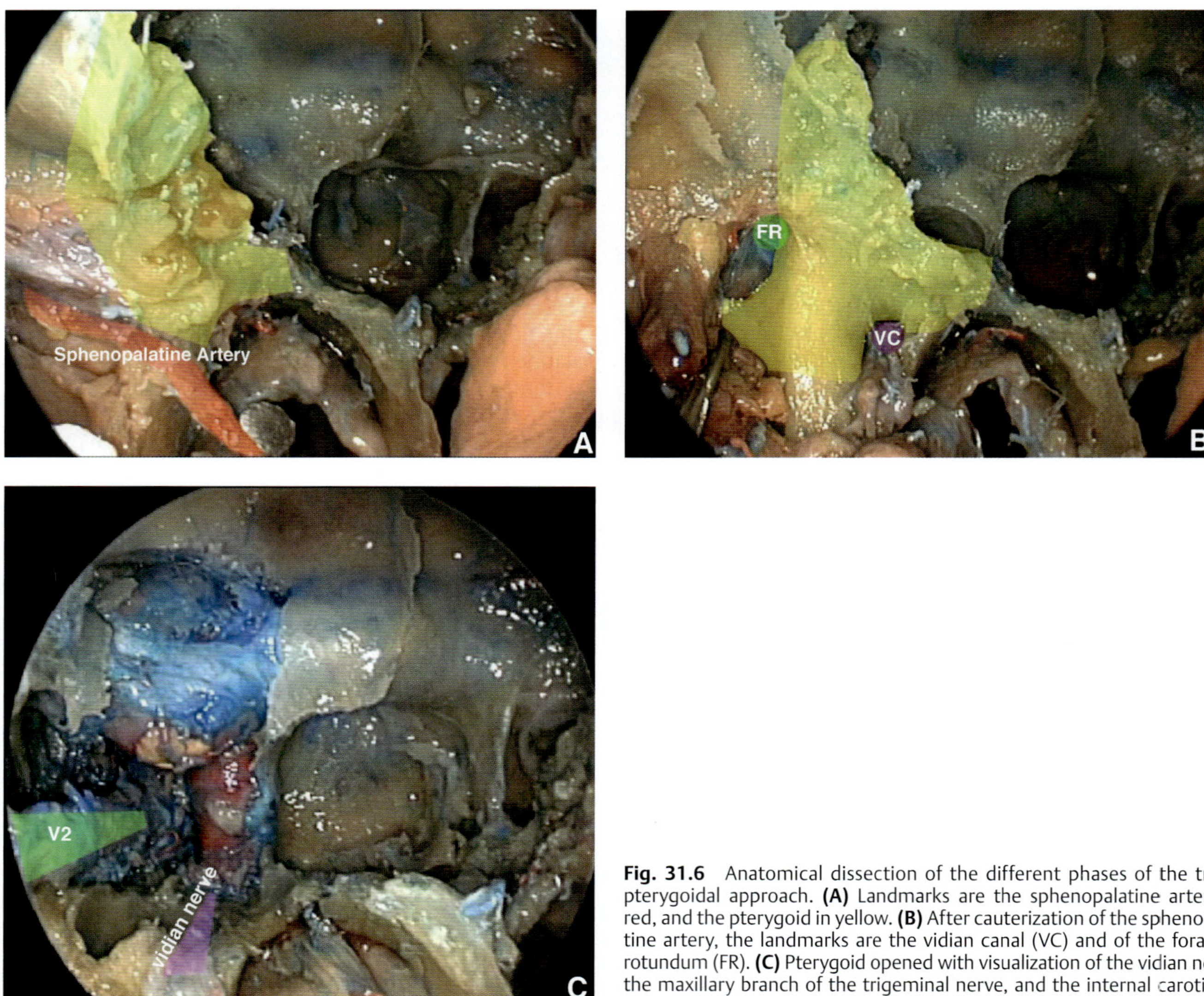

Fig. 31.6 Anatomical dissection of the different phases of the transpterygoidal approach. **(A)** Landmarks are the sphenopalatine artery in red, and the pterygoid in yellow. **(B)** After cauterization of the sphenopalatine artery, the landmarks are the vidian canal (VC) and of the foramen rotundum (FR). **(C)** Pterygoid opened with visualization of the vidian nerve, the maxillary branch of the trigeminal nerve, and the internal carotid artery (paraclival tract and cavernous sinus superiorly).

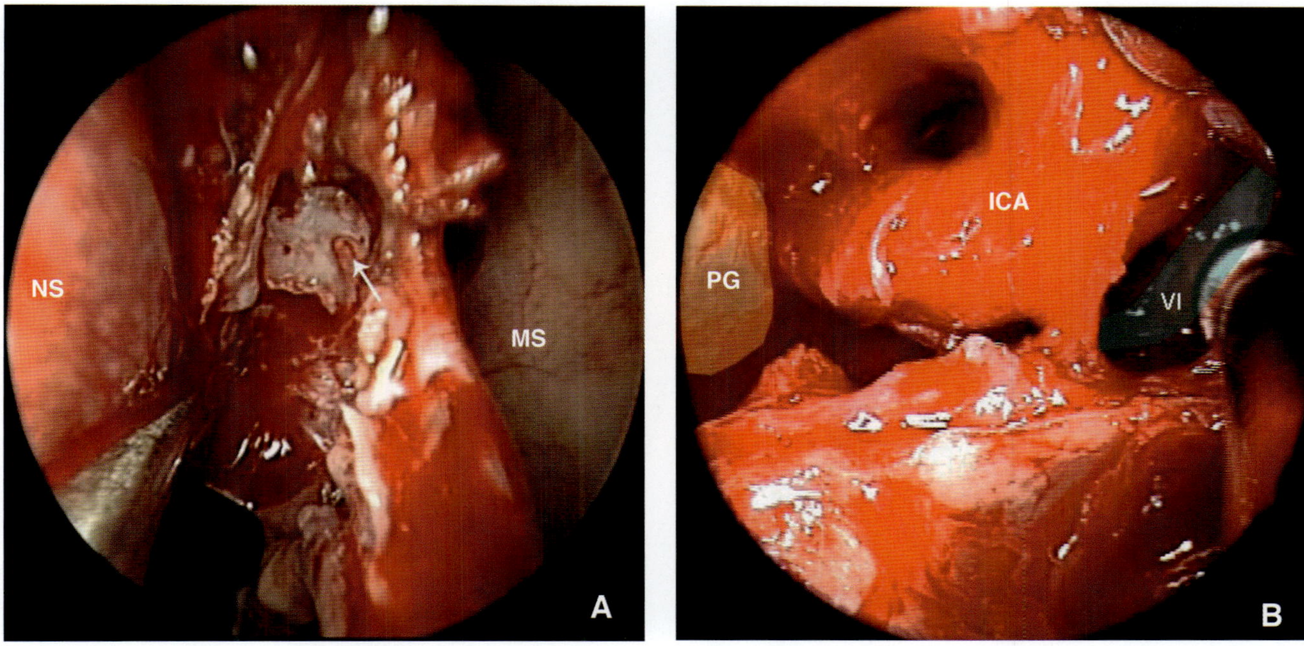

Fig. 31.7 Intraoperative images of the different phases of the transpterygoidal approach. **(A)** Landmark is the vidian artery during pterygoid opening. MS: maxillary sinus; NS: nasal septum. The arrow indicates the emergence of the vidian artery from the pterygoid. **(B)** Opening of the right cavernous sinus. ICA: internal carotid artery; PG: pituitary gland; VI: abducent nerve.

the pterygopalatine fossa and diseases located laterally to the borders of the intracavernous and paraclival carotid artery. The extent of resection varies according to the type and to the location of the lesion. The floor of the sphenoid sinus can be removed with an intranasal diamond burr drill beginning from the choana to its insertion into the clivus working in an anteroposterior and mediolateral direction medial to the vidian canal. The pterygoid process can be removed in a mediolateral and craniocaudal direction with the limit of the eustachian tube posteriorly and of the pterygoid muscles laterally. The vidian canal forms the upper boundary. If the vidian artery needs to be resected, the bony canal can be opened using a diamond burr drill starting below the vidian foramen and thus removing the superior and the lateral portion of the canal. If necessary, the superior wall of the pterygopalatine fossa, represented by the greater wing of the sphenoid bone, can be removed, opening a surgical route to the middle cranial fossa.[7]

In managing diseases of the pterygopalatine fossa, such as angiofibromas in the lateral wall of the sphenoid or CSF leaks of the Sternberg's canal, a monolateral transethmoid-pterygoid-sphenoid approach may be sufficient. The management of sellar lesions extending into the cavernous sinus or intracranially in the temporal fossa generally requires an enlargement of the surgical corridor using the contralateral nasal fossa.

The Intracavernous Step

The cavernous sinus extends on both sides of the sella from the superior orbital fissure to the petrous portion of the temporal bone. It is a venous compartment between two dural layers adhering to the body of the sphenoid bone and to the anterior and posterior clinoid processes. The internal carotid artery (ICA) with its intracavernous branches, the abducent nerve, and sympathetic nerve fibers sheathing the ICA course in the cavernous sinus. The oculomotor and trochlear nerves and trigeminal ophthalmic branch (V1) course along the lateral wall of the sinus in a dural fold. The trigeminal maxillary branch (V2) runs, posteriorly, along the lateral side, and, anteriorly, along the floor of the sinus (**Fig. 31.8**).

The meningohypophyseal trunk and inferior cavernous sinus artery are the intracavernous branches of the ICA. The meningohypophyseal trunk emerges in the medial compartment of the cavernous sinus from the posterior bend of the ICA and gives off three branches: the tentorial artery (Bernasconi-Cassinari); the inferior hypophysial artery, which runs medial to the pituitary gland; and the dorsal meningeal artery, leading to the dura of the superior clivus. The artery of the inferior cavernous sinus emerges in the lateral compartment of the cavernous sinus from the horizontal segment and runs above the abducent nerve.

The abducent nerve (VI) enters the cavernous sinus through a dural foramen coming from the Dorello's canal that is an osteofibrous conduit from the petrous apex to the Gruber's ligament. The nerve changes direction above the petrous apex to reach the ICA. Inside Dorello's canal, the nerve is anchored to the endosteum and connects to the artery in 80% of cases. In the sinus it courses the lateral wall of the ICA and sometimes subdivides into several bundles.

Surgical entry into these structures can use spaces created by the lesion to access the sinus, preserving anatomical

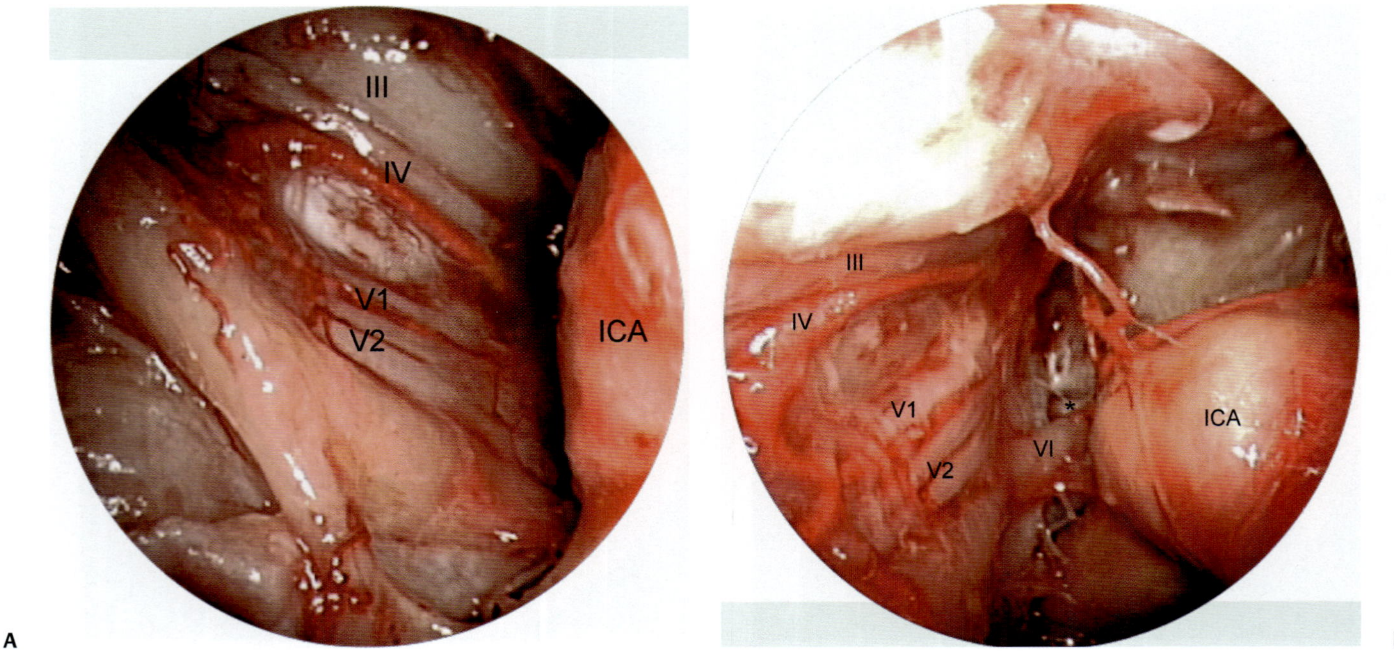

Fig. 31.8 (A,B) Anatomical dissection of the lateral compartment of the cavernous sinus. ICA: internal carotid artery; *: Gruber's ligament. *Nerves:* III: oculomotor nerve; IV: trochlear nerve; V1: ophthalmic branch of the trigeminal nerve; V2: maxillary branch of the trigeminal nerve; VI: abducent nerve.

structures. One technique we widely use is the "diving" technique, as described in the next section.

Diving Technique

Once the surgeon has removed a part of the lesion and a new cavity is visualized, continuous irrigation through the pump enables the surgeon to enter the space with the endoscope. Filling that dead space with saline solution allows the endoscope to be introduced into the tumor itself, providing an excellent "underwater" view of residual tumor, the capsule, normal pituitary tissue, and cavernous sinus walls. The removal of the tumor is completed with this "diving" technique, injecting saline solution into the cavity created after tumor resection and checking for the presence of residual tumor. Thanks to this technique, vision is not impaired by blood oozing from the cavernous sinus or from tumor residues, as we are able to dissect tiny residues.[8]

The advantages of this technique include the following:

- Final hydrodissection of the lesion and removal of microresidues
- Visualization of structures, fistulas, and perforations of the cavernous sinus walls, in the presence of bleeding, thanks to the flushing pressure
- Exploration of spaces hidden by the descent of the cistern, as the flow of saline solution reexpands the pseudocapsule through variations in pressure and direction
- Elimination of hematic residues and minimal bleeding that prevents clear visualization

Diving surgery can be performed in the sellar cavity, in the cavernous sinus, and at the level of the posterior cranial fossa in the cavity obtained after clivectomy[9–11] (**Fig. 31.9**).

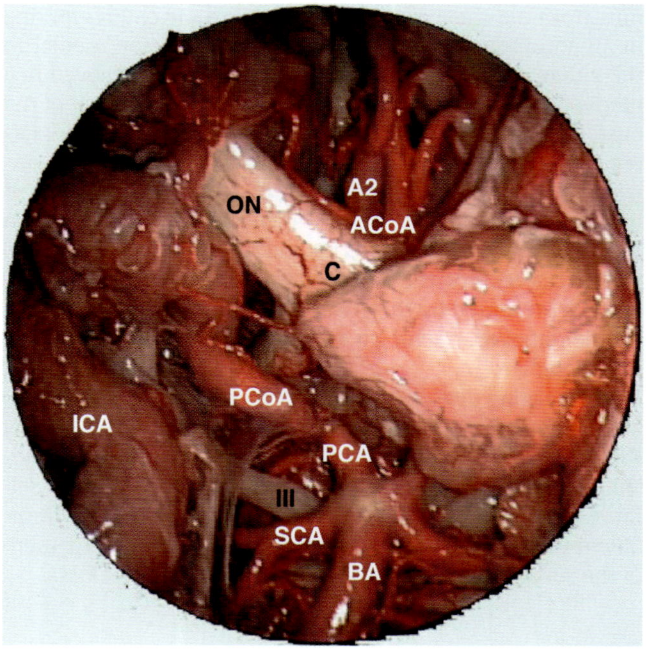

Fig. 31.9 Anatomical dissection of the parasellar spaces: A2: second tract of the anterior cerebral artery; ACoA: anterior communicating artery; BA: basilar artery; C: chiasm; ICA: internal carotid artery; ON: optic nerve; PCA: posterior cerebral artery; PCoA: posterior communicating artery; SCA: superior cerebellar artery; III: oculomotor nerve.

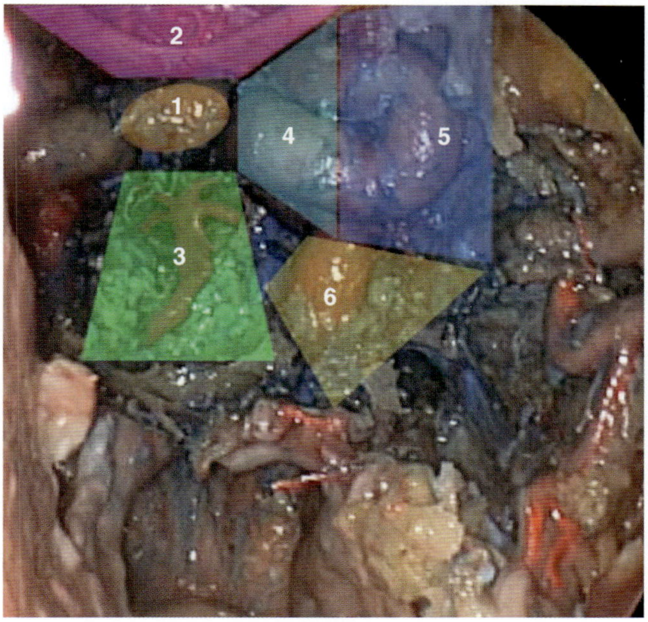

Fig. 31.10 Surgical targets. 1. Sellar region. The pituitary gland, stalk, inferior hypophyseal artery, intercavernous sinus, and diaphragma may be at risk. 2. Suprasellar region. The chiasm, optic nerves, superior hypophyseal artery (lesion of the perforating branches to the chiasm can lead to scotomas), olfactory nerves, frontal cerebral parenchyma, and anterior cerebral circulation may be at risk. 3. Posterior fossa. The posterior cerebral circulation, oculomotor nerve, brainstem, and dorsal clival sinus may be at risk. 4. Medial compartment of the cavernous sinus. The meningohypophyseal trunk and internal carotid artery may be at risk. 5. Lateral compartment of the cavernous sinus. The internal carotid artery, oculomotor nerve, trochlear nerve, trigeminal nerve, abducent nerve, and the artery of the inferior cavernous sinus may be at risk. 6. Middle cranial fossa. The paraclival carotid artery, vidian artery, vidian canal, and Gasser ganglion may be at risk.

Conclusion

The TPS approach provides a direct route for the endoscope to access the middle cranial fossa in the regions of the cavernous sinus and paraclival and infratemporal spaces. The various phases of the surgical approach require special care so as to avoid anatomical disorientation, which could lead to serious complications. Dedicated instruments must be used, as it is absolutely crucial to preserve vessels and nerves in the intracranial compartment and skull base.

Laboratory anatomical dissection and surgical practice are of the essence in acquiring a sound knowledge of the complex three-dimensional anatomy and endoscopic dissection skills. Neuronavigation and intraoperative Doppler sonography are effective complementary instruments but they cannot replace a surgeon's experience.[12,13]

In all cases, preoperative planning should take into consideration not only the patient's anatomy but also the anatomical characteristics of the lesion. Virtual anatomical spaces can become surgical pathways resulting from the development of the lesion (**Figs. 31.10** and **31.11**).

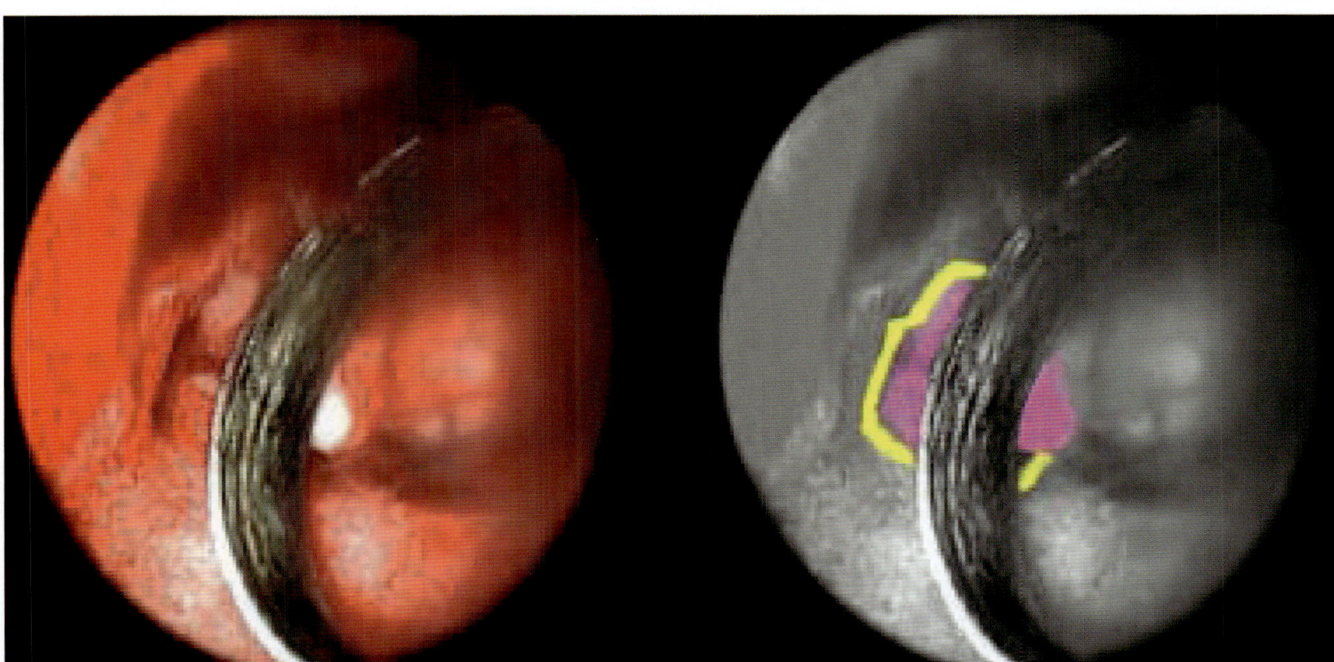

Fig. 31.11 Diving technique for the removal of a small tumor residue from the cavernous sinus. Better visualization of the cavernous wall is provided by the diving technique.

References

1. Castelnuovo P, Locatelli D. Endoscopic surgical management of cerebrospinal fluid rhinorrhea. Tuttlingen 2008:7–15
2. Locatelli D, Rampa F, Acchiardi I, Bignami M, De Bernardi F, Castelnuovo P. Endoscopic endonasal approaches for repair of cerebrospinal fluid leaks: nine-year experience. Neurosurgery 2006;58(4, suppl 2): ONS246–ONS257
3. Frank G, Pasquini E, Doglietto F, et al. The endoscopic extended transsphenoidal approach for craniopharyngiomas. Neurosurgery 2006; 59(1, Suppl 1):ONS75–ONS83, discussion ONS75–ONS83
4. Cavallo LM, Messina A, Cappabianca P, et al. Endoscopic endonasal surgery of the midline skull base: anatomical study and clinical considerations. Neurosurg Focus 2005;19:E2
5. Frank G, Pasquini E, Mazzatenta D. Extended transsphenoidal approach. J Neurosurg 2001;95:917–918
6. Kassam A, Snyderman CH, Mintz A, Gardner P, Carrau RL. Expanded endonasal approach: the rostrocaudal axis. Part I. Crista galli to the sella turcica. Neurosurg Focus 2005;19:E3
7. Cavallo LM, Messina A, Gardner P, et al. Extended endoscopic endonasal approach to the pterygopalatine fossa: anatomical study and clinical considerations. Neurosurg Focus 2005;19:E5
8. Locatelli D, Canevari FR, Acchiardi I, Castelnuovo P. The endoscopic diving technique in pituitary and cranial base surgery: technical note. Neurosurgery 2010;66:E400–E401, discussion E401
9. Cavallo LM, Cappabianca P, Messina A, et al. The extended endoscopic endonasal approach to the clivus and cranio-vertebral junction: anatomical study. Childs Nerv Syst 2007;23:665–671
10. Kassam A, Snyderman CH, Mintz A, Gardner P, Carrau RL. Expanded endonasal approach: the rostrocaudal axis. Part II. Posterior clinoids to the foramen magnum. Neurosurg Focus 2005;19:E4
11. Kassam AB, Gardner P, Snyderman C, Mintz A, Carrau RL. Expanded endonasal approach: fully endoscopic, completely transnasal approach to the middle third of the clivus, petrous bone, middle cranial fossa, and infratemporal fossa. Neurosurg Focus 2005;19:E6
12. Castelnuovo P, Locatelli D. "Two nostrils-four hands" endoscopic endonasal surgical technique. Silver book (informative publication) published by Karl Storz.
13. Castelnuovo P, Pistochini A, Locatelli D. Different surgical approaches to the sellar region: focusing on the "two nostrils four hands technique". Rhinology 2006;44:2–7

32 Pterygopalatine and Infratemporal Fossae

Marc A. Tewfik and Peter-John Wormald

Tips and Pearls

- The endoscopic approach to lesions in the pterygopalatine fossa (PPF) and infratemporal fossa (ITF) offers the advantages of a direct route of access, and the avoidance of facial scars, facial nerve dysfunction, conductive hearing loss, and dental malocclusion.
- A high level of endoscopic surgical experience, as well as detailed anatomical knowledge of these spaces, is necessary for the surgeon approaching these areas.
- The two-surgeon endoscopic technique offers the distinct advantages of providing a second surgeon for tumor retraction and additional assistance in the event of hemorrhage; access for the second surgeon can be transseptal or through a canine fossa trephine.
- Indications for approaching the PPF include internal maxillary artery ligation and vidian neurectomy; indications for approaching the ITF include resection of tumors and large meningoencephaloceles extending into this space.
- Tumors extension into the masseteric space, buccogingival sulcus, middle cranial fossa, parasellar region, and orbital apex present challenges to resection.
- Careful review of imaging is critical prior to any biopsy to rule out a highly vascular lesion or meningoencephalocele; computed tomography (CT) and magnetic resonance imaging (MRI) are necessary to characterize the bony anatomy and determine the relationship of tumors to critical structures, respectively.
- Preoperative arteriography and selective embolization of feeding vessels is performed for vascular tumors, and a repeat embolization may be beneficial for large tumors.
- Access to the PPF can be achieved through a large middle meatal antrostomy, whereas access laterally into the ITF requires an endoscopic medial maxillectomy.
- After debulking the nasal component of the tumor, the posterior wall of the maxillary sinus is removed with a Hajek-Koeffler punch, beginning at the sphenopalatine foramen.
- The second surgeon places traction on the tumor and rolls it out of the ITF, while the primary surgeon cauterizes or clips the feeding blood vessels.
- Following tumor removal, the vidian canal, clivus, nasopharynx, and pterygoid plates are carefully inspected to ensure that no residual extensions of tumor remain.
- Dural defects are repaired with two layers of fascia lata, a nasal septal flap, and fibrin glue; otherwise the maxillary sinus mucosa is redraped over the resection site.

Introduction

In the past, access to the pterygopalatine fossa (PPF) and infratemporal fossa (ITF) could only be achieved by either anterior or lateral approaches. Anterior approaches include midfacial degloving, lateral rhinotomy, extended maxillotomy/maxillectomy, facial translocation, and transantral maxillectomy approaches.[1–3] Although these all provide good exposure for procedures such as internal maxillary artery ligation, vidian neurectomy, and removal of tumors of the PPF and anteromedial ITF regions, they are often complicated by facial scars and deformity, facial and infraorbital nerve dysfunction, as well as lacrimal dysfunction.[2] Lateral approaches consist primarily of the Fisch C and D procedures,[4,5] which offer excellent access to structures within the ITF, as well as the basisphenoid, clivus, and intratemporal course of the internal carotid artery. However, adverse outcomes include dysfunction of the facial nerve, conductive hearing loss, and dental malocclusion.[3,6]

Recent advances in endoscopic sinus surgery, and in interventional radiology with preoperative embolization, have enabled endoscopic surgical access to tumors of the PPF and ITF. Among these advances are improved instrumentation, computer-based surgical navigation, as well as hypotensive anesthetic techniques. In addition, the development of the two-surgeon transnasal approach[7] has further facilitated access to the lateral ITF. However, an adequate level of experience in endoscopic sinus surgery as well as detailed knowledge of the endoscopic anatomy are necessary for any surgeon tackling pathology in these spaces. Although a comprehensive review of anatomy is beyond the scope of this chapter, the following pages provide an overview of the endoscopic transnasal approach to the PPF and ITF, beginning with a brief discussion of the structure and contents of these spaces.

Anatomy of the Pterygopalatine and Infratemporal Fossae

The PPF is a narrow space in the shape of an inverted cone, located between the posterior wall of the maxillary sinus and

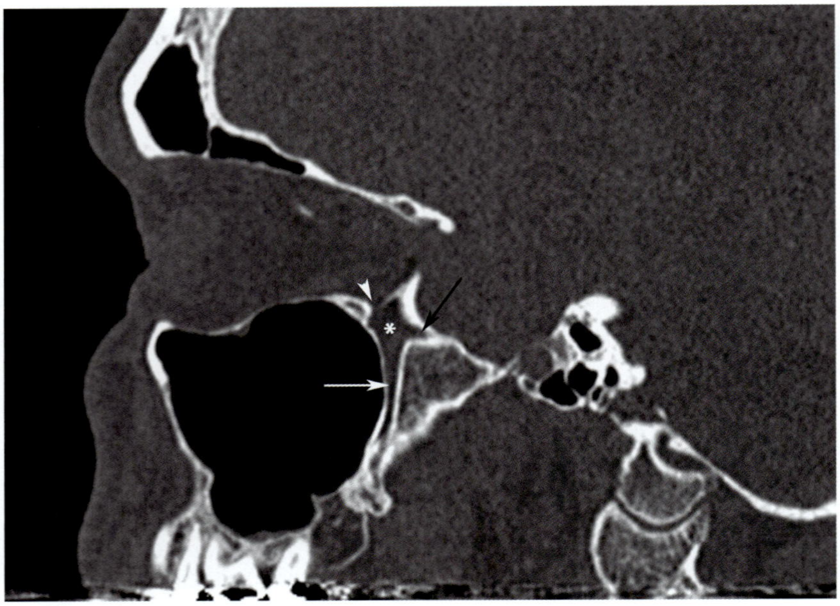

Fig. 32.1 Computed tomography (CT) scan of the sinuses, parasagittal cut, through the pterygopalatine fossa (PPF; *asterisk*), demonstrating the foramen rotundum (*black arrow*), descending palatine canal (*white arrow*), and inferior orbital fissure (*white arrowhead*).

the base of the pterygoid process (**Fig. 32.1**). Its contents consist of fat, the sphenopalatine ganglion, the vidian nerve, the maxillary division of the trigeminal nerve (V2), and terminal branches of the internal maxillary artery. The fat and blood vessels lie anteromedial to the neural structures, and are therefore encountered first during the endoscopic approach. The pterygoid or vidian canal opens into the posterior aspect of the fossa. The vidian canal starts at the anterior genu of the petrous carotid artery and carries the vidian nerve along the inferolateral border of the sphenoid sinus until it reaches the PPF. The palatovaginal or pharyngeal canal also opens into the posterior aspect of the fossa just medial to the vidian canal (**Fig. 32.2**). The apex of the PPF is continuous inferiorly with the descending palatine canal, which opens into the oral cavity via the greater and lesser palatine foramina. The superior border consists of the undersurface of the sphenoid bone and orbital process of the palatine bone. Cranial nerve V2 passes from the middle cranial fossa to the PPF through the foramen rotundum, before giving off connections to the sphenopalatine ganglion, as well as branches to the orbit via the inferior orbital fissure. Medially, the PPF is separated from the nasal cavity by the perpendicular plate of the palatine bone, which also constitutes the anterior and inferior borders of the sphenopalatine foramen. Endoscopically, the ethmoidal crest is a reliable landmark along the lateral nasal wall, lying immediately anterior to the sphenopalatine foramen and artery.

Laterally, the PPF is continuous with the ITF; they are divided by the pterygomaxillary fissure in the plane of the lateral pterygoid plate. The ITF is bordered laterally by the coronoid process, ramus of the mandible, and pterygoid muscles. As with the PPF, its anterior border is the posterior surface of the maxilla; however, its posterior border consists of the articular tubercle of the temporal bone and the spine of the sphenoid bone. The ITF is separated from the middle cranial fossa superiorly by the greater wing of the sphenoid bone,

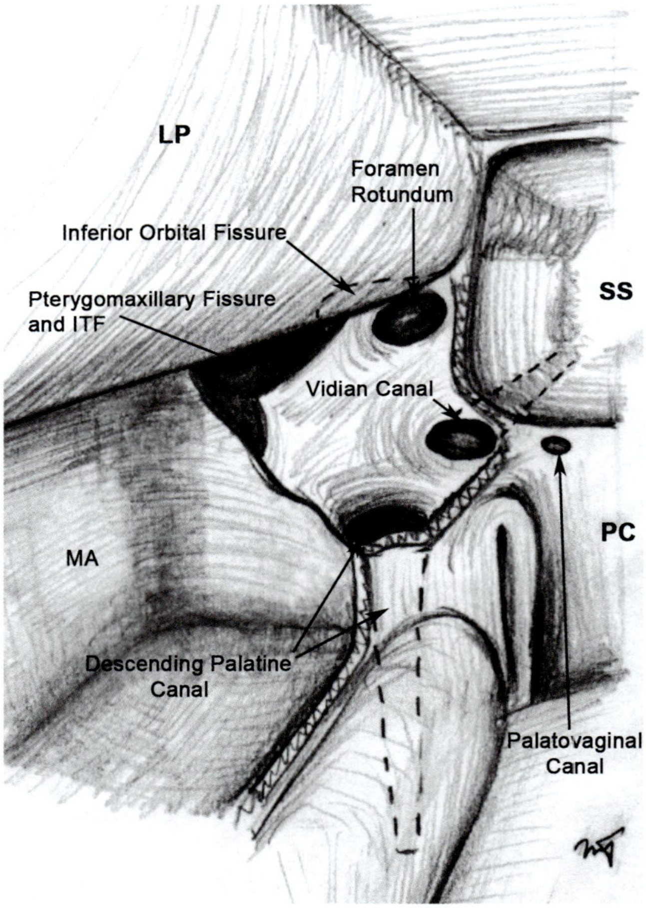

Fig. 32.2 Illustration depicting the PPF with the medial and anterior walls removed, demonstrating the foramina and openings along the inferior, posterior, superior, and lateral borders of the fossa. LP: lamina papyracea; MA: maxillary antrum; PC: posterior choana; SS: sphenoid sinus.

which contains the foramen ovale and foramen spinosum; they transmit the mandibular division of trigeminal (V3) and the middle meningeal artery, respectively. The alveolar border of the maxilla delineates the inferior margin of the ITF. The relationships between these various structures are important in helping the surgeon identify and preserve those that are normal, and fully remove pathologic tissue.

Indications and Advantages of the Endoscopic Approach

The endoscopic approach to the PPF is indicated for internal maxillary artery ligation in patients with uncontrolled posterior epistaxis and in whom ligation of the sphenopalatine and posterior nasal arteries has failed,[8] for vidian neurectomy in patients with refractory vasomotor rhinitis,[9] and for the repair of laterally based meningoencephaloceles.[10] Given that the PPF and ITF are adjacent and continuous spaces, masses that arise in one space can easily spread to the other. Such masses include juvenile nasopharyngeal angiofibromas (JNAs), maxillary nerve schwannomas, large inverting papillomas, and large temporal lobe meningoencephaloceles.[7]

The advantages of the endoscopic technique are numerous, including the avoidance of adverse outcomes associated with open approaches, such as facial incisions, hearing loss, and nerve dysfunction. Relatively straightforward access is achieved to the PPF and ITF, areas traditionally considered difficult to reach. The endoscope provides a magnified and multiangled view for more precise discrimination of the dissection planes between the tumor and the adjacent structures. Furthermore, the two-surgeon technique offers improved surgical control by providing a second surgeon for tumor retraction and additional assistance for suctioning in the event of brisk surgical bleeding.

Contraindications

Given the continual refinements in surgical technique and instrumentation, it is unlikely that the limits of endoscopic resection of tumors in the ITF have been achieved. Tumors extending into the masseteric space, buccogingival sulcus, middle cranial fossa, parasellar region, and cavernous sinus, as well as around the optic nerve and orbital apex, present challenges to endoscopic resection. However, these regions are also very difficult to access via open approaches, and in skilled hands these regions can all be approached endoscopically. There is an ongoing controversy over the role of endoscopic resection for malignant neoplasms; such an approach may be acceptable in select malignancies, as long as it does not compromise the completeness of oncologic resection. However, certain malignant tumors, such as squamous cell carcinoma, tend to fare poorly due to their extensively infiltrative nature, and so are not recommended for endoscopic resection.

Diagnostic Workup

Clinical Assessment

The clinical history and physical examination are important in obtaining the diagnosis of lesions extending from or into the ITF. The most common nasal tumor with ITF involvement is JNA. It has the classical presentation of recurrent unilateral epistaxis in teenage or young adult males. If it is suspected in a female patient, karyotyping should be obtained to rule out an androgen insensitivity syndrome. A history of seizures may be seen in tumors with significant intracranial extension via the foramen rotundum or in large meningoencephaloceles.

The physical examination should include assessment of cranial nerve function, along with extraocular movements and visual acuity. If any orbital or optic nerve involvement is suspected, a complete ophthalmologic evaluation is warranted. Rigid nasal endoscopy is performed to assess for masses with an intranasal component, as well as for the detection of septal deviation, unusual nasal anatomy, or other obstacles to endoscopic access.

In most cases, the diagnosis of these tumors is self-evident, without the need for histopathology. However, if there is significant doubt as to the diagnosis, then histologic confirmation may be required. Careful review of imaging is essential because biopsy of a highly vascular lesion may result in catastrophic hemorrhage.

Imaging Studies

Computed tomography (CT) provides useful information regarding bony sinus anatomy, the position and integrity of the lamina papyracea, as well as involvement of the ethmoid and sphenoid sinuses. Magnetic resonance imaging (MRI) is essential in determining the relationship of tumors to critical structures. Tumor extension through the inferior orbital fissure into the orbital apex and cavernous sinus needs to be identified and a plan developed for the removal of the tumor from this region (**Fig. 32.3**). The other critical region is the vidian canal. Tumor will often infiltrate the clivus, and occasionally reach the carotid artery by expanding along this canal (**Fig. 32.4**). Within the ITF, the relationship of the tumor to the middle cranial fossa, buccogingival sulcus, and masseteric space also needs to be ascertained, to decide whether this tumor can be safely resected using the endoscope and two-surgeon technique. High-resolution CT or MRI scans specifically suitable for image-guided surgical navigation should be obtained preoperatively.

During the 24 hours preceding surgery, an arteriogram is performed to establish if there are any significant feeders from the internal carotid or internal maxillary arteries. If this is the case, a highly selective embolization of all feeding vessels is performed. It is important that arteriography be performed bilaterally, as tumors can receive feeding vessels from both sides. With large tumors, a repeat arteriography and embolization of any remaining vessels may be useful immediately before surgery. We have found that this significantly

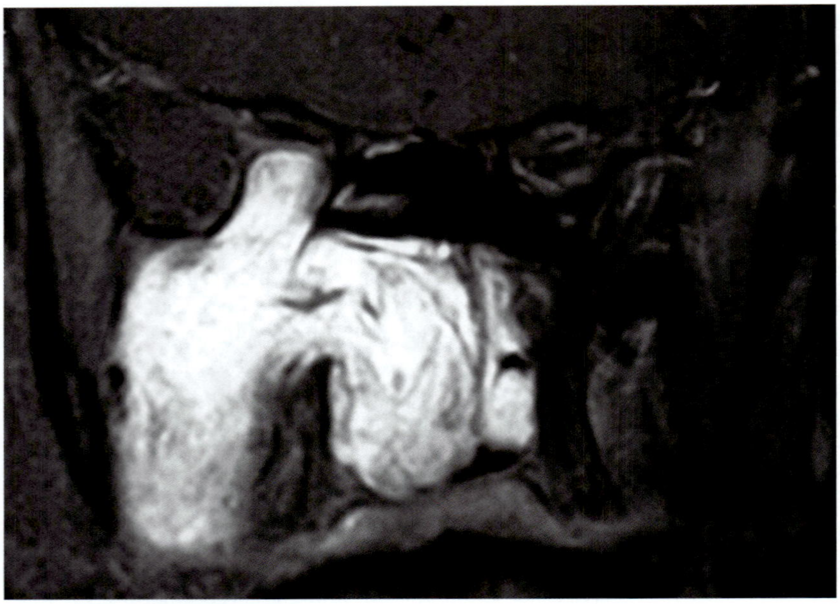

Fig. 32.3 T1-weighted magnetic resonance imaging (MRI) of the sinuses demonstrating a gadolinium-enhancing juvenile nasopharyngeal angiofibroma (JNA) extending superiorly from the PPF though the inferior orbital fissure and compressing the contents of the orbital apex.

reduces the vascularity and intraoperative bleeding in comparison to large tumors that had only been preoperatively embolized once.

Surgery

Instrumentation

In addition to standard functional endoscopic sinus surgery (FESS) equipment, including high-quality 0-, 30-, and 70-degree endoscopes, sharp through-biting instruments, a microdebrider, and a Hajek-Koeffler or Kerrison punch, several additional instruments are necessary. Malleable suction dissectors (both curette and Freer elevator; Medtronic ENT, Jacksonville, FL) are very useful in performing the dissection, and can be bent into the required angle needed to reach difficult areas. A dacryocystorhinostomy (DCR) spear knife (Medtronic ENT) is necessary to open the nasolacrimal sac in cases where a medial maxillectomy is performed. A 25-degree skull base diamond burr (Medtronic ENT) is needed when there is tumor extension through the inferior orbital fissure, to drill the medial pterygoid plate for better visualization. An endoscopic suction bipolar cautery (Medtronic ENT) or Ligar clips are necessary to deal with tumor feeding vessels and intraoperative bleeding. A Coblation plasma wand (ArthroCare ENT; Sunnyvale, CA) may also be useful in the resection of

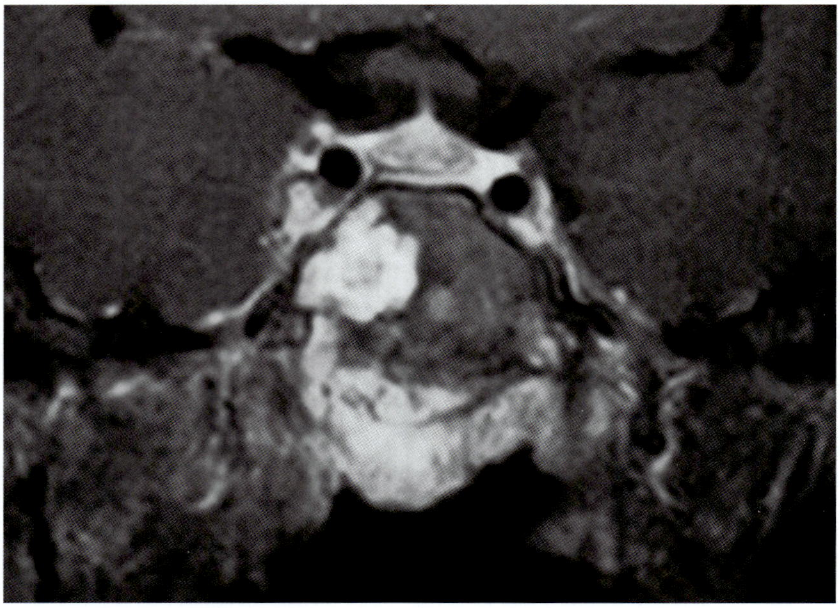

Fig. 32.4 T1-weighted MRI of the sinuses with gadolinium enhancement, demonstrating tumor extension along an expanded vidian canal, toward the internal carotid artery.

highly vascular lesions. Finally, the canine fossa trephination kit (Medtronic ENT)—consisting of an endoscope sheath with a protruding blade for soft tissue retraction, a reusable drill guide, as well as a 5-mm reusable drill bit that fits the microdebrider handpiece—can be used to create an additional port for the second surgeon in the anterior wall of the maxilla.

Operative Setup

Patients undergo total intravenous anesthesia and have local anesthetic agents injected into the lateral nasal wall and transorally through the greater palatine foramen.[11] Intraoperative antibiotics with gram-positive coverage are administered on induction of anesthesia.

Preparation

In cases where a dural defect is anticipated, such as in meningoencephalocele repair, a nasal septal flap is elevated off the side of the septum opposite to the defect. This is based on the contralateral sphenopalatine bundle to ensure that the pedicle is free of pathology and is not damaged during the dissection.

As a first step, a routine uncinectomy and large middle meatal antrostomy are performed. Anterior and posterior ethmoidectomies are performed on the side of the lesion, with removal of the lower half of the middle and superior turbinates. A large sphenoidotomy is then created to clearly identify the skull base. This also enables the tumor to be accurately defined, provides access over the top of the tumor, and enables any tumor extension into the sphenoid to be visualized. Frontal recess clearance is performed if there are inflammatory changes in this area.

If only limited exposure to the PPF and medial ITF is required, then the posterior wall of the maxillary sinus can be removed through a large middle meatal antrostomy alone.[12] However, if there is significant tumor within the ITF and gingivobuccal sulcus, then an endoscopic medial maxillectomy is necessary to allow complete access.

To perform the medial maxillectomy, the inferior turbinate is first crushed with a Tilley's packing forceps to devascularize it, and cut with a scissors at its anterior attachment to the lateral nasal wall (**Fig. 32.5A**). A mucosal incision is made from the middle meatal antrostomy to the floor of the nasal cavity and then extended posteriorly to the posterior end of the inferior turbinate (**Fig. 32.5B**). A chisel is then used to perform osteotomies along these mucosal incisions (**Fig. 32.5C**).[7] The nasolacrimal duct will tether the medial

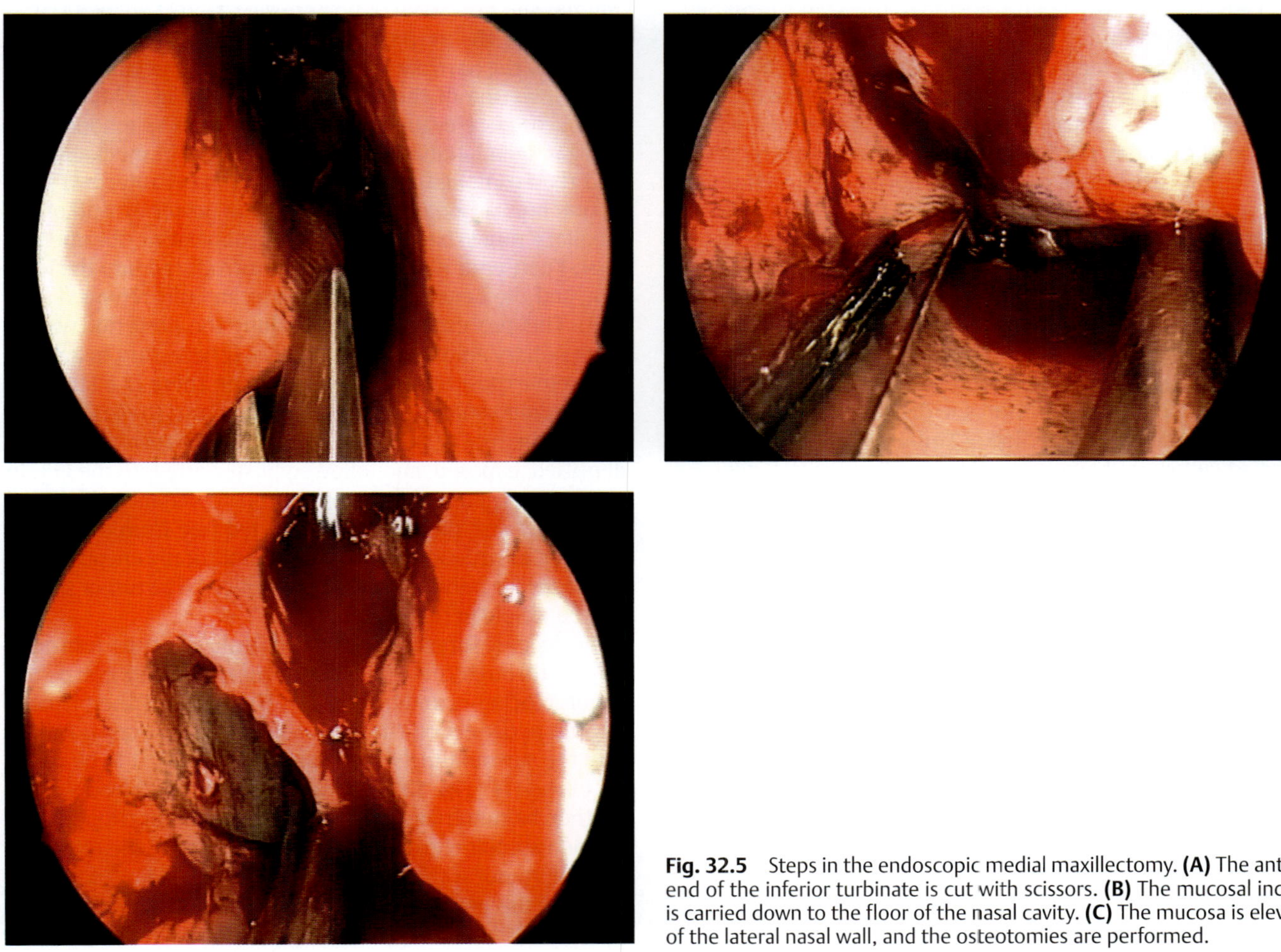

A B C

Fig. 32.5 Steps in the endoscopic medial maxillectomy. **(A)** The anterior end of the inferior turbinate is cut with scissors. **(B)** The mucosal incision is carried down to the floor of the nasal cavity. **(C)** The mucosa is elevated of the lateral nasal wall, and the osteotomies are performed.

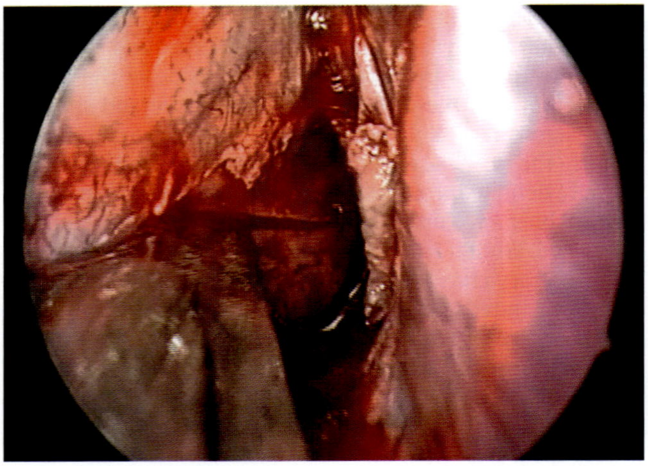

Fig. 32.6 Creation of the transseptal access port; endoscopic view through a left hemitransfixion incision, following removal of septal cartilage, and creation of the horizontal incision in the contralateral septal mucosal flap using a No. 15 blade.

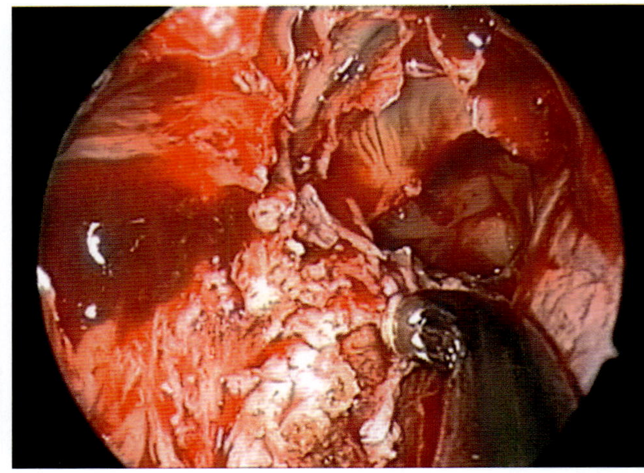

Fig. 32.7 Endoscopic view demonstrating a Coblation wand being used to separate the endonasal component of a JNA from the main tumor bulk within the PPF and infratemporal fossa (ITF).

wall of the maxillary sinus, and is cut with scissors or a scalpel to allow removal of the wall. At the end of the procedure, the lumen of the nasolacrimal sac is opened superiorly with the DCR spear knife, and the mucosal flaps are laid out on the lateral nasal wall. This prevents postoperative stenosis of the nasolacrimal system.

Transseptal access for a second surgeon is achieved by placing a hemi-transfixion incision through the opposite nostril to the lesion. If necessary, a septoplasty is performed with resection of the bony posterior septum; otherwise, a rectangular strip of cartilage is removed. A horizontal incision is made in the septal flap adjacent to the tumor (**Fig. 32.6**), enabling an instrument to be placed from the opposite nostril through the septum into the surgical field. This key step enables the second surgeon to place traction on the ITF component of tumors, facilitating their dissection and allowing them to be rolled out of the ITF. This way, the internal maxillary artery may be clipped and cauterized once encountered. Another excellent access option for the second surgeon is through a canine fossa trephine.[13] This access point has the added advantage of being separate from the nostrils, giving the second surgeon more space to maneuver the instrument without touching or bumping the primary surgeon.

Approach

In cases of ITF tumors, the nasal component of the tumor is removed first along with any extension of the tumor into the sphenoid. This allows for more exposure to the difficult areas of dissection in the ITF and inferior orbital fissure. The nasal component is mobilized with a suction Freer and separated from the septum and posterior bony choanae. If the tumor pushes through the floor of the sphenoid sinus, it is mobilized into the nasal cavity through the large sphenoidotomy. In vascular tumors, a Coblation wand is used to separate the endonasal component from the main ITF tumor bulk, and any bleeding from the surface is cauterized (**Fig. 32.7**). Once freed, the endonasal tumor component is delivered through the choana and removed transorally.

The mucosa of the posterior maxillary antrum is elevated laterally and preserved. A posteriorly based U-shaped flap is created over the perpendicular plate of palatine bone from just below the horizontal portion of the ground lamella down to the insertion of the inferior turbinate (**Fig. 32.8A**). Once the mucosa is elevated posteriorly and the sphenopalatine artery is seen emanating from its foramen immediately behind the ethmoidal crest (**Fig. 32.8B**), it is cauterized with suction bipolar forceps. Removal of the posterior wall of the maxillary sinus begins at the sphenopalatine foramen. A Hajek-Koeffler or Kerrison punch is introduced into the foramen, and the bone anterior to the foramen is removed (**Fig. 32.9**). This process is continued along the posterior wall of the maxillary sinus, as far laterally as is necessary to achieve complete exposure of the tumor. When there is a large ITF tumor component, the bone is removed down to the floor and up onto the roof of the sinus, where the infraorbital nerve is identified, exposed, and followed posteriorly into the PPF. In most cases, there is an anatomical plane between the nerve and tumor, and these can be dissected free from one other. However, in situations where the tumor totally encompasses or invades the nerve, the nerve is sacrificed. The tumor should now be visible in the PPF and ITF.

The second surgeon places a Blakesley forceps transseptally or through the canine fossa puncture and grasps the tumor, placing it under traction. This enables the primary surgeon to dissect on the capsule of the tumor, separating it from the surrounding structures, and allowing it to be rolled out of the ITF (**Fig. 32.10**). The tumor feeding blood vessels can then be cauterized with a suction bipolar or clipped with a small vascular clip applicator, further freeing the tumor.

As the tumor is rolled out of the ITF, the medial and lateral heads of the pterygoid muscles are seen. If the tumor extends into the inferior orbital fissure, the lateral sphenoid

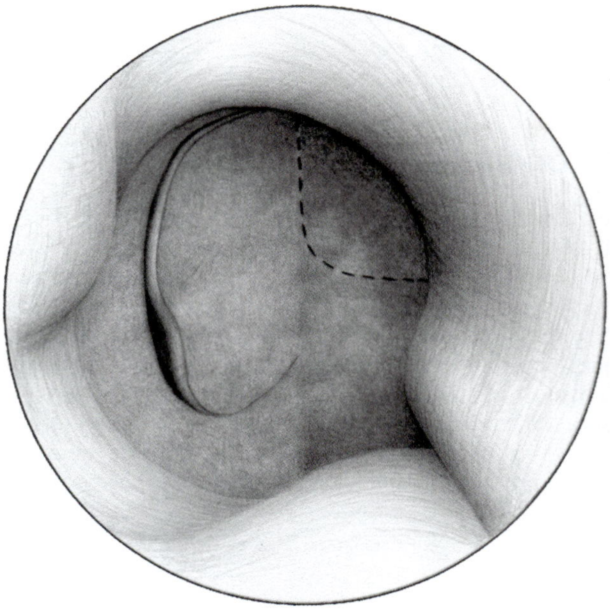

A

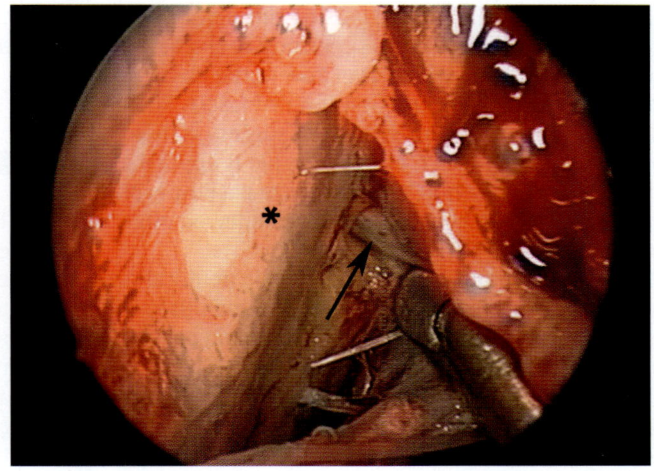

B

Fig. 32.8 **(A)** Illustration depicting the mucosal flap from just below the horizontal portion of the ground lamella of the middle turbinate down to the insertion of the inferior turbinate to uncover the sphenopalatine artery. **(B)** Intraoperative view of the right sphenopalatine artery (*black arrow*) and the vertical portion of palatine bone (*asterisk*).

bone should be removed using a diamond burr, opening up the inferior orbital fissure. The tumor will often widen the vidian canal, and tumor extensions can be followed along the canal in the floor of the sphenoid sinus for up to 2 cm before the internal carotid artery is reached.[14] In this region, tumor may push up against the cavernous sinus, and it is not uncommon to get profuse venous bleeding as the tumor is dissected from the sinus. This is best controlled by packing the area with Gelfoam (Pharmacia Corp.; Kalamazoo, MI) paste and applying pressure with a neuropatty.

Benign tumors that erode into the middle cranial fossa and push on the dura can usually be separated from the dura by gentle traction and staying in the plane directly adjacent to the tumor. If there is tumor invasion through the dura, dural incisions are best made with a No. 11 blade, incorporating a margin of normal dura around the tumor. The intradural portion of the dissection can then be performed with the neurosurgeon. Once the tumor has been completely removed from the ITF, the vidian canal, clivus, nasopharynx, and pterygoid plates are carefully checked to ensure that no small residual extensions of tumor remain. The mobilized tumor is then delivered through the nasopharynx and mouth. Hemostasis is achieved with a combination of Gelfoam paste and bipolar cautery.

Repair

In cases resulting in a dural defect, the dural repair is performed with two layers of fascia lata. The first layer is fashioned to

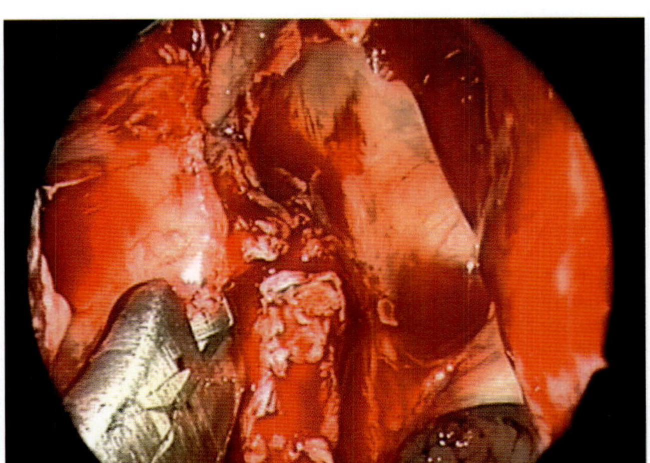

Fig. 32.9 Hajek-Koeffler punch used to remove bone of the posterior wall of the maxillary sinus, anterior to the sphenopalatine foramen and, in this instance, tumor.

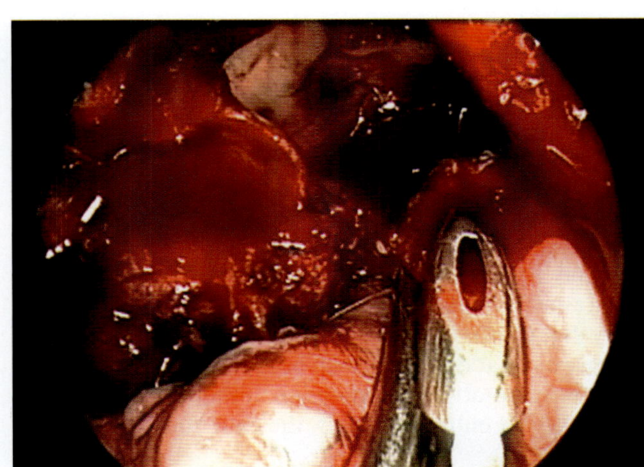

Fig. 32.10 Blakesley forceps placed transseptally by the second surgeon to grasps the tumor and place it under traction, so that it may be rolled out of the ITF.

slightly larger than the dimensions of the defect, and the edges of the fascia are tucked in superiorly to the bony margins of the defect. The second layer covers the nasal side of the defect and is laid over the first layer of fascia. The nasal septal flap harvested at the beginning of surgery is then used to cover the repaired defect, and fibrin glue is applied along the edges of the flap. Gentle Vaseline gauze packing is placed to support the dural reconstruction, and removed after 5 to 7 days.

In most benign tumor resections, there is no dural defect produced, and the nose is not packed. The maxillary antral mucosa preserved earlier in the approach is laid over the resection site. The septum is quilted with a Vicryl Rapide suture (Ethicon; Johnson & Johnson, Somerville, NJ), ensuring that the edges of the horizontal incision are brought together. The hemi-transfixion incision is sutured.

Complications

The complications of these techniques can be divided into several categories. Vascular complications may occur with hemorrhage from branches of the internal maxillary artery or feeding vessels off the internal carotid, as well as venous bleeding from the cavernous sinus. Neural injury may occur to branches of the maxillary nerve (V2) or sphenopalatine ganglion, causing facial paresthesias or dry eye, respectively. The chances of adverse orbital events increase with tumor extension through the inferior orbital fissure, and include transient or permanent visual loss, and extraocular muscle injury. Postoperative cerebrospinal fluid (CSF) leak or intracranial bleeding may also occur. Septal perforation may result from the creation of the transseptal access port. In cases where packing is used, dislodgment and aspiration, as well as toxic shock syndrome, may occur. Finally, residual or recurrent tumor may complicate the postoperative course.

Postoperative Care

Patients are placed on systemic broad-spectrum antibiotics for 5 days after surgery, and saline nasal douches are started the day after surgery. The first postoperative nasal debridement is performed at 2 weeks and repeated regularly until the nose stops crusting. In tumor cases, regular nasal endoscopy and a postoperative imaging are recommended. Magnetic resonance imaging is routinely performed at 6-month intervals for JNAs. Areas of enhancement are watched closely and measured at each follow-up because they may only represent postoperative inflammation. If there is clear growth of any of these enhancing areas, the patient is taken back to the operating room for surgical reexploration and removal of any tumor remnant.

Conclusion

The endoscopic approach to the PPF and the ITF offers several advantages over the traditional open techniques. However, a high level of endoscopic skill, as well as detailed anatomical knowledge of these spaces, is necessary to confidently utilize these techniques. The two-surgeon endoscopic technique allows improved surgical control for tumor retraction and hemostasis. Careful preoperative planning is necessary to ensure the feasibility of complete endoscopic resection, and the surgeon should obtain patient consent for the appropriate open procedure if the endoscopic approach becomes too difficult.

References

1. Hitotsumatsu T, Rhoton AL Jr. Unilateral upper and lower subtotal maxillectomy approaches to the cranial base: microsurgical anatomy. Neurosurgery 2000;46:1416–1452, discussion 1452–1453
2. Janecka IP. Classification of facial translocation approach to the skull base. Otolaryngol Head Neck Surg 1995;112:579–585
3. Sabit I, Schaefer SD, Couldwell WT. Modified infratemporal fossa approach via lateral transantral maxillotomy: a microsurgical model. Surg Neurol 2002;58:21–31, discussion 31
4. Fisch U. The infratemporal fossa approach for nasopharyngeal tumors. Laryngoscope 1983;93:36–44
5. Fisch U, Fagan P, Valavanis A. The infratemporal fossa approach for the lateral skull base. Otolaryngol Clin North Am 1984;17:513–552
6. Zhang M, Garvis W, Linder T, Fisch U. Update on the infratemporal fossa approaches to nasopharyngeal angiofibroma. Laryngoscope 1998;108 (11 Pt 1):1717–1723
7. Robinson S, Patel N, Wormald PJ. Endoscopic management of benign tumors extending into the infratemporal fossa: a two-surgeon transnasal approach. Laryngoscope 2005;115:1818–1822
8. Wormald PJ, Wee DT, van Hasselt CA. Endoscopic ligation of the sphenopalatine artery for refractory posterior epistaxis. Am J Rhinol 2000; 14:261–264
9. Robinson SR, Wormald PJ. Endoscopic vidian neurectomy. Am J Rhinol 2006;20:197–202
10. Wormald PJ, McDonogh M. The bath-plug closure of anterior skull base cerebrospinal fluid leaks. Am J Rhinol 2003;17:299–305
11. Wormald PJ, Athanasiadis T, Rees G, Robinson S. An evaluation of effect of pterygopalatine fossa injection with local anesthetic and adrenalin in the control of nasal bleeding during endoscopic sinus surgery. Am J Rhinol 2005;19:288–292
12. Wormald PJ, Ooi E, van Hasselt CA, Nair S. Endoscopic removal of sinonasal inverted papilloma including endoscopic medial maxillectomy. Laryngoscope 2003;113:867–873
13. Singhal D, Douglas R, Robinson S, Wormald PJ. The incidence of complications using new landmarks and a modified technique of canine fossa puncture. Am J Rhinol 2007;21:316–319
14. Kassam AB, Vescan AD, Carrau RL, et al. Expanded endonasal approach: vidian canal as a landmark to the petrous internal carotid artery. J Neurosurg 2008;108:177–183

33 Endoscopic Surgery for Juvenile Nasopharyngeal Angiofibroma

Paolo Castelnuovo, Andrea Pistochini, Francesca Simoncello, Ignazio Ermoli, Andrea Bolzoni Villaret, and Piero Nicolai

Tips and Pearls

- Juvenile nasopharyngeal angiofibroma (JNA) typically occurs in young males, and several studies demonstrated the association with chromosomal aberrations.[1,2]
- The diagnosis of JNA can be achieved by radiologic assessment. Computed tomography (CT) scans and magnetic resonance imaging (MRI) findings are specific. CT, in particular, demonstrates a pathognomonic enlargement of the sphenopalatine foramen, and MRI demonstrates an apparent widespread lack of signal (flow void) related to the presence of high-flow vessels. This makes biopsy unnecessary, thus avoiding the risk of severe bleeding.
- Preoperative embolization of the lesion, usually performed 24 to 48 hours before surgery, enables a minimally invasive endonasal endoscopic approach.
- The endonasal endoscopic surgical technique involves the use of a transethmoidal-pterygoidal-sphenoidal (TEPS) approach, which is often adequate to remove the lesion.
- Regardless of the approach and the extension of the lesion, it is important to drill into the cancellous bone of the base of the pterygoid process and on the sphenoidal floor along the vidian canal, the sites of onset of the disease.
- Follow-up includes periodic MRI in addition to routine endoscopic examinations.

Introduction

Until the 1980s, the surgical technique for juvenile nasopharyngeal angiofibroma (JNA) removal involved only external (transfacial and transcranial) approaches. Over the years, endoscopic endonasal surgery, introduced to treat inflammatory diseases of the nose and paranasal sinuses, gradually expanded its uses to include the removal of selected benign and malignant neoplasms, such as JNA.[3–18] This was made possible since the late 1990s by better assessment of the lesion due to improvements in imaging techniques (magnetic resonance imaging [MRI] and highly selective angiography), increased experience with embolization and endoscopic surgery, and the refinement of instrumentation.

Surgery is also considered an alternative therapy for JNA with intradural or intracavernous extension because of the possible complications of radiotherapy on intracranial structures and the side effects of chemotherapy.[19]

Indications and Contraindications

The classification used to preoperatively assess the extension of the lesion was proposed by Andrews and modified by Fisch (**Table 33.1**).[20] Based on this classification, the possibility of performing a purely endoscopic approach is evaluated.

In the first years of our experience, only type I and type II were purely endoscopically treated, rarely type IIIa. In recent years, thanks to the evolution of the technique, it has been possible to remove also a small number of type IIIb JNAs. Contraindications for endonasal endoscopic surgery alone include type IV JNAs, the presence of residual lesions involving critical areas with significant scarring, such as the internal carotid artery (ICA), optic nerve, and cavernous sinus; the extension to soft tissues of the zygomatic region and cheek and associated with scarring from previous surgery (**Fig. 33.1**); tumor extension encasing the ICA (**Fig. 33.2**); and blood supply from important branches of the ICA (vidian and ophthalmic arteries). In these cases, and in the setting of greater tumor extension, the endoscopic endonasal approach can be used in combination with more aggressive external approaches.

Table 33.1 Classification of Juvenile Nasopharyngeal Angiofibroma (JNA) by Andrews and Fisch[20]

Type	Tumor Extent
I	Limited to the nasopharynx and nasal cavity, with bone destruction negligible, or limited to the sphenopalatine foramen
II	Invades the pterygopalatine fossa or the maxillary, ethmoid, or sphenoid sinus with bone destruction
IIIa	Invades the infratemporal fossa or the orbital region without intracranial involvement
IIIb	Invades the infratemporal fossa or orbit with intracranial extradural (parasellar) involvement
IVa	Intracranial intradural tumor without infiltration of the cavernous sinus, pituitary fossa, or optic chiasm
IVb	Intracranial intradural tumor with infiltration of the cavernous sinus, pituitary fossa, or optic chiasm

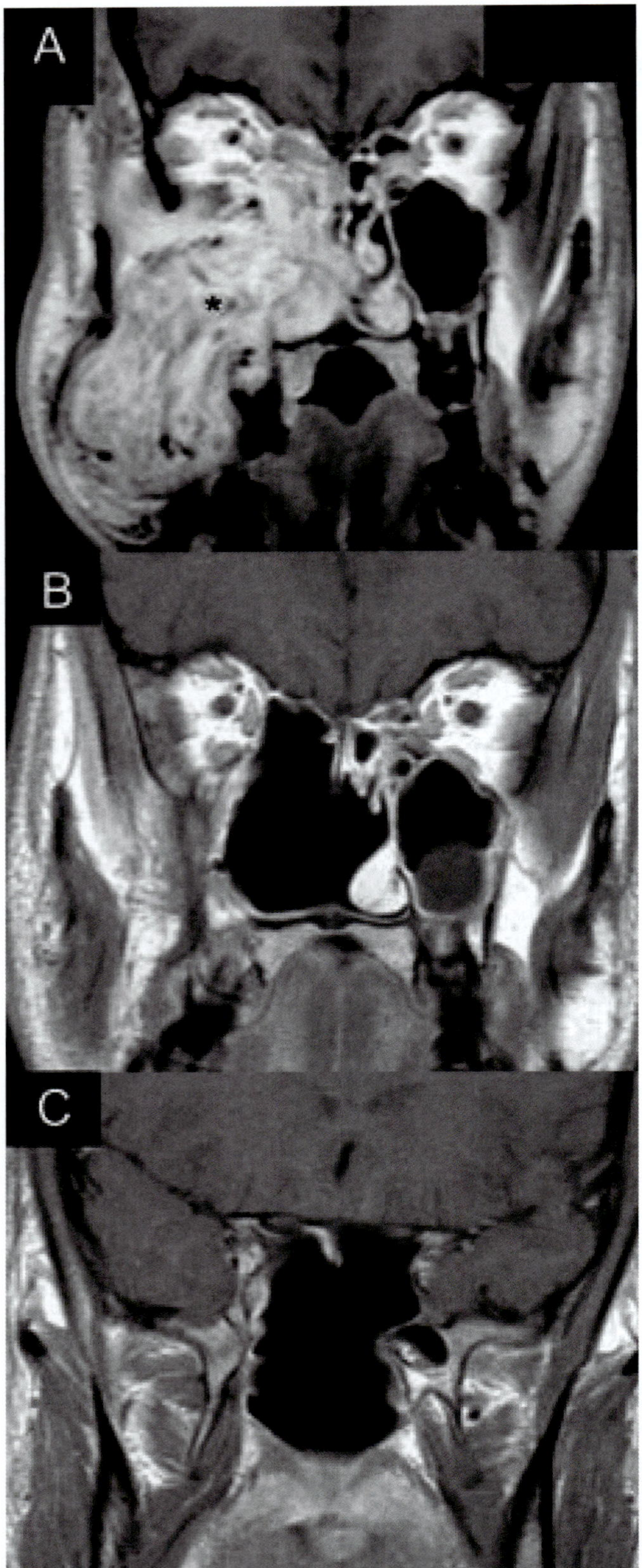

Fig. 33.1 **(A)** A case in which the lesion involved the whole maxillary sinus with erosion of its lateral wall and extension to the subcutaneous layer of the cheek. In cases like this, the extension of the tumor can be easily removed from the nose with a purely endoscopic approach if the patient has not undergone previous surgery. In cases of recurrence, scarring will hinder the endoscopic resection, and a combined external approach (midfacial degloving) is required. Asterisk indicates the juvenile nasopharyngeal angiofibroma (JNA). **(B,C)** Postoperative radiologic control (enhanced magnetic resonance imaging [MRI]) after 1 year, showing the complete removal of the lesion.

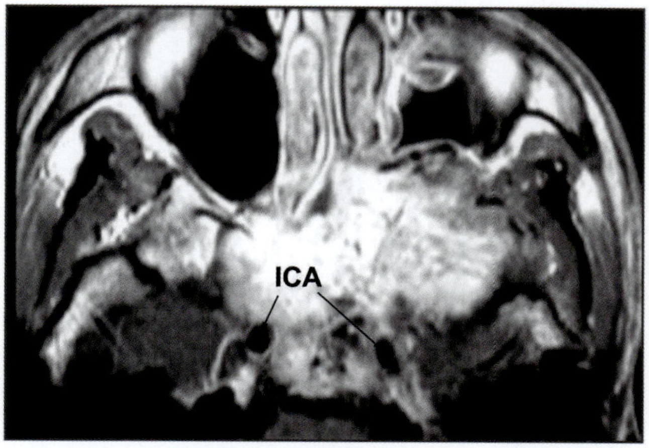

Fig. 33.2 Magnetic resonance imaging demonstrating the extension of the JNA from the pterygomaxillary region to include both cavernous sinuses, with tumor surrounding both paraclival tracts of the internal carotid artery (ICA) and also erosion of the clivus.

Diagnosis and Preoperative Workup

Diagnosis of JNA is made by the history, clinical features, and imaging findings. The lesion typically occurs in adolescent boys or young men complaining of nasal obstruction and epistaxis.[20] Nasal endoscopy reveals a multilobulated, dusky red lesion occupying the nasal fossa and nasopharynx (**Fig. 33.3**). CT and MRI facilitate identification of the characteristic features. Thus, a biopsy of the tumor is considered unnecessary; it is also risky.[21,22]

Specific goals of imaging include confirmation of the diagnosis; definition of the extension of the lesion, with particular interest in the study of the orbital region, infratemporal fossa, and intracranial invasion (cavernous sinus, ICA, dura mater); and evaluation of bone erosion.[19,23] Therefore, noninvasive imaging of JNA includes a bone window CT scan without contrast to look for bony modifications and an MRI with gadolinium to assess tumor enhancement, intralesional features, its relationship with perilesional soft tissues (periorbit, dura mater, ICA), and its extension.

On CT the pathognomonic sign is the enlargement of the anteroposterior diameter of the sphenopalatine fissure in the axial view (**Fig. 33.4**), which is also evident in an early lesion. From this area, through the sphenopalatine foramen, the JNA spreads toward the nasal fossa or into the diploe of the pterygopalatine process or to the basisphenoid enlarging the vidian canal.[24] The other important radiologic feature is the erosion of the base of the pterygoid process (Holman-Miller sign), which is evident in a coronal view (**Fig. 33.5**).[25]

The characteristic finding on MRI is the bright enhancement after gadolinium administration. The presence of high-

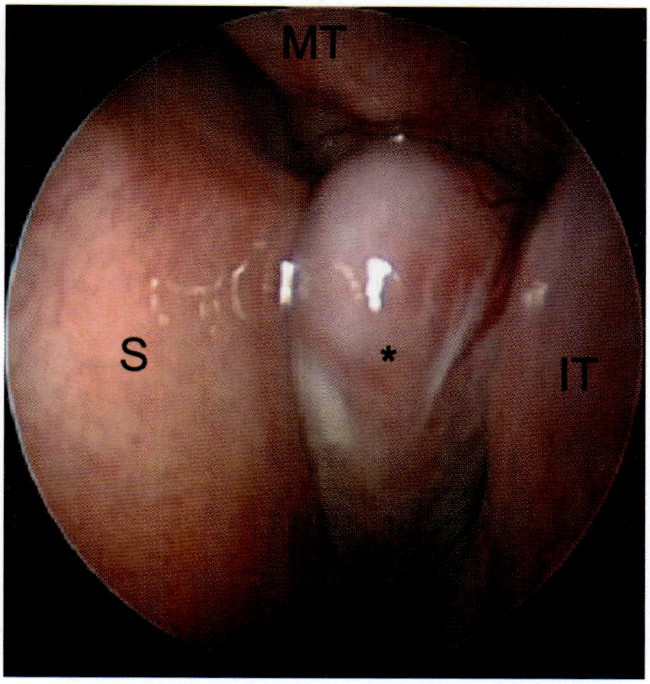

Fig. 33.3 Endoscopic endonasal image with a 0-degree endoscope showing a preoperative view of a JNA (*asterisk*) of the left nostril completely occluding the rhinopharynx. IT: inferior turbinate; MT: middle turbinate; S: septum.

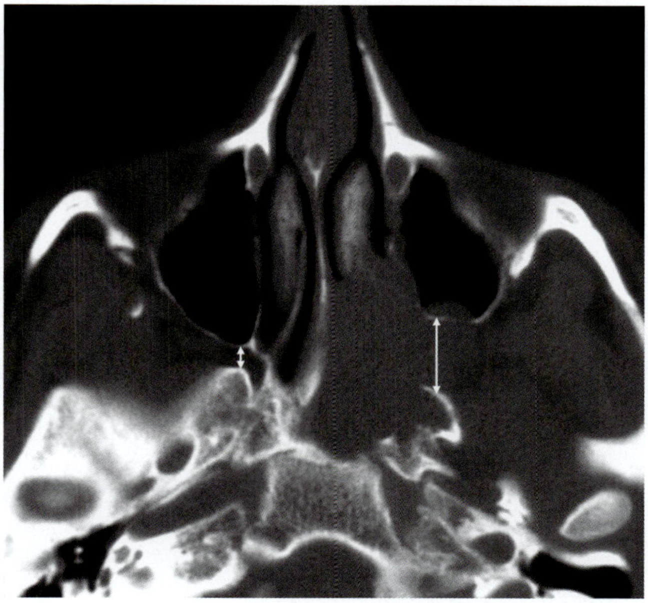

Fig. 33.4 The pathognomonic sign of JNA on an axial computed tomography (CT) scan is the enlargement of the sphenopalatine foramen and the erosion of the basisphenoid, with eventual obliteration of the vidian canal. The two white arrows show the different anteroposterior diameters of the foramen in the presence of a left JNA.

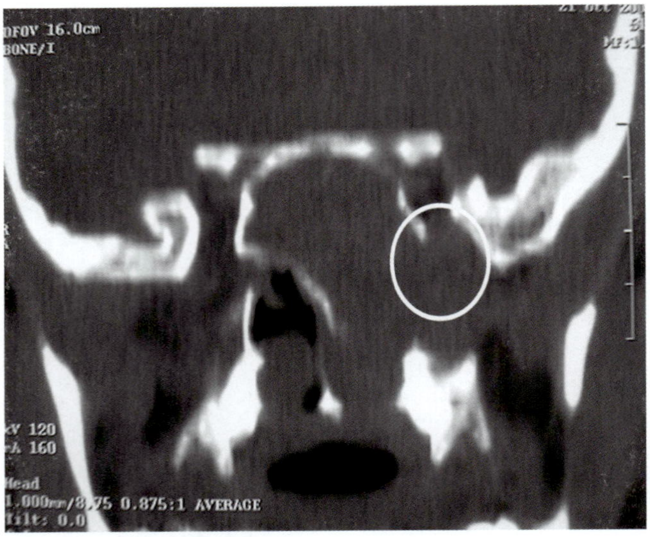

Fig. 33.5 Coronal view CT scan showing the erosion of the base of the pterygoid process (Holman-Miller sign) in the white circle.

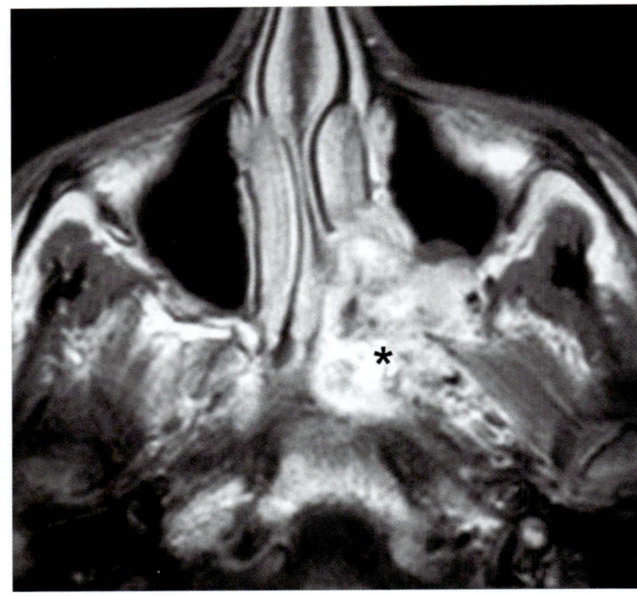

Fig. 33.6 On MRI the appearance of a JNA (*asterisk*) is typical, with dark spots on a bright matrix. This is due to the contrast between the high gadolinium enhancement and the signal voids caused by the presence of high flow vessels.

flow vessels, characterized by the absence of signal (flow void), can give the lesion its typical heterogeneous appearance (bright-dark contrast) (**Fig. 33.6**).[24]

The last examination of paramount importance in the preoperative workup is angiography, which has to be performed 24 to 48 hours before surgery. It must include the evaluation of both the carotid system (internal and external) and the vertebral arteries. In addition, it should be accompanied by a highly selective study of the most distal branches of the external carotid arteries (ECAs) to identify the afferent vessels and to reveal possible contralateral blood supply. The evaluation of the degree of vascularization coming from the ICA is crucial in determining the feasibility of the endoscopic endonasal approach. For this reason, the analysis of the images has to carefully assess the dimension of the vidian artery, the possible afferences from the cavernous system (rare), the contribution of ophthalmic arteries, and the presence of unknown arteriovenous fistulas. The assessment of the blood supply from the ICA system represents an important estimation of intraoperative bleeding (**Fig. 33.7**).

During angiography, the lesion has to be embolized, if possible, introducing a microcatheter to be selectively positioned

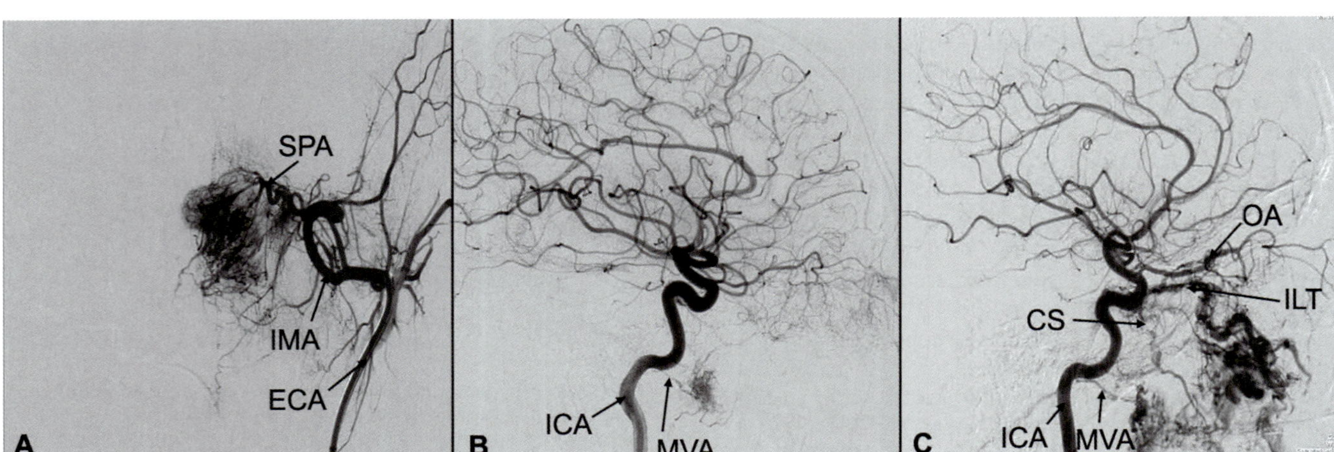

Fig. 33.7 **(A)** Left external carotid artery (ECA) selective injection. A pathologic blush reveals the angiofibromatous lesion. IMA: internal maxillary artery; SPA: sphenopalatine artery. **(B)** In this case the pathologic afference comes also from a mandibulovidian branch of the ICA (mandibulovidian artery [MVA]). **(C)** The afferent vessels to the lesion can originate also from multiple branches of the ICA: mandibulovidian trunk, inferolateral trunk (ILT), branches from the ophthalmic artery (OA), and minor multiple afferences from the carotid-cavernous branches. CS: cavernous sinus.

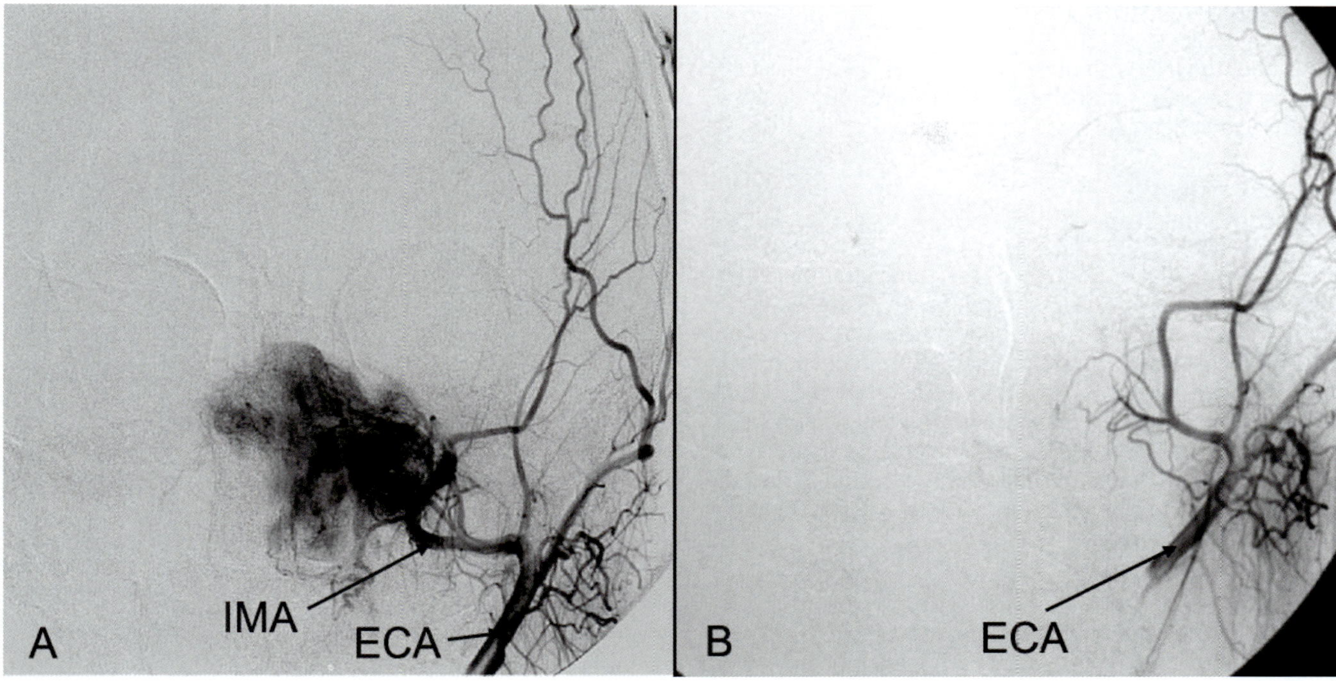

Fig. 33.8 **(A)** A guide catheter (5-French) is inserted in the ECA with continuous perfusion. Then, with coaxial system, a selective microcatheterism is performed (microcatheter: Tracher Excel 14; microguide: Transend 14; Boston Scientific, Natick, MA) to reach the left IMA. Microparticles (contour type; Boston Scientific) are injected until there is complete devascularization of the lesion. **(B)** The correct embolization of the afferent vessels 40 minutes later is evident.

at the level of the involved carotid districts. Polyvinyl alcohol (PVA) particles (150 to 200 µm in diameter) are used for embolization (**Fig. 33.8**). These diagnostic procedures combined with endoscopy can help to differentiate JNA from other sinonasal lesions (**Table 33.2**).

■ Surgical Procedure

Preparation of the Patient

Surgery is performed with the patient under general anesthesia and controlled hypotension. The patient is placed supine in an anti-Trendelenburg position (10 to 20 degrees). Both nostrils are decongested with cottonoids soaked in a solution composed of 20 mL of naphazoline nitrate, 20 mL of ossibuprocaine hydrochloride 1%, and 1 mg of adrenaline, left in place for several minutes.

Instrumentation

Surgery performed with the endoscopic endonasal technique requires 4-mm endoscopes with direct (0-degree) or angled (45-degree) vision, equipped with a cleaning system. For tumor removal, straight or curved instruments in combination with 0- or 45-degree endoscopes are used, making it possible to operate laterally. A drill with an intranasal long handle enables the removal of bony parts with a diamond or cutting burr. The use of a diode laser (25 to 30 W, pulsated) helps the surgeon to minimize bleeding.

Table 33.2 Differential Diagnosis Between Sinonasal Lesions Compared with JNA, Considering that All These Lesions Do Not Present the Pathognomonic Radiologic Signs of JNA

Lesions	Clinical Features
Antrochoanal polyp	Translucid appearance, exit from accessory maxillary ostium; T2-weighted MRI with homogeneous hyperintensity of the signal
Acute adenoiditis	Bilateral association with fever; benefits from antibiotic and antiinflammatory therapy
Lobular capillary hemangioma	Association with injury and hormonal factors; origin is from sinuses, nasal septum, and turbinates
Hemangiopericytoma	Slight female predominance, with a peak in the 7th decade
Benign schwannoma	Occurs in middle-aged adults; arises from branches of cranial nerve V; frequently located in the midline

Operative Technique

Removal of the JNA with the endoscopic technique basically includes three steps: nasoethmoidal, pterygo-infratemporal, and pterygo-sphenoidal.

Nasoethmoidal Step

The nasoethmoidal step involves the transnasal piecemeal removal of the lesion using a diode laser. In this way the endoluminal component, occupying the nasal cavity and the rhinopharynx, is removed. Then an ethmoidectomy is performed with partial or subtotal removal of the middle turbinate. The ethmoidectomy is performed in several steps: uncinectomy and enlarged medial antrostomy, exposure of the posterior wall of the maxillary sinus, removal of the ethmoidal bulla, and posterior ethmoid cells. A large sphenoidotomy is then performed.

Pterygo-Infratemporal Step

The pterygo-infratemporal step includes an endonasal endoscopic access to the sphenoethmoidal and pterygoidal compartment (preferred site of tumor growth). At this point the mass can be visualized and, after identification and closure of the afferent vessels, dissection from the surrounding structures can be performed. The exposure of the pterygopalatine fossa and of the pterygomaxillary fissure, obtained by removing the posterior wall of the maxillary sinus with the help of bone-cutting instruments, enables the surgeon to control the internal maxillary artery (IMA), which can be coagulated with bipolar forceps or clipped.

The tumor in the pterygomaxillary and infratemporal fossae is then dissected using blunt instruments. In performing this step, it is essential to drill the base of the pterygoid process, which makes it possible to mobilize the tumor and to dissect it from the pterygoid muscles and the infratemporal fossa fat tissue.

If needed, depending on the lateral extension of the tumor, the procedure may include a medial maxillectomy (modified Sturman-Canfield approach), with removal of the entire medial wall of the maxillary sinus, the lateral aspect of the piriform aperture (**Fig. 33.9**), and the inferior turbinate. Removal of the posterior aspect of the septum allows for a four-hand intranasal dissection, which is extremely helpful whenever the tumor is completely filling the nasopharynx. By using both nostrils, surgical maneuvers and in particular exposure of the posterior aspect of the lesion are made easier.[26]

Pterygo-Sphenoidal Step

For the pterygo-sphenoidal step, the surgeon completes the drilling of the pterygoid process and extends it to the basisphenoid along the vidian canal. This is necessary to reduce the risk of persistence (**Fig. 33.10**).[27] During this step the sphenoidal sinus, with its bony depressions and protrusions, is an important landmark that enables the surgeon to identify the ICA (petrous portion, paraclival, cavernous), the optic nerve, the cavernous sinus, and the foramen rotundum with the cleft containing V2. The surgeon has to identify all these structures before drilling the posterior part of the pterygoid root to reach the cavernous sinus and the dura of the middle cranial fossa to perform the removal of possible tumor digitations in this area.

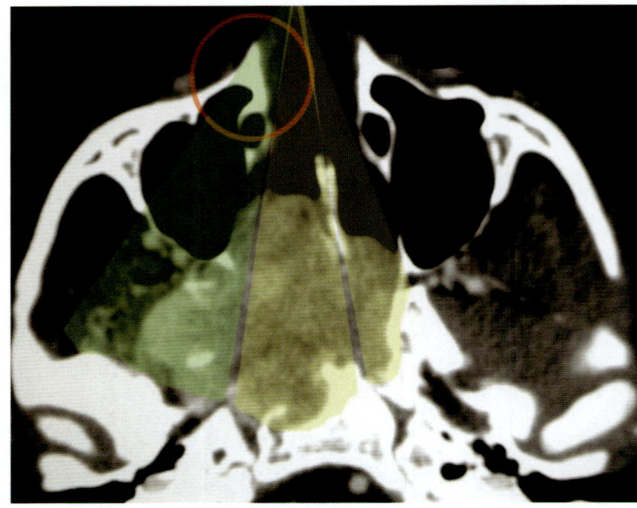

Fig. 33.9 Schematic demonstrating how the removal of the lateral aspect of the piriform overture (in the *red circle*) enables a wider approach (the *green cone* compared with the *yellow cone*) to the lateral regions (pterygopalatine and infratemporal fossa).

The nasopharyngeal portion of the tumor is removed with an incision of the adjacent pharyngobasilar fascia, which is performed behind the torus tubarius (when its preservation is possible) to reach the most medial extension of the neoplasm.

Multiple biopsies (V2, inferior orbital fissure, nasopharynx, infratemporal fossa) with frozen section examination enable the surgeon to assess the resection limits.

After careful inspection of the surgical field to perform a careful hemostasis, the surgical field is covered with hemostatic sponges and fibrin glue. Nasal packing is inserted in both nostrils.

■ Postoperative Management and Follow-Up

Depending on the amount of blood lost, postoperative care in the intensive care unit is advisable. Nasal packing can be removed on the first or second postoperative day, and the patient (considering the minimal invasiveness of the approach, which does not need external osteotomies) can be discharged usually within 3 to 5 days after surgery, provided no complications occur.

All patients need a prospective evaluation with periodic nasal endoscopies (after 3 months and then every 6 months

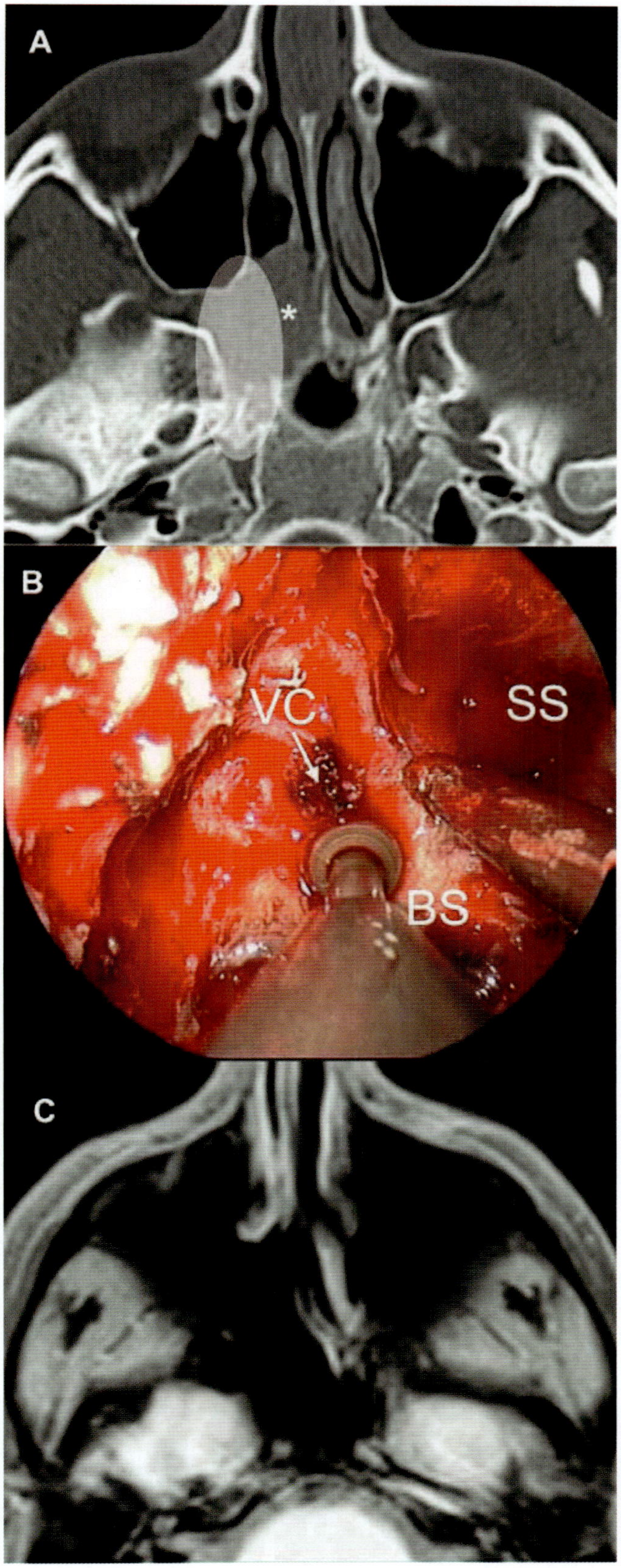

Fig. 33.10 **(A)** A CT scan in the axial plane demonstrates the presence of a JNA (*asterisk*), and the white circle indicates the area, along the TEPS approach and along the vidian canal, which has to be drilled for a radical excision of the tumor. **(B)** Endoscopic endonasal surgical image with 0-degree endoscope showing the drilling of the basisphenoid (BS) and of the vidian canal (VC). SS: sphenoidal sinus. **(C)** Postoperative MRI after 1 year with no evidence of disease.

for the first 3 years). An MRI should be obtained every 6 months during the first 2 years after surgery and then once a year for at least 5 years after surgery. Routine angiography is performed 1 year after surgery.

Results

The endoscopic endonasal approach facilitates exposure of tumor projections due to the angled view, encounters no interference from facial bone growth centers, causes less post-operative pain, shortens hospital stay, and avoids unsightly scars. The disadvantages are increased difficulty in controlling serious bleeding from intracranial circulation, and the need for longer training, especially with the four-hand technique.

In our series, 96.5% of patients were treated with a purely endoscopic approach and 3.5% with a combined (midfacial degloving, nasal-paralateral, craniotomy) approach (20% of type IIIb cases and one type IVb case). Recurrence was diagnosed on follow-up MRI (mean 58.5 months) in 9.68% of cases treated endoscopically (unpublished data), and only one patient needed a reintervention.

We have never used radiation therapy or chemotherapy. Radiation therapy is reserved for patients who refuse surgery, those with surgically inaccessible intracranial extensions of the tumor, and those with significant medical contraindications to surgical intervention. Chemotherapy is recommended only for recurrent lesions not amenable to surgery or radiation.[28]

Complications

Possible complications linked to angiographic procedure can be related to selective catheterism or to embolization.[29] A vessel dissection or the formation of an embolus can rarely occur. Even more rare is the occurrence of a vessel laceration. More frequently (especially in younger patients) a vasospasm can impair the continuation of the examination. During the injection of embolic material, which is performed under radioscopic control, a series of angiographic sequences has to be obtained to verify the possible opening of new shunts (with ICA or with the vertebrobasilar system), which can lead to embolism of the intracranial circulation.

Complications that may occur during surgery are related to the different areas involved by the dissection. During posterior ethmoidectomy, a lesion of the lamina papyracea/periorbit can occur, leading to orbital emphysema, which often has a spontaneous regression (it is imperative to tell patients not to blow their nose and to keep their mouth open when they sneeze). Even damage to the medial rectum muscle can occur with transient or permanent diplopia. Sphenoidotomy and drilling of the pterygoid-infratemporal region can lead to severe bleeding (sphenopalatine artery [SPA], internal maxillary artery [IMA], ICA), to cranial base defects (posterior portion of the olfactory cleft or lateral wall of the sphenoid sinus), and to nerve deficits (vidian, optic, V2). In cases of large blood loss, transfusion is often mandatory. In cases of cerebrospinal fluid (CSF) leak, a multilayer closure technique, which has to be performed during the same surgery, is recommended.

We did not observe any surgical complications (minor or major). In our experience we never needed to convert an endoscopic approach into an external approach, because of precise planning based on preoperative imaging. Surgery was never interrupted by excessive bleeding (intraoperative blood loss ranged from 80 to 1200 mL, with a mean of 410 mL).

References

1. Schick B, Brunner C, Praetorius M, Plinkert PK, Urbschat S. First evidence of genetic imbalances in angiofibromas. Laryngoscope 2002; 112:397–401
2. Schick B, Wemmert S, Bechtel U, et al. Comprehensive genomic analysis identifies MDM2 and AURKA as novel amplified genes in juvenile angiofibromas. Head Neck 2007;29:479–487
3. Kamel RH. Transnasal endoscopic surgery in juvenile nasopharyngeal angiofibroma. J Laryngol Otol 1996;110:962–968
4. Zicot AF, Daele J. Endoscopic surgery for nasal and sinusal vascular tumours: about two cases of nasopharyngeal angiofibromas and one case of turbinate angioma. Acta Otorhinolaryngol Belg 1996;50:177–182
5. Fagan JJ, Snyderman CH, Carrau RL, Janecka IP. Nasopharyngeal angiofibromas: selecting a surgical approach. Head Neck 1997;19:391–399
6. Tseng HZ, Chao WY. Transnasal endoscopic approach for juvenile nasopharyngeal angiofibroma. Am J Otolaryngol 1997;18:151–154
7. Bernal-Sprekelsen M, Vasquez AA, Pueyo J, Carbonell Casasus J. Die endoskopische Resektion juveniler Nasen-Rachen-Fibrome. HNO 1998; 46:172–174
8. Nakamura H, Kawasaki M, Higuchi Y, Seki S, Takahashi S. Transnasal endoscopic resection of juvenile nasopharyngeal angiofibroma with KTP laser. Eur Arch Otorhinolaryngol 1999;256:212–214
9. Herman P, Lot G, Chapot R, Salvan D, Huy PT. Long-term follow-up of juvenile nasopharyngeal angiofibromas: analysis of recurrences. Laryngoscope 1999;109:140–147
10. Newlands SD, Weymuller EA Jr. Endoscopic treatment of juvenile nasopharyngeal angiofibroma. Am J Rhinol 1999;13:213–219
11. Stammberger H, Anderhuber W, Walch C, Papaefthymiou G. Possibilities and limitations of endoscopic management of nasal and paranasal sinus malignancies. Acta Otorhinolaryngol Belg 1999;53:199–205
12. Jorissen M, Eloy PH, Rombaux PH, Bachert CL, Daele J. Endoscopic sinus surgery for juvenile nasopharyngeal angiofibroma. Acta Otorhinolaryngol Belg 2000;54:201–219
13. Sarria R, Capitan A, Sprekelsen C, Viviente E, Cuervo G, Ferran A. Chirurgia endoscopica del angiofibroma nasofaringeo mediante doble embolizacion. Acta Otorrinolaringol Esp 2000;51:259–262
14. Carrau RL, Snyderman CH, Kassam AB, Jungreis CA. Endoscopic and endoscopic-assisted surgery for juvenile angiofibroma. Laryngoscope 2001;111:483–487
15. Scholtz AW, Appenroth E, Kammen-Jolly K, Scholtz LU, Thumfart WF. Juvenile nasopharyngeal angiofibroma: management and therapy. Laryngoscope 2001;111(4 Pt 1):681–687
16. Hazarika P, Nayak DR, Balakrishnan R, Raj G, Pillai S. Endoscopic and KTP laser-assisted surgery for juvenile nasopharyngeal angiofibroma. Am J Otolaryngol 2002;23:282–286
17. Ochi K, Watanabe S, Miyabe S. Endoscopic transnasal resection of a juvenile angiofibroma using an ultrasonically activated scalpel. ORL J Otorhinolaryngol Relat Spec 2002;64:290–293
18. Roger G, Tran Ba Huy P, Froehlich P, et al. Exclusively endoscopic removal of juvenile nasopharyngeal angiofibroma: trends and limits. Arch Otolaryngol Head Neck Surg 2002;128:928–935
19. Danesi G, Panizza B, Mazzoni A, Calabrese V. Anterior approaches in juvenile nasopharyngeal angiofibromas with intracranial extension. Otolaryngol Head Neck Surg 2000;122:277–283

20. Andrews JC, Fisch U, Valavanis A, Aeppli U, Makek MS. The surgical management of extensive nasopharyngeal angiofibromas with the infratemporal fossa approach. Laryngoscope 1989;99:429–437

21. Schick B, Kahle G. Radiological findings in angiofibroma. Acta Radiol 2000;41:585–593

22. Lloyd G, Howard D, Lund VJ, Savy L. Imaging for juvenile angiofibroma. J Laryngol Otol 2000;114:727–730

23. Nicolai P, Berlucchi M, Tomenzoli D, et al. Endoscopic surgery for juvenile angiofibroma: when and how. Laryngoscope 2003;113:775–782

24. Lloyd G, Howard D, Phelps P, Cheesman A. Juvenile angiofibroma: the lessons of 20 years of modern imaging. J Laryngol Otol 1999;113:127–134

25. Ungkanont K, Byers RM, Weber RS, Callender DL, Wolf PF, Goepfert H. Juvenile nasopharyngeal angiofibroma: an update of therapeutic management. Head Neck 1996;18:60–66

26. Castelnuovo P, Pistochini A, Locatelli D. Different surgical approaches to the sellar region: focusing on the "two nostrils four hands technique". Rhinology 2006;44:2–7

27. Howard DJ, Lloyd G, Lund V. Recurrence and its avoidance in juvenile angiofibroma. Laryngoscope 2001;111:1509–1511

28. Mitskavich MT, Carrau RL, Snyderman CH, Weissman JL, Fagan JJ. Intranasal endoscopic excision of a juvenile angiofibroma. Auris Nasus Larynx 1998;25:39–44

29. Onerci M, Gumus K, Cil B, Eldem B. A rare complication of embolization in juvenile nasopharyngeal angiofibroma. Int J Pediatr Otorhinolaryngol 2005;69:423–428

34 Lesions of the Petrous Apex

Carl H. Snyderman, Emiro E. Caicedo, Daniel M. Prevedello, Ricardo L. Carrau, Paul A. Gardner, and Amin B. Kassam

Tips and Pearls

- A completely endoscopic endonasal approach provides direct access to the petrous apex for the treatment of cholesterol granulomas, petrous apicitis, and primary and metastatic neoplasms.
- The choice of a surgical approach depends on the relationship to the internal carotid artery (ICA) (medial or inferior), the degree of medial expansion, and the pathology.
- The petrous apex is accessible between the brainstem and the ICA at the level of the clival recess (medial approach).
- The petrous apex is accessible inferior to the petrous segment of the ICA (infrapetrous approach).
- Key landmarks for locating the ICA include the vidian artery and nerve.
- Potential advantages of an endoscopic endonasal approach include avoidance of a craniotomy, minimal postoperative symptoms, faster recovery, shorter hospitalization, and improved maintenance of a drainage pathway.
- In addition to injury to the ICA, potential risks of surgery include injury to the brainstem, second and third divisions of the trigeminal nerve, and the sixth cranial nerve.
- The endoscopic endonasal approach to the petrous apex should be considered as an alternative to lateral skull base approaches for selected patients

Introduction

Surgical approaches to the petrous apex include transtemporal, middle cranial fossa, and transsphenoidal approaches. Lateral transtemporal approaches to the petrous apex may not be possible when there is poor pneumatization of the temporal bone, and continued aeration of the petrous apex may be difficult to maintain. A transcranial middle fossa approach is technically difficult and also suffers from the lack of a permanent drainage pathway. Risks of lateral approaches include brain injury, facial paralysis, hearing loss, and vestibulopathy.

The transsphenoidal approach to the petrous apex was first described in 1977 by Montgomery.[1] Subsequent reports have established the utility of an endoscopic transsphenoidal approach in adult and pediatric patients, primarily for cholesterol granulomas.[2,3]

Indications and Advantages

A completely endoscopic endonasal approach provides direct access to the petrous apex for the treatment of cholesterol granulomas (**Fig. 34.1**), petrous apicitis, and primary (chondrosarcoma, chordoma, squamous cell carcinoma) and metastatic neoplasms.[4-8]

Potential advantages of an endonasal approach include avoidance of a craniotomy, minimal postoperative symptoms,

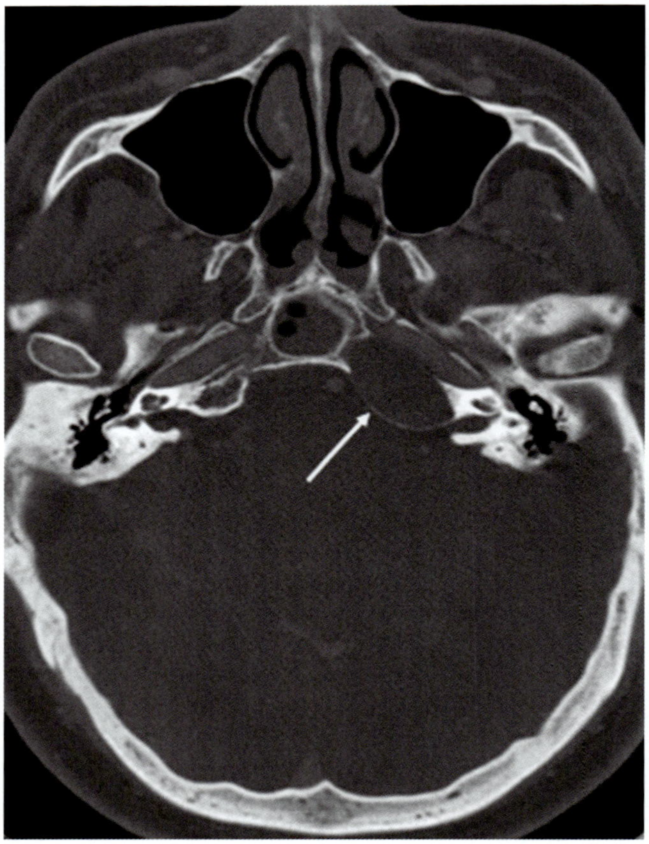

Fig. 34.1 Axial computed tomography (CT) angiography showing a left petrous apex lesion (*white arrow*) with expansion posteriorly and medially in the direction of the sphenoid sinus. It is an example of a cholesterol granuloma that can be resected by an endonasal endoscopic medial petrous apex approach.

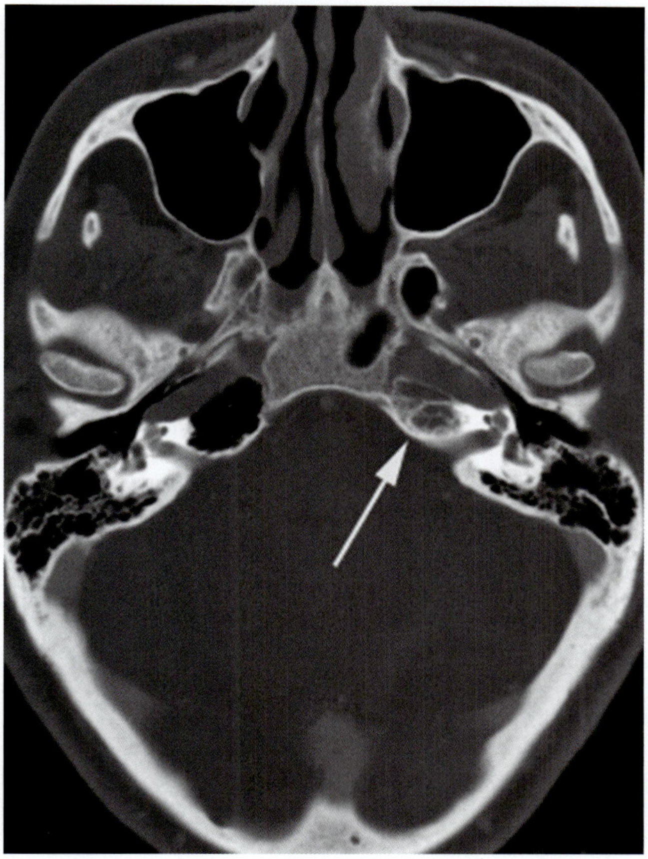

Fig. 34.2 Axial CT angiography showing a left petrous apex lesion (*white arrow*) with minimal expansion. This cholesterol granuloma is located behind the left internal carotid artery (ICA), and it would require an endoscopic endonasal infrapetrous approach for resection.

faster recovery, a cosmetically acceptable result, and shorter hospitalization. The risks of a lateral approach are avoided, and a permanent drainage pathway is created.

Contraindications

A medial approach to the petrous apex is contraindicated when there is no medial expansion of the lesion into the sphenoid sinus (**Fig. 34.2**) or the lesion is situated inferior to the plane of the petrous internal carotid artery (ICA). An infrapetrous approach should only be attempted by experienced endoscopic skull base surgeons with secure knowledge of the ICA's endonasal anatomy and with experience in exposing the petrous ICA.

Diagnostic Workup

Patients with petrous apex lesions often have nonspecific symptoms such as headache, disequilibrium, and tinnitus. A thorough evaluation including assessment of cranial nerve function, nasal endoscopy, audiogram, vestibular testing, and radiologic imaging should be performed when indicated to exclude other sources of the patient's symptoms. Referral to a neurologist for evaluation and treatment of headaches may be considered prior to surgery.

Imaging

Computed tomography (CT) and magnetic resonance imaging (MRI) provide complementary information and are often both necessary to establish a diagnosis. CT provides important information regarding sinus anatomy (pneumatization, variations), medial expansion into the sphenoid sinus, and bone erosion of the carotid canal. MRI helps establish a diagnosis, and differentiates among cholesterol granuloma, petrous apicitis, and neoplasia.

Surgery

Instrumentation

Essential equipment includes a standard array of endoscopic sinus surgery instruments, Kerrison rongeurs, endoscopic bipolar electrocautery, an endoscopic drill with 3- and 4-mm extended hybrid diamond bits, hemostatic materials, and a Silastic stent. A warm water bath maintained at 40°C provides warm saline for irrigation to promote hemostasis.

Operative Setup

The patient is placed in the supine position with neurophysiologic monitoring (somatosensory-evoked potentials) to measure cortical function in case there is injury to the ICA. The head is placed in a Mayfield holder, and registration of the image guidance system is performed. The surgical team is positioned on the right side of the patient, across from anesthesia.

Preparation

The nasal mucosa is decongested with pledgets soaked in 0.05% oxymetazoline and a third- or fourth-generation cephalosporin is administered intravenously for perioperative prophylaxis. The nasal vestibule is prepped with an iodine solution, and the abdomen is similarly prepped in case a fat graft is needed for reconstruction.

Medial Approach (Fig. 34.1)

A bilateral sphenoidotomy is performed with wide resection of the sphenoid rostrum and posterior septal attachment. This provides binostril access, with greater room for instrumentation and increased angles for viewing. The vascular

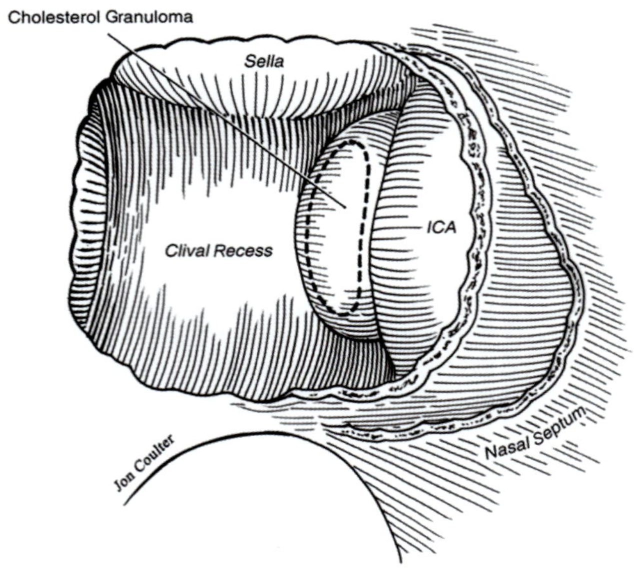

Fig. 34.3 Drawing demonstrating the medial projection of the petrous apex when it is expanded by a cholesterol granuloma immediately behind the ICA.

pedicle for a septal mucosal flap can be preserved on the side opposite the lesion in case it is needed. Sinus landmarks are identified and intrasinus septations are removed with the drill. Mucosa is stripped from the clival recess and lateral wall to fully visualize the bony anatomy. Usually the petrous apex lesion is readily apparent due to bony expansion medially at the level of the clival recess (**Fig. 34.3**).

The course of the paraclival ICA is verified with image guidance, and bone overlying the petrous apex lesion is carefully thinned with the drill parallel to the course of the ICA and equidistant between the ICA and the posterior wall of the clival recess (**Fig. 34.4**). A small opening is made and then enlarged with Kerrison rongeurs, being careful to work parallel to the course of the paraclival ICA. The opening is maximally enlarged with rongeurs. If necessary, bone overlying the brainstem can be thinned to the underlying dura to provide wider exposure. Drilling of bone laterally at the level of the sellar floor should be minimized to prevent thermal injury to cranial nerve VI.

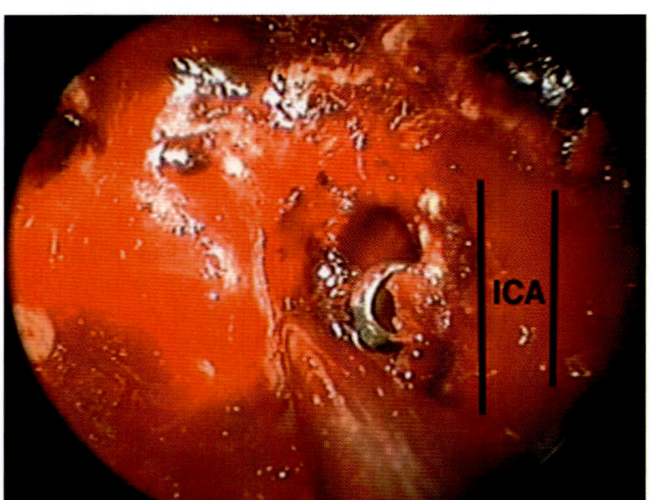

Fig. 34.4 Intraoperative picture during resection of a cholesterol granuloma that was located in the left petrous apex. Note the left internal carotid artery (ICA) immediately anterior in the field.

Infrapetrous Approach (Fig. 34.2)

A transpterygoid approach on the side of the lesion is performed in addition to bilateral sphenoidotomies. The sphenopalatine vessels are ligated, and the pterygopalatine space is exposed. The fascia is elevated along the inferior edge of the sphenoidotomy to expose the medial pterygoid plate. The contents of the pterygopalatine space are elevated from the underlying bone to expose the base of the pterygoid plates, and the pterygoid canal is identified inferolateral to the sphenoid sinus. The vidian artery and nerve are cauterized with bipolar electrocautery and transected; occasionally, the vividian nerve can be preserved.[9] The pterygoid bone surrounding the vidian artery is drilled until the plane of the anterior genu of the ICA is reached.

Increased infrapetrous exposure requires resection of nasopharyngeal soft tissues (mucosa, longus capitis muscle) and resection of the medial eustachian tube. This is done with endoscopic scissors angled away from the ICA at the foramen lacerum. The position of the parapharyngeal ICA should be verified with image guidance to avoid injury. Bone medial and inferior to the genu can then be drilled to provide both medial and inferior access to the petrous apex. It is important to remember that the anterior genu is the most anterior projection of the petrous ICA. If the patient has a cholesterol granuloma, the contents are evacuated with angled suctions and irrigation. Curetting of the posterior surface of the ICA should be avoided.

Repair

A Silastic stent is usually placed into the petrous apex cavity to maintain patency until healing is complete. Various stents have been used successfully including a rolled Silastic sheet, extraventricular drain catheter, and a Montgomery T-tube tracheal stent (**Fig. 34.5**). The stent is trimmed, leaving enough to enable endoscopic extraction in the clinic after several months (**Fig. 34.6**). If the ICA has been exposed, it is covered with a fat graft or septal mucosal flap.

■ Complications

Potential complications of a medial approach to the petrous apex include injury to the ICA, cranial nerve VI, and brainstem. All of these complications are avoidable with careful surgical technique.

With an infrapetrous approach, loss of vidian nerve function can occur and results in loss of emotional tearing on that

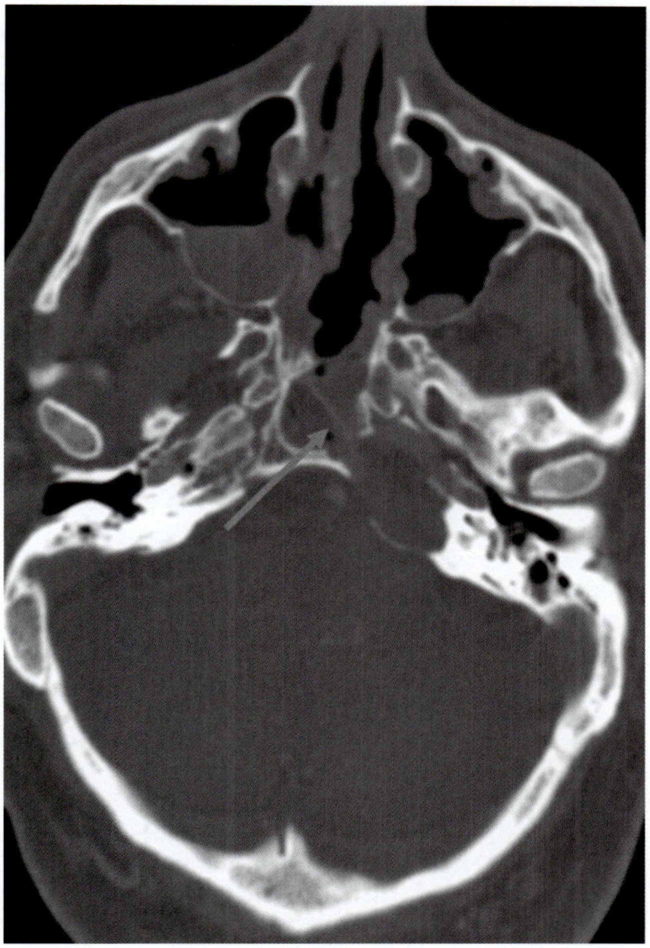

Fig. 34.5 Postoperative CT demonstrating the accomplished resection of a left cholesterol granuloma through an endonasal endoscopic medial petrous apex approach with a insertion of a stent into the cavity (*arrow*).

side. Vidian nerve function should not be sacrificed in someone with dry eyes or V1 hypesthesia. Resection of the medial eustachian tube results in a serous middle ear effusion that is treated with a tympanostomy tube. The risk of ICA injury is increased with an infrapetrous approach.

If a wide opening into the petrous apex is achieved, patency is usually maintained. If postoperative scarring results in obstruction of the petrous apex, patients often remain asymptomatic, and revision surgery is not performed unless symptoms return.

Postoperative Care

Routine postoperative care includes the use of saline nasal sprays and periodic debridement of crusts. Silastic stents are usually maintained for 3 to 4 months and removed endoscopically in the clinic. Patency of the opening can be verified with the endoscopic examination. Serial imaging is performed to detect recurrence if patency is not maintained.

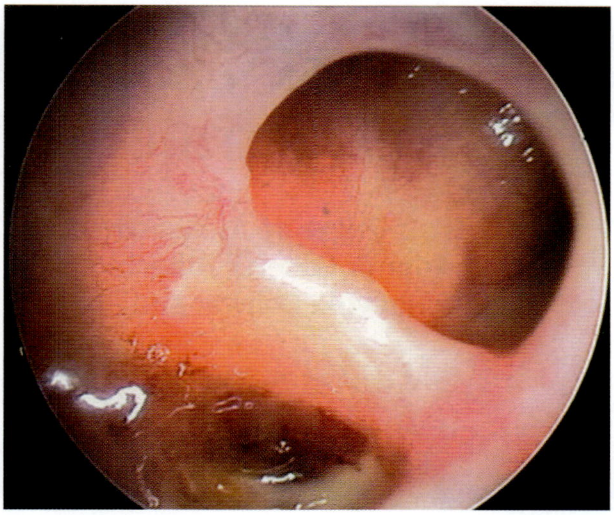

Fig. 34.6 Endoscopic visualization of the left petrous apex 3 months after evacuation of a cholesterol granuloma. Note that the stent was removed and epithelization has occurred.

Conclusion

Endoscopic endonasal approaches to the petrous apex can be classified based on their relationship to the petrous ICA. Knowledge of the anatomical landmarks and relationships of the ICA is necessary to avoid complications. Potential advantages of an endonasal approach include avoidance of a craniotomy, minimal postoperative symptoms, faster recovery, a cosmetically acceptable result, shorter hospitalization, and creation of a permanent drainage pathway.

References

1. Montgomery WW. Cystic lesions of the petrous apex: transsphenoid approach. Ann Otol Rhinol Laryngol 1977;86(4 Pt 1):429–435
2. Griffith AJ, Terrell JE. Transsphenoid endoscopic management of petrous apex cholesterol granuloma. Otolaryngol Head Neck Surg 1996;114: 91–94
3. Michaelson PG, Cable BB, Mair EA. Image-guided transsphenoidal drainage of a cholesterol granuloma of the petrous apex in a child. Int J Pediatr Otorhinolaryngol 2001;57:165–169
4. Kingdom TT, Delgaudio JM. Endoscopic approach to lesions of the sphenoid sinus, orbital apex, and clivus. Am J Otolaryngol 2003;24:317–322
5. DiNardo LJ, Pippin GW, Sismanis A. Image-guided endoscopic transsphenoidal drainage of select petrous apex cholesterol granulomas. Otol Neurotol 2003;24:939–941
6. Kassam AB, Gardner P, Snyderman CH, Mintz A, Carrau R. Expanded endonasal approach: fully endoscopic, completely transnasal approach to the middle third of the clivus, petrous bone, middle cranial fossa, and infratemporal fossa. Neurosurg Focus 2005;19:E6
7. Snyderman CH, Kassam AB, Carrau R, Mintz A. Endoscopic Approaches to the Petrous Apex. Op Tech Otolaryngol Head Neck Surg 2006;17: 168–173
8. Zanation AM, Snyderman CH, Carrau RL, Gardner PA, Prevedello DM, Kassam AB. Endoscopic endonasal surgery for petrous apex lesions. Laryngoscope 2009;119:19–25
9. Prevedello DM, Pinheiro-Neto CD, Fernandez-Miranda J, Carrau RL, Snyderman CH, Gardner P, Kassam AB. Videan Nerve Transportion for endoscopic endonasal middle fossa approaches. Neurosurgery 2010;67: 478–484

35 Transmaxillary Endoscopic Approach to Contralateral Parasellar Lesions

Luiz Felipe de Alencastro, Luiz Carlos de Alencastro, Carolina Martins, Ademir Lodetti, Alberto Carlos Capel Cardoso, Mario Faria, Kohei Inoue, Shigeyuki Osawa, and Albert L. Rhoton, Jr.

Tips and Pearls

- The transmaxillary endoscopic approach to contralateral parasellar lesions (TEACPS) technique favors the exposure of parasellar structures from the side opposite the maxillary entrance, with a better angle for visualization and manipulation.
- The technique facilitates simultaneous access and manipulation of surgical instruments from the nasal cavity and maxillary sinus.
- The technique enables facial submucosal dissection and maxillotomy without causing cosmetic defects.
- A closure mucosal flap needs to be planned on the side opposite the maxillary opening.

Introduction

From Bozzini's invention of the endoscope in the 18th century, to the neurosurgical application of endoscopic concepts by Guiot in the beginning of the 20th century, and to the use of the endoscope in endonasal surgery by Jankowski in the early 1990s, great technological and technical advances in endoscopic surgery have been observed[1]

Increasing effort has been focused on refining the anatomical, diagnostic, and surgical techniques, the indications for surgery, and the technologies used to resect tumors from the anterior skull base and their extensions. The pioneer work of Cushing has been furthered with the introduction of modern technology as well.[1,2]

Based on observations of the anatomy of the air cavities, it was recognized that craniectomies to access anterior base structures may be performed from alternative directions so as to facilitate the removal of the full extent of the tumor.

This chapter introduces the concept of radial endoscopic accesses to the skull base, focusing on a transmaxillary endoscopic approach to the contralateral structures that are involved with tumor, precluding in some cases the need for traditional extensive craniofacial approaches (**Fig. 35.1**).

As the sphenoid rostrum is opened bilaterally, simultaneous access through the nose and maxilla is obtained, offering surgeons the opportunity to dissect from different surgical routes at the same time and facilitating two-surgeon, four-hand techniques (**Fig. 35.2**).

Extensive knowledge of the anatomy is crucial to enable recognition of the anatomical landmarks in preoperative imaging studies, which is a fundamental prerequisite for performing surgery.

Technique Description

The transmaxillary endoscopic approach to contralateral parasellar lesions (TEACPS) technique is a multistep procedure to expose the parasellar structures from the side opposite the maxillary entrance. The cooperation of the neurosurgeon and the ear, nose, and throat (ENT) surgeon working together facilitates this approach and increases its safety. The technique entails the following steps:

1. Endonasal inspection
2. Preparation of the septal pediculated mucosal flap
3. Posterior nasal septostomy and anterior sphenoidal wall resection
4. Middle turbinectomy and maxillary medial wall initial resection
5. Opening of the anterior wall of the maxilla
6. Identification of maxillary sinus landmarks
7. Combined work through the maxillary sinus and nasal cavity

Step 1: Endonasal Inspection

This step entails identifying the anatomical landmarks in the nasal cavity. The major landmark is the nasal septum, extending from the nasal spine anteriorly to the rostrum of the sphenoid bone posteriorly.[3] The surgeon must inspect both nasal cavities; anatomical abnormalities, such as nasal septum deviation or spurs, must be corrected before continuing with the procedure. These corrections may be made either prior to or during the TEACPS surgery (**Fig. 35.3**).

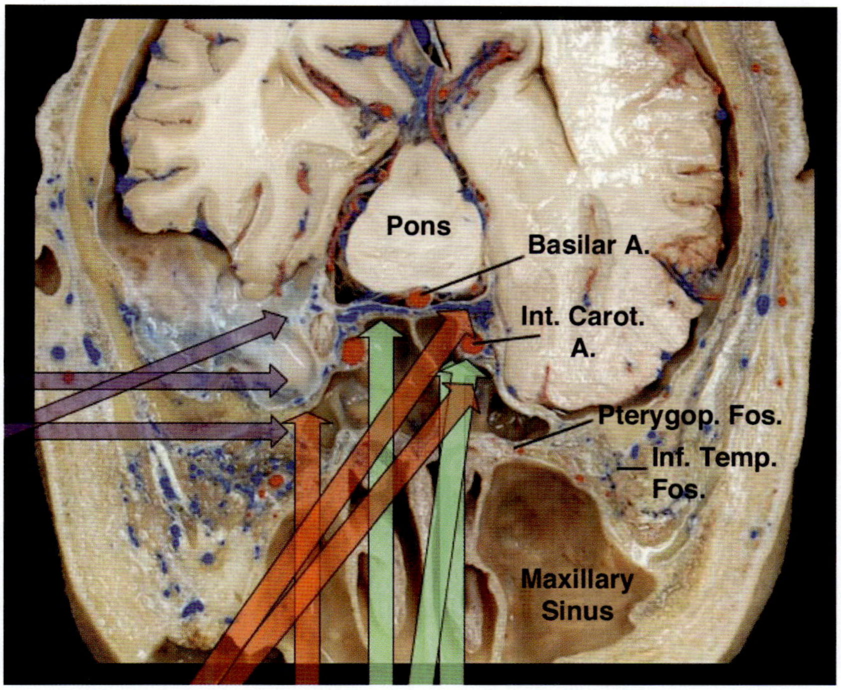

Fig. 35.1 Cranial base, axial superior view. General view of the radial endoscopic accesses to the skull base. The green arrows represent the endonasal approaches, the red arrows represent the transmaxillary approaches, and the purple arrows represent the subtemporal approaches. Note the multiple possibilities of combination of these approaches. A.: artery; Inf. Temp. Fos.: infratemporal fossa; Int. Carot. A.: internal carotid artery; Pterygop. Fos.: pterygopalatine fossa.

Special attention must be given to the nasal septum regarding closure at the end of the procedure. Covering the bone defect with pediculated septal mucosal flap is a reliable technique to avoid cerebrospinal fluid (CSF) fistulas. Usually this flap is racquet-shaped, with variable width and length, pediculated in the lateroposterior aspect of the nasal cavity, where the sphenopalatine artery enters from the pterygopalatine fossa through the sphenopalatine ostium. Once created, the mucosal flap can be moved to the pharynx to keep the surgical pathway clear[4] (**Figs. 35.4** and **35.5**).

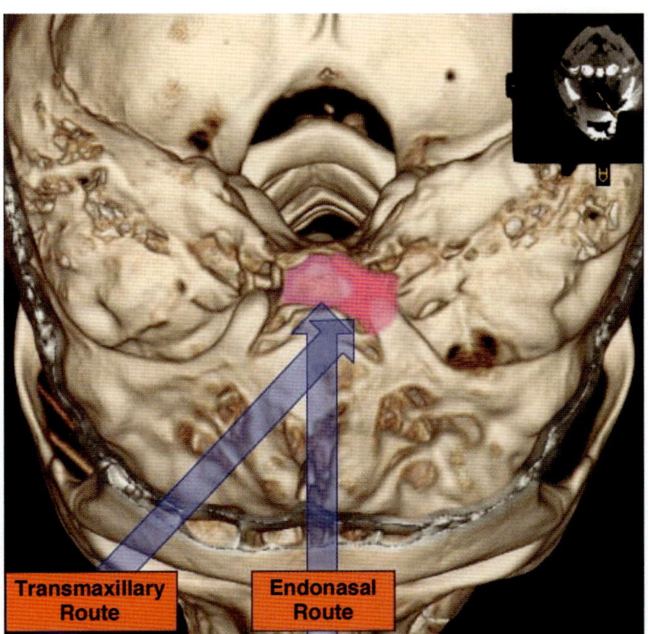

Fig. 35.2 Three-dimensional (3D) computed tomography (CT) scan of the cranial base. The arrows represent the different angles of approach from the endonasal and maxillary routes.

Another important landmark in the nasal cavity is the middle turbinate. Right after entering the nasal cavity, the surgeon must identify the head of the inferior and middle turbinates. The middle turbinate can be followed posteriorly from its head through its tail, ending just above the laterosuperior aspect of the choana. The sphenopalatine artery can be found a few millimeters superior, posterior, and lateral to the end of the middle turbinate tail. This is a useful landmark to help avoid major bleeding during this approach and preserve the vessels that irrigate the mucosal flap[3] (**Fig. 35.6**).

The middle turbinate also helps guide the surgeon to the sphenoid ostium, which is a notable landmark. From the end of the middle turbinate tail, the surgeon can move medially and then superiorly in the sphenoid rostrum until the sphenoidal ostium is found, usually 1.5 cm above the plane of the middle turbinate tail.[5]

Step 2: Preparation of the Septal Pediculated Mucosal Flap

Most skull base defects created during endoscopic endonasal surgery can be repaired with a pediculated septal mucosal flap, decreasing the incidence of CSF fistulas.[4,6]

The inferior incision of the mucosa should start by following a line inferior to the axis of the middle turbinate tail

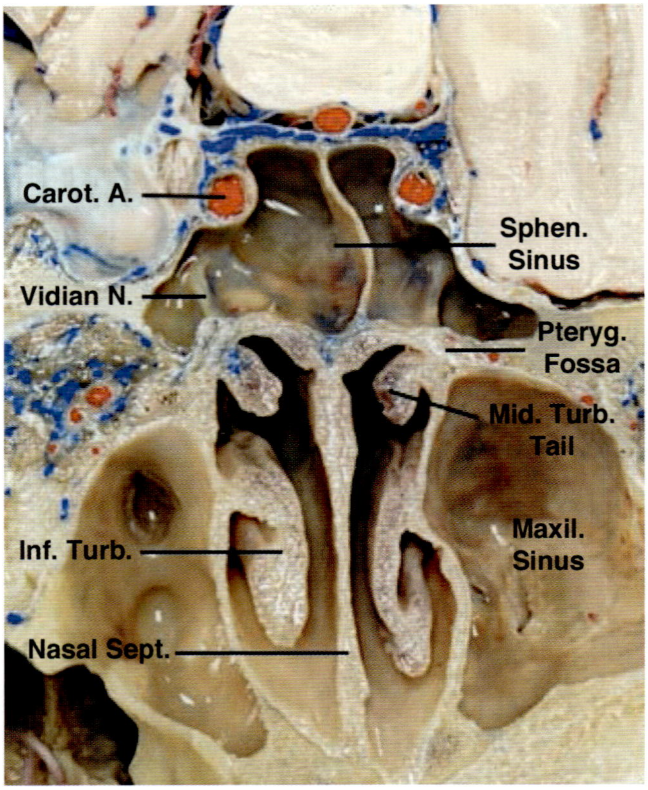

Fig. 35.3 Skull base, superior view. Entering through the nasal cavity, several structures can be identified as landmarks for safe navigation. The nasal septum in the midline is the first anatomical repair to be observed. Moving backward in a parallel trajectory to the nasal septum, the nasal choana and nasopharynx are identified. The middle turbinate is easy to identify and facilitates navigating in the nasal cavity. It is positioned in the lateral wall of the nasal cavity. Following the tail of the middle turbinate backward will lead to the most anteroinferior segment of the sphenoid rostrum. Just posterior, superior, and lateral to the end of the tail is the sphenopalatine foramen, a communication between the nasal cavity and the pterygopalatine fossa. Carot. A.: carotid artery; Inf.: inferior; Maxil.: maxillary; Mid.: middle; N.: nerve; Pteryg.: pterygoid; Sept.: septum; Sphen.: sphenoidal; Turb.: turbinate.

directly to the inferior border of the nasal septum, crossing just above the superior margin of the choana, beginning the incision at the most lateral point of this border, thus preserving vascularization of the flap. Once in the nasal septum, the incision line may go downward and follow the junction of the nasal septum and the nasal cavity floor. The incision progresses as anterior as necessary to the border of the mucosal/skin interface in the nasal cavity. The size of the flap is dependent on the predicted skull base defect.

After this anterior trajectory, the incision line must be directed upward in the nasal septum up to 1 to 2 cm of the junction of the nasal septum and the roof of the nasal cavity to prevent olfactory mucosa damage. The extension of the superior incision follows the septum posteriorly, turns laterally over the sphenoid rostrum, and progresses as laterally as possible, ending a few millimeters above the initial incision.

Once the incision is completed, the flap will have a racquet-like shape, being narrower in its posterolateral area. Then the

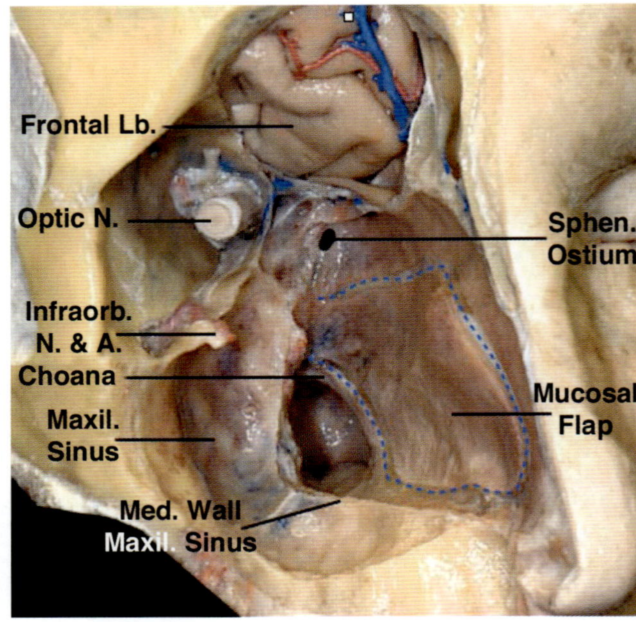

Fig. 35.4 Face, anterolateral view. Creating a septal pediculated mucosal flap is an extremely important initial step in endonasal cranial base approaches. The flap has a racquet-like shape, being pediculated posterolaterally. Terminal branches of the sphenopalatine artery irrigate the flap. A.: artery; Infraorb.: infraorbital; Lb.: lobe; Maxil.: maxillary; Med.: medial; N.: nerve; Sphen.: sphenoidal.

surgeon dissects the nasal mucosa from the bony and cartilaginous structures of the septum and sphenoidal rostrum. The dissected flap is reflected downward to the pharynx to keep the surgical route clear.

It is recommended that the mucosal flap in the nasal cavity be created on the side opposite the maxillary opening, to

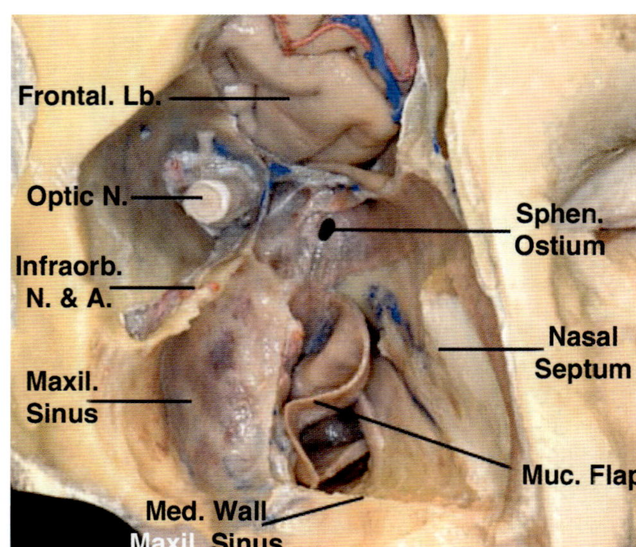

Fig. 35.5 After the dissection of the mucosal flap, it can be moved to the pharynx through the choana to keep the surgical route unobstructed. A.: artery; Lb.: lobe; Maxil.: maxillary; Med.: medial; Muc.: mucosal; N.: nerve; Sphen.: sphenoidal.

A

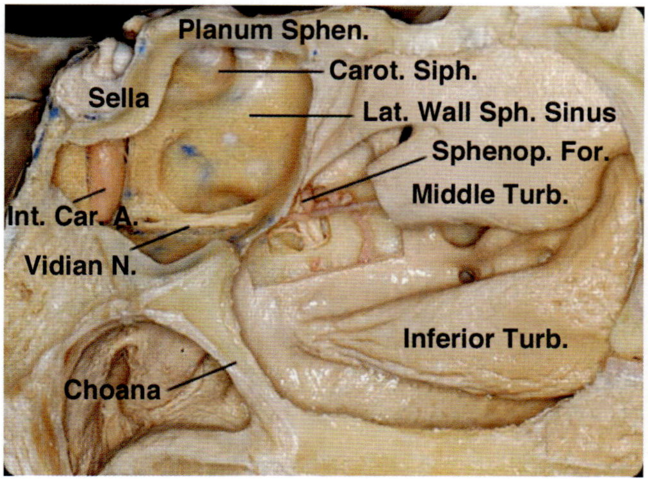

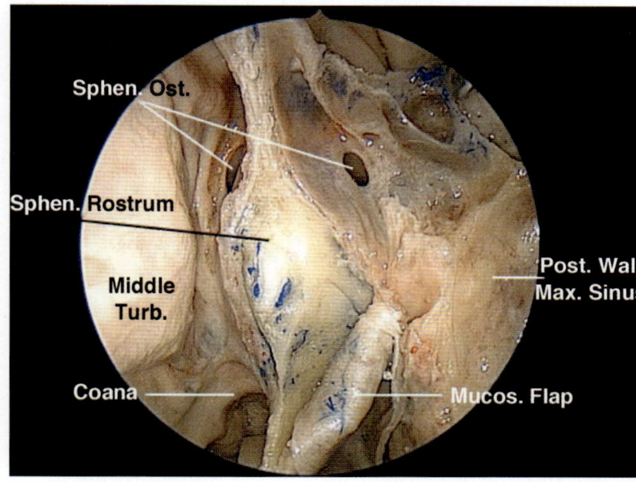

B

Fig. 35.6 **(A)** Nasal cavity, endoscopic view. The posterior segment of the nasal septum was resected. The mucosal flap is rotated downward to the pharynx. Both sphenoidal ostia are identified in the uppermost segment of the anterior wall of the sphenoid sinus. The tail of the middle turbinate of the contralateral nasal cavity is seen, ending just above the choana and hiding the sphenopalatine foramen. **(B)** Nasal cavity, sagittal view. The posterior segment of the middle turbinate tail was resected and the sphenopalatine foramen was enlarged, exposing the sphenopalatine artery and sphenopalatine ganglion. From the sphenopalatine ganglion, the vidian nerve can be followed backward in the floor of the sphenoid sinus, reaching the foramen lacerum. Carot.: carotid; Int. Car. A.: internal carotid artery; Lat.: lateral; Mucos: mucosal; N.: nerve; Ost.: ostium; Siph.: siphon; Sphen.: sphenoid; Sphenop.: sphenopalatine; Turb.: turbinate.

avoid damaging the flap pedicle vessels during the opening of the medial wall of the maxillary sinus (**Figs. 35.4** and **35.5**).

Step 3: Posterior Nasal Septostomy and Anterior Sphenoidal Wall Resection

After creating the mucosal flap, the posterior 2 cm of the bony nasal septum are resected to expose the rostrum of the sphenoid sinus. In creating this opening, it is extremely important to produce a wide exposure of the anterior wall of the sphenoid sinus. The surgeon must have access to the junction between the anterior wall of the sphenoid sinus and the roof of the nasal cavity above, resecting additionally the posterior ethmoid cells. The exposure must proceed downward to the junction of the anterior wall of the sphenoid sinus and the floor of the sphenoid sinus. At this point, the vomer should be removed as well at the junction of this bone with the sphenoid spine, at the anteroinferior part of the sphenoid rostrum (**Fig. 35.7**).

Resection of the posterior part of the nasal septum is essential to gain additional space for maneuvering surgical tools.

The next step is opening the anterior wall of the sphenoid sinus. This can be done from the ostia and then progressing both downward and upward. Alternatively, the anterior wall of the sphenoid sinus can be drilled off.

The opening of the anterior wall of the sphenoid sinus should progress to the sphenoidal plane. The anterior wall

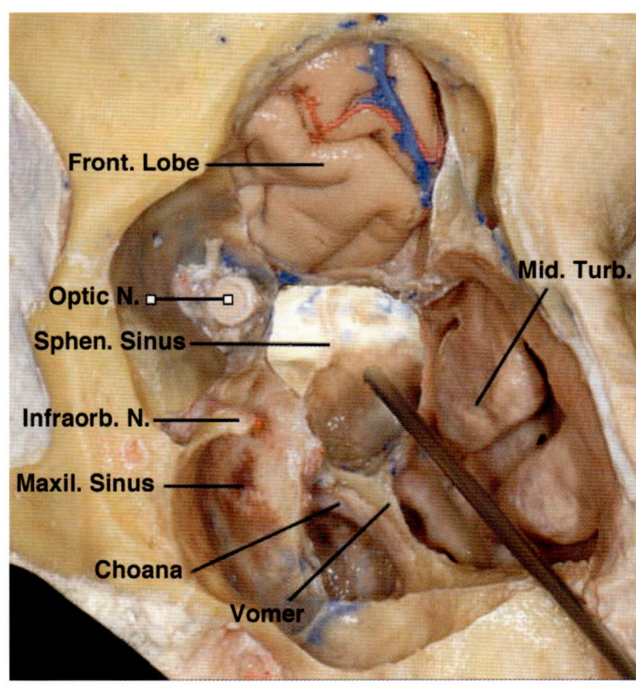

Fig. 35.7 Facial oblique view. The orbit and maxillary sinus walls were removed. The frontal lobe is exposed by removal of the floor of the anterior cranial base. Most of the nasal septum was resected, exposing the structures in the contralateral nasal cavity. The endoscope is introduced in the nasal cavity, crossing its extension and entering the sphenoid sinus. The sphenoid rostrum was widely resected. It is possible to observe the relationship of the surrounding structures with the sphenoid sinus. Front. Lobe: frontal lobe; Infraorbit. N.: infraorbital nerve; Maxil. Sinus: maxillary sinus; Mid. Turb.: middle turbinate; Optic N.: optic nerve; Sphen. Sinus: sphenoidal sinus.

should be removed as far laterally as the orbital medial wall. Specific attention must be given to the lateral border of this resection to avoid damaging the medial wall of the orbit, which is thin and can be mistaken for lateral ethmoid air cells.

Step 4: Middle Turbinectomy and Maxillary Medial Wall Initial Resection

The communication of the nasal cavity with the maxillary sinus begins with opening the medial wall of the maxillary sinus through the nasal cavity.

Initially, the posterior two thirds of the middle turbinate must be removed. In some cases, it is also necessary to remove the posterior segment of the inferior turbinate to produce a wide communication between the nasal cavity and the maxillary sinus[7] (**Figs. 35.8** and **35.9**).

When the turbinectomy is done, the maxillary ostium is identified and the maxillary cavity can be inspected with angled lens scopes. The opening of the medial wall of the maxilla begins through the ostium, progressing upward, downward, and posteriorly. In most cases it is not necessary to open the maxillary wall anterior to the maxillary ostium, but if necessary it can be accomplished respecting the borders of the nasociliary duct.

The posterior border when opening the medial wall of the maxillary sinus is the interface of this wall with the posterior wall of the maxillary sinus. It is very important to avoid damaging the posterior wall, because just behind this thin layer of bone is the pterygopalatine fossa, which is rich in fat tissue and neurovascular structures[8] (**Figs. 35.10** and **35.11**),

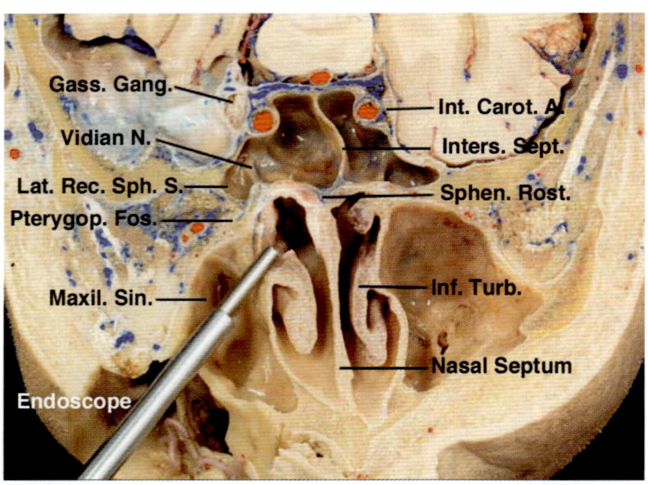

Fig. 35.8 Cranial base, inferior view. The transmaxillary approach is demonstrated. With partial resection, the anterior and medial walls of the maxillary sinus were removed, enabling the endoscope to progress to the nasal cavity and sphenoidal sinus. The posterior of the maxillary sinus must remain untouched to avoid damaging the neurovascular structures of the pterygopalatine fossa. Gass. Gang.: gasserian ganglion; Inf. Turb.: inferior turbinate; Int. Carot. A.: internal carotid artery; Inters. Sept.: intersinus septum; Lat. Rec. Sph. S.: lateral recess sphenoidal sinus; Maxil. Sin.: maxillary sinus; N.: nerve; Pterygop. Fos.: pterygopalatine fossa; Sphen. Rost.: sphenoidal rostrum.

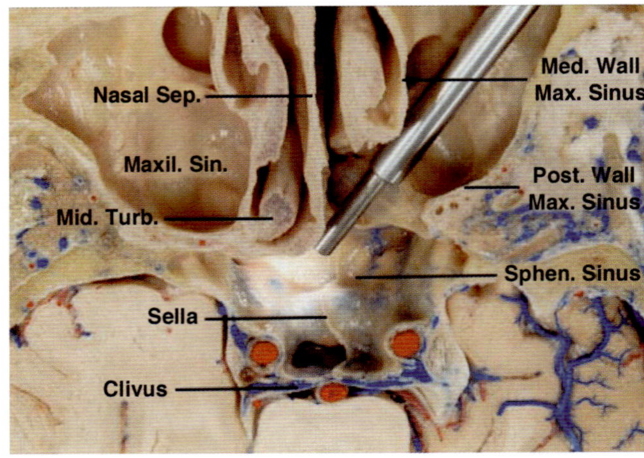

Fig. 35.9 Cranial base, superior view. The sella is posterior and superior to the tip of the endoscope. The same resection as in **Fig. 35.8** is demonstrated from an inferior perspective.

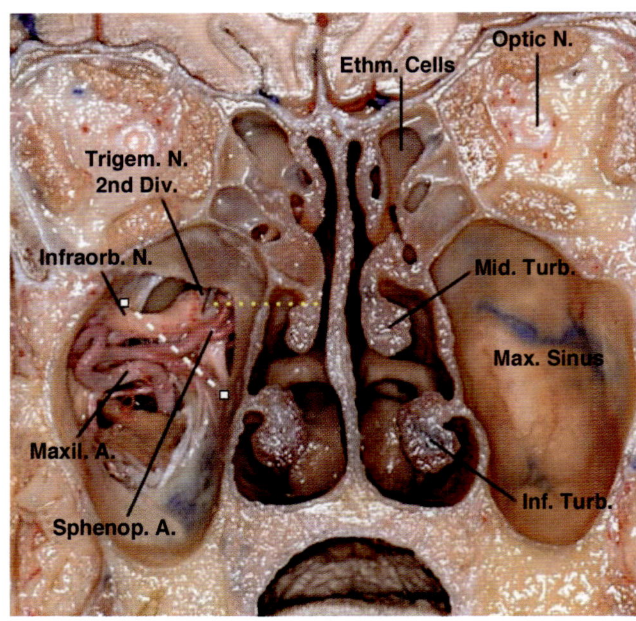

Fig. 35.10 Cranial base, coronal view. The posterior wall of the right maxillary sinus was removed, exposing the subtemporal fossa laterally, and the pterygopalatine fossa medially. The maxillary division of the trigeminal nerve is exiting the sphenoid bone through the foramen rotundum and running in the superior wall of the maxillary sinus as the infraorbital nerve. The maxillary artery loops in the subtemporal fossa, entering the pterygopalatine fossa and giving its terminal branches. The yellow line demonstrates the relationship of the axis of the middle turbinate tail and the sphenopalatine foramen. The white line represents the transition from the subtemporal fossa laterally, to the pterygopalatine fossa medially. Ethm.: ethmoidal; Sphenop.: sphenopalatine; Trigem.: trigeminal.

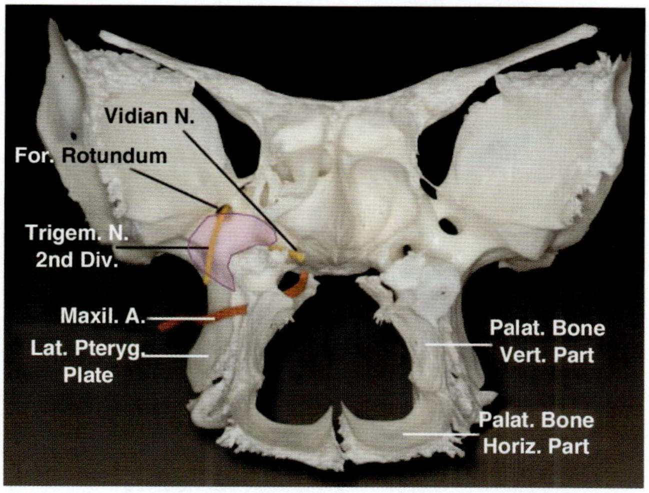

Fig. 35.11 Sphenoid bone and palatine bone, coronal view. The main neurovascular structures that lie behind the posterior maxillary wall (removed) are observed. The maxillary division of the trigeminal nerve exits the sphenoid bone through the foramen rotundum, entering the pterygopalatine fossa. The vidian nerve is demonstrated leaving the anterior opening of the vidian canal, joining the pterygopalatine fossa. The maxillary artery gives rise to its main terminal branch, the sphenopalatine artery, which pierces the sphenopalatine foramen to enter in the nasal cavity. For.: foramen; Horiz.: horizontal; Palat.: palatine; Vert.: vertical.

After opening the anterior wall of the maxilla, additional resection of the medial wall may be necessary.

Step 5: Opening of the Anterior Wall of the Maxilla

At this point the surgeon leave the nasal cavity and starts working through the maxilla.

After sublabial retraction, the oral mucosa is exposed 2 to 3 cm laterally from the midline. A horizontal mucosal incision is done in the transition of the gingival and oral mucosa, exposing the anterior wall of the maxillary sinus and the canine jugum. The mucosa is dissected from the bone as far as necessary. The superior border of the dissection is indicated by the infraorbital foramen and nerve. The medial border is the canine jugum[9] (**Fig. 35.12**).

After the anterior wall of the maxillary sinus is exposed, a high-speed drill is used to perform the maxillotomy. The canine fossa and canine jugum are the medial borders for the osteotomy. Progressing beyond this point may cause a lesion to the innervation of the teeth. Superiorly, the infraorbital nerve limits the resection. Laterally, the anterior wall of the maxillary sinus may be exposed as far as the intersection with the lateral wall of the maxilla. The size of the osteotomy will depend on the patient's anatomy and on the need for exposure regarding the lesion to be resected. Usually, a 1-cm-high and 2-cm-wide opening is appropriate in most cases.

Step 6: Recognition of Maxillary Sinus Landmarks

The 0-degree lens endoscope is inserted in the maxillary sinus, through which the surgeon can identify the anatomical landmarks. The maxillary sinus is pyramidal in shape, and the lateral, superior, medial, and inferior walls must be identified.[10]

At this point, the opening created in the medial maxillary wall from the nasal cavity is clearly observed, and it facilitates the surgeon's orientation. Looking upward, the infraorbital nerve can be visualized clearly in the superior maxillary wall. This nerve points to the pterygopalatine fossa when followed posteriorly.[9]

Another important structure is the nasociliary duct, crossing from superior to inferior on the most anterior aspect of the medial wall of the maxillary sinus. The duct is the anterior limit of the opening between the maxillary sinus and the nasal cavity[3] (**Fig. 35.12**).

Entering the maxillary sinus, in this lateral to medial pathway, the medial wall of the cavernous sinus on the contralateral

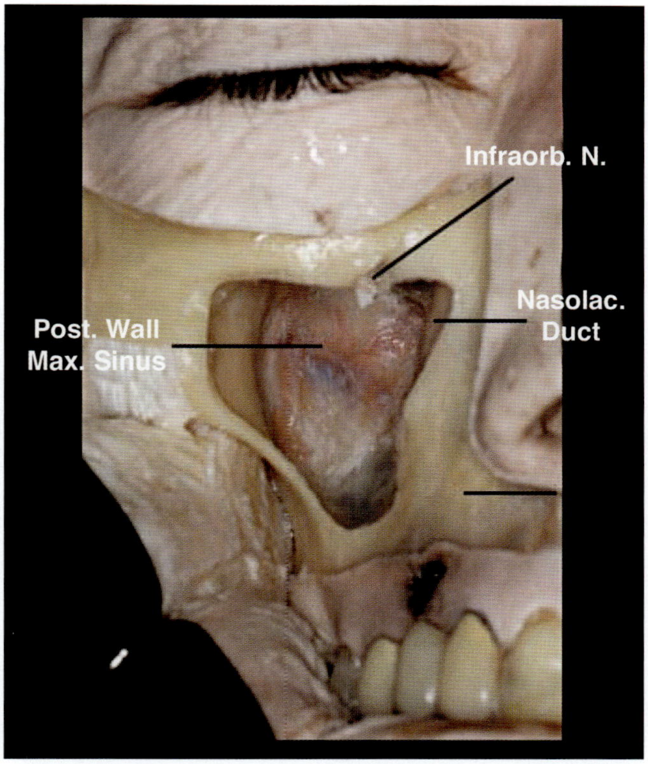

Fig. 35.12 Maxillary sinus, anterior view. The anterior wall of the maxillary sinus was resected. The uppermost limit of this resection is the infraorbital nerve. The medial limits are the canine fossa and jugum. The nasolacrimal duct is visualized in the medial wall of the maxillary sinus, and represents the anterior limit for resection of the medial wall during transmaxillary approach. The posterior wall of the maxillary sinus remains intact, hiding the pterygopalatine fossa. Nasolac.: nasolacrimal.

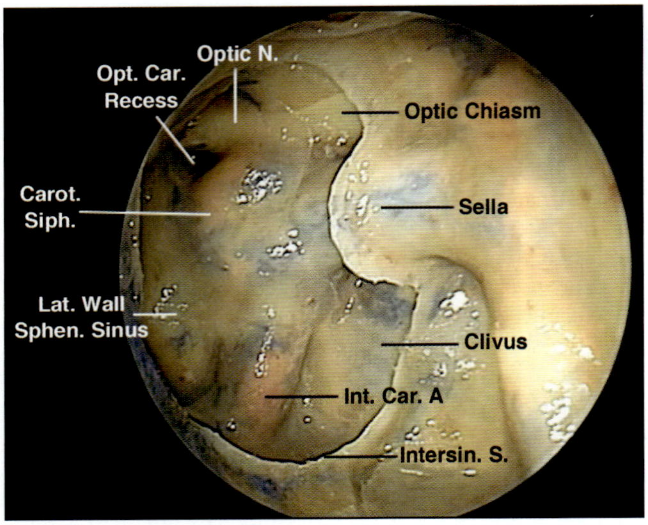

Fig. 35.13 Sphenoid sinus, from the maxillary sinus, endoscopic view. From the transmaxillary approach, the structures in the sphenoid sinus are observed obliquely. The intersinusal sinus was partially resected, demonstrating the internal carotid artery, optic-carotid recess, and lateral wall of the sphenoid sinus in the contralateral side.

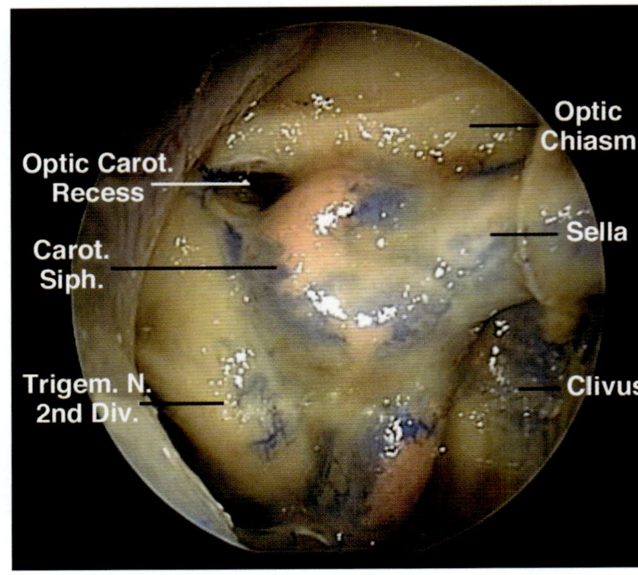

Fig. 35.14 Close-up view of the same structures as in Fig. 35.13. The impression of the maxillary division of the trigeminal nerve is seen in the lateral wall of the sphenoid sinus.

side is seen in a perpendicular view. Based on the tumor extension, it may be possible to widen the aperture in the medial wall of the maxillary sinus as was already done through the nasal cavity.

As the sphenoidal wall was properly opened, the structures in the sphenoid sinus can be observed, such as the optic nerve impression, the sellar protrusion, the optic-carotid recess, and, in same cases, the vidian nerve impression (**Figs. 35.13, 35.14,** and **35.15**).

The need for expansion of the fenestration of the medial wall of the maxilla takes into consideration the following landmarks: (1) the pterygopalatine fossa constitutes the pos-

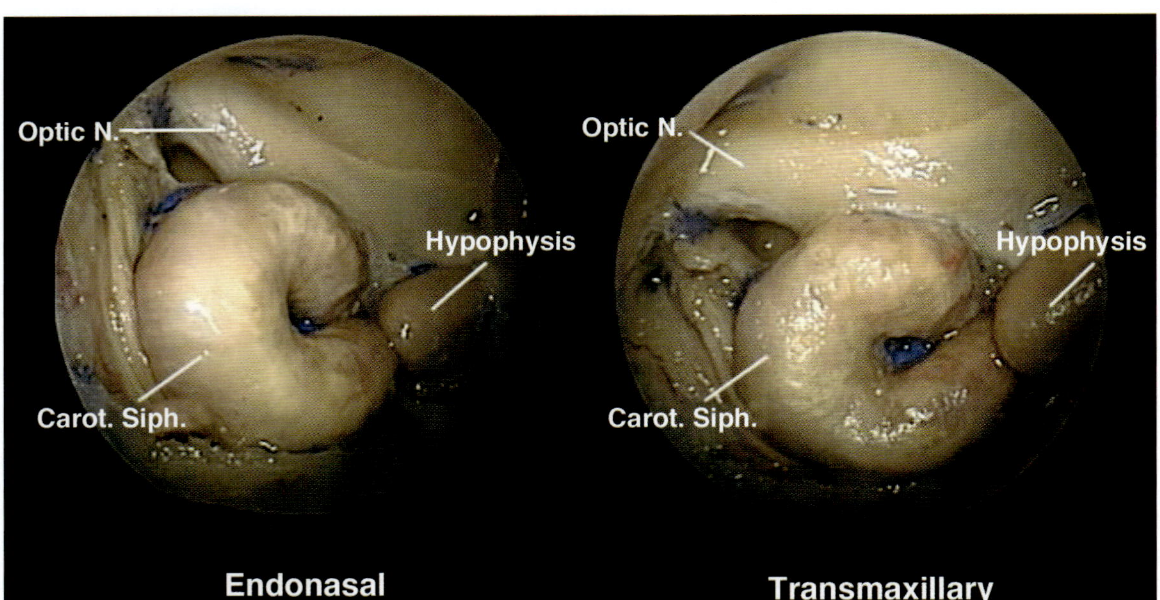

Fig. 35.15 Sphenoid sinus, endoscopic view. Endonasal and transmaxillary endoscopic approaches to the sphenoid sinus, demonstrating different angles of vision. Note that in the transmaxillary approach the structures in the lateral wall of the sphenoid sinus are seen in a more perpendicular way, facilitating dissection of this region.

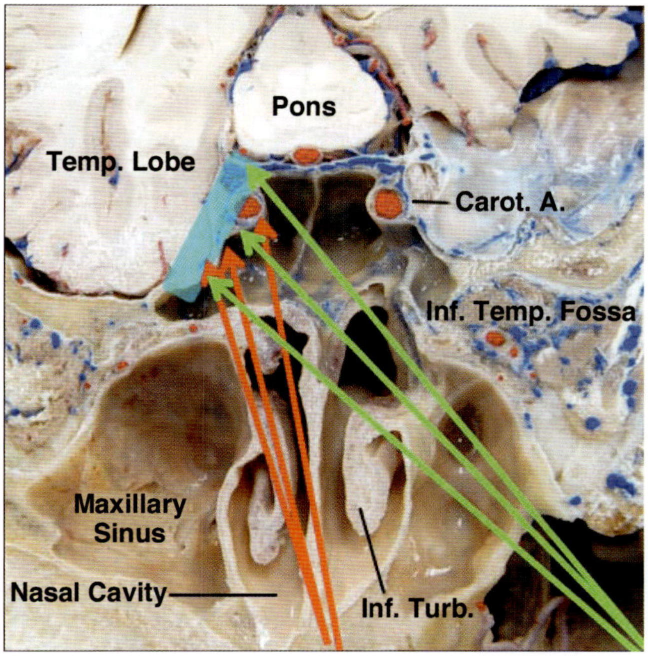

Fig. 35.16 Cranial base, superior view. The red arrows demonstrate the endonasal approach, and the green arrows represents the transmaxillary approach. The blue rectangle shows the parasellar structures. A more perpendicular angle of attack is achieved in the transmaxillary approach, and the distance to the target from this route is equal to or smaller than that in the endonasal approach. Temp.: temporal.

terior limit, 2) the vidian nerve is the inferior limit, (3) the nasolacrimal duct is the anterior limit, and (4) the floor of the anterior cranial base the superior limit.[11]

Step 7: Combined Work Through Maxillary Sinus and Nasal Cavity

Once the proper communication among the maxillary sinus, nasal cavity, and sphenoid sinus is established, the surgeon is ready to approach the lesion in the sellar and parasellar area. Based on the circumstances, a biportal or triportal approach can be elected, accessing the target area through both nasal cavities and the maxillary sinus.

The objective of this combined approach is to provide better exposure and easier manipulation of structures that lie lateral to the midline in the parasellar area, especially those that compromise the cavernous sinus and the retrocarotid spaces. Operating on lesions involving the medial wall of the cavernous sinus near the nose obligates the surgeon to use surgical instruments in a narrow angle of attack to the cavernous sinus wall; the endonasal axis of approach is very similar to the axis of the medial wall of the cavernous sinus (**Fig. 35.16**).

Conversely, introducing the surgical tools from the maxillary route enables the surgeon to face the cavernous sinus wall in an almost perpendicular axis. A more comfortable and accurate manipulation of instruments can be achieved in this way. In addition, two instruments can be handled and manipulated more easily and with more comfort from the maxillary approach than from the nasal cavity, which is tighter (**Figs. 35.16** and **35.17**).

The endoscope is introduced preferably through one of the nasal cavities, mainly the one ipsilateral to the lesion. Usually, 30-degree lens scopes are selected because they may produce better visualization of the structures in the sphenoid sinus lateral wall. In some circumstances, 0-degree lenses can be useful (**Fig. 35.18**).

The surgeon can choose many combinations of endoscope position and surgical instruments. In some cases, the endoscope may be introduced through the maxilla and the surgical tools from both nasal cavities. Alternative options may yield better visualization and dissection (**Figs. 35.19, 35.20, 35.21, 35.22,** and **35.23**).

Compared with the endonasal approach, the transmaxillary route is shorter in length in two thirds of cases and equal in length in one third.

Radiologic Investigation

Detailed image acquisition is mandatory due to frequent anatomical variations. Accurate understanding of the patient's anatomy can prevent problems from occurring in the surgery.

Awareness of the aeration of the maxillary sinus is crucial. It should be noted that some sinuses might be very tight,

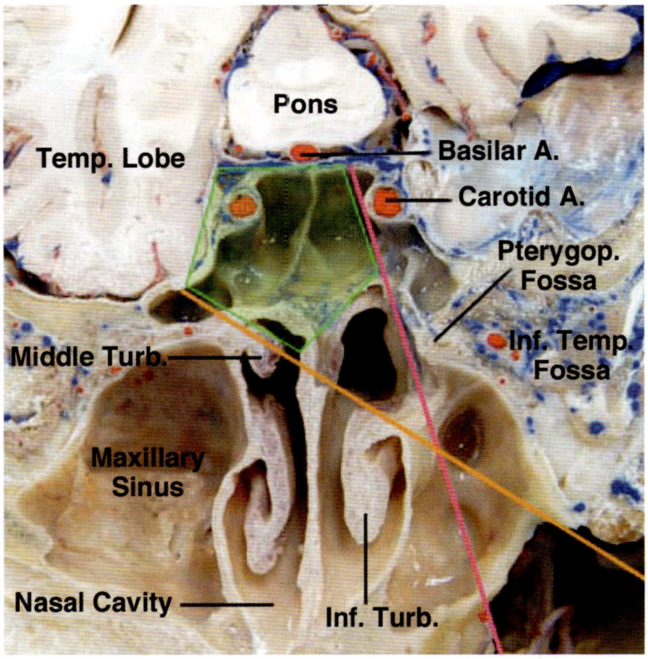

Fig. 35.17 Cranial base, superior view. The pink and orange lines demonstrate the possible angles of maneuver in transmaxillary approach. In green is emphasized the possibilities of resection through transmaxillary approach.

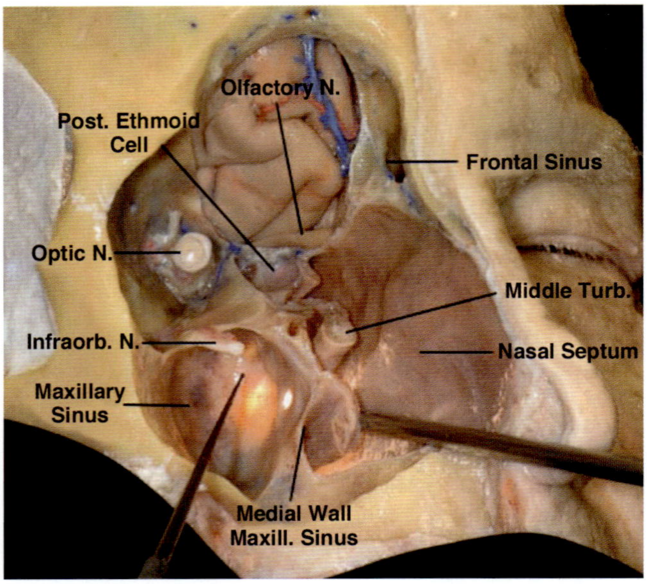

Fig. 35.18 Face, oblique view. Demonstration of possible usage of surgical instruments and endoscope through combined transmaxillary and endonasal approaches. Many different combinations of maneuvering surgical tools are possible, using biportal or triportal approaches.

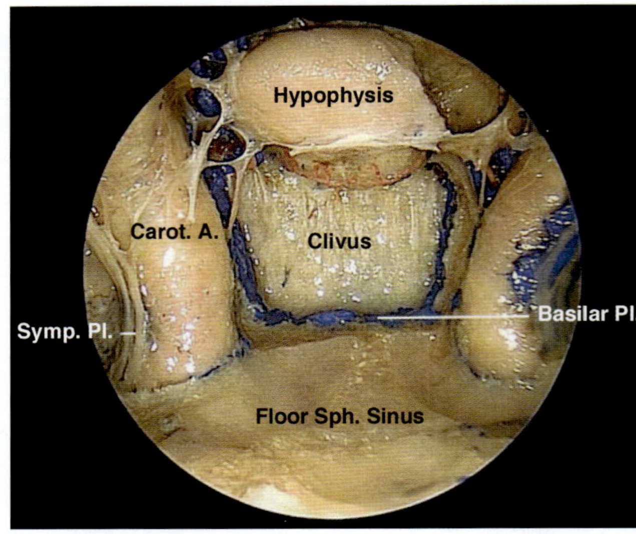

Fig. 35.19 Sphenoid sinus, endonasal view. The intersinusal septum was removed. Both vertical segments of the internal carotid artery are seen. The pituitary gland (anterior and posterior lobes) lies in the central part of the surgical field, with multiple trabeculae giving support to the gland. The posterior wall of the sphenoid sinus was resected, exposing the dura mater of the posterior fossa. Pl.: plexus; Symp.: sympathetic.

proving to be too narrow even for endoscopic navigation (**Fig. 35.24**).

Although high-quality gadolinium-enhanced magnetic resonance imaging (MRI) is elementary for understanding the characteristics of the lesion, the volumetric computed tomography (CT) scan will effectively help the surgeon to decide if this surgical approach is applicable or not. The CT workstation facilitates planning the route of approach in a three-dimensional fashion.

Special attention must be given to the necessary alignments to facilitate this approach. The main alignment is that of the anteromedial margin of the maxillary sinus with the

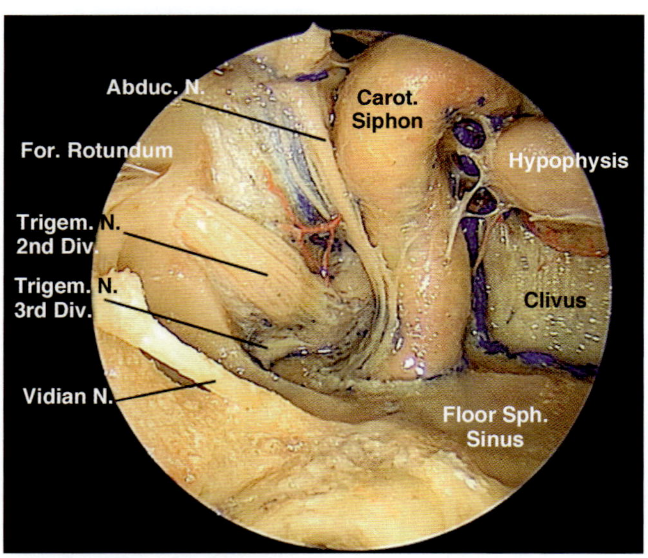

Fig. 35.20 Medial wall of the cavernous sinus, transmaxillary approach. The medial wall of the cavernous sinus was resected and the blue silicone of the venous channels was removed. All segments of the intracavernous carotid artery are visualized. The gasserian ganglion is seen in the center of the surgical view, and all three branches of the trigeminal nerve are demonstrated. The vidian nerve is shown crossing through the floor of the sphenoid sinus. Abduc. N.: abducens nerve.

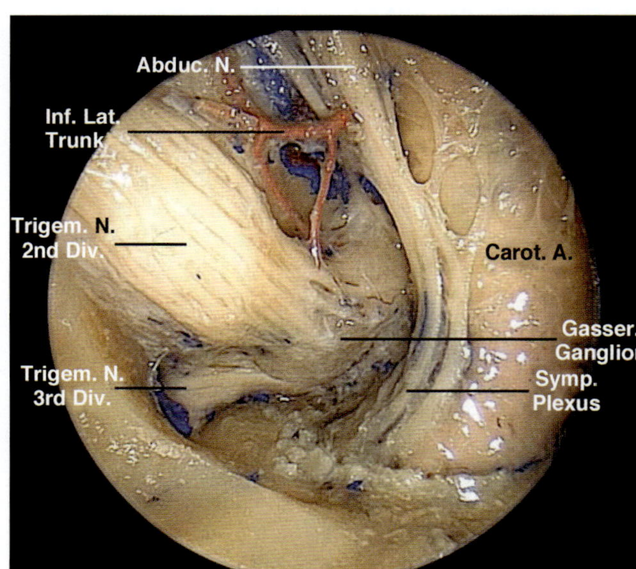

Fig. 35.21 Close-up view of the cavernous sinus through the transmaxillary approach. Gasser.: gasserian.

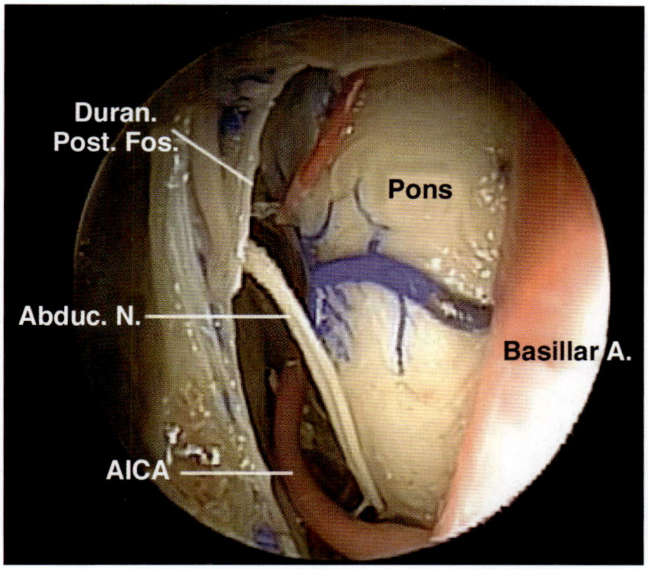

Fig. 35.22 Clivus, transmaxillary approach. The clival bone and dura of the posterior fossa were removed. The angle of approach of the transmaxillary route enables the visualization of the structures into the cerebellopontine angle. At the first plane, the abducens nerve crosses the prepontine cistern, pierces the posterior fossa dura, and runs upward to Dorello's channel. AICA: anterior inferior cerebellar artery; Duram.: dura mater.

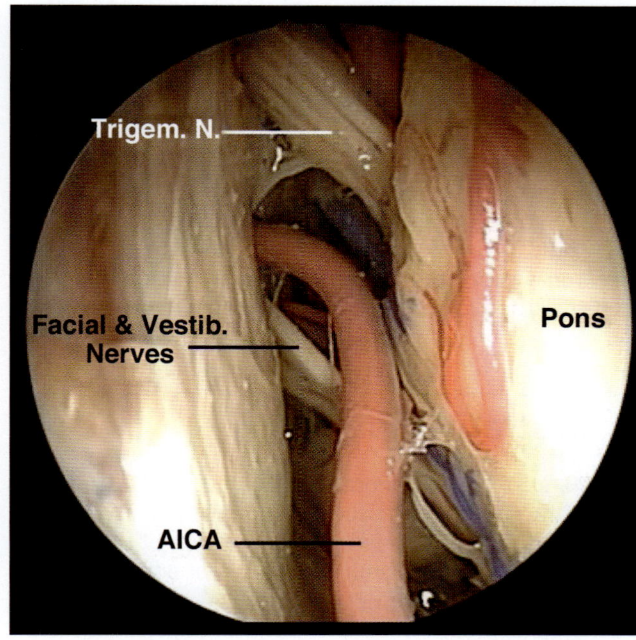

Fig. 35.23 A close-up view from the structures of Fig. 35.22. The anterior-inferior cerebellar artery crosses from medial to lateral toward the cerebellopontine angle, superior to the facial, vestibular, and cochlear nerves, and inferior to the trigeminal nerve. Vestib.: vestibular.

junction of the maxillary medial and posterior walls. The projection of this axis must allow the visualization of the most posterior segment of the lateral wall of the sphenoid sinus. Similarly, the alignment of the anterolateral border of the maxillary sinus with the junction of the medial and posterior wall of this sinus may produce an access projection that facilitates the visualization of the anterior border of the lateral sphenoidal wall (**Fig. 35.17**).

It is very important to observe the distance between the nasolacrimal duct and the junction of the medial and lateral

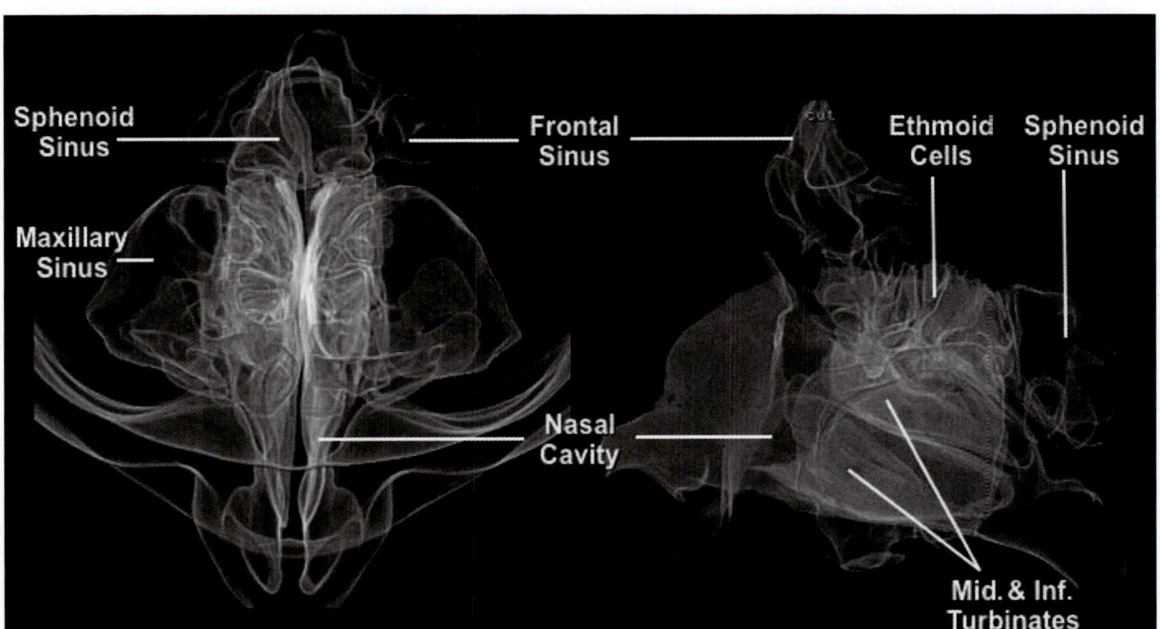

Fig. 35.24 A 3D CT scan, air reconstruction. In the preoperative planning, it is very important to understand the aeration of the natural cavities of the anterior cranial base to establish safe routes for navigation.

walls of the maxillary sinus. This information confirms how far anteriorly the medial wall of the maxillary sinus can be opened.

Several key points must be observed in a three-dimensional (3D) CT investigation, such as the alignment of the nasal septum, the size and position of the posterior ethmoid cells, the nasolacrimal duct, the maxillary ostium, the middle turbinate, the sphenopalatine ostium, and the sphenoidal intersinusal and intrasinusal septa.

Neuronavigation can contribute to the approach, but it cannot be used as a substitute for careful preoperative planning.

Illustrative Case

In 2009, a 31-year-old woman presented with acromegaly, with characteristic soft tissue enlargement and acromegalic facies. In 2005 she first noticed enlargement of the nose. In 2006 she observed thickening of fingers of both hands. She was surgically treated in 2006 and 2008 through a transsphenoidal approach in another surgical department, without control of the growth hormone (GH) levels. In this previous surgery the tumor was described as extremely hard.

In 2009 she consulted in our neurosurgical department with the same complaints and a GH level of 90 µg/dL. MRI scanning was performed, demonstrating a heterogeneous lesion, highly enhanced by gadolinium, located inside the sella with extensions to the suprasellar space and toward the right cavernous sinus (**Fig. 35.25**). An endonasal endoscopic approach was proposed, combined with a transmaxillary contralateral approach to reach the extension to the cavernous sinus.

The surgery was performed through both routes in complementary fashion. The transmaxillary extension of the approach enabled a very wide visualization of the lateral extension of the tumor, with comfortable maneuverability of the surgical instruments and endoscope through the nasal cavity and maxilla (**Figs. 35.26. 35.27,** and **35.28**). Neuronavigation proved to be very helpful in this case, not only for dissecting the tumor but also for planning the transmaxillary route (**Fig. 35.29**).

Postsurgery, the patient was treated with radiotherapy.

At 6-month follow-up, she demonstrated clear reduction of the acromegalic characteristics, especially in the face. The GH decreased to 8 µg/dL.

Discussion

Dissecting tumors projecting toward the parasellar area, especially those extending into the cavernous sinus, constitutes a technical challenge in endonasal approaches. The modular classification of the possible approaches to this area helps to identify the best operative approach. Surgeons must have extensive knowledge of the anatomy.[2,12]

The transmaxillary access provides a straightforward view to the medial wall of the contralateral cavernous sinus, being especially useful in cases where the tumor insinuates between the horizontal segments of the intracavernous carotid artery.

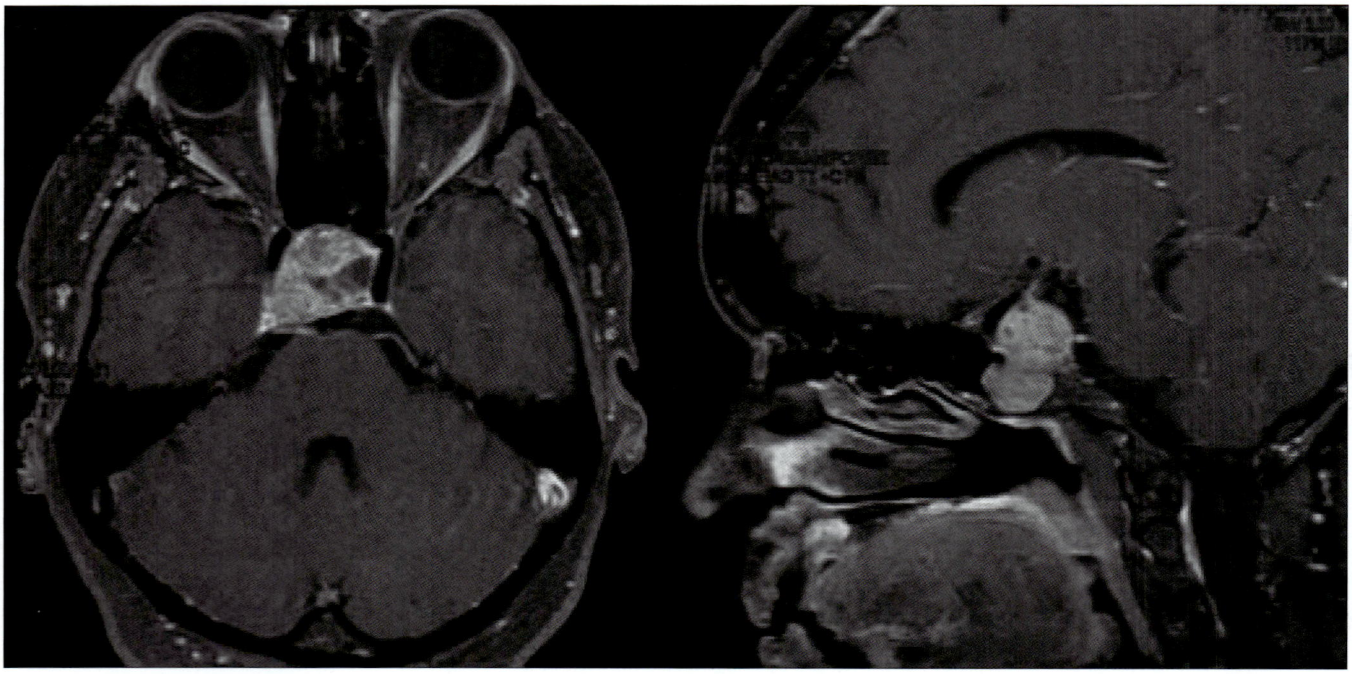

Fig. 35.25 Illustrative case, preoperative MRI. A heterogeneous lesion, highly enhanced by gadolinium, is located inside the sella with extensions to the suprasellar space and toward the right cavernous sinus.

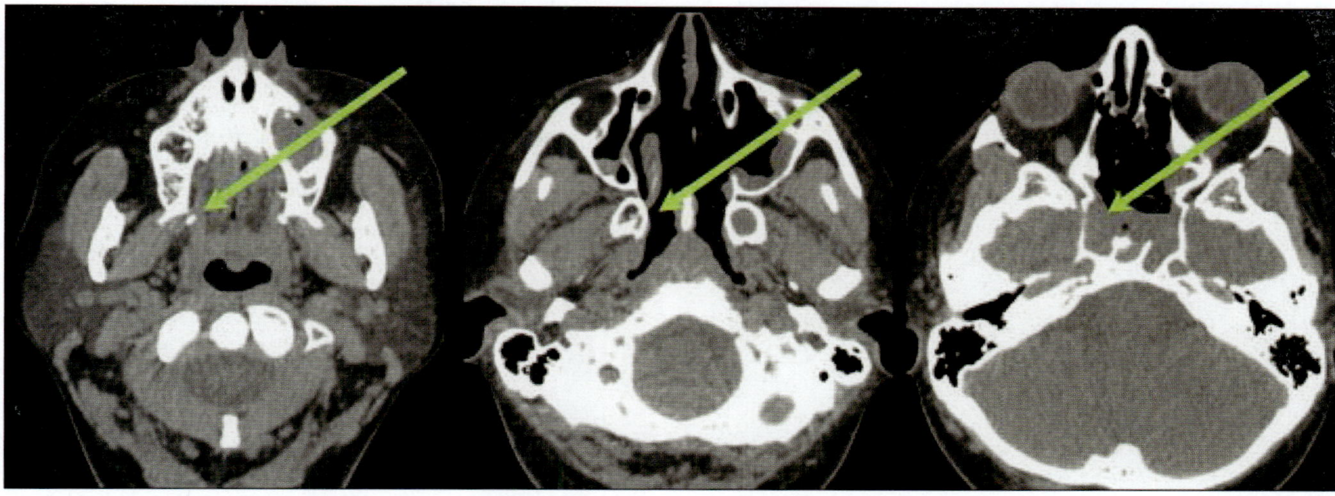

Fig. 35.26 Illustrative case, postoperative CT scan. The trajectory of the transmaxillary approach is outlined. The opening of the anterior and medial walls of the maxillary sinus is clearly observed. The direct and perpendicular trajectory from the maxillary sinus to the contralateral parasellar area is evident.

The possibility of using a combined endonasal and transmaxillary approach gives the surgeon the option of working through both pathways simultaneously, which facilitates the dissection, and the option of driving one instrument through the nose and the other from the maxillary sinus.

Thorough knowledge of the complex anatomy of this region is mandatory, as well as understanding the patient's specific anatomy and its variations before surgery. Although the transmaxillary approach is a low-risk technique, complications such as facial numbness and teeth denervation may be avoided by analyzing the volumetric information from MRI and CT scans.

The straight angle view to the medial wall of the contralateral cavernous sinus enables tumor removal from the sinus, leaving the nerves in the lateral wall undisturbed.

The transmaxillary approach represents a combined access to the endonasal approach and does not significantly lengthen the surgical time. No cosmetic or functional defects are expected.

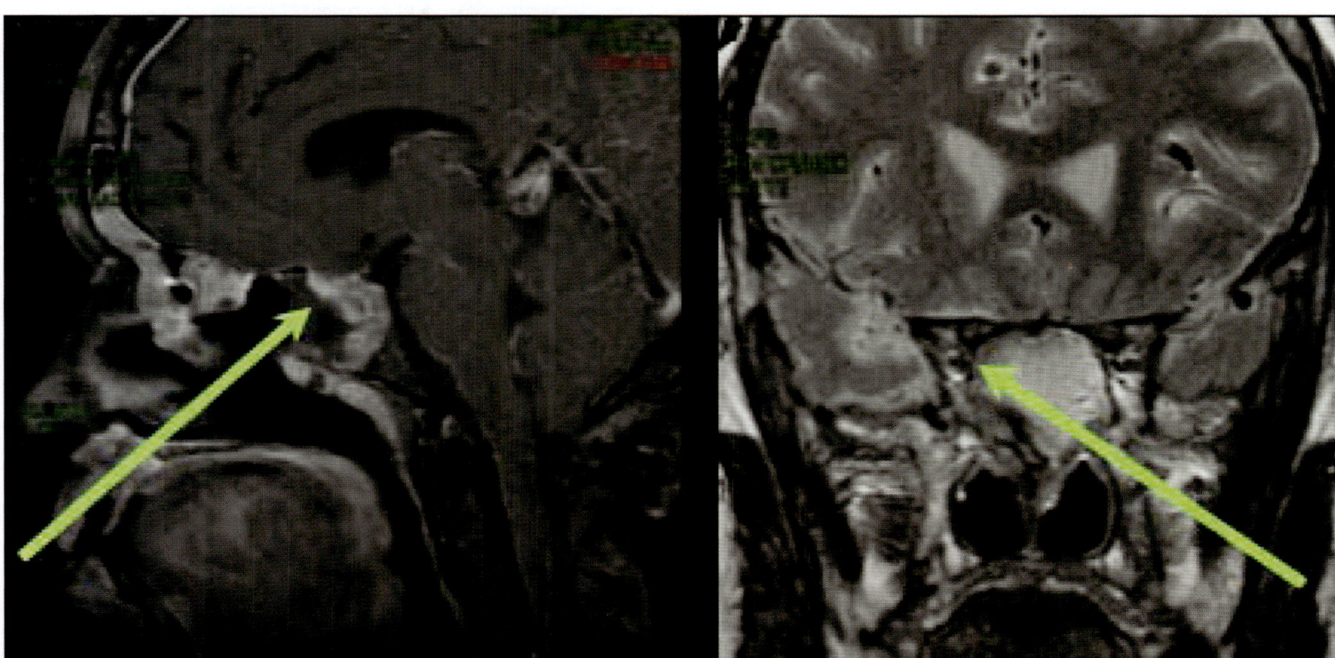

Fig. 35.27 Illustrative case, early postoperative MRI.

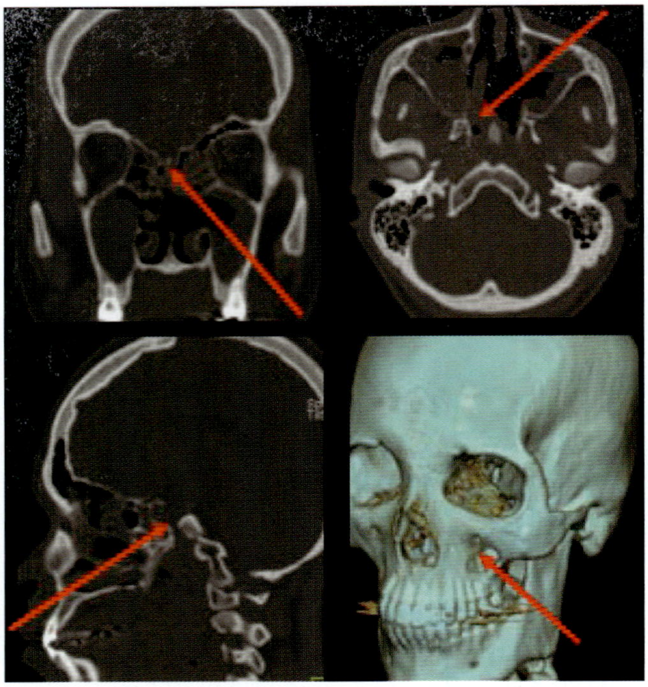

Fig. 35.28 Illustrative case, postoperative CT scan. The transmaxillary approach can be understood as an inferior to superior and lateral to medial approach. The volume reconstruction of the face shows the opening in the anterior maxillary wall.

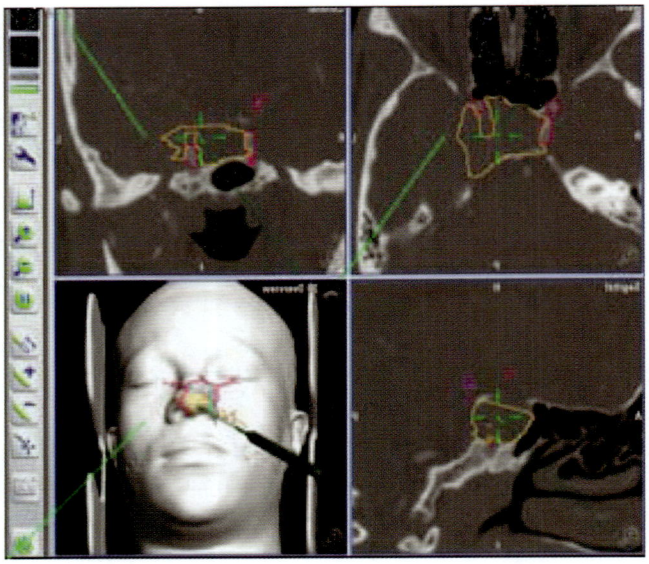

Fig. 35.29 Illustrative case, neuronavigation.

The transmaxillary endoscopic approach to contralateral parasellar lesions offers a complementary opportunity for tumor removal in selected cases.

References

1. Doglietto F, Prevedello DM, Jane JA Jr, Han J, Laws ER Jr. Brief history of endoscopic transsphenoidal surgery—from Philipp Bozzini to the First World Congress of Endoscopic Skull Base Surgery. Neurosurg Focus 2005;19:E3
2. Prevedello DM, Kassam AB, Snyderman C, et al. Endoscopic cranial base surgery: ready for prime time? Clin Neurosurg 2007;54:48–57
3. Rhoton AL Jr. The sellar region. Neurosurgery 2002;51(4, Suppl): S335–S374
4. Hadad G, Bassagasteguy L, Carrau RL, et al. A novel reconstructive technique after endoscopic expanded endonasal approaches: vascular pedicle nasoseptal flap. Laryngoscope 2006;116:1882–1886
5. Kassam AB, Vescan AD, Carrau RL, et al. Expanded endonasal approach: vidian canal as a landmark to the petrous internal carotid artery. J Neurosurg 2008;108:177–183
6. Harvey RJ, Nogueira JF, Schlosser RJ, Patel SJ, Vellutini E, Stamm AC. Closure of large skull base defects after endoscopic transnasal craniotomy. Clinical article. J Neurosurg 2009;111:371–379
7. Theodosopoulos PV, Guthikonda B, Brescia A, Keller JT, Zimmer LA. Endoscopic approach to the infratemporal fossa: anatomic study. Neurosurgery 2010;66:196–202, discussion 202–203
8. Solari D, Magro F, Cappabianca P, et al. Anatomical study of the pterygopalatine fossa using an endoscopic endonasal approach: spatial relations and distances between surgical landmarks. J Neurosurg 2007; 106:157–163
9. Couldwell WT, Sabit I, Weiss MH, Giannotta SL, Rice D. Transmaxillary approach to the anterior cavernous sinus: a microanatomic study. Neurosurgery 1997;40:1307–1311
10. Moore CC, Bromwich M, Roth K, Matic DB. Endoscopic anatomy of the orbital floor and maxillary sinus. J Craniofac Surg 2008;19:271–276
11. Fortes FS, Sennes LU, Carrau RL, et al. Endoscopic anatomy of the pterygopalatine fossa and the transpterygoid approach: development of a surgical instruction model. Laryngoscope 2008;118:44–49
12. Schwartz TH, Fraser JF, Brown S, Tabaee A, Kacker A, Anand VK. Endoscopic cranial base surgery: classification of operative approaches. Neurosurgery 2008;62:991–1002, discussion 1002–1005

36 Suprapetrous Approach to Meckel's Cave and Temporal Fossa

Daniel M. Prevedello, Amin B. Kassam, Ricardo L. Carrau, Juan C. Fernandez-Miranda, Paul A. Gardner, and Carl H. Snyderman

Tips and Pearls

- Endonasal endoscopic surgery of middle fossa lesions requires a multidisciplinary team.
- Common current indications for an endoscopic endonasal approach to the middle cranial fossa are trigeminal schwannomas, meningiomas, encephaloceles with or without cerebrospinal fluid (CSF) leaks, juvenile angiofibromas, invasive pituitary adenomas, and perineural invasion (trigeminal) by intermediate and low-grade tumors.
- An important advantage of the endoscopic endonasal approach is the avoidance of temporal lobe retraction.
- Contraindications to this approach include patient comorbidities, unfavorable anatomy, lack of availability of a multidisciplinary team, and lack of specialized equipment/instruments.
- Careful preoperative evaluation, including a physical examination and imaging studies, is critical.
- Preoperative computed tomographic angiography (CTA) and magnetic resonance imaging (MRI) are complementary and can be fused for image guidance.
- A pedicle nasoseptal flap (if available) is harvested on the contralateral side at the beginning of the surgery.
- The vidian nerve is followed posteriorly to reach and identify the petrous internal carotid artery (ICA). It can be preserved in selected cases.
- Drilling of the internal carotid canal is technically difficult and requires the use of diamond or hybrid drill bits. Cutting drill bits should never be used for this purpose.
- The anteromedial and lateral triangles of the cavernous sinus are used to reach the middle fossa.
- The area medial to the gasserian ganglion is reached through the quadrangular space, which is limited inferiorly and medially by the ICA, laterally by V2, and superiorly by cranial nerve VI.
- Electrophysiologic monitoring with electromyogram (EMG) of cranial nerve VI and the motor branch of V3 helps to gauge the delicate dissection and preserve function.
- Zero-degree and angled endoscopes should be used to appreciate the anatomy of the region as well as to identify any residual disease. The posterior fossa can be approached in selected cases.
- The resultant dural defect is repaired with the pedicle nasoseptal flap, which should also cover the exposed ICA. Packing is used to buttress the reconstruction, and septal silicone splints are placed to prevent synechiae.

Introduction

Meckel's cave represents a diverticulum of the dura mater within the middle cranial fossa. The periosteum layer of the dura mater maintains its dense attachment with the middle fossa bone, and the meningeal layer separates to form the space for the trigeminal nerve and Meckel's cave. The trigeminal nerve leaves the brainstem toward the middle fossa, where it forms the gasserian ganglion and divides into three segmental branches; therefore, Meckel's cave is also known as the trigeminal cave.[1–4]

Various pathologies can be encountered in Meckel's cave. Trigeminal schwannomas and meningiomas are the most common.[5–7] Other lesions include juvenile nasopharyngeal angiofibromas, chondrosarcomas, chordomas, and sinonasal malignancies, such as adenoid cystic carcinoma, which commonly spreads through the perineurium of cranial nerves.[7–11]

Many surgical approaches have been described to access lesions located in Meckel's cave.[1–3,12–14] These approaches can be divided in three main groups according to their anatomical route into: anterolateral, lateral, and posterolateral. None of these approaches is ideally suited to reach the entire Meckel's cave.[15] The expanded endonasal approach to the middle fossa is an alternative surgical approach that offers direct access without brain retraction.[15]

Indications and Advantages

The expanded endoscopic endonasal approach provides a direct route to the anteromedial region of Meckel's cave. Its primary advantage is that it facilitates the dissection between the trigeminal nerve and the periosteal layer of the dura mater for lesions within the inferomedial component of Meckel's cave. Lesions located lateral to the gasserian ganglion can also be accessed through the endonasal route using the anteromedial (V1-V2) and anterolateral (V2-V3) triangles of the middle fossa (cavernous sinus). Posterior fossa extensions can be resected in selected cases.[15]

The main advantage of the endonasal route is the possibility of resecting large temporal fossa/Meckel's cave lesions without temporal lobe brain retraction.

Contraindications

Complex lesions with involvement of multiple fossas or regions need to be thoroughly evaluated. If the main tumoral component of the lesion is located in the posterior fossa, then a retrosigmoid-suprameatal approach may be more appropriate. The same is valid for lesions that occupy the lateral aspect of the middle cranial or infratemporal fossa. In those cases, an open middle cranial/infratemporal approach may be more appropriate. Each patient is evaluated individually, and commonly there is a need for combining approaches to optimize the resection without transgressing the plane of cranial nerves.

Diagnostic Workup

The physical examination includes a neurologic assessment, with special focus on cranial nerve function. Trigeminal sensory and motor function must be studied in detail. An ophthalmologic examination including a visual field examination is advocated for patients presenting optic nerve or orbital compromise. Endoscopic assessment of the nasal cavity is recommended to identify any nasal lesions and to document septal integrity, deviations, and other anatomical variants.

Imaging

All patients undergo a preoperative computed tomographic angiography (CTA) and magnetic resonance imaging (MRI), which are fused for intraoperative frameless stereotactic image guidance (Stryker-Leibinger Corp., Kalamazoo, MI).

Surgery

Instrumentation

Appropriate instrumentation is vital for the endonasal endoscopic approach to the infratemporal fossa and Meckel's cave. Necessary equipment includes high-quality endoscopes (0- and 45-degree); videocamera and monitor; long endonasal endoscopic bipolar electrocautery; long and delicate endonasal drills with 3- and 4-mm hybrid drill tips; long dissection instruments; and hemostatic materials.

Operative Setup

Following orotracheal intubation, the patient is placed in a three-pin head holder, positioned with the head turned to the right and slightly tilted to the left.

Nasal Preparation

The nose is decongested with topical 0.05% oxymetazoline applied using ½" × 3" cottonoids. A povidone solution is

Fig. 36.1 (*opposite*) Meckel's cave approach. **(A)** A general overview of the endonasal approach to Meckel's cave. The maxillary sinus lies anterior to the pterygopalatine fossa. Removal of the posterior wall of the maxillary sinus exposes the pterygopalatine fossa, where the vidian canal and foramen rotundum can be identified. The pterygoid process has to be drilled out to access the lateral recess of the sphenoid sinus. The vidian nerve runs in the floor of the lateral recess, and the maxillary nerve (V2) courses in the lateral wall. Both nerves tend to converge as they travel posteriorly, and are used as surgical landmarks that guide the approach. The vidian nerve, which can be preserved in selected cases, is followed posteriorly until it meets the lateral aspect of the internal carotid artery at the foramen lacerum, and the maxillary nerve is followed posteriorly where it joins the trigeminal ganglion, located posterolateral to the paraclival segment of the internal carotid artery. The superior orbital fissure, which is the anterior continuation of the cavernous sinus, is located anterosuperior to Meckel's cave and anterolateral to the parasellar segment of the internal carotid artery. **(B–F)** Stepwise approach to Meckel's cave. **(B)** After identifying the vidian nerve at the pterygopalatine fossa, the vidian canal is drilled out in an anteroposterior direction toward the internal carotid artery. Drilling the inferior wall of the vidian canal, pterygoid process, and upper portion of the medial pterygoid plate exposes the upper wall of the eustachian tube, which represents another important surgical landmark. Both the vidian nerve and the eustachian tube converge at the lower (or fibrocartilaginous) portion of the foramen lacerum. Remarkably, the anterior genu of the internal carotid artery (petrous-paraclival transition) occupies the upper (or vascular) portion of the foramen lacerum. Once the carotid artery has been exposed at this level, complete exposure of the paraclival and parasellar segments of the internal carotid artery is achieved. **(C)** Drilling now continues lateral to the paraclival carotid artery, exposing the dura of the middle fossa. The mandibular nerve and foramen ovale are identified after drilling the floor of the middle fossa. **(D)** The dura of the middle fossa has been opened to expose the three branches of the trigeminal nerve. The abducens nerve runs medial to the ophthalmic nerve (V1) from the cavernous sinus to the superior orbital fissure. The carotid nerve, which is a sympathetic nerve extending upward from the superior cervical ganglion along the internal carotid artery, joins the abducens nerve at the cavernous sinus. **(E)** An angled scope is used to inspect the regional anatomy in a different anatomical specimen. The extradural portion of the endonasal approach to Meckel's cave has been completed. The dura covering the V2 and V3 branches remains intact. Further drilling has been performed at the anterolateral triangle of the middle fossa (between V2 and V3), whereas the osseus covering of the anteromedial triangle has not been removed. Note the confluence of the vidian nerve and the eustachian tube at the lower portion of the foramen lacerum. **(F)** Close-up view of Meckel's cave. The dura that lies over the trigeminal ganglion has been opened to expose the medial aspect of Meckel's cave. The abducens and carotid nerves are clearly identified and should be preserved during the surgical procedure. Ant.: anterior; Car.: carotid; Cav.: cavernous; Eust.: eustachian; For.: foramen; Fos.: fossa; Gan.: ganglion; ICA: internal carotid artery; Lac.: lacerum; Lat.: lateral; Max.: maxillary; Med.: medial; Mid.: middle; N.: nerve; Pal.: palatine; Paracl.: paraclival; Parasel.: parasellar; Pit.: pituitary; Pter.: pterygoid; Sin.: sinus; SOF: superior orbital fissure; Tr.: triangle; Trig.: trigeminal; Vid.: vidian.

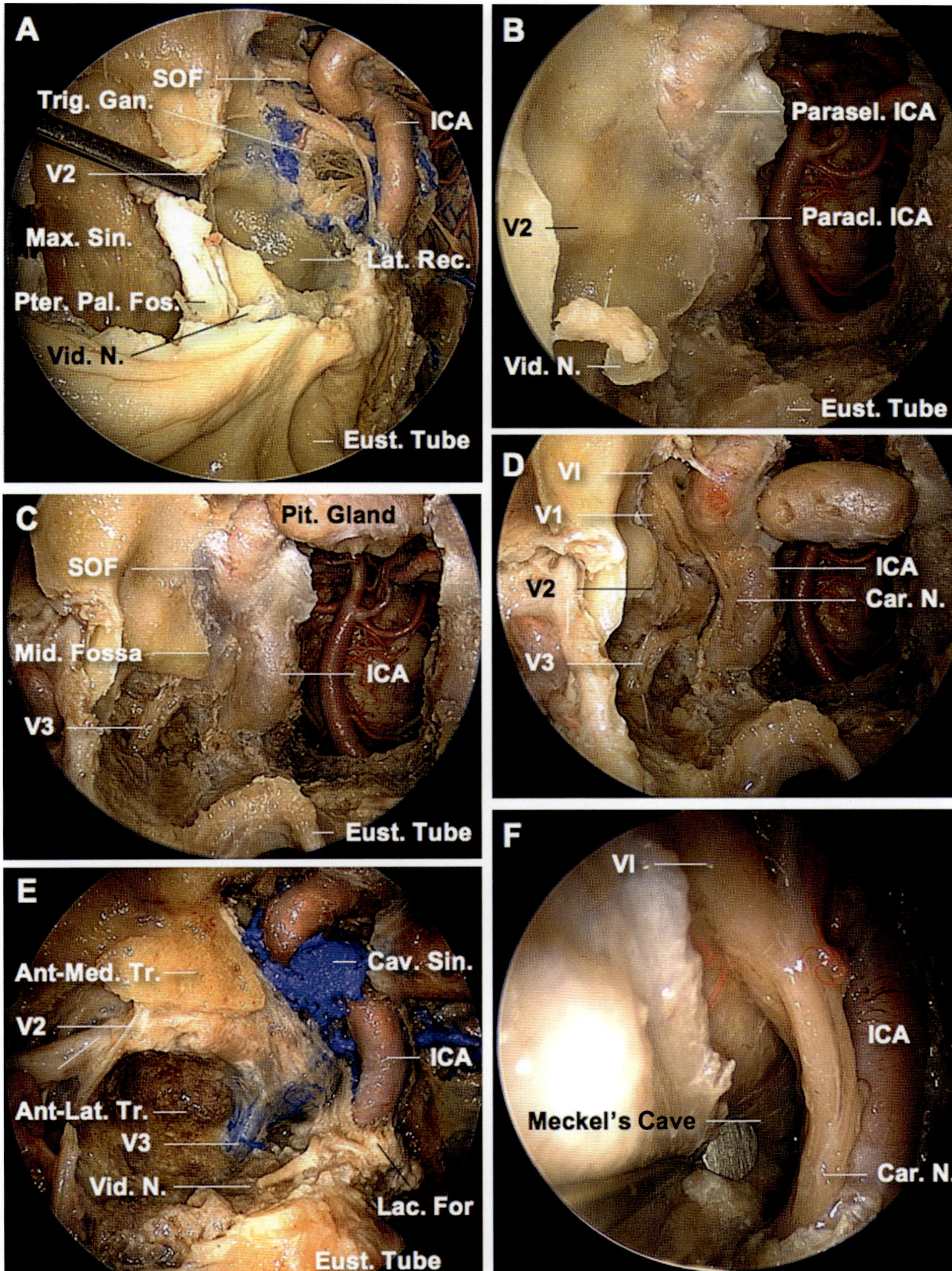
A
SOF
Trig. Gan.
ICA
V2
Max. Sin.
Lat. Rec.
Pter. Pal. Fos.
Vid. N.
Eust. Tube
B
Parasel. ICA
Paracl. ICA
V2
Vid. N.
Eust. Tube
C
Pit. Gland
SOF
Mid. Fossa
ICA
V3
Eust. Tube
D
VI
V1
ICA
V2
Car. N.
V3
E
Cav. Sin.
Ant-Med. Tr.
V2
ICA
Ant-Lat. Tr.
V3
Vid. N.
Lac. For
Eust. Tube
F
VI
ICA
Meckel's Cave
Car. N.

applied to the perinasal and periumbilical areas (in case an autologous fat free graft is necessary for reconstruction).

Approach

The exposure is initiated using a zero-degree rod lens endoscope (Karl Storz Endoscopy; Culver City, CA). We use an irrigating system, in the form of an endoscopic sheath or by manual irrigation with a 60-cc syringe, to clean the endoscope lens and maintain visualization. Lateralization of the inferior turbinates increases the space for the insertion and manipulation of the instruments. In select cases the inferior turbinate can be resected as part of a medial maxillectomy with or without a Denker's extension to provide access to lesions located laterally in the infratemporal fossa. We also resect the middle turbinate that is ipsilateral to the lesion and, hence, the involved Meckel's cave. The contralateral middle turbinate is out-fractured. At this point, we harvest a nasoseptal flap pedicled on the posterior septal arteries of the contralateral side. It is used to reconstruct the skull base defect and cover an exposed internal carotid artery at the end of the procedure.[16] The flap is stored either in the nasopharynx or in the maxillary sinus during extirpative phase of the surgery.

A posterior nasal septectomy in addition to wide bilateral sphenoidotomies and ipsilateral posterior ethmoidectomies complete the nasal corridor. This corridor is then expanded laterally adding a transpterygoid approach ipsilateral to the involved Meckel's cave, creating a direct access to the lateral recess of the sphenoid sinus.[15,17] This requires removal of the posterior wall of the antrum using a 1- to 2-mm Kerrison rongeur, following the sphenopalatine artery and exposing the pterygopalatine fossa (PPF) (**Fig. 36.1A**). Once the exposure is completed, the soft tissue contents of the fossa can be retracted laterally after the palatovaginal and vidian nerves are transected. This provides access to the entire base of the pterygoid plates. In select cases that do not require extreme lateralization of the PPF, the vidian nerve can be preserved. Image guidance may be used to confirm the adequacy of the exposure and to confirm the identification of the vidian canal and foramen rotundum.

The vidian canal and its neurovascular bundle are then followed posteriorly to identify the petrous internal carotid artery (ICA) and the V2 to reach Meckel's cave. Drilling must occur along the inferior hemicircumference of the vidian canal, as the ICA is located along the superior margin.[17–19] The foramen rotundum is identified directly or following the infraorbital nerve proximally. Bone around V2 is removed until it pierces the dura mater of the middle cranial fossa.[15,17–19] If the vidian nerve is preserved, it needs to be completely freed from its canal to allow lateral mobilization and transposition.

Once identified, the bone over the ICA is drilled (**Fig. 36.1B**), thus achieving proximal and distal control of the ICA. Subsequently, the bone lateral to the clival ICA is also drilled out, completely exposing the periosteum of the middle fossa (**Fig. 36.1C–E**).

The dura, or periosteal layer, is opened within the quadrangular space, which is bound by the ICA medially, V2 laterally, and the horizontal petrous ICA inferiorly. Its superior boundary is the abducens nerve that runs obliquely and superiorly. The abducens nerve runs at the level of V1 (the ophthalmic branch of the trigeminal nerve) within the cavernous sinus along its inferior margin as it extends into the superior orbital fissure.[20–22] By maintaining the dissection at the upper level of V2, cranial nerve VI is preserved (**Fig. 36.1F**).[15]

In patients with lesions that infiltrate the gasserian ganglion producing hypesthesia, such as adenoid cystic carcinoma, the trigeminal nerve is sacrificed and the resection of the tumor includes those trigeminal nerve segments that are infiltrated. Intraoperative frozen section analysis is necessary to confirm a complete resection (margins). In patients presenting with benign lesions that occupy the medial inferior compartment of Meckel's cave, the trigeminal nerve is preserved and most often displaced superolaterally against the middle fossa dura. In rare situations the ganglion may be displaced medially and the lesion located laterally. In these cases the anteromedial (between V1 and V2) and anterolateral (between V2 and V3) middle fossa triangles are utilized to reach the lateral aspect of Meckel's cave. Using these landmarks the meningeal layer of the dura can be opened along these corridors to expose the subarachnoid space of the anterior temporal fossa. Electrophysiologic monitoring is used to determine the position of the motor V3 and cranial nerve VI, enabling a safer dissection.

Repair

Dural repair includes a multilayer technique that begins with an inlay graft of collagen matrix (Duragen; Integra Life Sciences Corp., Plainsboro, NJ). The pedicled nasoseptal flap is moved from its stored position to cover the middle fossa and the exposed ICA. It is then secured with oxidized methylcellulose and a synthetic glue (Duraseal). Should the defect be larger than the previously elevated flap, the reconstruction is augmented by the addition of a free mucosal graft from the middle turbinate, a free fat graft from the periumbilical area, or acellular dermis. Expandable sponge packing or the balloon of a Foley catheter is used to buttress the reconstruction and avoid tissue displacement. If a Foley balloon is used, it must be positioned and inflated under direct visualization. Packing is removed 3 to 5 days later. Silicone septal splints are inserted bilaterally to prevent synechia. Broad-spectrum antibiotics are used while the packing is in position.

Complications

In our series, 12.5% (5/40) of patients experienced a new postoperative hypesthesia, which was permanent in 5% (2/40). There were no additional long-term morbidities, cerebrospinal fluid (CSF) leaks, or mortality.[15]

Postoperative Care

In our series, nine of 30 patients (30%) recovered preexistent cranial nerve deficits (cranial nerves III, IV, V, VI) related to lesions in Meckel's cave. We believe that the cavernous sinus decompression led to the recovery of the cranial neuropathies.[15]

Conclusion

Surgical access to Meckel's cave is challenging, as it is guarded by critical structures. No single surgical approach provides unlimited access; therefore, each specific lesion requires a customized approach that takes into account its location and extension, and which pathway would require the smallest amount of manipulation of neurovascular structures. Mastery of multiple corridors (open and endoscopic) is often required, in isolation or combination, for the adequate treatment of lesions located in Meckel's cave and infratemporal fossa; therefore, the operating surgeon must be well versed in multiple if not all approaches. It is critical to offer the approach or combination of approaches that better suits each patient. The endoscopic endonasal approach provides an important anterior, inferior, and medial corridor that in select patients offers adequate exposure to Meckel's cave with low morbidity, thus complementing the standard open approaches and providing the modern skull base surgeon with 360-degree access to Meckel's cave.

References

1. Inoue T, Rhoton AL Jr, Theele D, Barry ME. Surgical approaches to the cavernous sinus: a microsurgical study. Neurosurgery 1990;26:903–932
2. Seoane E, Rhoton AL Jr. Suprameatal extension of the retrosigmoid approach: microsurgical anatomy. Neurosurgery 1999;44:553–560
3. Yasuda A, Campero A, Martins C, Rhoton AL Jr, de Oliveira E, Ribas GC. Microsurgical anatomy and approaches to the cavernous sinus. Neurosurgery 2005;56(1, Suppl):4–27, discussion 4–27
4. Yasuda A, Campero A, Martins C, Rhoton AL Jr, Ribas GC. The medial wall of the cavernous sinus: microsurgical anatomy. Neurosurgery 2004;55:179–189, discussion 189–190
5. Kouyialis AT, Stranjalis G, Papadogiorgakis N, et al. Giant dumbbell-shaped middle cranial fossa trigeminal schwannoma with extension to the infratemporal and posterior fossae. Acta Neurochir (Wien) 2007;149:959–963, discussion 964
6. Verstappen CC, Beems T, Erasmus CE, van Lindert EJ. Dumbbell trigeminal schwannoma in a child: complete removal by a one-stage pterional surgical approach. Childs Nerv Syst 2005;21:1008–1011
7. Yuh WT, Wright DC, Barloon TJ, Schultz DH, Sato Y, Cervantes CA. MR imaging of primary tumors of trigeminal nerve and Meckel's cave. AJR Am J Roentgenol 1988;151:577–582
8. Dolan EJ, Schwartz ML, Lewis AJ, Kassel EE, Cooper PW. Adenoid cystic carcinoma: an unusual neurosurgical entity. Can J Neurol Sci 1985;12:65–68
9. Fowler BZ, Crocker IR, Johnstone PA. Perineural spread of cutaneous malignancy to the brain: a review of the literature and five patients treated with stereotactic radiotherapy. Cancer 2005;103:2143–2153
10. Ginsberg LE, DeMonte F. Imaging of perineural tumor spread from palatal carcinoma. AJNR Am J Neuroradiol 1998;19:1417–1422
11. Zhu JJ, Padillo O, Duff J, Hsi BL, Fletcher JA, Querfurth H. Cavernous sinus and leptomeningeal metastases arising from a squamous cell carcinoma of the face: case report. Neurosurgery 2004;54:492–498, discussion 498–499
12. Taha JM, Tew JM Jr, van Loveren HR, Keller JT, el-Kalliny M. Comparison of conventional and skull base surgical approaches for the excision of trigeminal neurinomas. J Neurosurg 1995;82:719–725
13. Samii M, Carvalho GA, Tatagiba M, Matthies C. Surgical management of meningiomas originating in Meckel's cave. Neurosurgery 1997;41:767–774, discussion 774–775
14. Samii M, Tatagiba M, Carvalho GA. Retrosigmoid intradural suprameatal approach to Meckel's cave and the middle fossa: surgical technique and outcome. J Neurosurg 2000;92:235–241
15. Kassam AB, Prevedello DM, Carrau RL, et al. The front door to Meckel's cave: an anteromedial corridor via expanded endoscopic endonasal approach- technical considerations and clinical series. Neurosurgery 2009;64(3, Suppl):71–82, discussion 82–83
16. Hadad G, Bassagasteguy L, Carrau RL, et al. A novel reconstructive technique after endoscopic expanded endonasal approaches: vascular pedicle nasoseptal flap. Laryngoscope 2006;116:1882–1886
17. Vescan AD, Snyderman CH, Carrau RL, et al. Vidian canal: analysis and relationship to the internal carotid artery. Laryngoscope 2007;117:1338–1342
18. Fortes FS, Sennes LU, Carrau RL, et al. Endoscopic anatomy of the pterygopalatine fossa and the transpterygoid approach: development of a surgical instruction model. Laryngoscope 2008;118:44–49
19. Kassam AB, Vescan AD, Carrau RL, et al. Expanded endonasal approach: vidian canal as a landmark to the petrous internal carotid artery. J Neurosurg 2008;108:177–183
20. Iaconetta G, Fusco M, Cavallo LM, Cappabianca P, Samii M, Tschabitscher M. The abducens nerve: microanatomic and endoscopic study. Neurosurgery 2007;61(3, Suppl):7–14, discussion 14
21. Cavallo LM, Cappabianca P, Galzio R, Iaconetta G, de Divitiis E, Tschabitscher M. Endoscopic transnasal approach to the cavernous sinus versus transcranial route: anatomic study. Neurosurgery 2005;56(2, Suppl):379–389, discussion 379–389
22. Alfieri A, Jho HD. Endoscopic endonasal approaches to the cavernous sinus: surgical approaches. Neurosurgery 2001;49:354–360, discussion 360–362

37 How to Manage Lateral Sphenoid Cerebrospinal Fluid Leaks

Emiro E. Caicedo, Alfredo Herrera, Ricardo L. Carrau, Carl H. Snyderman, Amin B. Kassam, Daniel M. Prevedello, Paul A. Gardner, Juan C. Fernandez-Miranda, and Victor Morera

Tips and Pearls

- The lateral recess of the sphenoid sinus represents an extension of the pneumatization of the sphenoid sinus into the base of the pterygoid plates and may extend from the pterygoid canal to areas lateral to the foramen rotundum (i.e., sphenoid wing) (**Fig. 37.1**).[1]
- Cerebrospinal fluid (CSF) leaks at the lateral recess of the sphenoid sinus have been associated with arachnoid granulations of the middle cranial fossa, patent craniopharyngeal (Sternberg's) canal, and benign ventricular hypertension and trauma.[2,3]
- Preoperative evaluation includes a complete history, physical examination with emphasis on cranial nerve function, and imaging studies including high-resolution computed tomography (CT) and contrast-enhanced magnetic resonance imaging (MRI) for those patients presenting with spontaneous leaks or meningoencephaloceles (**Fig. 37.2**).
- Understanding the endoscopic anatomy of the pterygopalatine fossa and lateral recess of the sphenoid is critical to approach and repair these CSF leaks. The transantral-transpterygoid approach provides a wide and direct approach to the lateral recess of the sphenoid sinus with less morbidity than a transcranial or transfacial approach (**Fig. 37.3**).[4]
- The success rate for endoscopic repair of CSF leaks is reported to be 85 to 100%. A significant subpopulation of patients remains at high risk for failure after an adequate repair when high ventricular pressure is present.[5]
- Patients at risk for high ventricular pressure include those with a subarachnoid hemorrhage secondary to trauma or hemorrhagic stroke, those with intracranial tumors, and those with spontaneous CSF leaks.[5]

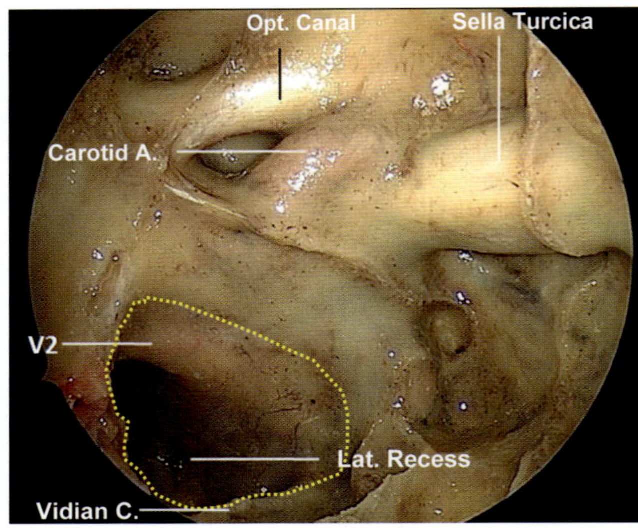

Fig. 37.1 Right sphenoid sinus lateral recess. The dotted line marks the entrance to the right lateral recess of the sphenoid sinus, which is bounded by the vidian canal and V2. A.: artery; C.: canal; Lat.: lateral; Opt.: optical.

Introduction

Pneumatization of the sphenoid sinus into the pterygoid process creates the lateral sphenoid recess. Pathologies of the lateral sphenoid recess include space-occupying lesions of a benign or malignant nature as well as cerebrospinal fluid (CSF) leaks and meningoencephaloceles.[6,7] CSF leaks of the lateral sphenoid recess are both a diagnostic and a therapeutic challenge. Traditional transseptal or transethmoidal approaches to the sphenoid sinus do not provide direct access to the lateral recess of the sphenoid. This limitation has been overcome with the use of endoscopic techniques that create a corridor through the pterygopalatine fossa, such as the endoscopic transpterygoid approach that can access lesions of the lateral sphenoid recess safely and efficiently.[6] This chapter describes the pearls and pitfalls to consider when treating CSF leaks and other lesions at the lateral recess of the sphenoid sinus.

Patient Selection

Indications for an endoscopic transpterygoid approach include lesions located in the lateral sphenoid recess, pterygopalatine fossa, and infratemporal skull base (base of the middle cranial fossa). It is important to identify the extension of the disease preoperatively by means of physical examination, contrast-enhanced high-resolution computed tomogra-

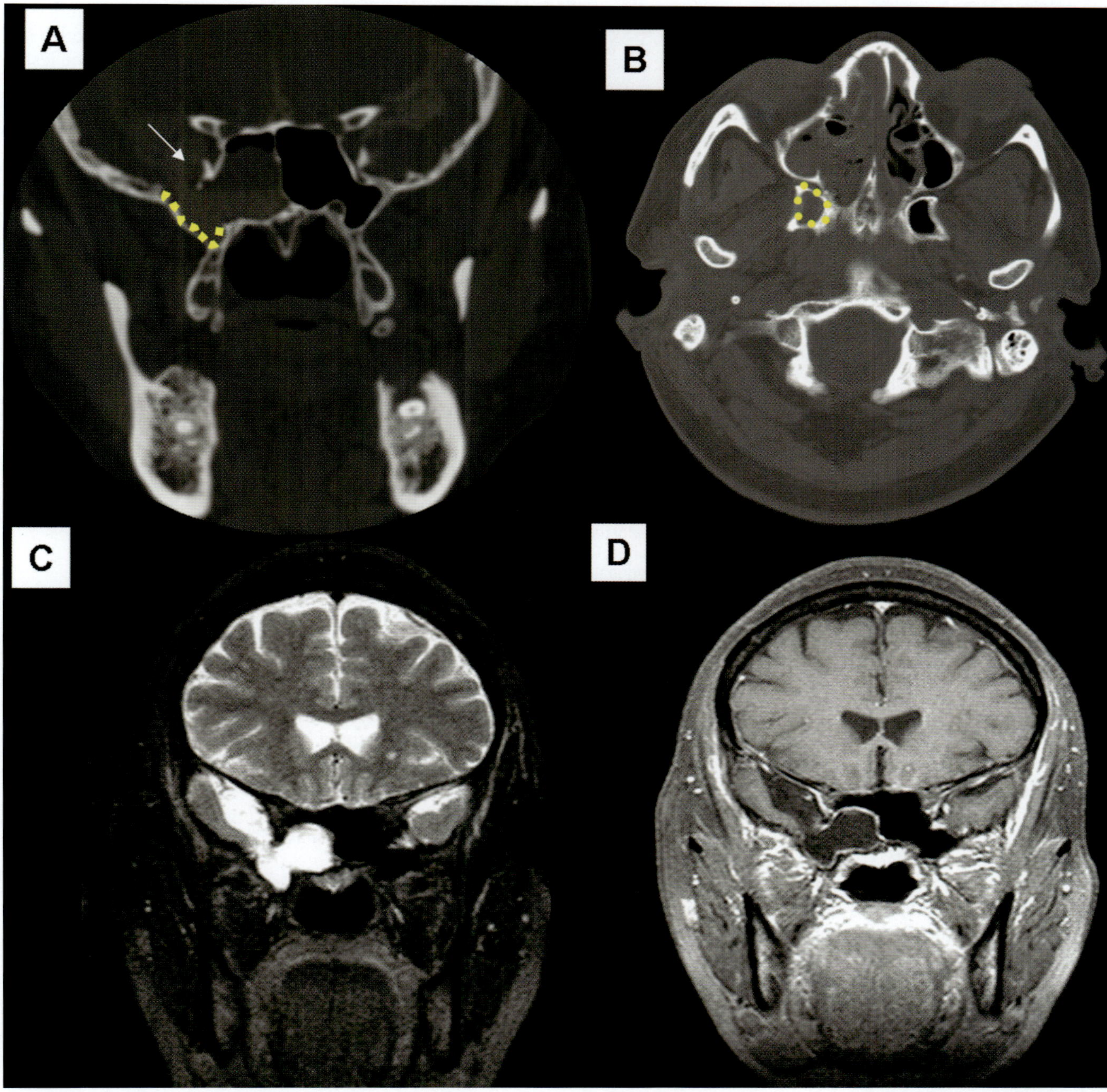

Fig. 37.2 Imaging studies of the lateral sphenoid recess. **(A)** Coronal high-resolution computed tomography (CT) showing a bony defect indicated by the arrowhead at the lateral recess of the sphenoid sinus (*yellow dotted line*). **(B)** Axial high-resolution CT showing the lateral recess of the sphenoid sinus (*yellow dotted line*). The opposite lateral recess of the sphenoid sinus is normal. **(C)** T2-weighted magnetic resonance imaging (MRI) showing hyperintense signal in the lateral recess of the sphenoid sinus compatible with cerebrospinal fluid (CSF). **(D)** T1-weighted MRI with fat suppression showing a low-density lesion in the lateral recess of the sphenoid sinus.

phy (CT) and magnetic resonance imaging (MRI).[6] When treating patients with CSF leaks, it is important to differentiate CSF leak from other sources of rhinorrhea, locating the specific site of the leak and ruling out the presence of increased intracranial pressure. β_2-transferrin and to even a greater extent β-trace protein are reliable chemical markers for the presence of CSF.[5]

The endoscopic transpterygoid approach addresses lesions that extend to the pterygomaxillary fissure and medial aspect of the middle cranial fossa and infratemporal fossa. An extended lateral reach is possible with the use of an endoscopic Denker's procedure. This procedure includes an endoscopic medial maxillectomy and the removal of the inferior pyriform aperture and medial maxillary buttress. It is

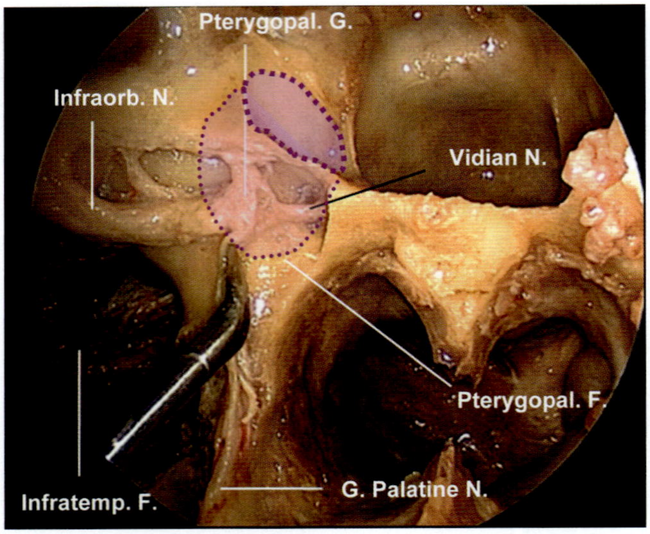

Fig. 37.3 Pterygopalatine fossa contents and location of the lateral recess of the sphenoid. Anatomical dissection shows the contents of the pterygopalatine fossa. The thinner dotted line shows the location of the lateral recess of the sphenoid sinus. The thicker dotted line shows the entrance to the lateral recess of the sphenoid sinus. F.: fossa; G.: ganglion, great; Infraorb.: infraorbital; N.: nerve; Pterygopal.: pterygopalatine.

important to have a clear understanding regarding the extension of the lesion (**Fig. 37.4**).

Preoperative Planning

Preoperative antibiotic prophylaxis providing coverage against flora of the upper aerodigestive tract and with good blood–brain barrier penetration is administered 1 to 2 hours before surgery and continued for 48 hours after surgery. Patients are placed in a supine position with the neck slightly turned to the right and slightly tilted to the left. In our practice we use stereotactic image guidance for every case, although it is not critical for obtaining an adequate outcome. If the lesion is intimately related to the adjacent neurovascular structures, the patient is monitored intraoperatively using somatosensory evoked potentials and electromyography of the extraocular muscles as indicated. Patients who present such a lesion should also be evaluated with a CT angiography. High-resolution computed tomography (HRCT) is the preferred initial imaging study to help identify the site of the leak or the extent of a lesion. In addition, HRCT can be used in conjunction with intrathecal injection of contrast to identify the CSF leak (CT cysternography) (**Fig. 37.5**). However, identification of CSF leaks with contrast-enhanced HRCT requires the presence of an active CSF leak.

Surgical Technique

- The nasal cavity is decongested with oxymetazoline 0.5% solution and the middle meatus is injected with lidocaine 1% with epinephrine 1:100,000.
- Uncinectomy
- Maxillary antrostomy extended posteriorly to the level of the posterior wall of the maxillary sinus and inferiorly to the inferior turbinate (**Fig. 37.6**)
- Anterior and posterior ethmoidectomy with identification of the skull base
- Bilateral wide sphenoidotomy
- Posterior septectomy to provide binarial access (the procedure may be done using an ipsilateral corridor but we prefer a binarial as we also advocate a vascularized pedicled nasoseptal flap)
- Identify the sphenopalatine foramen posterior to the crista ethmoidalis.
- Remove posterior wall of maxillary sinus using Kerrison rongeurs, angulated forceps, or a drill exposing the superior pterygopalatine fossa.

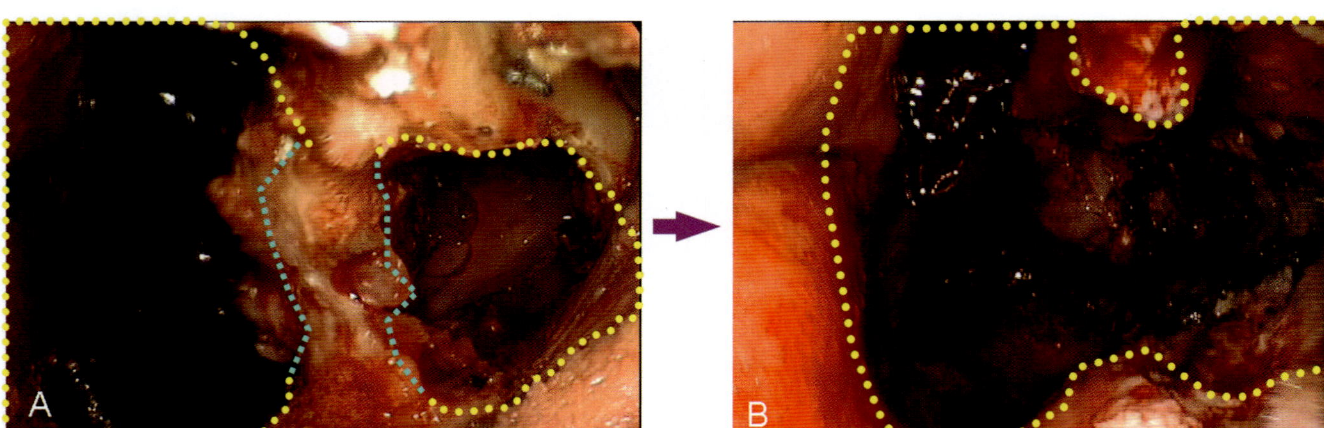

Fig. 37.4 Endoscopic Denker's procedure. **(A)** Blue dotted line shows the medial maxillary wall. **(B)** Panoramic view after removing the medial maxillary wall. Yellow dotted line shows the connected nasal cavity with the maxillary sinus. Notice the wide lateral exposure obtained with this approach.

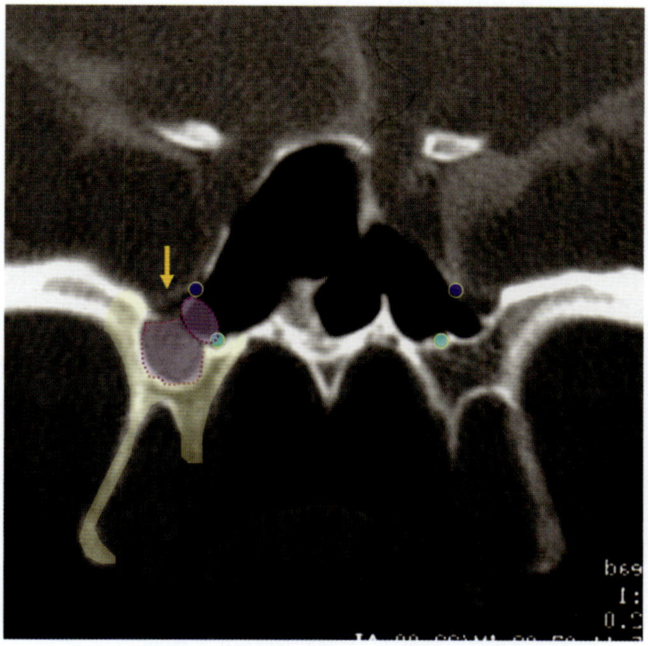

Fig. 37.5 Computed tomography cisternography. High-resolution CT cisternography shows a CSF fistula (*arrow*) at the lateral recess of the sphenoid sinus (red dotted line). The vidian nerve (*green dot*) and V2 (*blue dot*) are depicted here.

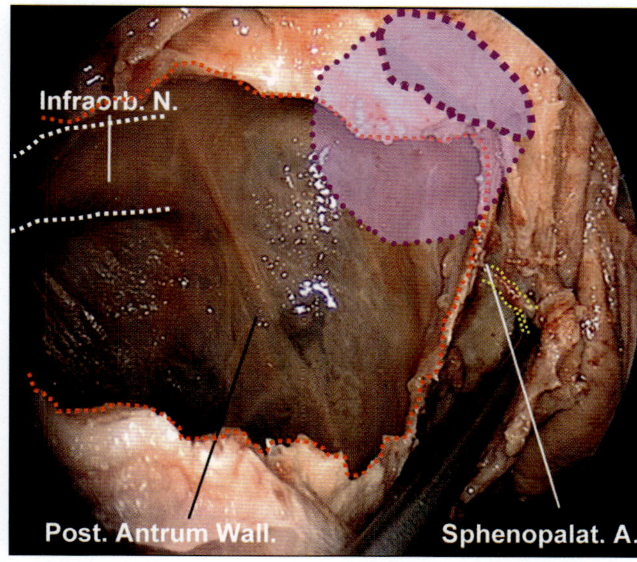

Fig. 37.6 Exposure of posterior maxillary wall. Wide maxillary antrostomy shown by the red dotted line and sphenopalatine artery shown by the yellow dotted line are depicted here. The posterior wall of the maxillary sinus is clearly seen as well as the infraorbital nerve (*white dotted line*). The location of the lateral recess of the sphenoid sinus is shown as the purple thin dotted line. The thicker dotted line represents the entrance to the lateral recess of the sphenoid sinus. Post.: posterior; Sphenopalat.: sphenopalatine.

- Coagulate and divide the posterior nasal artery.
- Identify the vidian nerve, sphenopalatine ganglion, descending palatine nerve, and V2 (**Fig. 37.7**)
- Elevate the soft tissue from the base of the pterygoid plates in a medial to lateral and superior to inferior direction, preserving the above-mentioned structures.
- At this point the lateral recess of the sphenoid is widely exposed.
- An endoscopic Denker's increases the lateral angle of the approach and allows endoscopic access to the most lateral aspect of the infratemporal and middle cranial fossa.
- Extend the sphenoidotomy toward the pterygopalatine fossa, above the vidian nerve and artery.
- CSF leak repair is accomplished using a multilayer technique with an inlay collagen matrix. Then we use an onlay free mucosal graft or vascularized nasoseptal or inferior turbinate flap. As previously stated, we prefer the pedicled nasoseptal flap.
- Removal of space-occupying lesions within the lateral sphenoid recess and base of the middle cranial fossa is accomplished using a bimanual technique.

Complications

Complications of the transpterygoid approach can be classified as sinonasal, neural, or vascular. Sinonasal complications include sinusitis, chronic rhinitis, crusting, nasal synechiae, nasal obstruction, epistaxis, and loss of olfaction. These complications are relatively minor but can impact the patient's quality of life substantially. Neural complications include symptoms related to the loss of vidian nerve function. The patients complain of diminished tearing during cold or windy weather and emotional situations. When dissecting the pterygopalatine fossa, the descending palatine nerve can be injured, resulting in palatal hypoesthesia.[8] In addition, the

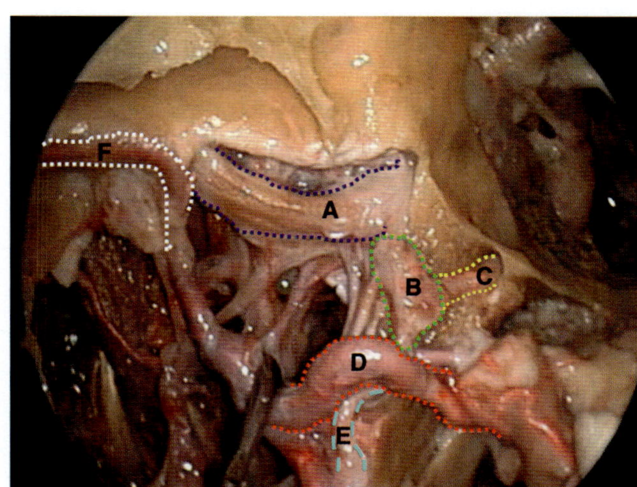

Fig. 37.7 Pterygopalatine fossa. A, V2 (*blue dotted line*) coming out from the foramen rotundum; B, green-yellow dotted line shows the pterygopalatine ganglion; C, yellow dotted line shows the vidian nerve; D, red dotted line shows the sphenopalatine artery; E, light blue dotted line shows the great palatine nerve; F, white dotted line showing the infraorbital artery.

infraorbital nerve and V2 are at risk of injury when dissecting the pterygopalatine fossa and the region of the foramen rotundum.[9]

Vascular complications include injury to the carotid artery and internal maxillary artery. These complications are best avoided if the surgeon possesses precise knowledge of the anatomy in this region. The vidian artery is a very reliable landmark to identify the location of the petrous carotid artery and the second genu. Injury to the internal maxillary artery is controlled with bipolar cautery or Ligaclips.

Postoperative Management

The patient is admitted to the intensive care unit or stepdown setting, and serial neurologic examinations are performed for the first 24 hours postoperatively. A head CT is obtained postoperatively to search for intracranial complications. Nasal packing is removed 5 to 7 days after a CSF leak repair. We favor the use of perioperative prophylactic antibiotics during CSF leak repair, and they are continued until the nasal packing is removed. After the nasal packing is removed, the patient initiates normal saline solution nasal sprays and irrigations. The patient is instructed to avoid strenuous activities, nose blowing, bending, and lifting any weight for 4 to 6 weeks. Other measures include bed rest, stool softeners, head of bed elevation to 30 to 45 degrees, and instructing patients to keep the mouth open when sneezing. If a pedicled nasal-septal flap was used for reconstruction, septal splints are maintained for 3 weeks; otherwise, splints are removed 1 week postoperatively. Endoscopic debridement of crusts is performed in the office until healing is complete. A lumbar drain is used only on those patients suspected of having high-pressure hydrocephalus (HPH), which is defined as sustained or intermittent CSF pressure of over 20 H_2O. If HPH is suspected, a lumbar drain is placed at the time of the CSF repair.[5] Three to 5 days after surgery the lumbar drain is clamped. If no CSF leak is identified in the next 24 hours, the lumbar drain is removed; 24 to 48 hours later, a lumbar puncture is performed to measure CSF opening pressure. If the opening pressure is elevated, a ventriculoperitoneal shunt is recommended. If the CSF opening pressure is normal, the patient is discharged and a head CT is obtained 6 weeks after surgery to search for ventriculomegalia and transependymal edema, which are signs of HPH. Patients with CSF leak without risk factors for HPH are repaired endoscopically without the use of a lumbar drain.[5]

Conclusion

The pterygopalatine fossa approach provides a safe, wide, and direct approach to the lateral recess of the sphenoid. The excellent visualization and space provided by this approach is advantageous in the treatment of CSF leaks or when dealing with space-occupying lesions confined to this area. The morbidity of the transpterygoid approach is lower than that of transcranial or transfacial approaches. Management of lesions located in the lateral sphenoid recess requires a team familiar with the challenging anatomy of this region.

References

1. Fortes FS, Sennes LU, Carrau RL, et al. Endoscopic anatomy of the pterygopalatine fossa and the transpterygoid approach: development of a surgical instruction model. Laryngoscope 2008;118:44–49
2. Castelnuovo P, Dallan I, Pistochini A, Battaglia P, Locatelli D, Bignami M. Endonasal endoscopic repair of Sternberg's canal cerebrospinal fluid leaks. Laryngoscope 2007;117:345–349
3. Schick B, Brors D, Prescher A. Sternberg's canal—cause of congenital sphenoidal meningocele. Eur Arch Otorhinolaryngol 2000;257:430–432
4. Tosun F, Carrau RL, Snyderman CH, Kassam A, Celin S, Schaitkin B. Endonasal endoscopic repair of cerebrospinal fluid leaks of the sphenoid sinus. Arch Otolaryngol Head Neck Surg 2003;129:576–580
5. Carrau RL, Snyderman CH, Kassam AB. The management of cerebrospinal fluid leaks in patients at risk for high-pressure hydrocephalus. Laryngoscope 2005;115:205–212
6. Al-Nashar IS, Carrau RL, Herrera A, Snyderman CH. Endoscopic transnasal transpterygopalatine fossa approach to the lateral recess of the sphenoid sinus. Laryngoscope 2004;114:528–532
7. Lai SY, Kennedy DW, Bolger WE. Sphenoid encephaloceles: disease management and identification of lesions within the lateral recess of the sphenoid sinus. Laryngoscope 2002;112:1800–1805
8. Tami TA. Surgical management of lesions of the sphenoid lateral recess. Am J Rhinol 2006;20:412–416
9. Bolger WE. Endoscopic transpterygoid approach to the lateral sphenoid recess: surgical approach and clinical experience. Otolaryngol Head Neck Surg 2005;133:20–26

X Tips and Pearls in Endoscopic Surgery for Malignancies

38 Endonasal Surgery of Malignancies of the Sinus and Skull Base

Paolo Castelnuovo, Maurizio Bignami, Paolo Battaglia, Andrea Bolzoni Villaret, and Piero Nicolai

Tips and Pearls

- Endoscopic endonasal surgery for sinonasal and adjacent skull base malignancies is a relatively recent advance, and its results need to be validated by statistically comparing them with those of the standard anterior craniofacial resection.
- A multidisciplinary skull base team is mandatory.
- The main advantages include magnified visualization of the site of origin of the tumor after central debulking, a very limited morbidity, and the possibility of avoiding any brain retraction related to external craniotomy.
- The contraindications are tumors involving the brain, orbit, frontal sinus, maxillary sinus (except the medial wall), lacrimal system, or palate.
- Careful preoperative imaging evaluation is crucial to properly select the surgical approach.
- Piecemeal resection is very often required.
- Tumor removal is planned as a step-by-step procedure until achieving free surgical margins; multiple frozen sections are mandatory.
- Experience in skull base reconstruction and advanced instrumentation are prerequisites for performing this surgery.

Introduction

The application of endoscopic surgery for the management of sinonasal malignancies emerged in the last 10 years as a valid and safe alternative to the gold standard represented by anterior craniofacial resection (ACFR).[1–6] This application was made by four factors: the creation of a multidisciplinary skull base team of an otolaryngologist and a neurosurgeons, the experience acquired with endoscopic procedures in the treatment of benign lesions and skull base defects, technical improvements in surgery and radiology, and the acceptance of piecemeal resection.

Indication and Advantages

Indications for an endoscopic endonasal approach (EEA) have been modified by our group over a 10-year period.[6] Up to 2003, only patients with limited nasoethmoidal lesions that did not infiltrate the external bony boundaries of the ethmoid (i.e., lamina papyracea, cribriform plate, ethmoid roof), with minimal extension into the maxillary or frontal sinus, were considered eligible for EEA. From 2004, the indications have been extended to include advanced lesions in contact with or minimally infiltrating the dura. In the last 2 years, selected intradural lesions without brain infiltration also have been treated.[7]

The advantages of endoscopic techniques include avoidance of facial incisions and osteotomies, short hospitalization, a very limited morbidity, and the possibility of avoiding any brain retraction. The major advantage lies in the outstanding magnified visualization of the site of origin as well as of the areas involved by the tumor. The use of angled telescopes permits viewing behind the corner, providing better visualization of the structures involved by the tumor.

Contraindications

An EEA is contraindicated if there is a lateral extension over the orbital roof, or extensive involvement of the brain; in these situations, a cranioendoscopic or a standard ACFR is performed. Other contraindications for EEA are extensive lacrimal pathway infiltration, involvement of the anterior wall and lateral portion of the frontal sinus, infiltration of the bony walls of the maxillary sinus with the exception of the medial one, infiltration of the hard palate, and erosion of the nasal bones.

Diagnostic Workup

The preoperative diagnostic workup includes endoscopic examination of the nasal cavity to evaluate the borders and the features of the lesion as well as the sinonasal and septal anatomical variations, and magnetic resonance imaging (MRI) with gadolinium enhancement, except with uncooperative patients, in which case computed tomography (CT) with contrast medium is performed instead. MRI with gadolinium enhancement is preferable to CT because it provides better delineation of the interface between the tumor and the surrounding soft tissues (periorbita, orbital content, dura).

In very aggressive histologies (e.g., malignant melanoma, malignant schwannoma, neuroendocrine carcinoma, undifferentiated carcinoma) a positron emission tomography (PET)-CT is included in the preoperative assessment to evaluate the presence of systemic dissemination of the disease. All patients should be informed that it might be necessary to switch intraoperatively to a transfacial or transcranial approach in case any unexpected contraindication is found during the surgery.

Surgery

Instrumentation

The following instrumentation is required for the endoscopic approach to sinonasal malignancies of the sinonasal tract and the anterior skull base: high-quality 0- and 45-degree endoscopes; video equipment (camera and monitors); a recording system; long-handle endoscopic bipolar forceps; curved and double-curved cutting instruments; diode laser supports; long stem and curved drills; long dissection instruments and dural reconstruction instruments; and intranasal vascular Doppler. The use of a microdebrider is strongly recommended. Cavitron and ENT navigation systems can be helpful.

Operative Setup

The patient is placed in a supine, 10- to 20-degree reverse-Trendelenburg position, with the head slightly hyperextended. The surgeon stands on the right side of the patient and the assistant stands on the left side. The nurse stands on the right of the operating surgeon. The anesthesiologist stands on the patient's left side with the anesthesiology equipment, next to the assistant. Hypotensive general anesthesia is required.[4] The nasal cavity is decongested with topical application of oxymetazoline chlorohydrate (10 mL), mixed with oxybuprocaine (10 mL) and adrenaline (1 mL).

Approach

The approach consists of six main steps (**Fig. 38.1**):

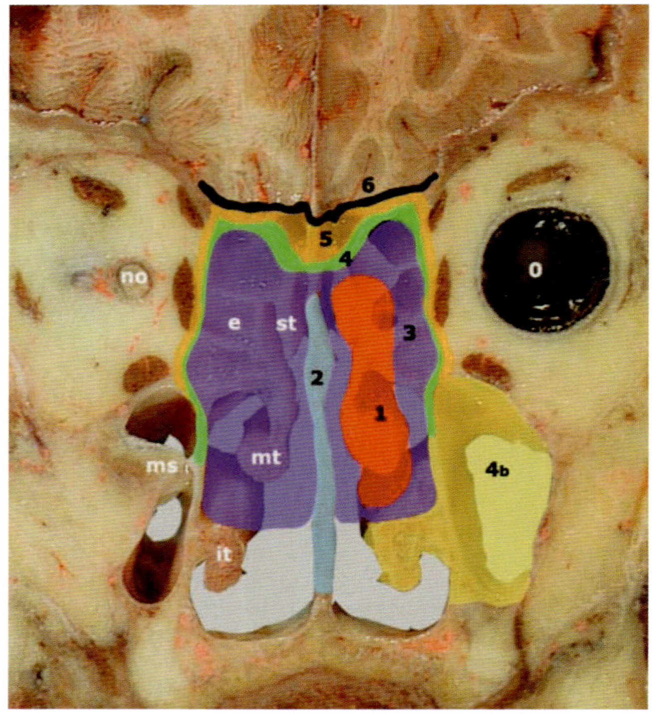

Fig. 38.1 The six main steps of the endoscopic endonasal approach (EEA) are presented schematically on a cadaveric specimen: 1, tumor debulking; 2, removal of the septum; 3, Draf III, with centripetal removal of the ethmoidosphenoidal "box"; 4, removal of bone/cartilage in contact with the tumor; 5, removal of connective tissue around the tumor; 6, skull base duraplasty. E: ethmoid; it.:inferior turbinate; ms.: maxillary sinus; mt.: middle turbinate; no.: optic nerve; o: orbit; st.: superior turbinate.

1. The tumor is debulked through cutting instruments, powered instruments (microdebrider or ultrasonic aspiration, high-speed burrs), or angled and malleable instruments, to clearly identify the possible site of origin of the lesion. En-bloc resection can be achieved only in small tumors.
2. The nasal branch of the sphenopalatine artery is cauterized by bipolar instrumentation. The vomer is detached from the sphenoidal rostrum using an intranasal drill, and a large sphenoidotomy is performed. A diode laser is used to remove the posterior two thirds of the septum. These first two steps widen the surgical field and enable both surgeons to work together through both nostrils. Using aspirators and grasping instruments, the second operating surgeon can help in controlling bleeding as well.
3. A Draf III frontal sinusotomy is performed, a subperiosteal dissection of the nasoethmoidosphenoidal complex (mono- or bilateral) is performed, and the surgical specimen is removed either transnasally or transorally. If necessary, this step can include medial maxillectomy and resection of the nasolacrimal duct. Multiple biopsies from the surgical margins are routinely sent to the laboratory for frozen sections.
4. The lamina papyracea and the ethmoid roof, including the cribriform plate, need to be removed only when the lesions involve their mucosal covering.
5. Radiologic or intraoperative findings of any suspicious contact or infiltration of the dura or periorbita require their resection and frozen sections at this site to evaluate margins. A diagnosis of olfactory neuroblastoma (ONB) also requires dura and olfactory bulb resection due to its high propensity to spread along the olfactory phyla. It is better to dissect the dura from the underlying ethmoidal roof with dedicated instrumentation before opening the dura. The dissection of the epidural space is a key point in EEA.
6. Duraplasty with a "three-layer" technique is preferably performed using autologous material: fascia lata or an

iliotibial tract both for the intradural and intracranial extradural layers (underlay) and for the extracranial layer (overlay), stabilized with fat tissue and fibrin glue. No bone or cartilage graft is used to repair the skull base to avoid radionecrosis and infection after postoperative radiotherapy. If possible, a vascularized septal flap pedicled on the nasal branch of the sphenopalatine artery[8,9] can be used as a third layer. Our group usually does not utilize this flap because of the frequent involvement by the tumor of the septum.

Postoperative Care

Nasal packing is removed on the second postoperative day, and nasal cavities are endoscopically suctioned. The patient is instructed to perform nasal irrigations with 0.9% saline solution and topic antibiotics. If dural repair was performed, the patient must avoid nose blowing, sneezing with a closed mouth, and physical efforts at least for 1 month after surgery.

The follow-up includes monthly endoscopic examinations and MRI every 4 months during the first year; endoscopic examination and MRI every 3 and 6 months, respectively, during the second year; and both examinations at 6-month intervals after the second year.

Results

Our group treated 190 patients with EEA from 1996 to 2008 (**Fig. 38.2**). The 5-year overall, disease-specific, and recurrence-free survival rates were 88.1%, 83.9%, and 82.1%, respectively (unpublished data).

Complications

Complications that can occur in the management of sinonasal tumors can be divided into five main groups: systemic (e.g., sepsis), central nervous system (meningitis, brain

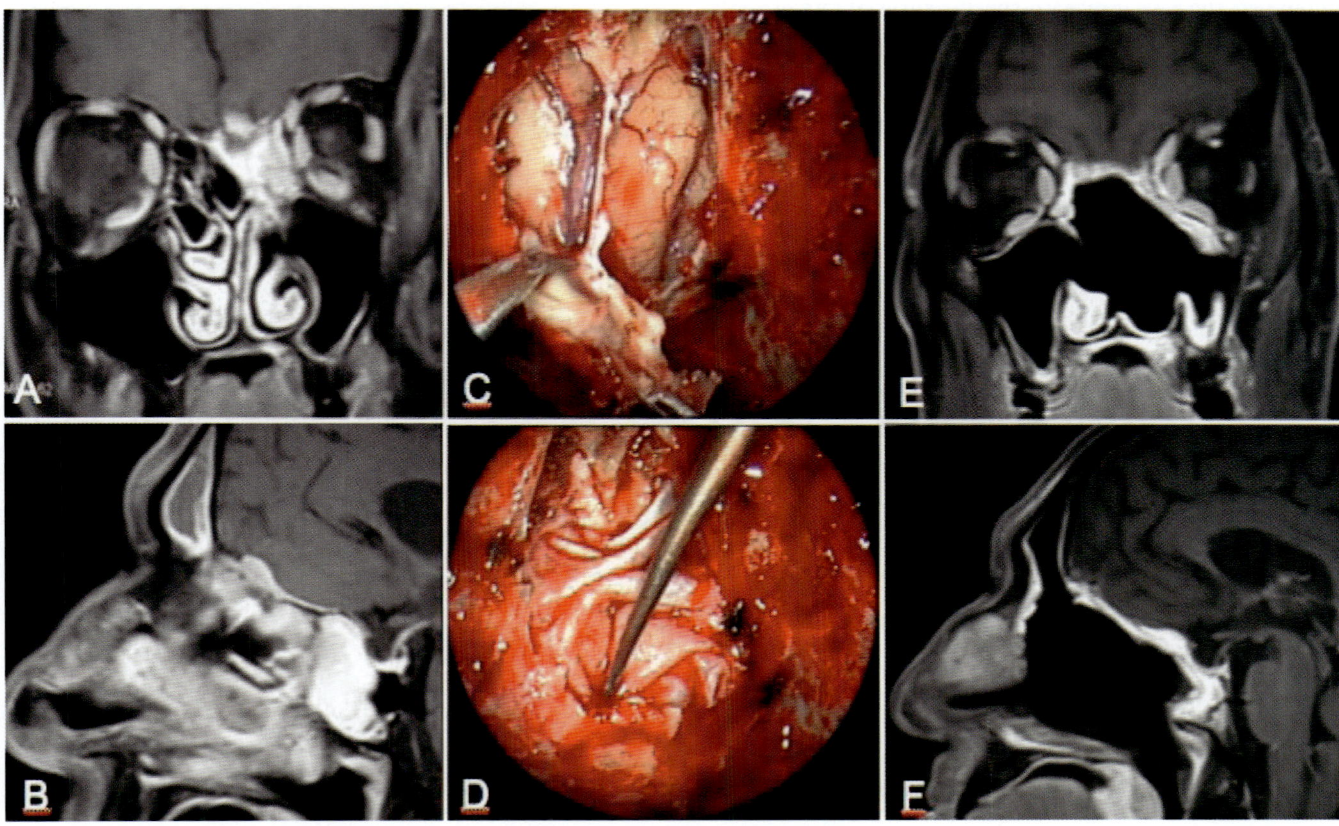

Fig. 38.2 **(A)** Enhanced T1-weighted magnetic resonance imaging (MRI) coronal section demonstrates a left nasoethmoidal lesion (esthesioneuroblastoma) with an intradural extension through the ethmoidal roof. The right olfactory bulb is involved. **(B)** Enhanced T1-weighted MRI, sagittal section. The lesion involves the olfactory bulb without an invasion of the brain parenchyma above. **(C)** Intraoperative endoscopic image shows removal of the dura and the olfactory bulb bilaterally, with the lesion involving these structures. **(D)** Intraoperative endoscopic image shows skull base reconstruction with the iliotibial tract (intradural layer). **(E)** Enhanced T1-weighted MRI, coronal section, 1 year after surgery. The lesion is totally removed. **(F)** Enhanced T1-weighted MRI, sagittal section, 1 year after surgery. The Draf III frontal sinusotomy appears well calibrated, with no evidence of disease or any skull base defects.

abscess, pneumocephalus, cranial nerves injuries, etc.), orbital (orbital hematoma, pneumorbit, epiphora, etc.) vascular (bleeding from internal carotid artery, nasal bleeding after nasal packing removal), and skull base defects after duraplasty. In our series overall postoperative complications occurred in 6.9% of patients. The most frequent was a cerebrospinal fluid (CSF) leak in 3.1%.

Conclusion

The EEA for malignancies of the sinonasal tract should be performed only in specialized centers by surgeons with extensive experience in advanced endonasal procedures. It requires long surgical training, including extensive experience in anatomical dissection and performing a large number of endoscopic operations (treatment of inflammatory diseases and benign tumors). Another requirement is multidisciplinary skull base teams consisting of otorhinolaryngologists, neurosurgeons, neuroradiologists, pathologists, and anesthesiologists.

Even though our series, reported above, suffers from some common limitations (e.g., histologic heterogeneity, limited follow-up), the 5-year disease-specific survival rate of 83.9% for EEA suggests that endoscopic surgery may be an effective alternative to standard approaches in the management of malignancies of the sinonasal tract. This technique is safe and has a low complication rate. Experience is needed to improve the techniques of skull base reconstruction and to reduce the occurrence of CSF leak, which is the major complication in our series. A longer follow-up and a larger number of patients are needed to definitively validate EEA.

References

1. Stammberger H, Anderhuber W, Walch C, Papaefthymiou G. Possibilities and limitations of endoscopic management of nasal and paranasal sinus malignancies. Acta Otorhinolaryngol Belg 1999;53:199–205
2. Goffart Y, Jorissen M, Daele J, et al. Minimally invasive endoscopic management of malignant sinonasal tumours. Acta Otorhinolaryngol Belg 2000;54:221–232
3. Dave SP, Bared A, Casiano RR. Surgical outcomes and safety of transnasal endoscopic resection for anterior skull tumors. Otolaryngol Head Neck Surg 2007;136:920–927
4. Castelnuovo P, Battaglia P, Locatelli D, et al. Endonasal micro-endoscopic treatment of the malignant tumors of paranasal sinuses and anterior skull base. Op Tech Otolaryngol 2006;17:152–167
5. Nicolai P, Castelnuovo P, Lombardi D, et al. Role of endoscopic surgery in the management of selected malignant epithelial neoplasms of the naso-ethmoidal complex. Head Neck 2007;29:1075–1082
6. Nicolai P, Battaglia P, Bignami M, et al. Endoscopic surgery for malignant tumors of the sinonasal tract and adjacent skull base: a 10-year experience. Am J Rhinol 2008;22:308–316
7. Villaret AB, Yakirevitch A, Bizzoni A, et al. Endoscopic transnasal craniectomy in the management of selected sinonasal malignancies. Am J Rhinol Allergy 2010;24:60–65
8. Carrau R, Kassam A, Snyderman C, Duvvuri U, Mintz A, Gardner P. Endoscopic transnasal anterior skull base resection for the management of sinonasal malignancies. Op Tech Otolaryngol 2006;17:102–110
9. Hadad G, Bassagasteguy L, Carrau RL, et al. A novel reconstructive technique after endoscopic expanded endonasal approaches: vascular pedicle nasoseptal flap. Laryngoscope 2006;116:1882–1886

39 Endoscopic-Assisted Transnasal Craniectomy Approach to Esthesioneuroblastoma

Aldo Cassol Stamm, Larry H. Kalish, Fernando Oto Balieiro, Iulo Barauna, and David W. Kennedy

Tips and Pearls

- Carefully assess the tumor size and site for potential endoscopic respectability.
- Endoscopic resection of these tumors requires a team approach with neurosurgery and significant endoscopic expertise.
- Current staging systems lack appropriate differentiation for surgical decision making. A revised staging system more suited to endoscopic assisted transnasal craniectomy is suggested.
- These tumors are malignant, and they require an oncologic resection with a clear tissue margin.
- The oncologic resection should never be compromised for the sake of performing the surgery endoscopically.
- The site of tumor attachment must be carefully identified after the tumor is debulked.
- The dura and olfactory bulb should be resected on the affected side, along with the tumor.
- Frozen section is utilized to ensure a tumor-free margin.
- Unless it would compromise tumor resection, a sphenopalatine flap is the preferred method of closure, typically with a multilayer closure.
- Postoperative radiation therapy or proton beam therapy is recommended for larger tumors, and in some cases chemotherapy also remains a perioperative consideration.

Introduction

Esthesioneuroblastoma (ENB) is a rare, malignant tumor of neural crest origin arising from neurosensory receptor cells of the olfactory epithelium, lying in the nasal cavity and paranasal sinuses. It is also referred to as an olfactory neuroblastoma, which better describes the origin and nature of the tumor. It accounts for 3 to 5% of cancers of the nasal cavity[1] and has a wide age range (3–90 years) with a bimodal age distribution with peaks in the second and fifth decades.[2–4] Both sexes are equally affected, and there is no apparent racial predilection.

Etiology

The basal cells of the olfactory neuroepithelium are presumably the progenitors of the esthesioneuroblastoma. No known causal factor exists for this tumor, and no hereditary patterns have been described for this neoplasm.[1]

Pathology

Hyams[5] developed a pathology grading system with four grades to classify esthesioneuroblastomas based on their histologic features (**Table 39.1**). The utility of this grading system has been questioned. Some studies have correlated it with survival and prognosis,[1,6–8] whereas others have failed to show any useful correlation.[9,10] Many studies have combined grades 1 and 2 into low grade and grades 3 and 4 into high grade.[6]

These tumors have a tendency to spread locally through the submucosal plane of the paranasal sinuses and invade the anterior cranial base. Extension to the brain and subarachnoid space may follow.[11] Hematogenous spread and lymphatic spread have also been well described with locoregional metastases to cervical lymph nodes seen in 10% to 30% of patients with esthesioneuroblastoma,[2,12] and distant metastases to the lung, bone, and other atypical sites have been reported less frequently.[11,13–17]

Clinical

The most common presenting symptoms include unilateral nasal obstruction, recurrent epistaxis, and anosmia.[18,19] The presenting symptoms are related to the site and local invasion of the tumor, so that occasionally these tumors may present with eustachian tube obstruction and a unilateral middle ear

Table 39.1 Hyams Histologic Grading System

Microscopic Feature	Grade 1	Grade 2	Grade 3	Grade 4
Architecture	Lobular	Lobular	±Lobular	±Lobular
Nuclear pleomorphism	Absent to slight	Present	Prominent	Marked
Neurofibrillary matrix	Prominent	Present	May be present	Absent
Rosettes	Homer-Wright pseudorosettes	Homer-Wright pseudorosettes	Flexner-Wintersteiner true neural rosettes	Flexner-Wintersteiner true neural rosettes
Mitoses	Absent	Present	Prominent	Marked
Necrosis	Absent	Absent	Present	Prominent
Glands	May be present	May be present	May be present	May be present
Calcification	Variable	Variable	Absent	Absent

Source: From Hyams VJ. Tumors of the upper respiratory tract and ear. In: Atlas of Tumor Pathology, 2nd series, fascicle 25. Washington, DC: Armed Forces Institute of Pathology; 1988:240–248. Reprinted with permission.

effusion, or diplopia with a rapid proptosis and visual loss.[18] They may also be associated with hormone excess syndromes such as Cushing syndrome[20,21] or the syndrome of inappropriate antidiuretic hormone secretion (SIADH).[22]

Treatment

Although there is no consensus about the treatment of these tumors, many clinicians believe that control is best achieved by combining surgery with adjuvant therapy, such as radiotherapy and chemotherapy.[23–27]

Craniofacial resection with or without bifrontal craniotomy has been considered the standard surgical approach to ENB, and must be considered the gold standard with which all other treatments are compared.[28] Craniofacial resection has the advantage of providing excellent intradural and extradural exposure of the structures of the anterior cranial fossa, and facilitates a multilayered reconstruction. The associated surgical morbidity includes postoperative cerebrospinal fluid (CSF) leak, meningitis, bone flap infection, wound infection, hemorrhage, and symptomatic pneumocephalus. Many series have reported a relatively low incidence of complications (22–30%), with some complications resulting from postoperative radiotherapy. Many studies, however, do not address the effects related to retraction of the frontal lobes and the high incidence of anosmia seen even in unilateral tumors.[23,24,26,28,29] Complications have improved over time with the advances in perioperative care, but are higher in older patients and in centers performing fewer procedures[30,31]

Endoscopic technology, techniques, and instrumentation have all evolved significantly, and the visualization provided by the use of endoscopes during tumor resection is unsurpassed, resulting in more frequent utilization of an endoscopic approach in the resection of these tumors.[24,26,32,33] This approach may be limited to assisting in the nasal component of the craniofacial resection (endoscopic-assisted craniofacial resection) to complete the tumor resection using a solely endoscopic access. Whichever technique is employed, it is critical that the important precepts of oncologic resection be maintained.

The debate as to the best technique continues; however, a recent meta-analysis supports endoscopic approaches.[34] Surgery was clearly shown to be superior to nonsurgical treatment modalities. Endoscopic surgery produced better survival rates than open surgery, but this is confounded by the larger number of patients with more advanced tumors undergoing open surgery compared with endoscopic. There is also considerable interinstitution and intersurgeon discrepancy and potential publication bias.[34]

Staging

When deciding on the approach, the stage of the tumor must be carefully considered. Kadish et al[35] in 1976 designed the most widely used pretreatment staging system for ENB This system divides patients into three groups: group A, tumor strictly confined to the nasal cavity; group B, tumor involving the nasal cavity and the paranasal sinuses; and group C, tumor extending beyond the nasal cavity and the paranasal sinuses into the intracranial compartment. The more advanced the Kadish staging, the worse the outcome; however, this staging system does not address the issue of tumor metastasis or extension to extracranial sites.[6,8] A fourth group, group D, tumor with cervical nodes or distant metastasis, is frequently added to this staging system.[36] Biller et al[37] devised a tumor-node-metastasis classification for esthesioneuroblastoma, whereby tumor extension was more clearly defined. Although more detailed than the Kadish system, it requires a craniotomy for staging and assumes universal cribriform plate involvement. Dulguerov and Calcaterra[23] modified this tumor-node-metastasis classification system, but the Kadish system is still more widely used due to its simplicity and prognostic value.

We believe that an additional shortcoming of the Kadish system is its inability to provide significant guidance with regard to surgical expectations and appropriate treatment modality, and that the stages are not fully applicable to the concepts of endoscopic transnasal resections.

Whereas the Kadish system differentiates between tumors confined to the nose and those involving the sinuses, with endoscopic-assisted transnasal craniectomy (EATNC), this differentiation is of limited importance in terms of surgical approach, and probably also is of limited prognostic importance. But for tumors that extend beyond the nose and paranasal sinuses, it becomes critically important to differentiate whether the tumor involves the dura or the orbit, because the appropriate surgical approach would differ markedly, and this differentiation is not achieved by the Kadish staging.[32,38,39] Similarly, it appears reasonable that, over time and given a sufficiently large series, differences in survival rates may also become evident between these two involvement sites. In terms of dural involvement, we believe, as do many surgical oncologic centers, that it is also important to determine whether the tumor involves just the dura or extends intracranially, and, if it does extend intradurally, whether it is still a tumor that can be resected with EATNC or will require a craniofacial approach.

We use the following staging system: stage 1, tumor confined to the nose and paranasal sinuses; stage 2, dural involvement; stage 3, orbital involvement; stage 4, intracranial involvement; stage 5, regional or distant metastases (**Fig. 39.1**).

Differential Diagnosis

Esthesioneuroblastoma can often be confused with the following neoplasms:

- Sinonasal undifferentiated carcinoma
- Neuroendocrine carcinoma
- Melanoma
- Lymphoma
- Plasmacytoma
- Embryonal rhabdomyosarcoma
- Ewing sarcoma
- Peripheral primitive neuroectodermal tumors
- Vascular tumors, e.g., hemangiopericytomas

Imaging

Computed tomography (CT) and magnetic resonance imaging (MRI) are complementary imaging modalities that are both routinely performed. Fine-cut CT scan (1- to 2-mm slice thickness) with direct coronal reconstruction or coronal CT sections highlights the sinus anatomy and enables the surgeon to look for erosion of the lamina papyracea, cribriform

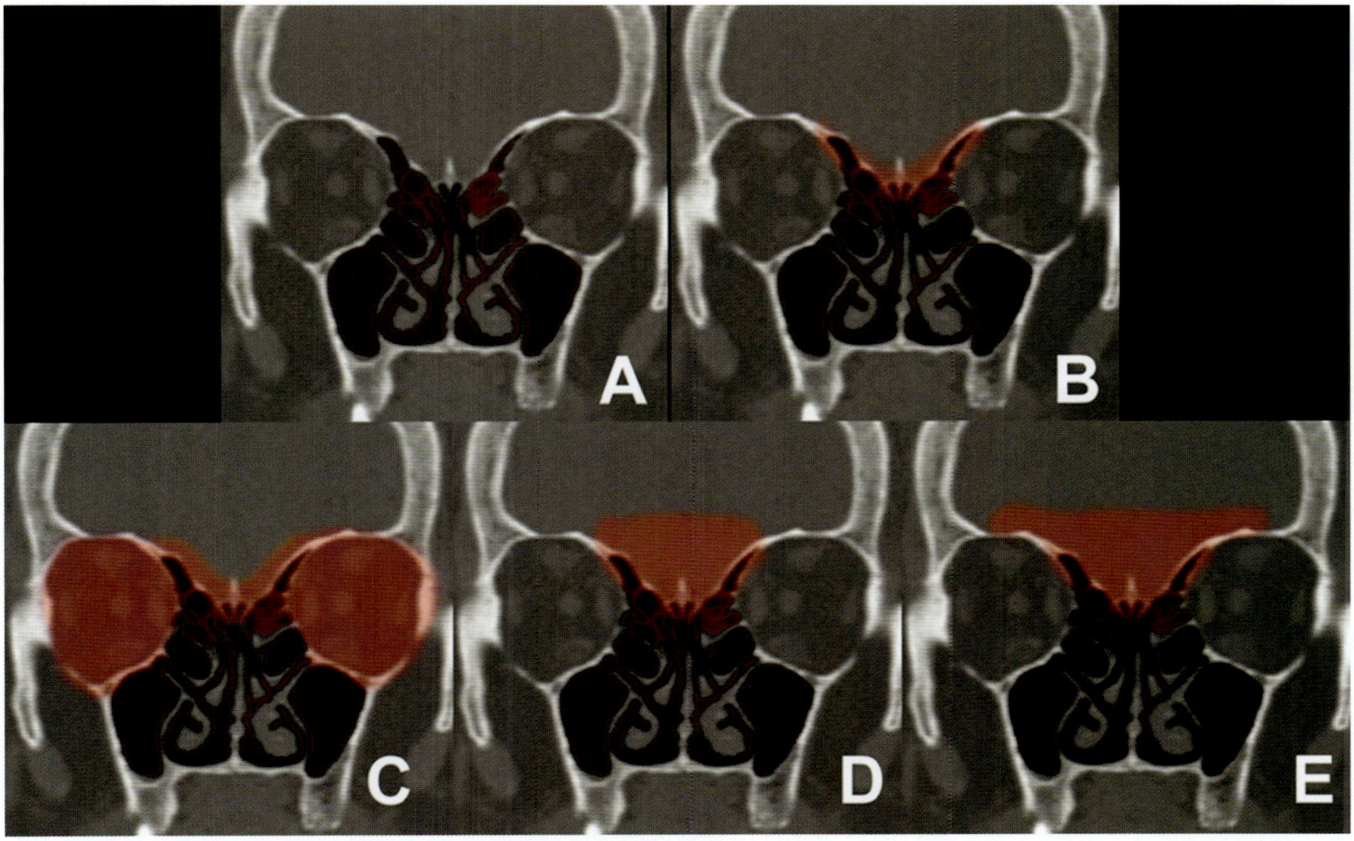

Fig. 39.1 Normal coronal computed tomography (CT) painted with the novel Stamm-Kennedy esthesioneuroblastoma staging system. **(A)** Stage 1. **(B)** Stage 2. **(C)** Stage 3. **(D)** Stage 4A. **(E)** Stage 4B.

plate, and fovea ethmoidalis. MRI provides a better estimate of tumor spread into surrounding soft tissue areas, especially breaching of the periorbita or dura, and it can differentiate mucus from tumor.

Preoperative Assessment

Included in a thorough examination assessing the patient's suitability for surgery should also be an ophthalmology assessment to exclude eye involvement, cranial nerve assessment, and documentation of the sense of smell in unilateral tumors if it is the surgeon's intention to preserve this sense. Multidisciplinary review including a neurosurgical review is important even if the patient is undergoing an endoscopic resection.

Surgical Overview

All procedures are performed under controlled hypotensive general anesthesia. The patient is placed in the supine position on the operating table in reverse Trendelenburg of up to 30 degrees, with the head slightly extended and turned toward the surgeon. Cottonoids (neuropatties) containing adrenaline, 1:1000, are placed in the nasal cavity, primarily in the areas of surgical access, for example, the axillae of the middle turbinates, the inferior and medial meatus, over the inferior turbinates, and between the mass and surrounding mucosal surfaces, and then left in place for at least 10 minutes.

The main principle in EATNC is resection of all involved structures of the skull base, including the nasal mucosa, bone, and the underlying dura. For large tumors and those with involvement of the dura or near the midline, surgery is performed through both sides of the nasal cavity. The extent of bone removal varies according to the relationship of the tumor to the crista galli.

Tumors Located Unilaterally with Respect to the Crista-Galli

In unilateral tumor cases, the surgery begins with a wide middle meatal antrostomy. The tumor is debulked sufficiently to enable identification of the relevant anatomy, and any sites of attachment are carefully identified for subsequent wide resection. The middle and superior turbinates are removed to the level of the skull base and a complete spheno-ethmoidectomy is performed, including removal of the lateral wall of the orbit, exposing the periorbita. Next, the frontal recess and then the frontal sinus are exposed. The anterior and posterior ethmoid arteries are identified, coagulated, and divided. The bone of the roof of the ethmoid sinus is removed, completely exposing the dura. The medial dissection is accomplished by removing the posterior and superior portions of the ipsilateral nasal septum. Perichondrium and periosteum of the contralateral side are preserved to be used in the reconstruction.

After skeletonization of the skull base, the roof of the ethmoid sinus is removed including the ipsilateral cribriform plate, using either a diamond burr or a micro-Kerrison punch. The dura of the olfactory region including the ipsilateral olfactory nerve filaments are resected so that the tumor attachment could be removed en bloc. The olfactory bulb is also resected at the affected side. Frozen sections of the margins are obtained to validate the oncologic resection.

Following the tumor removal, the dural defect is reconstructed with two layers of fascia lata harvested from the quadriceps muscle (one placed intradurally and the other extradurally), covered with the contralateral nasal septal mucoperiosteum graft or flap. The latter, pedunculated at the sphenopalatine artery, is currently the closure of choice.[40,41] Fibrin glue and nasal packing are used to secure these grafts in place (**Fig. 39.2**).

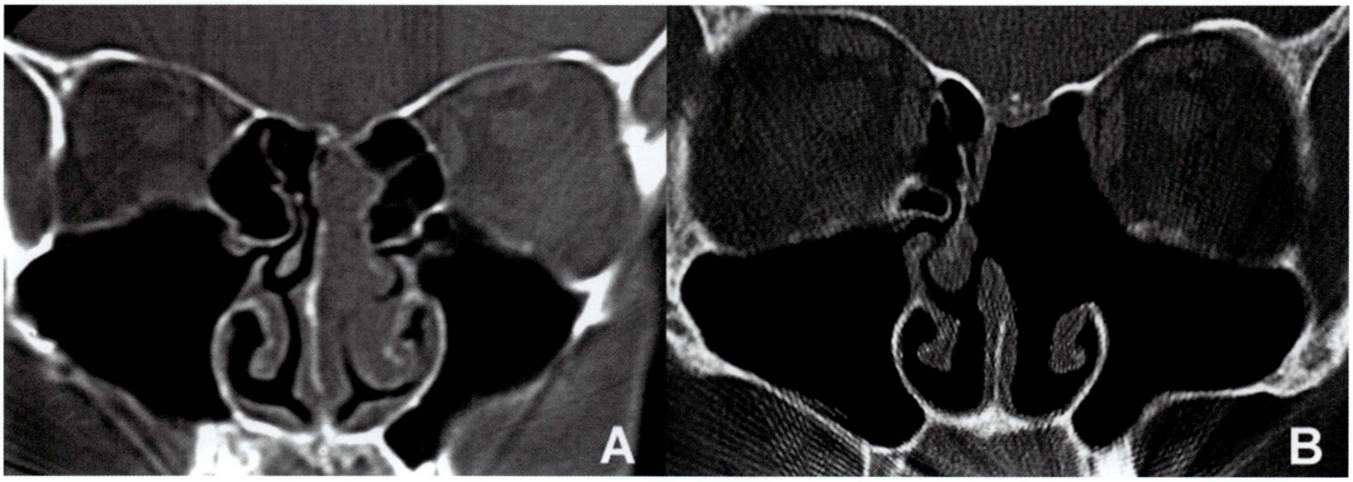

Fig. 39.2 Coronal CT of a patient with a unilateral tumor before **(A)** and after **(B)** an endoscopic assisted transnasal craniotomy approach.

Tumors Crossing the Crista Galli (Midline)

In the case of bilateral disease (**Fig. 39.3**), we also perform a Draf III frontal sinus approach[42] to widely expose the frontal sinus in addition to the exposure described above. As previously described, the craniotomy is initiated with a diamond drill and completed with micro-Kerrison forceps, preserving the underlying dura, and creating an osteotomy limited by the sphenoid planum posteriorly, the medial wall of orbits laterally, and the posterior wall of frontal sinus anteriorly.

The dura is opened with an incision at the margin of the craniotomy window. It is important to identify the falx cerebri at the very anterior region of the skull base dissection; any bleeding that occurs from the sagittal sinus can be controlled with local measures such as Surgicel packing. The falx is then detached from the crista galli, and the tumor removed en bloc along with the underlying dura. Freeing the tumor from the frontal lobe requires meticulous dissection.

The dural defect is reconstructed in the same way as in the unilateral approach described above, with two layers of fascia lata (one placed intradurally and the other extradurally), and a vascular pedicle nasal flap including mucoperiosteum/mucoperichondrium to cover the grafts. If a vascular pedicle flap is not available because of nasal septal involvement by the tumor, a mucoperiosteal flap from the floor of the nasal cavity can be used.

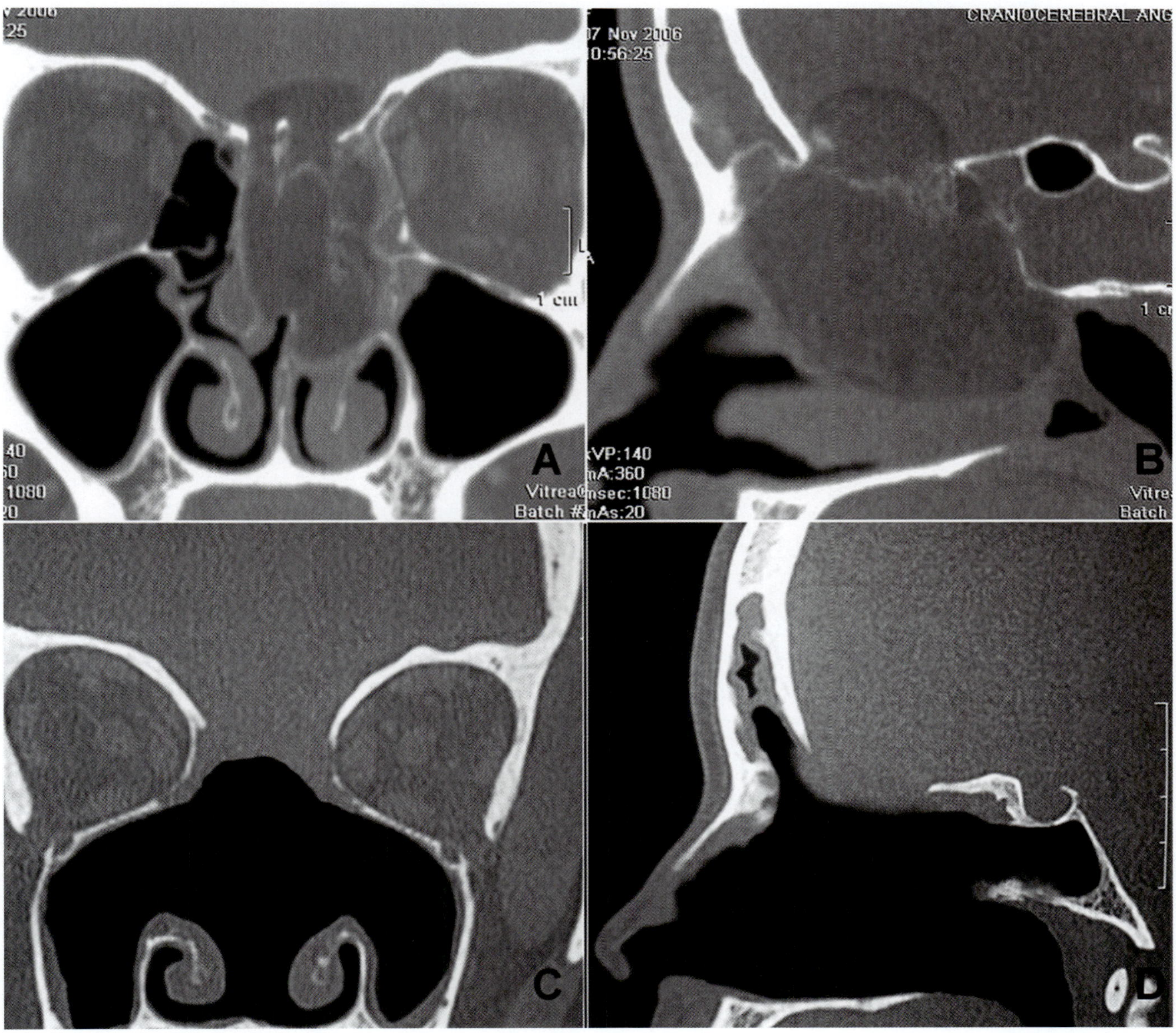

Fig. 39.3 Endoscopic assisted transnasal-craniotomy approach in a 26-year-old woman with recurrent epistaxes and nasal obstruction. A bilateral approach was performed. **(A)** Coronal CT image showing bilateral tumor arising from the olfactory vault. **(B)** Sagittal reconstruction. **(C)** Postoperative coronal CT image showing the complete endoscopic removal of the tumor. **(D)** Sagittal reconstruction.

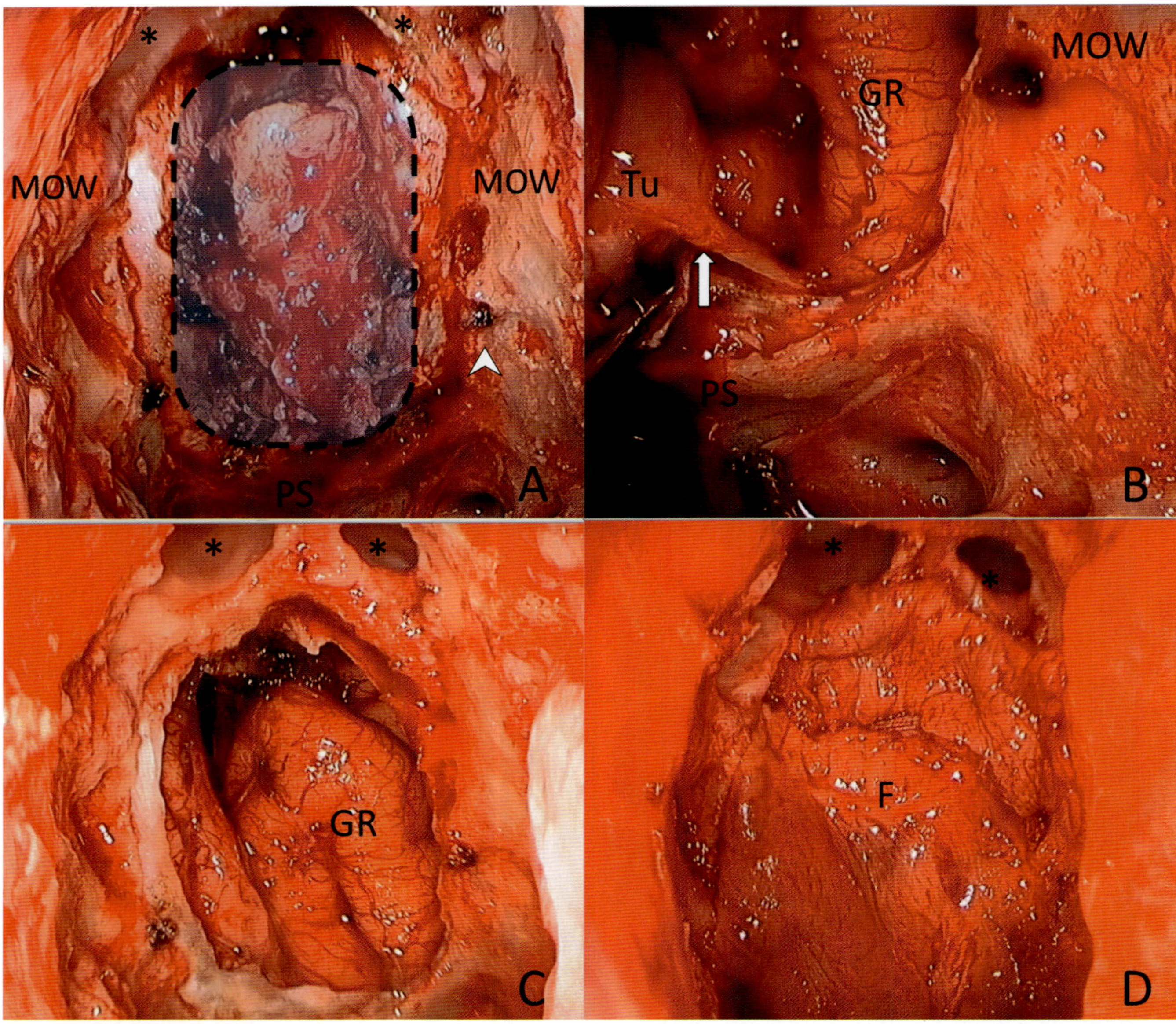

Fig. 39.4 A endoscopic-assisted transnasal/transcribriform craniectomy approach to resect a Stamm-Kennedy stage 4A esthesioneuroblastoma. **(A)** The dotted line indicates the extention of dural opening. **(B)** After the dural opening, image shows the relation between the tumor and the olfactory bulb (*white arrow*). **(C)** Final aspect of transnasal craniectomy after the tumor removal. **(D)** The skull base reconstruciton with a large pedicled vascular nasoseptal flap. MOW: medial orbital wall; PS: planum sphenoidale; Tu: tumor; GR; gyrus rectus; F: nasoseptal flap; (*): frontal sinus; arrowhead: anterior ethmoidal artery coagulated.

Free mucosal grafts are utilized to cover fascia and the defect, but pedicled vascular mucosal flaps are preferable whenever possible, although they can be supplemented with a free graft as required for very extensive skull base defects (**Fig. 39.4**).

Postoperative Care

Patients are nursed in a high dependency ward with neurosurgical nursing staff. The nasal packs are removed. If there is no evidence of CSF leak, early mobilization is encouraged and patients are often discharged in 5 days. Patients then return weekly for the first month to remove crusts and granulation tissues. After the first month, they are followed biweekly or monthly, depending on the healing progress. MRI and CT scans, along with endoscopic examinations, are performed at 6 months and 1 year following surgery.

References

1. Dulguerov P, Allal AS, Calcaterra TC. Esthesioneuroblastoma: a meta-analysis and review. Lancet Oncol 2001;2:683–690

2. Ferlito A, Rinaldo A, Rhys-Evans PH. Contemporary clinical commentary: esthesioneuroblastoma: an update on management of the neck. Laryngoscope 2003;113:1935–1938

3. Cohen ZR, Marmor E, Fuller GN, DeMonte F. Misdiagnosis of olfactory neuroblastoma. Neurosurg Focus 2002;12:e3

4. Hwang SK, Paek SH, Kim DG, Jeon YK, Chi JG, Jung HW. Olfactory neuroblastomas: survival rate and prognostic factor. J Neurooncol 2002; 59:217–226

5. Hyams VJ. Tumors of the upper respiratory tract and ear. In: Atlas of Tumor Pathology, 2nd series, fascicle 25. Washington, DC: Armed Forces Institute of Pathology; 1988:240–248

6. Constantinidis J, Steinhart H, Koch M, et al. Olfactory neuroblastoma: the University of Erlangen-Nuremberg experience 1975-2000. Otolaryngol Head Neck Surg 2004;130:567–574

7. Nakao K, Watanabe K, Fujishiro Y, et al. Olfactory neuroblastoma: long-term clinical outcome at a single institute between 1979 and 2003. Acta Otolaryngol Suppl 2007;559:113–117

8. Miyamoto RC, Gleich LL, Biddinger PW, Gluckman JL. Esthesioneuroblastoma and sinonasal undifferentiated carcinoma: impact of histological grading and clinical staging on survival and prognosis. Laryngoscope 2000;110:1262–1265

9. Ingeholm P, Theilgaard SA, Buchwald C, Hansen HS, Francis D. Esthesioneuroblastoma: a Danish clinicopathological study of 40 consecutive cases. APMIS 2002;110:639–645

10. Weinreb I, Goldstein D, Irish J, Perez-Ordonez B. Expression patterns of Trk-A, Trk-B, GRP78, and p75NRT in olfactory neuroblastoma. Hum Pathol 2009;40:1330–1335

11. Oskouian RJJ Jr, Jane JAS Sr, Dumont AS, Sheehan JM, Laurent JJ, Levine PA. Esthesioneuroblastoma: clinical presentation, radiological, and pathological features, treatment, review of the literature, and the University of Virginia experience. Neurosurg Focus 2002;12:e4

12. Jethanamest D, Morris LG, Sikora AG, Kutler DI. Esthesioneuroblastoma: a population-based analysis of survival and prognostic factors. Arch Otolaryngol Head Neck Surg 2007;133:276–280

13. Davis RE, Weissler MC. Esthesioneuroblastoma and neck metastasis. Head Neck 1992;14:477–482

14. Franklin D, Miller RH, Bloom MG, Easley J, Stiernberg CM. Esthesioneuroblastoma metastatic to the trachea. Head Neck Surg 1987;10: 102–106

15. Logrono R, Futoran RM, Hartig G, Inhorn SL. Olfactory neuroblastoma (esthesioneuroblastoma): appearance on fine-needle aspiration: report of a case. Diagn Cytopathol 1997;17:205–208

16. Zollinger LV, Wiggins RH III, Cornelius RS, Phillips CD. Retropharyngeal lymph node metastasis from esthesioneuroblastoma: a review of the therapeutic and prognostic implications. AJNR Am J Neuroradiol 2008; 29:1561–1563

17. Koka VN, Julieron M, Bourhis J, et al. Aesthesioneuroblastoma. J Laryngol Otol 1998;112:628–633

18. Sharma S, Sharma MC, Johnson MH, Lou M, Thakar A, Sarkar C. Esthesioneuroblastoma—a clinicopathologic study and role of DNA topoisomerase alpha. Pathol Oncol Res 2007;13:123–129

19. Nichols AC, Chan AW, Curry WT, Barker FG, Deschler DG, Lin DT. Esthesioneuroblastoma: the Massachusetts eye and ear infirmary and Massachusetts general hospital experience with craniofacial resection, proton beam radiation, and chemotherapy. Skull Base 2008;18: 327–337

20. Arnesen MA, Scheithauer BW, Freeman S. Cushing's syndrome secondary to olfactory neuroblastoma. Ultrastruct Pathol 1994;18:61–68

21. Kanno K, Morokuma Y, Tateno T, et al. Olfactory neuroblastoma causing ectopic ACTH syndrome. Endocr J 2005;52:675–681

22. Plasencia YL, Cortés MB, Arencibia DM, et al. Esthesioneuroblastoma recurrence presenting as a syndrome of inappropriate antidiuretic hormone secretion. Head Neck 2006;28:1142–1146

23. Dulguerov P, Calcaterra T. Esthesioneuroblastoma: the UCLA experience 1970-1990. Laryngoscope 1992;102:843–849

24. Liu JK, O'Neill B, Orlandi RR, Moscatello AL, Jensen RL, Couldwell WT. Endoscopic-assisted craniofacial resection of esthesioneuroblastoma: minimizing facial incisions—technical note and report of 3 cases. Minim Invasive Neurosurg 2003;46:310–315

25. Lund VJ, Milroy C. Olfactory neuroblastoma: clinical and pathological aspects. Rhinology 1993;31:1–6

26. Stammberger H, Anderhuber W, Walch C, Papaefthymiou G. Possibilities and limitations of endoscopic management of nasal and paranasal sinus malignancies. Acta Otorhinolaryngol Belg 1999;53: 199–205

27. Walch C, Stammberger H, Anderhuber W, Unger F, Köle W, Feichtinger K. The minimally invasive approach to olfactory neuroblastoma: combined endoscopic and stereotactic treatment. Laryngoscope 2000;110: 635–640

28. Lund VJ, Howard DJ, Wei WI, Cheesman AD. Craniofacial resection for tumors of the nasal cavity and paranasal sinuses—a 17-year experience. Head Neck 1998;20:97–105

29. Kryzanski JT, Annino DJ, Gopal H, Heilman CB. Low complication rates of cranial and craniofacial approaches to midline anterior skull base lesions. Skull Base 2008;18:229–241

30. Gil Z, Patel SG, Bilsky M, Shah JP, Kraus DH. Complications after craniofacial resection for malignant tumors: are complication trends changing? Otolaryngol Head Neck Surg 2009;140:218–223

31. Ganly I, Gross ND, Patel SG, Bilsky MH, Shah JP, Kraus DH. Outcome of craniofacial resection in patients 70 years of age and older. Head Neck 2007;29:89–94

32. Svane-Knudsen V, Jørgensen KE, Hansen O, Lindgren A, Marker P. Cancer of the nasal cavity and paranasal sinuses: a series of 115 patients. Rhinology 1998;36:12–14

33. Lund VJ, Howard D, Wei W, Spittle M. Olfactory neuroblastoma: past, present, and future? Laryngoscope 2003;113:502–507

34. Devaiah AK, Andreoli MT. Treatment of esthesioneuroblastoma: a 16-year meta-analysis of 361 patients. Laryngoscope 2009;119:1412–1416

35. Kadish S, Goodman M, Wang CC. Olfactory neuroblastoma. A clinical analysis of 17 cases. Cancer 1976;37:1571–1576

36. Morita A, Ebersold MJ, Olsen KD, Foote RL, Lewis JE, Quast LM. Esthesioneuroblastoma: prognosis and management. Neurosurgery 1993;32: 706–714, discussion 714–715

37. Biller HF, Lawson W, Sachdev VP, Som P. Esthesioneuroblastoma: surgical treatment without radiation. Laryngoscope 1990;100:1199–1201

38. Vrionis FD, Kienstra MA, Rivera M, Padhya TA. Malignant tumors of the anterior skull base. Cancer Contr 2004;11:144–151

39. Zumegen C, Michel O. [Classification and prognosis of esthesioneuroblastoma based on 7 treated cases]. Laryngorhinootologie 2000;79: 736–742

40. Hadad G, Bassagasteguy L, Carrau RL, et al. A novel reconstructive technique after endoscopic expanded endonasal approaches: vascular pedicle nasoseptal flap. Laryngoscope 2006;116):1882–1886

41. Stamm AC, Pignatari S, Vellutini E, Harvey RJ, Nogueira JFJ Jr. A novel approach allowing binostril work to the sphenoid sinus. Otolaryngol Head Neck Surg 2008;138:531–532

42. Draf W. Endonasal micro-endoscopic frontal sinus surgery: the Fulda concept. Oper Tech Otolaryngol—Head Neck Surg 1991;2:234–240

40 Combined Cranioendoscopic Approach

Piero Nicolai, Arkadi Yakirevitch, Andrea Bolzoni Villaret, Paolo Battaglia, Davide Locatelli, and Paolo Castelnuovo

Tips and Pearls

- This approach is indicated for sinonasal lesions with endonasal and endocranial extension requiring a dural resection extending over the orbital roof(s) or with extensive brain contact/involvement that are not suitable for a purely endoscopic resection.
- The availability in the operating room of multiple screens enables a panoramic view of the surgical field, more accurate control of the resection margins, and better interaction between the neurosurgical and ear, nose, and throat (ENT) surgical teams.
- During the endoscopic phase the "ethmoidal box" is isolated from the walls of the nasal cavity and periorbit. If necessary, this phase may include medial maxillectomy and resection of the nasolacrimal duct and the periorbit.
- The transcranial phase exposes the superior part of the tumor through a subfrontal approach and entails dissecting it from the uninvolved dura and brain. The anterior skull base is drilled around the tumor to complete the "ethmoidal box" mobilization.
- Central debulking of the tumor may be utilized in both the endoscopic and transcranial phases.
- The skull base is reconstructed with an intradural graft of pericranium or temporal fascia and an extradural pedicled pericranial flap. The accuracy of reconstruction is verified endoscopically.
- Brain computed tomography (CT) scan is obtained on the first postoperative day to rule out early complications.

Introduction

During the past 40 years, anterior craniofacial resection followed by radiotherapy has been considered the gold standard in the treatment of malignancies of the sinonasal tract encroaching upon the anterior skull base. In 1997, Yuen et al[1] pioneered the so-called cranionasal resection for treatment of malignant sinonasal tumors involving the anterior skull base, combining traditional frontal craniotomy with a transnasal endoscopic approach. Our group began to use this technique, called the cranioendoscopic approach (CEA), in 1996, and our preliminary results have been published.[2,3] The main advantage offered by this combined surgical technique over standard craniofacial resection is the multiperspective visualization afforded by straight and angled rigid telescopes. Tumor margins can be determined with greater confidence and magnification at the level of the sphenoid sinus, the medial maxillary wall, the pterygopalatine fossa, and especially at the sinonasal–orbital interface when orbital clearance is not needed. The technique also avoids facial incisions with additional pain, swelling, scar, and deformity.

Indications

The CEA is recommended for removal of sinonasal lesions with endonasal and endocranial extension requiring a dural resection extending over the orbital roof(s) (**Fig. 40.1**) or with extensive brain contact/involvement (**Fig. 40.2**).

Contraindications

The contraindications for CEA are summarized in **Table 40.1**. It is noteworthy that Batra et al[4] consider the need for orbital clearance, lateral tumor extension with invasion of the pterygopalatine space, and infratemporal fossa to be relative contraindications. In our experience, these situations cannot be safely managed with a purely endoscopic approach.

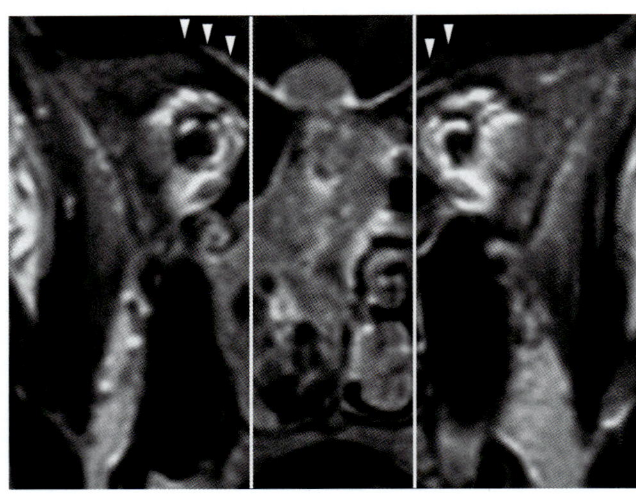

Fig. 40.1 Enhanced T1-weighted magnetic resonance imaging (MRI), coronal section demonstrates a right nasoethmoidal lesion (adenocarcinoma) with an "hourglass" intradural extension through the ethmoidal roof. Diffuse enhancement of the dural layer (*arrowheads*) over the orbital roof is suspicious for neoplastic spread. The vertical lines limit the area of the dura safely resectable by a pure endoscopic approach.

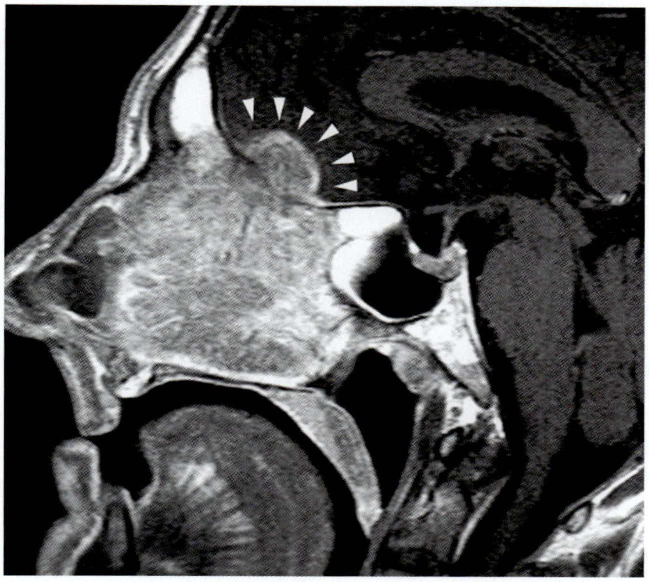

Fig. 40.2 Enhanced T1-weighted MRI, sagittal section demonstrates an ethmoidal squamous cell carcinoma with significant intracranial extension involving the brain parenchyma (*arrowheads*).

Diagnostic Workup

The preoperative diagnostic workup includes physical examination with a special focus on neurologic and ophthalmologic assessment; endoscopic examination with preoperative biopsies is always performed after the imaging studies. Magnetic resonance imaging (MRI) with gadolinium enhancement is preferred to computed tomography (CT) for its better definition in evaluating tumor spread in soft tissues, particularly at the interface of the orbital content and the brain. When required (in the presence of nodal disease or in a case of aggressive lesions such as malignant melanoma and sinonasal undifferentiated carcinoma), distant metastatic dissemination of the disease is excluded by total-body positron emission tomography (PET)-CT. Moreover, a 6-foot anterior-posterior x-ray of the skull is performed to obtain a template reproducing the projection of the frontal sinus on the anterior cranial wall. All patients should be informed that it might be necessary to switch intraoperatively to a transfacial approach in case any unexpected contraindication is found during the surgery.

Table 40.1 Contraindications for a Cranioendoscopic Approach

Lacrimal sac involvement
Involvement of the orbital content
Involvement of the bony walls of the maxillary sinus (except of the medial wall)
Extension into the pterygopalatine or infratemporal fossa
Posterior wall of the sphenoid sinus
Extension to the hard palate
Nasal pyramid involvement

Operative Setup

The surgery requires a double surgical team (neurosurgical and ear, nose, and throat [ENT]), an operating room nurse, and an anesthesiologist. The staff and equipment layout in the operating room is illustrated in **Fig. 40.3**. The presence of multiple screens (for the microscope and the endoscope) enables a panoramic view of the specimen, provides more accurate control of the resection margins, and facilitates interaction between the two surgical teams.

Endoscopic Phase

This phase requires the use of straight and angled rigid telescopes and dedicated instruments. If the neoplasm significantly obstructs the nasal fossa, it is necessary to perform tumor central debulking, usually with powered instruments, to allow centripetal collapse of the specimen walls and to facilitate identification of the lesion origin. The sphenopalatine artery is isolated and coagulated bilaterally, thus reducing bleeding during the entire procedure. The nasal septum is cut on its base parallel to the nasal floor, and then frontally with a vertical incision that reaches the nasal vault at the

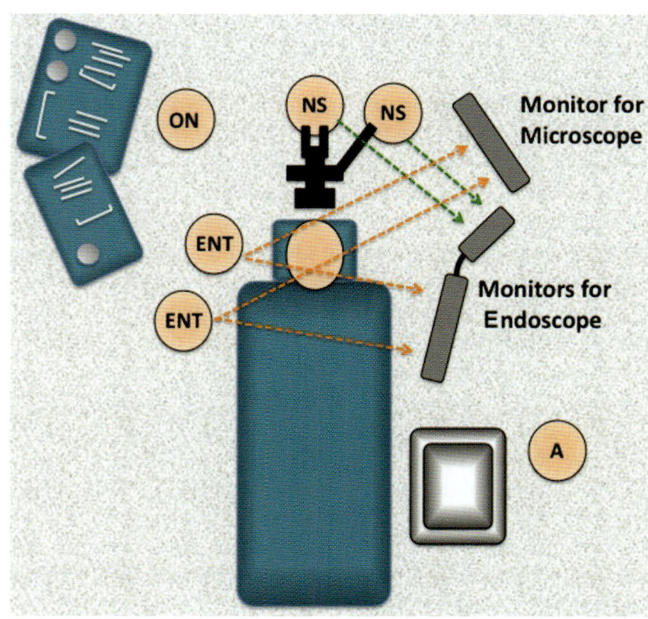

Fig. 40.3 Layout of the surgical teams and instrumentation during a combined cranioendoscopic resection. All the surgeons are able to control both the transnasal and transcranial aspects of the approach with multiple monitors. A: anesthesiologist; ENT: otorhinolaryngologist; NS: neurosurgeon; ON: operating nurse.

height of the frontal beak. Posterior mobilization of the nasal septum is obtained by performing wide bilateral sinusotomy and resecting the sphenoid rostrum to better define the posterior margin of resection.

The lamina papyracea is dissected on one or both sides from the periorbit based on the extent of the lesion, starting with the anterior margin back to the orbital apex. At this moment, it is important for the other team members to interact correctly with the neurosurgeon, who cauterizes the ethmoidal arteries from above and helps the otorhinolaryngologist to medialize the residual lamina papyracea. Har-El and Casiano[5] described the "next compartment principle," according to which a surgeon dissects at least one compartment away from the tumor. For example, for a lesion involving the superior meatus and the superior nasal septum, the surgeon should enter the middle meatus on both sides and dissect the ethmoid complex superiorly toward the ethmoid roof.

In regard to tumor extension, this surgical phase may be associated with medial maxillectomy, nasolacrimal duct exposure and removal below the lacrimal sac, or resection of the periorbit. At the end of the endoscopic phase, multiple biopsies are sent to the laboratory for frozen sections.

Transcranial Phase

This phase is initialized with a coronal flap and a subfrontal craniotomy variable in size and shape depending on the surgical needs and anatomical variants. The incision starts just anteriorly to the tragus at the level of zygomatic arch and is enlarged superiorly and posteriorly at the level of the vertex to enable harvesting of a very long pedicled pericranial flap. Careful attention is paid to preserving the frontal branch of the facial nerve, which is achieved by incising the superficial temporal fascia 3 cm posteriorly to the orbitozygomatic arch and elevating it with the flap. The coronal flap is raised in the subgaleal plane. The pericranium is incised even more posteriorly to the skin incision and raised anteriorly until the glabella and the supraorbital rims are exposed. The supraorbital foramen/incisure is bilaterally identified and its neurovascular bundle is preserved. To facilitate maximal inferior displacement of the orbital content on both sides, the inferior portion of the supraorbital foramina (if not dehiscent) is resected with a small chisel.

A subfrontal approach, first described by Raveh et al[6] in 1993 is always preferred to the classic frontal craniotomy because it minimizes brain retraction and therefore decreases the risk of neurologic complications (**Fig. 40.4**). With the help of a frontal template or intraoperative navigation system, as described by Schipper et al,[7] osteotomies are performed along the superolateral borders of both frontal sinuses, with the oscillating saw properly angled (approximately 45 degrees) toward the frontal sinuses. A frontal bone flap including the anterior wall of the frontal sinuses and the superomedial contour of the orbits is removed after preplating. The inferior border of the volet is the nasion. The posterior wall of the frontal sinuses is drilled out (**Fig. 40.5**).

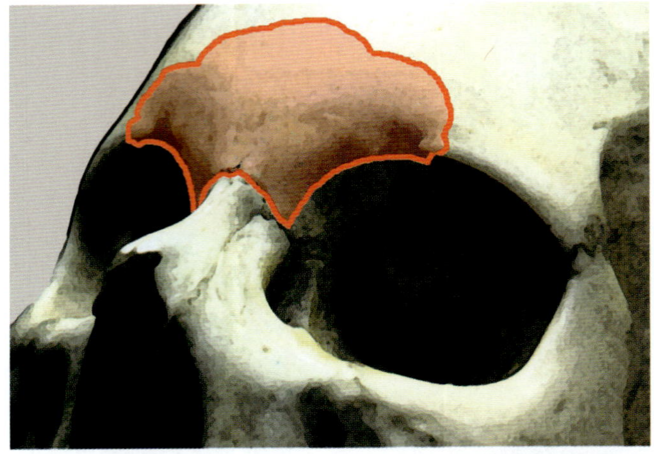

A

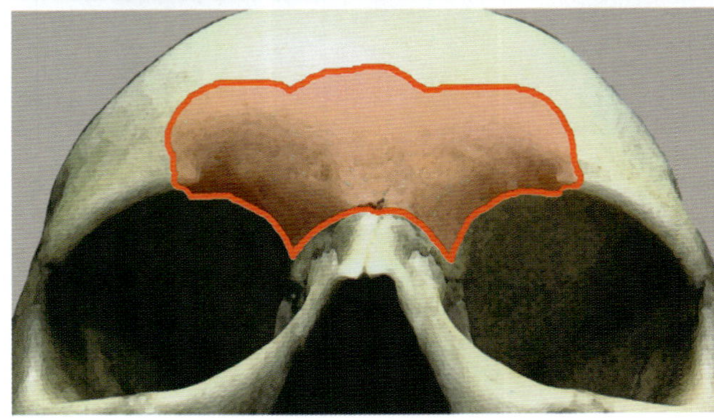

B

Fig. 40.4 (A,B) Subfrontal craniotomy.

The dura of the anterior skull base is extensively lifted from the orbital roof. The exposed dura is incised transversally and then longitudinally on both sides along the junction between the lamina papyracea and the orbital roof to check the intradural extension of the lesion. The frontal lobes are carefully retracted with the visualization of olfactory bulbs and tracts over the inner aspect of the resected dura. If the intracranial part of the tumor is bulky, it can be collapsed with initial central cavitation to allow its mobilization. Next, it is gradually isolated from the healthy brain parenchyma and optic nerves while progressively interposing protective cottonoids. With a diamond burr, the "ethmoidal box" is isolated. The olfactory tracts are transected posteriorly to the tumor, the dura incised, and the planum sphenoidale drilled to complete the resection.

Simultaneous Removal of the Ethmoidal Box

This phase is a crucial aspect of CEA when the two teams (ENT and neurosurgical) interact the most. Simultaneous visualization through a microscope and endoscopes enables observation of all the margins of the ethmoidal box during its resection. The box is always removed transcranially.

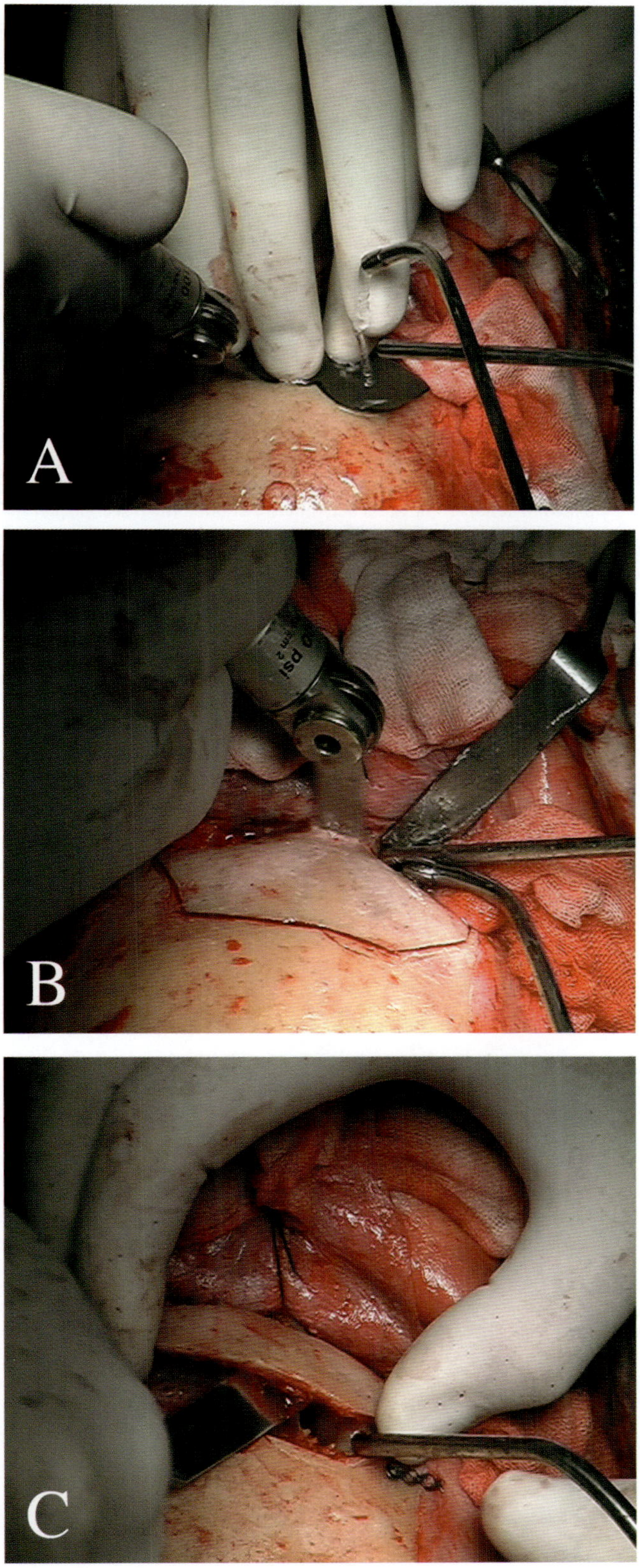

Fig. 40.5 Subfrontal craniotomy. **(A)** Osteotomies are performed based on a frontal template. **(B)** The bony volet is completed by dividing the frontal bone from the nasal pyramid with a horizontal cut. **(C)** After preplating, the bony volet is removed with exposure of the posterior wall of both frontal sinuses.

Reconstruction

The dural defect is repaired with an intradural graft of pericranium or temporal fascia, which should exceed the size of the defect by 30%. A pedicled pericranial flap is then inserted between the residual skull base and the dura, preferably in two layers. It can be fixed with stitches posteriorly to the planum sphenoidale and laterally to the ethmoidal roof when available. The accuracy of pericranial flap positioning is verified endoscopically. The frontal lobes are delicately extended above the flap that is fixed from below with fibrin glue. The bony volet is repositioned and fixed with titanium plates and screws. The galeal skin flap is then relocated, and the wound is sutured in layers after drainage positioning. Finally, the endonasal surgical cavity is packed.

Some authors advocate placing nasal trumpets in the inferior meatus below nasal packing. These help prevent immediate postoperative intracranial air-trapping that can occur as patients produce positive pharyngeal pressure by coughing and gagging on extubation.[8,9]

Postoperative Care

The patient is kept ventilated for 8 to 12 hours and in full bed rest in a 30-degree upright position until the third postoperative day. The patient is instructed to avoid straining and to keep the mouth open when sneezing. There is usually no need for lumbar drainage. A brain CT scan is obtained on the first postoperative day to rule out early complications. Nasal packing is gradually removed within 48 hours. Intravenous antibiotic therapy is started 1 day before surgery and continued for at least 5 days. Intravenous hyperhydration is usually administered. Gentle nasal irrigation with saline solution and application of bacitracin ointment twice daily is recommended for at least 2 months.

Results

The 5-year overall, disease-specific, and recurrence-free survival rates in our CEA group were 56.6%, 69.7%, and 56.6%, respectively (unpublished data), whereas in a large cohort of patients after craniofacial resection the rates were 48.3%, 53.3%, and 45.8%, respectively, as reported by Ganly et al.[10]

Complications

Cerebrospinal fluid leak can be resolved with lumbar drainage placement or with endoscopic revision of the duraplasty, under local or general anesthesia according to the site and size of the defect. Some degree of pneumocephalus is always detected on CT scan after craniotomy. It is crucial to exclude progression and brain compression. In extreme cases, the revision of duraplasty is required. Meningitis is prevented in most cases with perioperative antibiotic therapy. Brain edema, intracranial abscess, and hematoma result in neurologic changes, and are diagnosed by imaging and managed in close cooperation with a neurosurgeon.

Neurogenic adult respiratory distress syndrome was described in patients managed with lumbar drainage and responded within a few hours to the cessation of drainage.[9] Frontal bone osteomyelitis, due to radiotherapy frequently applied in this patient population, is a late complication requiring long-term antibiotic therapy and surgical debridement in persistent cases. Other possible complications include visual disorders, supraorbital anesthesia, and epistaxis. Perioperative mortality cases were also reported: in our series the rate was 4%,[3] similar to that in the craniofacial resection series.[11] The overall rate of complications after CEA in our experience is 16%,[3] being substantially lower than that reported after craniofacial resection.[11]

References

1. Yuen AP, Fung CF, Hung KN. Endoscopic cranionasal resection of anterior skull base tumor. Am J Otolaryngol 1997;18:431–433
2. Castelnuovo PG, Belli E, Bignami M, Battaglia P, Sberze F, Tomei G. Endoscopic nasal and anterior craniotomy resection for malignant naso-ethmoid tumors involving the anterior skull base. Skull Base 2006;16:15–18
3. Nicolai P, Battaglia P, Bignami M, et al. Endoscopic surgery for malignant tumors of the sinonasal tract and adjacent skull base: a 10-year experience. Am J Rhinol 2008;22:308–316
4. Batra PS, Citardi MJ, Worley S, Lee J, Lanza DC. Resection of anterior skull base tumors: comparison of combined traditional and endoscopic techniques. Am J Rhinol 2005;19:521–528
5. Har-El G, Casiano RR. Endoscopic management of anterior skull base tumors. Otolaryngol Clin North Am 2005;38:133–144, ix ix
6. Raveh J, Laedrach K, Speiser M, et al. The subcranial approach for fronto-orbital and anteroposterior skull-base tumors. Arch Otolaryngol Head Neck Surg 1993;119:385–393
7. Schipper J, Maier W, Arapakis I, Spetzger U, Laszig R. Navigation as a tool to visualize bone-covered hidden structures in transfrontal approaches. J Laryngol Otol 2004;118:849–856
8. Buchmann L, Larsen C, Pollack A, Tawfik O, Sykes K, Hoover LA. Endoscopic techniques in resection of anterior skull base/paranasal sinus malignancies. Laryngoscope 2006;116:1749–1754
9. Devaiah AK, Larsen C, Tawfik O, O'Boynick P, Hoover LA. Esthesioneuroblastoma: endoscopic nasal and anterior craniotomy resection. Laryngoscope 2003;113:2086–2090
10. Ganly I, Patel SG, Singh B, et al. Craniofacial resection for malignant paranasal sinus tumors: Report of an International Collaborative Study. Head Neck 2005;27:575–584
11. Ganly I, Patel SG, Singh B, et al. Complications of craniofacial resection for malignant tumors of the skull base: report of an International Collaborative Study. Head Neck 2005;27:445–451

41 External Versus Endoscopic Approaches for Skull Base Malignancies

Valerie J. Lund and David J. Howard

Tips and Pearls

- The extent and nature of the tumor must determine the choice of surgical approach, not the other way around.
- Surgeons undertaking endoscopic approaches for malignant tumors must be familiar with the natural history of the specific histopathologies and be able to offer the full range of surgical options.
- Patients must be fully informed about the available treatment options.
- Patients undergoing both external and endoscopic approaches must be available for the same rigorous long-term follow-up.
- Some tumors (e.g., olfactory neuroblastomas) are more suitable for curative endoscopic resection than others (e.g., squamous cell carcinomas).
- Endoscopic resection should be undertaken with the same curative aims as external approaches. It should not be regarded as a "debulking" except where treatment is palliative.
- The principal advantage of endoscopic resection is reduced morbidity, but serious complications (e.g., severe hemorrhage) can occur and prove difficult to manage.
- Accurate long-term collection of data will facilitate comparison of the various surgical approaches in the management of these rare tumors.

Introduction

Malignant tumors in the nose and paranasal sinuses affecting the skull base present some of the most challenging problems in head and neck cancer. Because they are rare, it is difficult for any one practitioner or institution to accrue large numbers of patients and extensive expertise in their management. This is further complicated by their enormous histologic diversity, with every tissue type represented.

The majority of tumors are managed by surgery alone or in combination with radiotherapy and/or chemotherapy, but because patients have relatively mild symptoms at the start, they often present when the tumor is quite extensive and has invaded adjacent structures, such as the intracranial cavity and orbit. This may compromise the surgical approaches that can be undertaken with curative intention. Although endoscopic techniques (endoscopic sinus surgery [ESS]) are being increasingly employed, the results must be compared with those of established external surgery such as craniofacial resection (CFR). At present that comparison is difficult, as the number of patients, by tumor and length of follow-up, are all significantly less in the endoscopically treated group. This is particularly important when some sinonasal malignancies can recur many years later. However, some information is emerging as to the selection of patients, and this chapter discusses that information.

Which Tumor?

As previously mentioned, histologic diversity is the norm in this area, and each tumor has its own natural history that may influence the choice of procedure. Some, for example squamous cell carcinoma, are much more infiltrative than others, such as adenocarcinoma, which often has a well-defined plane of cleavage from normal tissue, making an endoscopic approach a better choice in the latter rather than the former.

In olfactory neuroblastoma (ON), we know that microscopic disease can be found in the olfactory bulbs and tracts even when it is not apparent on the most detailed preoperative imaging. This was the tumor par excellence for which CFR was devised, as it enabled complete resection of these areas, providing accurate staging for the first time.[1] However, it is now technically possible to undertake this resection by an endonasal endoscopic approach, so this alone does not invalidate ESS for resection of ON.[2–6]

Interestingly, the accurate staging of disease extent provided by CFR led initially to radiotherapy being offered only to those with disease in the olfactory tract and bulbs, but in due course it became apparent that recurrence was higher in those individuals who did not receive radiotherapy (28% versus 4%), even though they had the smaller tumors.[7] This has confirmed the need for combined therapy irrespective of tumor extent, and has given further reassurance to those undertaking ESS that they were not committing their patients to additional oncologic treatment; the addition treatment is required irrespective of the surgical procedure.

Another epithelial tumor with a fascinating natural history is adenoid cystic carcinoma, which is well known to follow perineural lymphatics, sometimes embolically spreading widely and placing patients at risk of primary and secondary recurrence throughout their lifetime. It could be argued that patients should undergo the most radical surgery possible, yet long-term studies have still shown recurrence many years or even decades later. Thus, a more tempered approach associated with lower morbidity, for example ESS, could be supported by the published research.[6]

Malignant melanoma of the sinonasal mucosa is also an unpredictable and capricious tumor, overwhelming some individuals in a matter of weeks or living in symbiosis for many years with others. Overall the largest cohort study demonstrated a depressing 5-year actuarial survival of 28%,[8] and suggested that this occurred irrespective of surgical treatment, though patients undergoing craniofacial seemed to do particularly badly, which was not necessarily related to the extent of the disease. As a consequence, this tumor has been approached endoscopically for some time,[4,6] occurring as it does in elderly individuals with other comorbidities.

Chondrosarcoma is an indolent but inexorable tumor that is difficult to extirpate whatever the approach. It can also be multifocal, which explains why recurrence may occur many years later in relatively distant parts of the skull base from the original lesion. Thus survival figures fall from 94% at 5 years to 37% at 15 years.[9] This might seem a good reason to undertake a craniofacial approach, but one could equally argue that the improved magnification combined with the use of accurate high-speed drills actually supports ESS in accessible cases, especially when the orbital apex is involved, another area where ESS has shown itself to be of value.[10]

What Is the Site of the Tumor?

One of the most interesting aspects of ESS has been the appreciation of where tumors arise. A seemingly large tumor filling the nasal cavity and eroding the skull base on imaging may sometimes prove to originate from a small area of mucosa that can be readily resected. Endoscopic surgery has challenged some preconceptions regarding the usual site of origin.[11]

Combined computed tomography (CT) and magnetic resonance imaging (MRI) offers a high degree of accuracy, distinguishing tumor from inflammation, fibrosis, and secretion,[12] but it is only at surgery that this finding can be macroscopically confirmed and may often require frozen section corroboration. It therefore seems entirely reasonable, assuming local facilities allow, to have the patient sign a consent form for both ESS and CFR, and then begin operating endoscopically but with the option of converting to the external approach if required. With good patient selection, the number of occasions when this is required will remain very small.

How Extensive a Tumor?

When we talk about an endoscopic resection of a sinonasal malignancy affecting the skull base, we should be clear that this is not a debulking procedure but rather a genuine attempt at a curative resection. This means total excision of the tumor together with margins of normal tissue. The main advantage of CFR over the techniques that preceded it, such as lateral rhinotomy, is the ability to undertake an en-bloc resection of the ethmoids, including the cribriform niche and adjacent structures, as determined by the tumor extent.[9] One of the criticisms leveled against ESS has been the fact that this is inevitably a piecemeal removal. However, in reality CFR is often piecemeal, and once the main specimen was removed, further clearance of the cavity was undertaken to ensure clear margins. Thus, the principle of en-bloc resection has been shown to be far less important than the complete removal of a tumor, given the specific constraints imposed by the complex anatomy in this area.

There are technical limitations to the areas that can be accessed by an entirely endoscopic approach, and these relate mainly to lateral extension over the roofs of the orbit. A rule of thumb is that pathology extending (or arising) lateral to a line drawn through the midpoint of the orbit cannot safely be reached via an endonasal endoscopic approach, and this would therefore need to be combined with or supplanted by an external procedure. Posteriorly and inferiorly, the endoscope has shown itself to be a reasonable alternative to external procedures, though again extension to involve the anterior and lateral wall of the maxillary sinus can be inaccessible in some individuals. This is particularly the case with squamous cell carcinoma of the maxilla, where infiltration beyond the bony confines is especially challenging. Achieving clear margins in these circumstances by an endoscopic approach alone can be technically impossible, and combined techniques such as an extended maxillectomy via a midfacial degloving together with endoscopic control may be employed.

It has been shown by many years of experience with endoscopic orbital decompression[13] that significant portions of orbital periosteum can be removed endonasally, and our experience with preservation of the eye in CFR, as long as the tumor has not spread into the orbital contents, suggests that this approach can be safely undertaken in many patients who hitherto would have had their eye removed on oncologic grounds.[14] Thus, involvement of the periosteum per se would not be a contraindication to endoscopic surgery, but should be determined by frozen section, and the endoscopic surgery might then need to be accompanied by orbital clearance in selected cases.

Superior extension through the skull base and dura and into brain is the subject of other chapters in this book. How aggressively a tumor is pursued will depend on many factors, not least the experience of the surgeons, the tumor type, and patient comorbidities. These limits remain a matter of debate. What constitutes the superior extent for one team may not be deemed so by another.

Dealing with Complications and Minimizing Morbidity

The main reasons for selecting an external approach over an endoscopic one are the morbidity associated with the procedures and the ability to control potential complications. The high long-term success rates for endoscopic repair of cerebrospinal fluid (CSF) leaks and skull base defects irrespective of the repair material used paved the way for extended endoscopic resection of neoplasms in this region.[15,16] However, the resection of more and more extensive lesions resulted in defects that limited the utilization of some repair materials and led to the development of other techniques, including the pedicled septal flap, which increased the size of the dural defect that could be repaired endoscopically.[17] Nonetheless, CSF leaks remain a potential problem and may necessitate a large piece of fascia lata or a pericranial flap, best encompassed via an external approach.

The complication that is most difficult to deal with endoscopically is bleeding. This may be anticipated because of the tumor type, for example, olfactory neuroblastomas, malignant melanomas, or involvement of major vessels, and in selected cases may benefit from preoperative embolization. However, in the majority of cases CFR provides greater access if severe bleeding occurs, and for many surgeons concerns about bleeding from the internal carotid may prompt the use of this approach.[18] Nonetheless, some centers have published strategies for dealing with this eventuality endoscopically, so this may come to be regarded as a relative rather than an absolute contraindication to ESS.[19]

Both external and endoscopic procedures themselves can be associated with complications, which in theory are the same but in practice are significantly less using ESS.[4,6] Some series of CFR have shown very low mortality and morbidity,[9,20] but overall ESS intrinsically is less traumatic even though the amount of tissue removed is comparable, as there is less collateral damage resulting in shorter operating time and hospital stay.[4,21] Nonetheless, we should be very aware of the prognostic factors that determine outcome in these patients for whom the first treatment is the best treatment. Multivariate analyses consistently show that involvement of the dura and brain, involvement of the orbit, and the type of malignancy are the most important factors when large prospective long-term CFR series have been analyzed, and we must therefore choose the approach that best allows us to deal with them.[20] If both ESS and an external approach fulfill these criteria, then either may be chosen, but if we are in any doubt, we should be able to make the transition from one to another, combining conventional craniotomy with endoscopic resection from below.[22–24]

Adjunctive Medical Oncology

Chemoradiation is often given to patients with sinonasal malignancy and, depending on the center, may be given before or after surgery. It has been our experience that it is advisable to delay this treatment when it is used after a craniofacial approach to minimize problems with the skull base repair.[9] This may not be a constraint with ESS if the area of skull base repair is commensurately smaller. Whether this makes a difference to prognosis is unknown.

Table 41.1 Postoperative Follow-Up Protocol for Sinonasal Malignancy

Every 4 months for first 2 years, then every 6 months thereafter depending on histology:
Endoscopic examination under anesthesia
Magnetic resonance imaging: coronal, axial, and sagittal T1-weighted sequences, pre- and postgadolinium–diethylenetriamine pentaacetic acid (DTPA), and axial T2-weighted sequences

Source: Modified from Howard DJ, Lund VJ, Wei WI. Craniofacial resection for tumors of the nasal cavity and paranasal sinuses: a 25-year experience. Head Neck 2006;28:867–873.

Postoperative Follow-Up

Descriptions of the respective techniques are beyond the scope of this chapter and are described in detail elsewhere.[25] However, in all cases, irrespective of the surgical approach, patients must be submitted to rigorous long-term follow-up to ensure that residual or recurrent disease is found early. This may allow endoscopic resection even after CFR. Patients should be available for regular endoscopic examination in an outpatient setting, and posttherapy imaging, usually multiplanar contrast-enhanced MRI, combined with formal examination under anesthesia as indicated by the tumor type and imaging findings. Various protocols have been devised; an example of the one used by the authors is shown in **Table 41.1**.

Outcomes

Craniofacial resection has dramatically improved the outcome for malignant sinonasal tumors affecting the anterior skull base, doubling the survival in many cases (**Tables 41.2**

Table 41.2 Craniofacial Resection: Actuarial Survival for Whole Group and Individual Histologies

Histology	5 Years (%)	10 Years (%)	15 Years (%)	No. of Patients
Malignant	59	40	33	259
Adenocarcinoma	58	40	33	62
Olfactory neuroblastoma	74	50	40	56
Squamous cell carcinoma	53	35	35	34
Chondrosarcoma	94	56	37	24
Adenoid cystic carcinoma	61	31	31	19

Source: Modified from Howard DJ, Lund VJ, Wei WI. Craniofacial resection for tumors of the nasal cavity and paranasal sinuses: a 25-year experience. Head Neck 2006;28:867–873.

Table 41.3 Endoscopic Resection: Actuarial Survival for Whole Group and Individual Histologies in Two Series

Histology	5 Years (%)		No. of Patients	
	Lund[4]	Nicolai[6]	Lund[4]	Nicolai[6]
Malignant	88	91	49	134
Adenocarcinoma	83	94	15	44
Olfactory neuroblastoma	89	100	11	19
Malignant melanoma	80	0	11	14

and **41.3**). However, late recurrence is a feature of these tumors, emphasizing the fallibility of 5-year actuarial survival in predicting cure. Indeed with some tumors (e.g., adenoid cystic carcinoma), the patient will most probably die from the disease unless some other event intervenes. This, together with the rarity, range, and different extents of tumors, makes a direct comparison with endoscopic techniques difficult at present but speaks to the need for collaborative collection of accurate data.[26] Nonetheless, as indicated, there are an increasing number of patients who can be equally well treated with a curative endoscopic resection.[2-6,21] Ultimately the issue is not external versus endoscopic techniques but rather a strategy based on many factors, the most important of which is completely removing the tumor.

References

1. Dulguerov P, Allal AS, Calcaterra TC. Esthesioneuroblastoma: a meta-analysis and review. Lancet Oncol 2001;2:683–690
2. Walch C, Stammberger H, Anderhuber W, Unger F, Köle W, Feichtinger K. The minimally invasive approach to olfactory neuroblastoma: combined endoscopic and stereotactic treatment. Laryngoscope 2000;110:635–640
3. Dave SP, Bared A, Casiano RR. Surgical outcomes and safety of transnasal endoscopic resection for anterior skull tumors. Otolaryngol Head Neck Surg 2007;136:920–927
4. Lund VJ, Howard DJ, Wei WI. Endoscopic resection of malignant tumors of the nose and sinuses. Am J Rhinol 2007;21:89–94
5. Podboj J, Smid L. Endoscopic surgery with curative intent for malignant tumors of the nose and paranasal sinuses. Eur J Surg Oncol 2007;33:1081–1086
6. Nicolai P, Battaglia P, Bignami M, et al. Endoscopic surgery for malignant tumors of the sinonasal tract and adjacent skull base: a 10-year experience. Am J Rhinol 2008;22:308–316
7. Lund VJ, Howard D, Wei W, Spittle M. Olfactory neuroblastoma: past, present, and future? Laryngoscope 2003;113:502–507
8. Lund VJ, Howard DJ, Harding L, Wei WI. Management options and survival in malignant melanoma of the sinonasal mucosa. Laryngoscope 1999;109(2 Pt 1):208–211
9. Howard DJ, Lund VJ, Wei WI. Craniofacial resection for tumors of the nasal cavity and paranasal sinuses: a 25-year experience. Head Neck 2006;28:867–873
10. Lund VJ, Rose GE. Endoscopic transnasal orbital decompression for visual failure due to sphenoid wing meningioma. Eye (Lond) 2006;20:1213–1219
11. Jankowski R, Georgel T, Vignaud JM, et al. Endoscopic surgery reveals that woodworkers' adenocarcinomas originate in the olfactory cleft. Rhinology 2007;45:308–314
12. Madani G, Beale TJ, Lund VJ. Imaging of sinonasal tumors. Semin Ultrasound CT MR 2009;30:25–38
13. Lund VJ, Larkin G, Fells P, Adams G. Orbital decompression for thyroid eye disease: a comparison of external and endoscopic techniques. J Laryngol Otol 1997;111:1051–1055
14. Suárez C, Ferlito A, Lund VJ, et al. Management of the orbit in malignant sinonasal tumors. Head Neck 2008;30:242–250
15. Lund VJ. Endoscopic management of cerebrospinal fluid leaks. Am J Rhinol 2002;16:17–23
16. Zuckerman J, Stankiewicz JA, Chow JM. Long-term outcomes of endoscopic repair of cerebrospinal fluid leaks and meningoencephaloceles. Am J Rhinol 2005;19:582–587
17. Pinheiro-Neto CD, Prevedello DM, Carrau RL, et al. Improving the design of the pedicled nasoseptal flap for skull base reconstruction: a radioanatomic study. Laryngoscope 2007;117:1560–1569
18. Ganly I, Patel SG, Singh B, et al. Complications of craniofacial resection for malignant tumors of the skull base: report of an International Collaborative Study. Head Neck 2005;27:445–451
19. Kassam A, Snyderman CH, Carrau RL, Gardner P, Mintz A. Endoneurosurgical hemostasis techniques: lessons learned from 400 cases. Neurosurg Focus 2005;19:E7 10.3171/foc.2005.19.1.8
20. Ganly I, Patel SG, Singh B, et al. Craniofacial resection for malignant paranasal sinus tumors: report of an international collaborative study. Head Neck 2005;27:575–584
21. Eloy JA, Vivero RJ, Hoang K, et al. Comparison of transnasal endoscopic and open craniofacial resection for malignant tumors of the anterior skull base. Laryngoscope 2009;119:834–840
22. Thaler ER, Kotapka M, Lanza DC, Kennedy DW. Endoscopically assisted anterior cranial skull base resection of sinonasal tumors. Am J Rhinol 1999;13:303–310
23. Batra PS, Citardi MJ, Worley S, Lee J, Lanza DC. Resection of anterior skull base tumors: comparison of combined traditional and endoscopic techniques. Am J Rhinol 2005;19:521–528
24. Yuen AP, Fan YW, Fung CF, Hung KN. Endoscopic-assisted cranionasal resection of olfactory neuroblastoma. Head Neck 2005;27:488–493
25. Lund VJ, Howard DJ. Nose and sinuses. In: Watkinson J, Gilbert R, eds. Stell and Maran's Textbook of Head and Neck Surgery and Oncology. London: Hodder Arnold; 2010: in press
26. Trimarchi M, Lund VJ, Nicolai P, Pini M, Senna M, Howard DJ. Database for the collection and analysis of clinical data and images of neoplasms of the sinonasal tract. Ann Otol Rhinol Laryngol 2004;113:335–337

XI Tips and Pearls in Endoscopic Craniocervical Junction Surgery

42 Microendoscopic Anatomy of the Craniocervical Junction

Alberto Carlos Capel Cardoso, Roger S. Brock, Carolina Martins, Luiz Felipe de Alencastro, and Albert L. Rhoton, Jr.

Tips and Pearls

- Anatomical references are used for bone resections of the clivus:
  - The most critical structure is the internal carotid artery, located in the posterolateral corner of the nasopharynx (fossa of Rosenmüller).
- Extending a line from the hard palate will reach the odontoid apex. After removing the mucosa of the nasopharynx and the atlanto-occipital membrane, the anterior arch of the atlas and the body of the axis are exposed.
- The odontoid resection causes instability of the craniocervical junction. In those situations an occipital-cervical fusion is mandatory.
- The approach for intradural lesions requires special attention, because the basilar plexus hemostasis of this region can be difficult.

Introduction

The craniocervical junction (CVJ) is a complex transition between the skull and the upper cervical spine (**Fig. 42.1**). It comprises the basiocciput, the atlas, and the axis, forming a funnel that provides stability and motion.[1,2] It is a mobile junction responsible for more than a half of spinal axial rotation.[3,4]

The craniocervical junction is located immediately behind the nasopharynx, which can be directly accessed transnasally (**Figs. 42.2, 42.3,** and **42.4**).

An understanding of the bony configuration, joint articulations, ligamentous attachments, and vascular supply is necessary when attempting to reach this unique region through an anterior endoscopic approach.

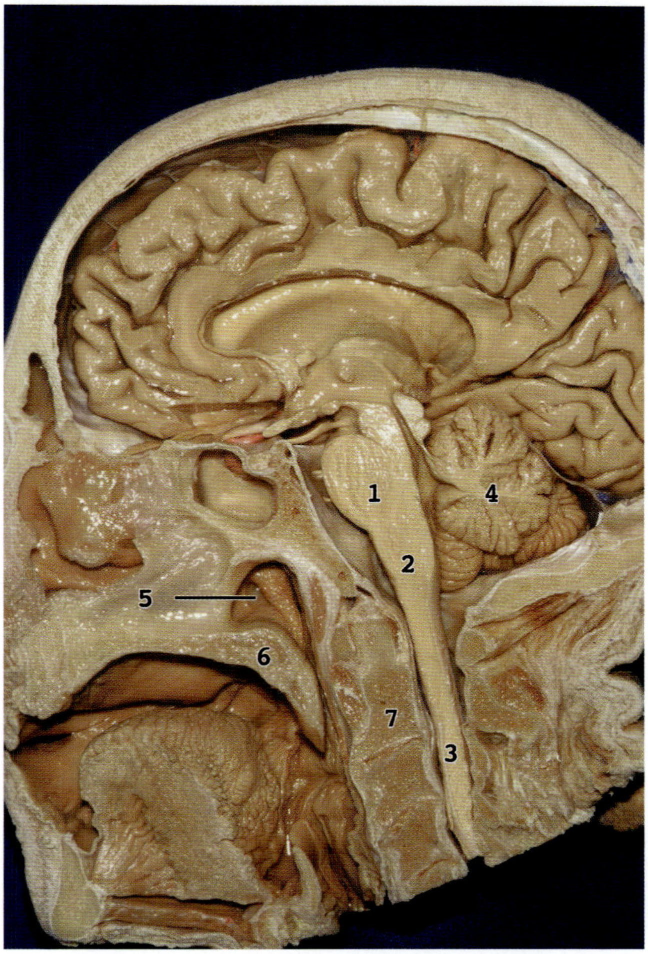

Fig. 42.1 Medial surface of the head. 1, pons; 2, medulla; 3, spinal cord; 4, cerebellum; 5, eustachian tube; 6, soft palate; 7, axis.

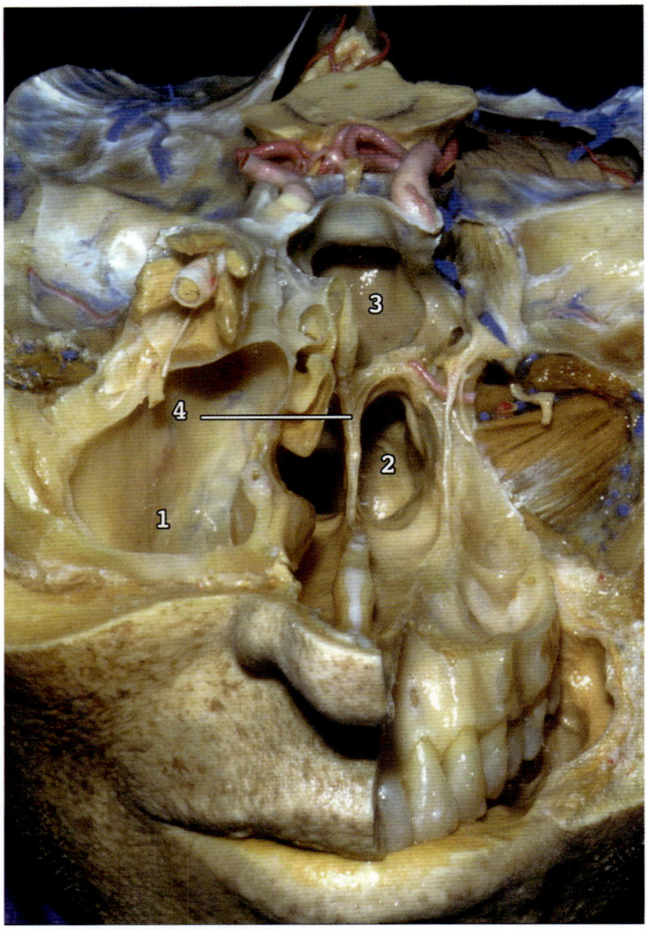

Fig. 42.2 Nasal pathway to the clivus. Dissection shows the structures that form the lateral limit of the transnasal route to the clivus. 1, maxillary sinus; 2, posterior nasopharyngeal wall; 3, sphenoid sinus; 4, vomer.

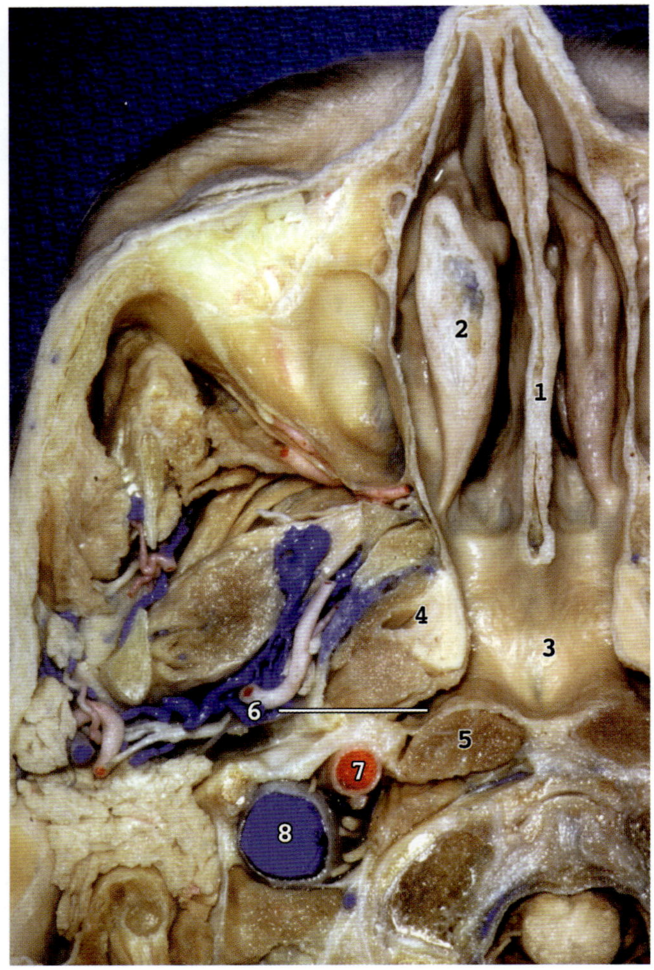

Fig. 42.3 Inferior view of an axial section of the skull base. 1, nasal septum; 2, middle concha; 3, posterior nasopharyngeal wall, which is separated from the lower clivus by the longus capitis muscle and the nasopharyngeal space; 4, eustachian tube; 5, longus capitis muscle; 6, pharyngeal recess (fossa of Rosenmüller), which projects laterally from the posterolateral corner of the nasopharynx with its lateral apex facing the internal carotid artery laterally and the foramen lacerum above; 7, carotid artery; 8, jugular vein.

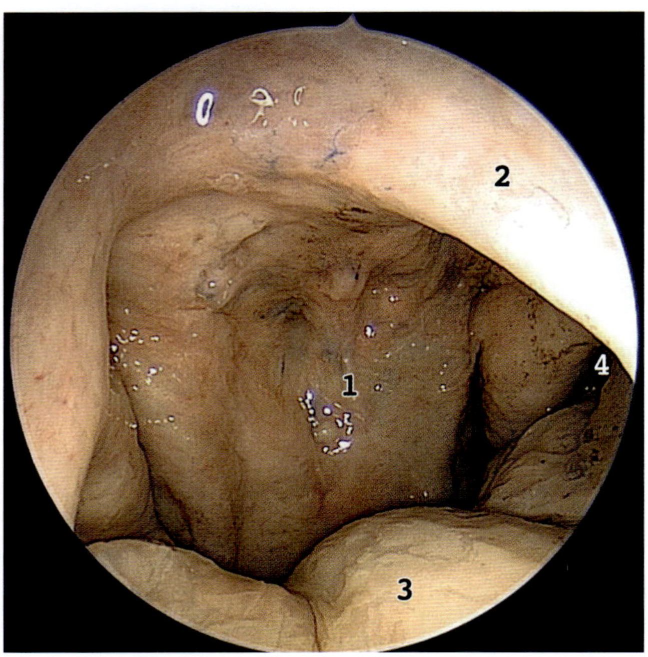

Fig. 42.4 View of the nasal cavity. 1, posterior nasopharyngeal wall; 2, nasal septum; 3, soft palate; 4, eustachian tube.

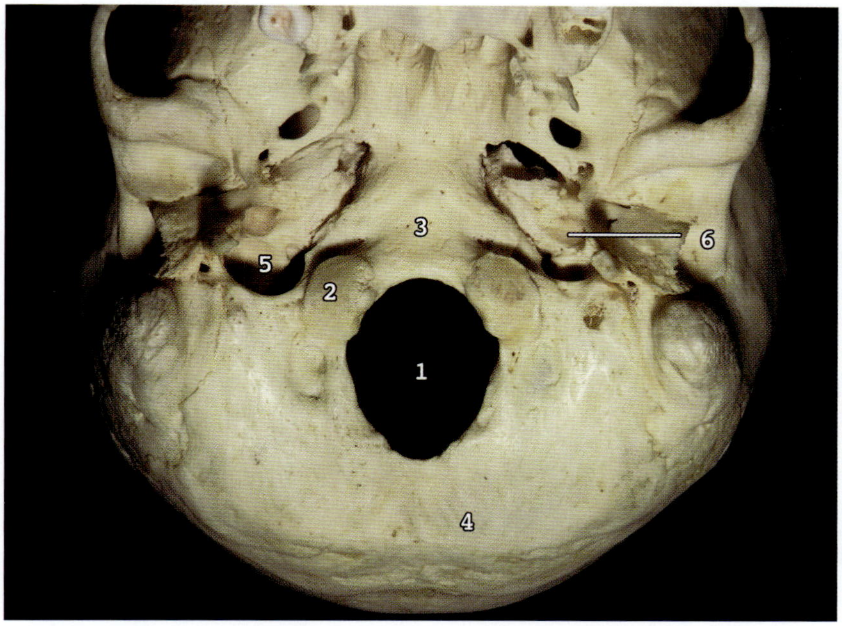

Fig. 42.5 Occipital one and foramen magnum, inferior view. The occipital bone surrounds the oval-shaped foramen magnum, which is wider posteriorly than anteriorly. The occipital bone is divided into a basal (clival) part situated in front of the foramen magnum; a paired condylar part located lateral to the foramen magnum; and a squamosal part located above and behind the foramen magnum. 1, foramen magnum; 2, occipital condyle; 3, clivus; 4, squamous part of the occipital bone; 5, jugular foramen; 6, carotid canal.

Bone Elements

Occipital Bone

The occipital bone can be divided into a basal part situated in front of the foramen magnum, a squamosal part located above and behind the foramen magnum, and paired condylar parts located lateral to the foramen magnum (**Figs. 42.5, 42.6, 42.7,** and **42.8**).

The Atlas

The atlas, the first cervical vertebra, differs from the other cervical vertebrae by being ring shaped and by lacking a vertebra body and a spinous process. It consists of two thick lateral masses connected in front by a short anterior arch and behind by a longer curved posterior arch. The position of the usual vertebral body is occupied by the odontoid process of the axis (**Fig. 42.9**). The upper surface of each lateral mass has an oval concave facet that articulates with the occipital

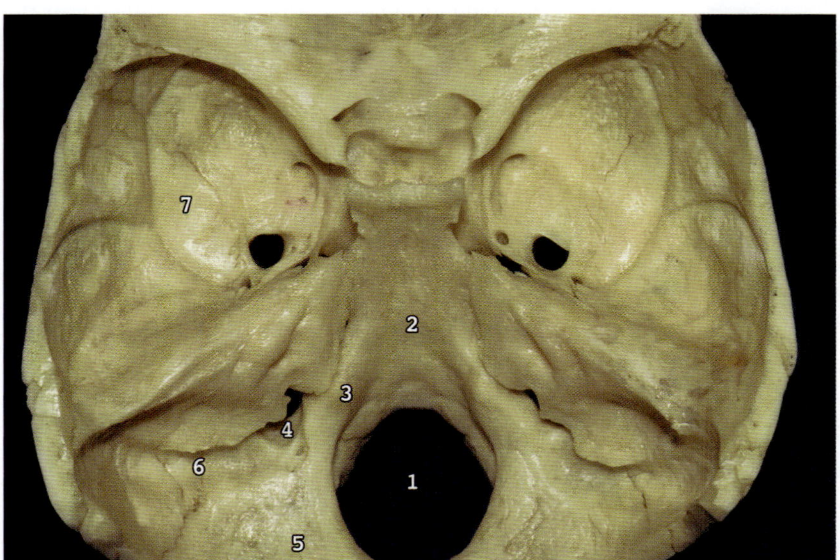

Fig. 42.6 Superior view of the occipital bone. 1, foramen magnum; 2, clivus, which is separated on each side from the petrous part of the temporal bone by the petroclival fissure; 3, jugular process of the occipital bone, which extends laterally from the posterior half of the condyle and articulates with the jugular surface of the temporal bone; 4, jugular foramen, which is bordered posteriorly by the jugular process of the occipital bone and anteriorly by the jugular fossa of the petrous temporal bone; 5, squamous part of the occipital bone; 6, sulcus of the sigmoid sinus, which crosses the superior surface of the jugular process; 7, temporal fossa.

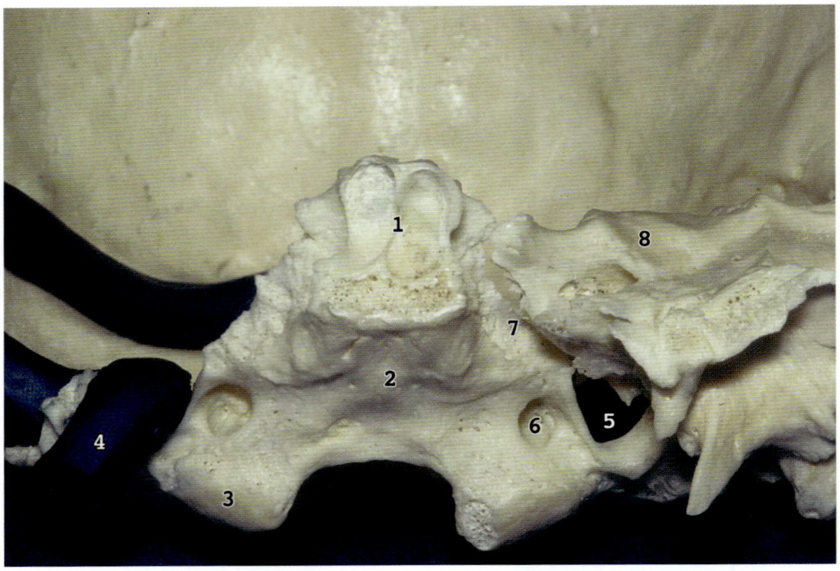

Fig. 42.7 Anterior view of the occipital bone. 1, sphenoid sinus; 2, pharyngeal tubercle, which gives attachment to the fibrous raphe of the pharynx; 3, occipital condyle; 4, jugular vein; 5, jugular foramen; 6, hypoglossal canal, which is situated above the condyle; 7, petroclival fissure; 8, temporal bone.

condyle. The inferior surface of each lateral mass has a circular slightly concave facet that articulates with the superior articular facet of the axis (**Fig. 42.10**).

The Axis

The axis is the second cervical vertebra. It forms a pivot for the atlas and the head to rotate. The axis is distinguished by the odontoid process (dens), which projects upward from the body. The dens and body are flanked by a pair of large oval facets that extend laterally from the body and articulate with the inferior facets of the atlas. The transverse process of the axis is small (**Fig. 42.11**).

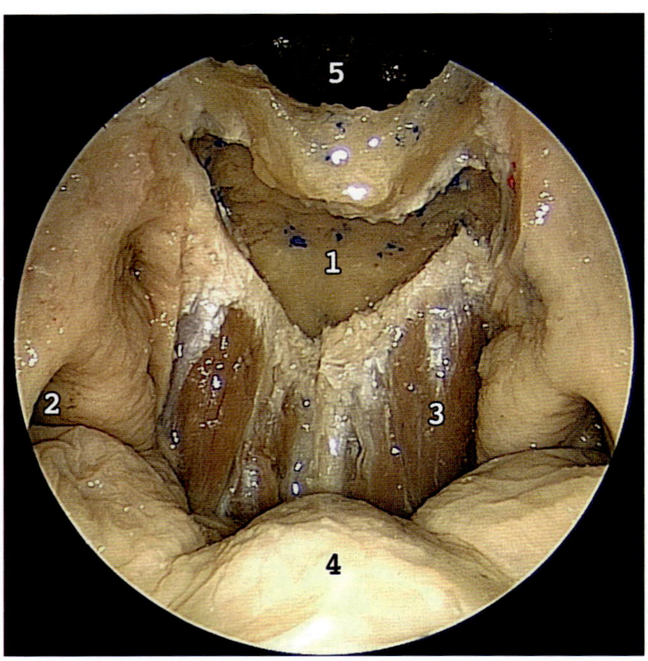

Fig. 42.8 Anterior view. The nasal septum has been removed. 1, clivus; 2, eustachian tube; 3, longus capitis muscle; 4, soft palate; 5, sphenoid sinus.

Ligamentous Anatomy

The special arrangements of the craniocervical junction ligaments are remarkable, allowing a complex motion and provide stability.[5]

The cruciform ligament and alar ligament are the most important for CVJ stability.

Cruciform Ligament

The cruciform ligament has transverse and vertical parts that form a cross behind the dens. The cranial extension of the vertical part is attached to the upper surface of the clivus between the apical ligament of the dens and the tectorial membrane. The lower band is attached to the posterior surface of the body of the axis.

The transverse part, called the transverse ligament, is one of the most important ligaments of the body. It is a thick strong band that arches across the ring of the atlas. The neck of the dens is constricted where it is embraced posteriorly by the transverse ligament (**Figs. 42.12, 42.13,** and **42.14**).

The biomechanical role of the cruciform ligament is to limit the anterior movement of the atlas on the axis, preventing anterior translation and flexion. Disruption of these ligamentous structures destabilizes the craniocervical junction.[6]

Alar Ligaments

The alar ligaments are two strong bands that arise on each side of the upper part of the dens and extend obliquely su-

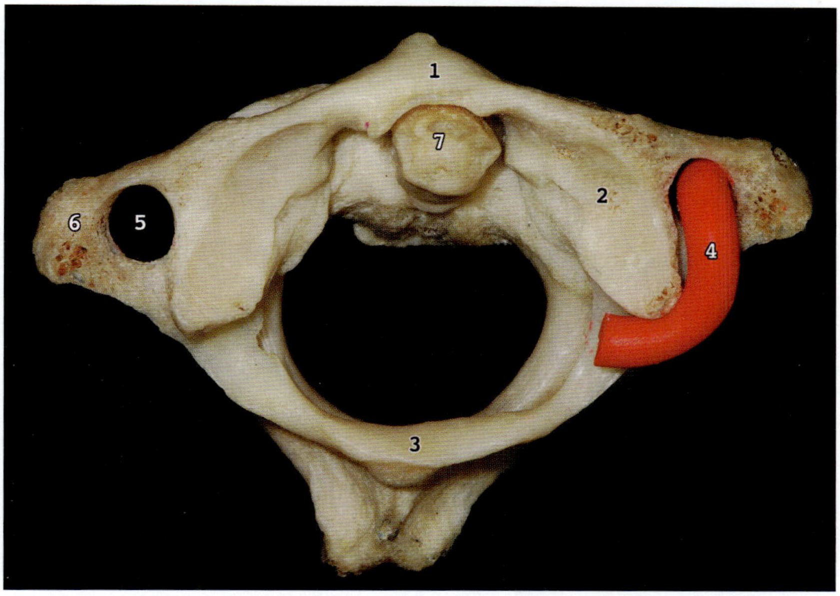

Fig. 42.9 Superior view of the atlas and the axis. The atlas consists of two thick lateral masses situated at the anteromedial part of the ring, which are connected in front by a short anterior arch and posteriorly by a longer curved posterior arch. 1, anterior arch of the atlas; 2, superior articular facet is an oval, concave facet that articulates with the occipital condyle; 3, posterior arch of the atlas; 4, vertebral artery (VA); 5, transverse foramina; 6, transverse process; 7, dens of the axis.

perolateral to attach to the medial surfaces of the occipital (**Figs. 42.14, 42.15,** and **42.16**). Their function is to limit axial rotation between the atlas and the skull.

Apical Ligament

The apical ligament of the odontoid process extends from the tip of the dens to the anterior margin of the foramen magnum and is situated between the anterior atlanto-occipital membrane and the superior prolongation of the cruciform ligament (**Figs. 42.12** and **42.14**).

Tectorial Membrane

The tectorial membrane is a cephalic extension of the posterior longitudinal ligament that covers the dens and cruciform

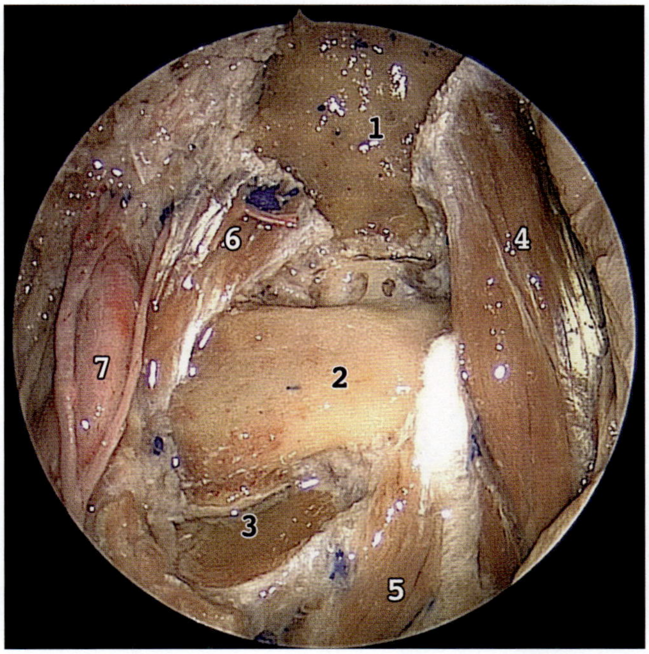

Fig. 42.10 Anterior view. The right longus capitis muscle has been removed. 1, clivus; 2, anterior arch of the atlas; 3, atlantoaxial joint; 4, left longus capitis muscle; 5, longus colli muscle; 6, rectus capitis anterior muscle; 7, carotid artery.

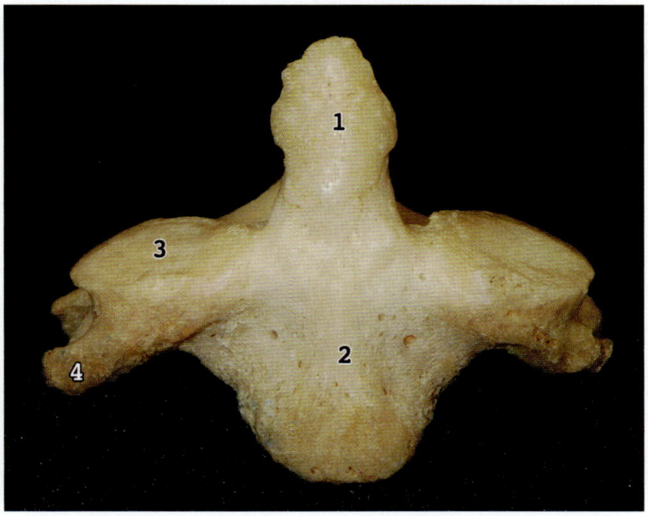

Fig. 42.11 The anterior view of the axis. The axis is distinguished by the odontoid process (dens), which projects upward from the body. 1, the dens, which is 1.0 to 1.5 cm long, and about 1 cm wide; 2, the body; 3, superior articular facet, which articulates with the inferior facet of the atlas; 4, transverse process of the axis is small.

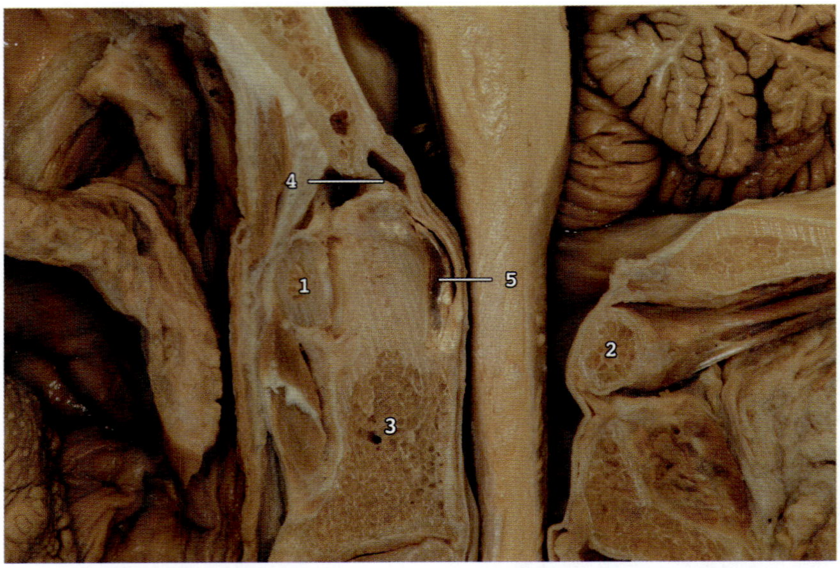

Fig. 42.12 Medial surface of the craniocervical junction. 1, anterior arch of the atlas, which is located anterior to the dens; 2, posterior arch of the atlas; 3, body of the axis; 4, apical ligament of the odontoid process; 5, transverse ligament, which is located behind the dens and divides the vertebral canal into a larger posterior compartment containing the dura and the spinal cord, and a smaller anterior compartment containing the odontoid process.

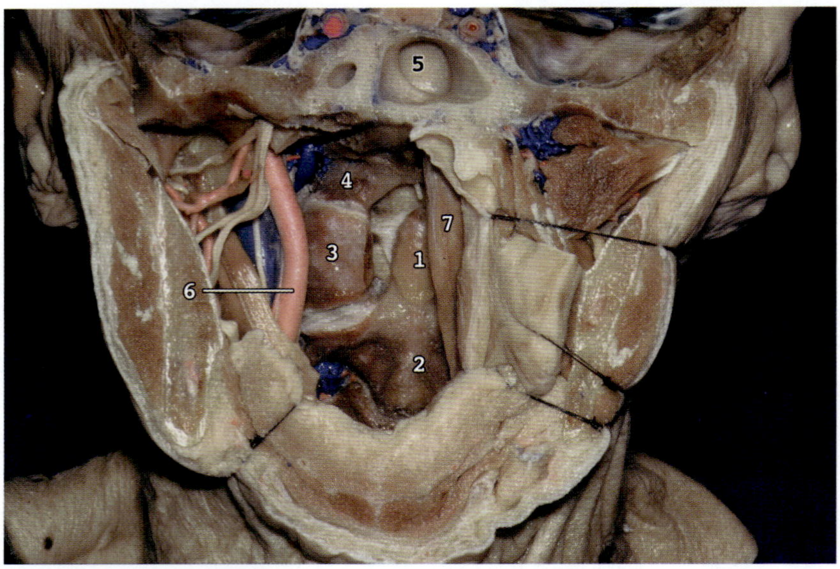

Fig. 42.13 Anterior view of a coronal section showing the relationship of the foramen magnum and clivus to the nasal an oral cavities, pharynx, and infratemporal fossa. 1, odontoid tip; 2, axis body; 3, lateral mass of the atlas; 4, occipital condyle; 5, sphenoid sinus; 6, carotid artery; 7, longus capitis muscle.

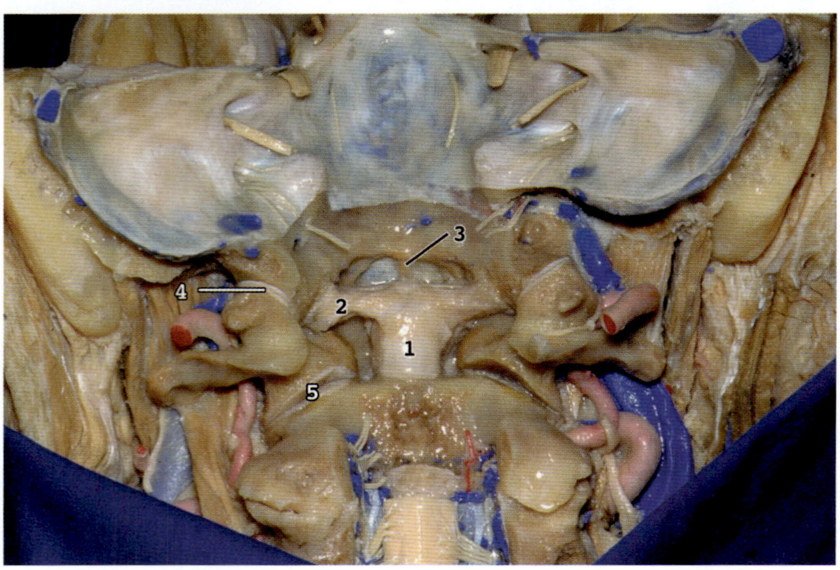

Fig. 42.14 Posterior view of the craniocervical junction. 1, odontoid process; 2, alar ligament, which arises on each side of the upper part of the dens and extends obliquely superolateral to attach to the medial surfaces of the occipital condyles; 3, apical ligament of the odontoid process, which extends from the tip of the dens to the anterior margin of the foramen magnum; 4, atlanto-occipital joint of the left side; 5, atlantoaxial joint of the left side.

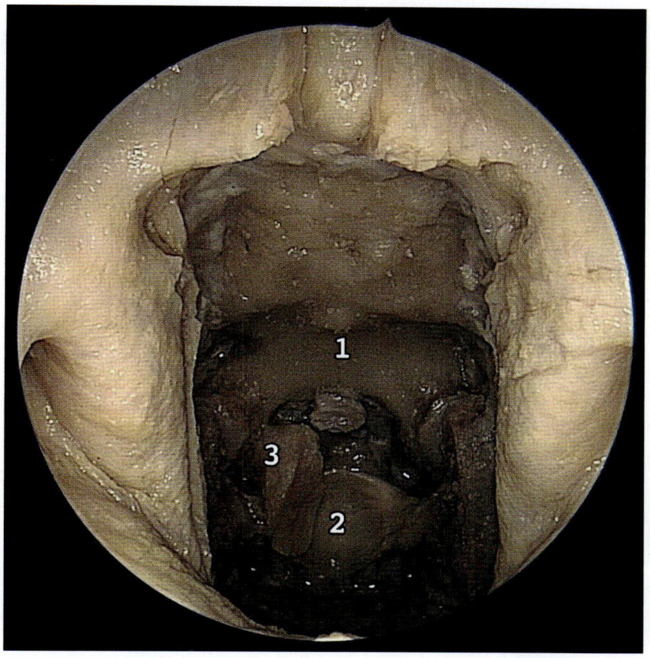

Fig. 42.15 Anterior view. The anterior arch of the atlas and the dens have been removed. 1, clivus; 2, transverse ligament, which is a thick strong band that arches across the ring of the atlas behind the dens; 3, right alar ligament, which has been detached from the dens.

ligament. It is attached below to the posterior surface of the body of the axis, above to the upper surface of the occipital bone in front of the foramen magnum, and laterally to the medial sides of the atlanto-occipital joints.

Neural Structures

The neural structures situated in the region of the craniocervical junction are the caudal part of the brainstem, cerebellum, and fourth ventricle, the rostral part of the spinal cord, and the lower cranial and upper cervical nerves (**Fig. 42.17**).

The anterior surface of the medulla is formed by the medullary pyramids, which face the clivus, the anterior edge of the foramen magnum, and the rostral part of the odontoid process.

The glossopharyngeal nerve arises from the upper medulla posterior to the upper one third of the olive, just caudal to the origin of the facial nerve and above the origin of the rostral rootlets of the vagus nerve.[7]

The accessory nerve is the only cranial nerve that passes through the foramen magnum. It has a cranial part composed of the rootlets that arise from the medulla and join the vagus nerve, and a spinal portion formed by the union of a series of rootlets that arise from the lower medulla and upper spinal cord (**Fig. 42.18**). The lowest level of origin of the rootlets contributing to the accessory nerves is at the C7 root level.

The hypoglossal nerve arises along the front of the inferior olive as a series of rootlets that converge on the dural orifice of the hypoglossal canal.

Arterial Structures

The major arteries related to the craniocervical junction are the vertebral artery, the posteroinferior cerebellar artery (PICA), and the anterior spinal artery.[8]

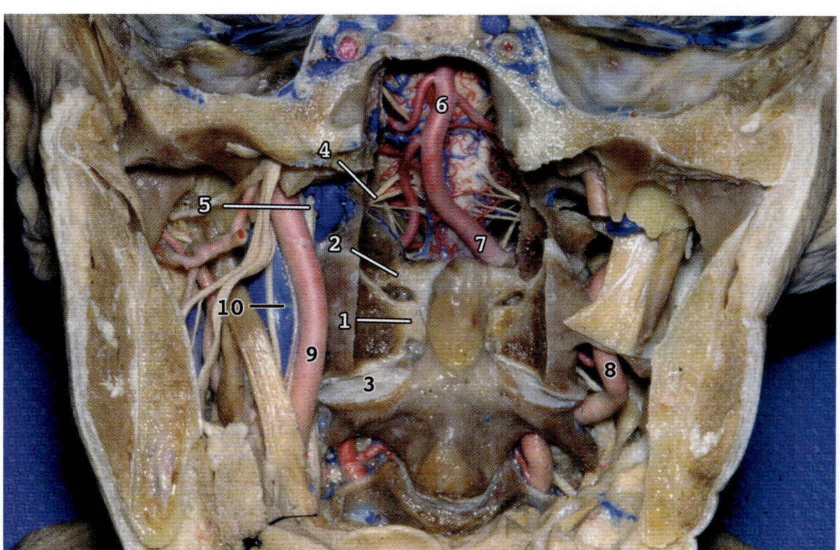

Fig. 42.16 The clivus and anterior arch of C1 have been removed. The dura has been opened to expose the vertebral and basilar arteries. The dens has been preserved. 1, transverse part of the cruciform ligament, called the transverse ligament, which extends across the back of the dens and attaches to a tubercle on the medial side of each lateral mass of the axis; 2, alar ligament, which attaches to the lateral edges of the foramen; 3, atlantoaxial joint; 4, hypoglossal nerve, which enters the hypoglossal canal; 5, hypoglossal nerve, which exits the inferolateral part of the hypoglossal canal and descends between the internal carotid artery and the internal jugular vein; 6, basilar artery; 7, intradural part of the vertebral artery; 8, extradural part of the vertebral artery; 9, internal carotid artery; 10, internal jugular vein.

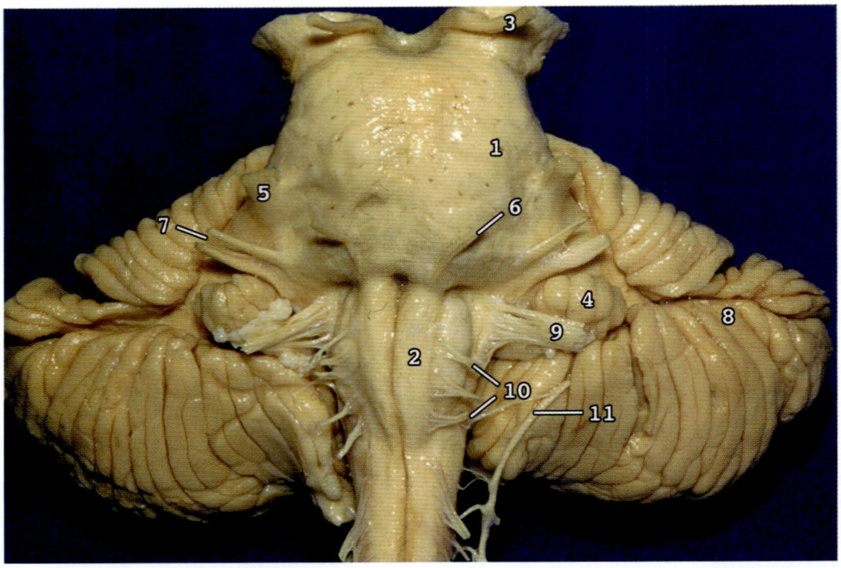

Fig. 42.17 Petrosal cerebellar surface. 1, pons; 2, medulla. The pons and medulla are separated by the pontomedullary sulcus, rostral to the medullary pyramids. 3, oculomotor nerve; 4, flocculus; 5, trigeminal nerve, which arises from the midpons; 6, abducens nerve, which arises in the medial part of the pontomedullary sulcus, rostral to the medullary pyramids; 7, facial and vestibulocochlear nerves, which arise at the lateral end of the pontomedullary sulcus immediately rostral to the foramen of Luschka; 8, inferior petrous surface of the cerebellum; 9, glossopharyngeal, vagus, and accessory nerves, which arise posterior to the olives; 10, hypoglossal nerve, which arises anterior to the olives; 11, cervical rootlets of the accessory nerve.

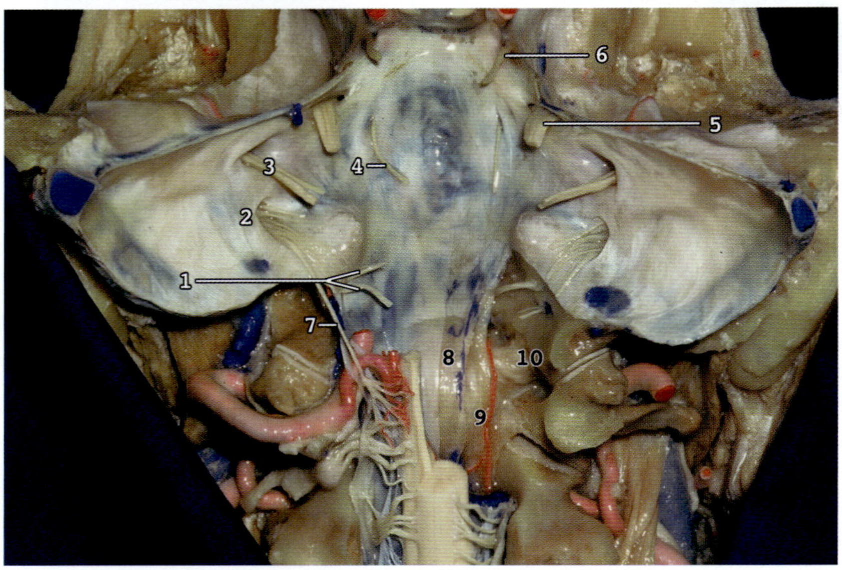

Fig. 42.18 Posterior view of the cranial base with the cranial nerves. 1, hypoglossal nerve; 2, glossopharyngeal, vagus, and accessory nerves; 3, facial and vestibular nerves; 4, abducens nerve; 5, trigeminal nerve; 6, oculomotor nerve; 7, spinal portion of the accessory nerve; 8, tectorial membrane; 9, cruciform ligament; 10, alar ligament.

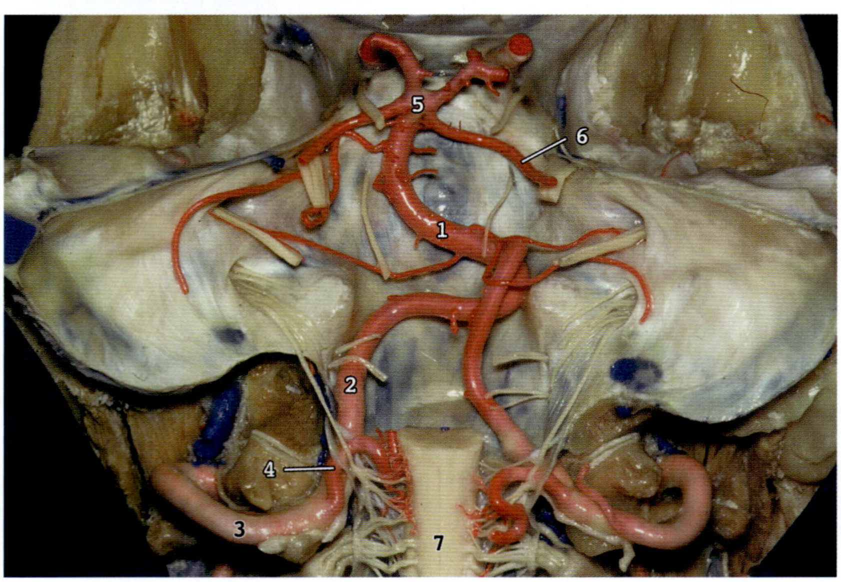

Fig. 42.19 Posterior view of the cranial base with the cranial nerves and arteries preserved. 1, basilar artery; 2, intradural segment of the vertebral artery; 3, third segment of the VA, which passes medially behind the lateral mass of the atlas and atlanto-occipital joint; 4, posteroinferior cerebellar artery (PICA) with an extradural origin, which passes through the dura and courses along the side of the medulla in front of the rootlets of the accessory nerve; 5, basilar apex, which is located behind the dorsum sellae; 6, superior cerebellar artery (SCA), which arises from the basilar artery near the apex, and passes below the oculomotor nerve and above the trigeminal nerve; 7, upper spinal cord.

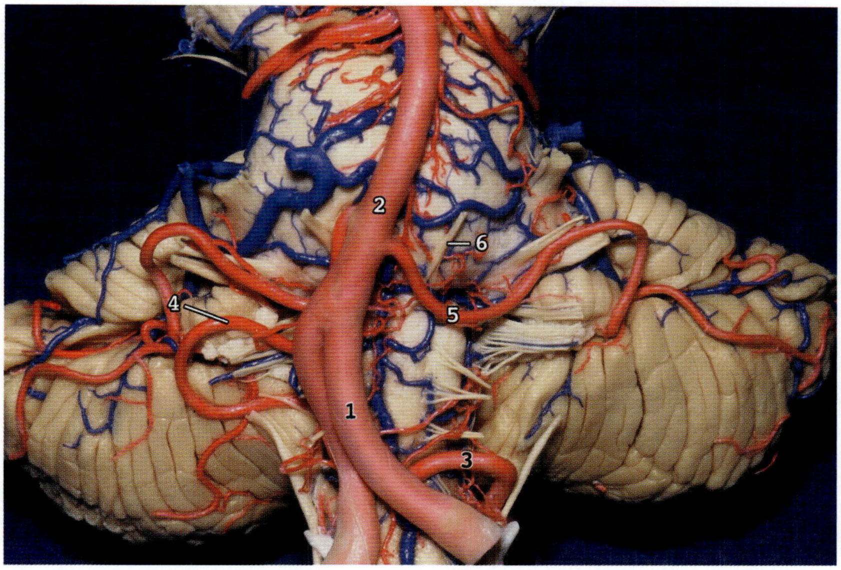

Fig. 42.20 Anterior view of the brainstem and cerebellar arteries. 1, vertebral artery (VA), which ascends from the lower to the upper anterior surface of the medulla. The VA joins with the other VAs at or near the pontomedullary sulcus to form the basilar artery. 2, basilar artery (BA). The PICA is the largest branch that arises from the vertebral artery that supplies the posteroinferior part of the cerebellum. 3, PICA of the left side, which arises inferior to the hypoglossal rootlets; 4, right PICA origins, which are located at level of the exits of the hypoglossal rootlets from the medulla; 5, left anteroinferior cerebellar artery (AICA), which passes below the abducens and between the facial and vestibulocochlear nerves before reaching the cerebellopontine fissure and petrosal cerebellar surface; 6, abducens nerve.

Vertebral Artery

The paired vertebral arteries pass behind the lateral masses of the axis, enter the dura mater behind the occipital condyles, ascend through the foramen magnum to the front of the medulla, and join to form the basilar artery at the pontomedullary junction (**Figs. 42.19** and **42.20**).

The intradural segment begins at the dural foramina just inferior to the lateral edge of the foramen magnum. Once inside the dura mater, the artery ascends from the lower lateral to the upper anterior surface of the medulla. It courses in front of, or between, the hypoglossal rootlets, and crosses the pyramid to join with the other vertebral artery at or near the pontomedullary sulcus to form the basilar artery.[9] The branches arising from the vertebral artery in the region of the foramen magnum are the posterior spinal, anterior spinal, PICA, and anterior and posterior meningeal arteries. Surgeons should pay attention to the anterior spinal artery when performing an anterior approach.[10]

Posteroinferior Cerebellar Artery

The posteroinferior cerebellar artery (PICA) is the largest branch of the vertebral artery that supplies the posteroinferior part of the cerebellum (**Figs. 42.20** and **42.21**). It usually originates with the dura mater, but it may infrequently originate from the terminal extradural part of the vertebral artery.

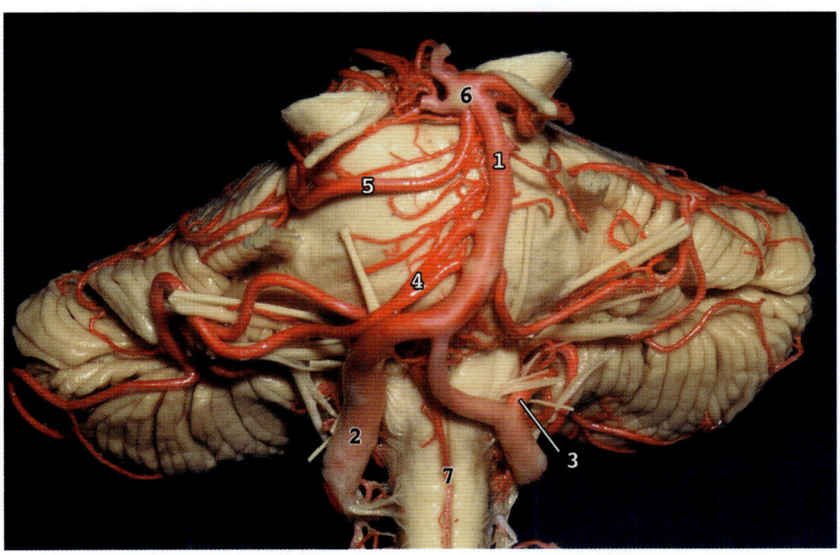

Fig. 42.21 Brainstem and petrous surface. 1, basilar artery (BA); 2, VA of the right side, which courses in front of the hypoglossal rootlets before joining with the other vertebral artery to form the BA; 3, PICA; 4, duplicate AICA; 5, superior cerebellar artery (SCA), which arises in front of the midbrain from the VA and passes below the oculomotor nerve, and encircles the brainstem near the pontomesencephalic junction and above the trigeminal nerve; 6, basilar apex; 7, anterior spinal artery, which is formed by the union of the paired anterior ventral spinal arteries, which originate from the vertebral arteries near the origin of the basilar artery. The anterior spinal artery descends through the foramen magnum on the anterior surface of the medulla and the spinal cord. On the medulla, it supplies the pyramids and their decussation.

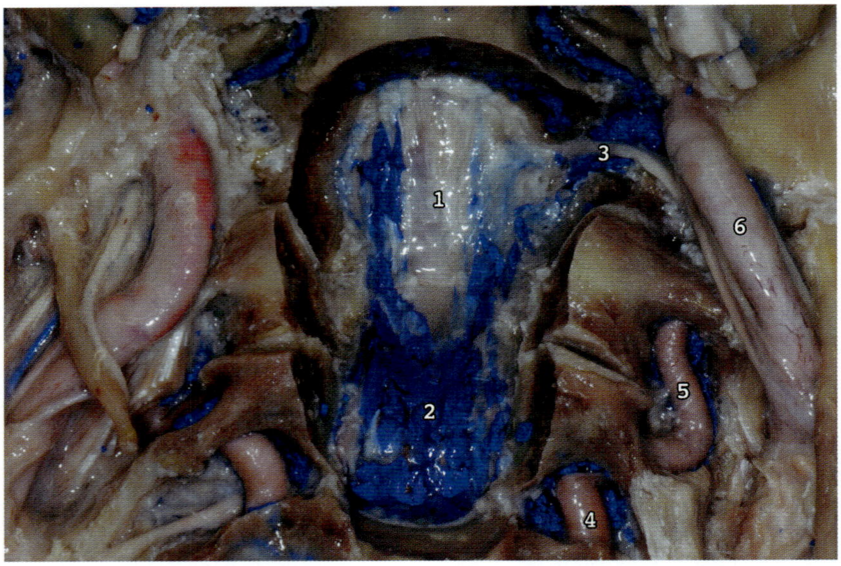

Fig. 42.22 Anterior view. The inferior clivus, anterior arch of the atlas, the dens, and the body of the axis have been removed. The transverse, the apical, the pair of alar ligaments, and the tectorial membrane have been detached. 1, dura of the craniocervical junction; 2, basilar plexus; 3, hypoglossal nerve; 4, VA between the axis and C3; 5, VA between the axis and the atlas; 6, carotid artery.

Anterior Spinal Artery

The anterior spinal artery descends through the foramen magnum on the anterior surface of the medulla and the spinal cord in or near the anteromedian fissure (**Fig. 42.21**). On the medulla, it supplies the pyramids and their decussation, the hypoglossal nuclei and nerves, and the posterior longitudinal fasciculus.

Venous Plexus

The basilar venous plexus is located between the layers of the dura mater on the upper clivus (**Fig. 42.22**). It is formed by interconnecting venous channels that anastomose with the inferior petrosal sinuses laterally, the cavernous sinuses superiorly, and the marginal sinus and epidural venous plexus inferiorly. The inferior petrosal sinuses extend along the petroclival fissure and communicate above with the basilar sinus and below with the jugular bulb. The sigmoid sinus descends along the sigmoid groove and exits the cranium through the sigmoid part of the jugular foramen.

References

1. Rhoton AL Jr. The foramen magnum. Neurosurgery 2000;47(3, Suppl): S155–S193
2. Menezes AH, Traynelis VC. Anatomy and biomechanics of normal craniovertebral junction (a) and biomechanics of stabilization (b). Childs Nerv Syst 2008;24:1091–1100
3. Dickman CA, Lekovic GP. Biomechanical considerations for stabilization of the craniovertebral junction. Clin Neurosurg 2005;52:205–213
4. White AA III, Panjabi MM. The clinical biomechanics of the occipito-atlantoaxial complex. Orthop Clin North Am 1978;9:867–878
5. Crawford NR, Hurlbert RJ. Anatomy and biomechanics of the craniocervical junction. Semin Neurosurg 2002;13:101–110
6. Menezes AH. Developmental abnormalities of the craniocervical junction. In: Winn RH, ed. Youmans Neurological Surgery, 5th ed. Philadelphia: Saunders, 2004:3331–3345
7. Katsuta T, Rhoton AL Jr, Matsushima T. The jugular foramen: microsurgical anatomy and operative approaches. Neurosurgery 1997;41: 149–201, discussion 201–202
8. Lister JR, Rhoton AL Jr, Matsushima T, Peace DA. Microsurgical anatomy of the posterior inferior cerebellar artery. Neurosurgery 1982;10: 170–199
9. Matsushima T, Rhoton AL Jr, de Oliveira E, Peace DA. Microsurgical anatomy of the veins of the posterior fossa. J Neurosurg 1983;59:63–105
10. de Oliveira E, Rhoton AL Jr, Peace DA. Microsurgical anatomy of the region of the foramen magnum. Surg Neurol 1985;24:293–352

43 Craniocervical Junction: Endoscopic Endonasal Approach

Paul A. Gardner, Daniel M. Prevedello, Amin B. Kassam, Carl H. Snyderman, and Ricardo L. Carrau

Tips and Pearls

- The soft palate is never affected due to the rostral to caudal angle of approach.
- The angle of approach and the caudal limit of access for the endoscopic endonasal approach (EEA) to the upper cervical spine is determined by the nasopalatine (Kassam) line.
- Disease into and below the body of C2 in the absence of basilar invagination requires either a transoral or transcervical approach.
- If there is an arthritic pannus with minimal or no neural compression, an isolate posterior fusion is adequate for treatment.
- Radiographic evaluation usually consists of both computed tomography angiography (CTA) and magnetic resonance imaging (MRI). CTA demonstrates the bony disease and anatomy while evaluating the presence of an ectatic parapharyngeal internal carotid artery (ICA). MRI better evaluates tumor involvement, soft tissue disease, and neural compression.
- Patients with cervicomedullary compression have somatosensory evoked potential (SSEP) monitoring before, during, and after positioning.
- To widen the corridor, the inferior turbinates can be lateralized.
- The ring of C1 is resected with a high-speed drill or Kerrison rongeur.
- The dens should be drilled from the tip downward to avoid leaving a free-floating bony fragment to be detached from the apical and transverse ligaments.
- To expand the approach laterally, particularly for tumors, the medial aspect of the occipital condyle can be drilled. The drilling process can be extended up to the hypoglossal canal.
- If there is pannus present, it should be resected until the underlying dura is observed to be pulsatile, confirming decompression.
- Simple odontoid resections are reconstructed by merely applying fibrin glue to the defect.
- If there is a dural defect, vascularized tissue provides the lowest rates of postoperative cerebrospinal fluid (CSF) leak and often requires fat graft augmentation.

Introduction

The craniocervical junction presents a surgical challenge because of the complexity of its anatomy and the difficulty accessing it. This region contains critical mobile joints that enable the majority of movement of the head relative to the neck and body in all directions. It also integrates the vertebral arteries, lower cranial nerves, and upper spinal nerves. The parapharyngeal internal carotid arteries (ICAs) limit access depending on the corridor of approach chosen. Anterior approaches for ventral pathology of the craniocervical junction present difficulties due to the craniofacial structures that must be transgressed. Traditional strategies for addressing this include facial, sublabial, or oropharyngeal incisions, which can require palatal or mandibular splitting. All of these strategies introduce morbidity related to the structures that are affected. The endoscopic endonasal approach (EEA) provides an anterior corridor that avoids many of these morbidities.

Advantages and Limitations

The main advantages of the EEA to the craniocervical junction result from the angle of approach and the fact that it is the nasopharynx and not the oropharynx that is transgressed. The nose and paranasal sinuses provide rostral access and a rostral-to-caudal angle that provides excellent access to the majority of pathologies at the craniocervical junction. This is especially true in cases with any degree of basilar invagination.

The foramen magnum and upper cervical spine are located immediately behind the nasopharynx, which can be easily and directly accessed transnasally. The nasopharynx has significantly fewer and less virulent bacterial flora than the oropharynx.[1] The palate is never affected by the approach, as the rostral-to-caudal angle of approach is parallel to the angle of the soft palate, thereby never transgressing it.

The angle of approach and the caudal limit of access for EEA to the upper cervical spine is determined by the nasopalatine (Kassam) line. This line is drawn on a midsagittal image (typically computed tomography [CT]) from the bony nasal bridge to the bony hard palate and extended into the depth (**Fig. 43.1**). Where this line crosses the second cervical vertebrae predicts the caudal limit of access. In our early clinical series, the actual point reached was an average of 12.7 mm rostral to the point predicted by the nasopalatine line.[2] The difference is likely due to soft tissues, which are accounted for by the bony landmarks, variability in midsagittal

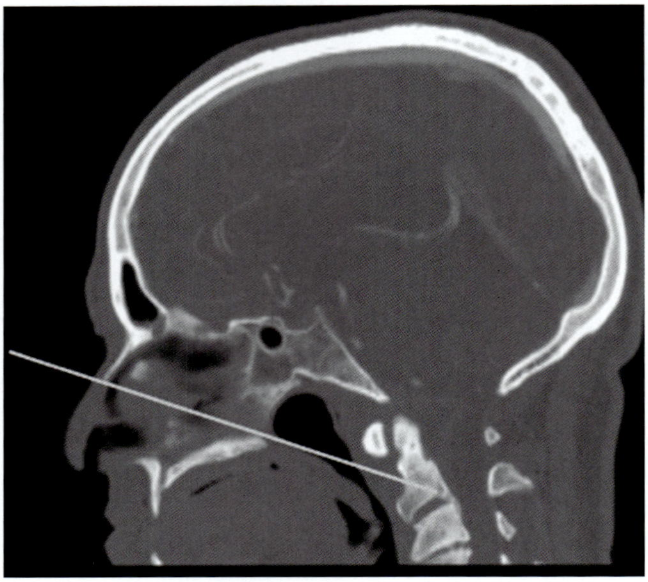

Fig. 43.1 Midsagittal computed tomography (CT) reconstruction showing the nasopalatine line, drawn from the bony nasal bridge to the hard palate and extended into the depth. This approximates the caudal extent of access via an endonasal approach.

imaging, and the fact that most cases do not require that the lowest possible point be decompressed.

With the above caudal access as the main limitation, we have never encountered a case of degenerative pannus or os odontoideum compression that could not be accessed transnasally. Caudal access does become an issue when addressing tumors. Foramen magnum meningiomas may have disease that extends below the endonasal reach. In addition, bony tumors such as chordomas or sarcomas often are encountered below that level, and the approach must not limit the degree of resection. Often, the entire C2 body is involved, and this cannot be completely resected via an EEA. Disease into and below the body of C2 in the absence of basilar invagination requires either a transoral or transcervical approach.

Laterally, access is limited by the parapharyngeal ICAs and jugular foramen. Especially when dealing with disease in and around the ICAs, proximal vascular control becomes difficult or impossible. It is often necessary to add a cervical approach for both lower pole tumor dissection and proper ICA control in the event of an injury.

Indications and Preoperative Evaluation

The common disease processes treated at the cervicomedullary junction are degenerative (rheumatoid and osteoarthritis) or posttraumatic atlantoaxial disease, meningiomas, and chordomas and other rare bony tumors. In the case of degenerative disease or benign tumors, the indications for EEA are no different from those for traditional anterior approaches. For example, if there is an arthritic pannus with minimal or no neural compression, a posterior fusion is adequate for treatment. However, if there is significant neural compression, especially if caused by bone rather than soft pannus, resection of the odontoid usually provides the quickest and most effective decompression.

With malignancy, accurate tissue diagnosis and, depending upon the tumor type, complete resection are usually the goals. If biopsy or palliation is the only goal, an EEA can provide a low morbidity corridor. However, all approaches must be considered when attempting gross total resection to ensure that the EEA is not being used by default. The limitations discussed above must be carefully evaluated prior to choosing an endonasal route.

Radiographic evaluation usually consists of both CT angiography (CTA) and magnetic resonance imaging (MRI). CTA shows the bony disease and involvement while evaluating limitations that may exist due to vascular involvement or anomalies (e.g., ectatic parapharyngeal ICA). MRI may better determine the extent of tumor involvement, soft tissue disease, and neural compression.

Other than radiographic and comorbidity evaluations to determine the goals of surgery and best approach, there are specific clinical symptoms that require careful preoperative evaluation when addressing disease of the craniocervical junction. Patients should be questioned closely for symptoms of dysphagia, aspiration, or voice changes. If these symptoms are present, they should undergo evaluation by an otolaryngologist to determine vocal cord function. If there is vocal fold paresis or paralysis, regardless of the approach being used, prophylactic tracheostomy should be strongly considered. This can greatly ease perioperative care and avoid further worsening caused by oral intubation.

Finally, range of motion should be evaluated preoperatively. This is helpful both for determining safe movement of the patient once under anesthesia as well as to guide clinical decision making related to the reducibility of compression and fixation options and consequences.

Surgical Technique

Perhaps the most critical part of a successful endonasal surgery is the development of a team of surgeons who can work together. We perform all surgeries with a team consisting of an otolaryngologist trained in open skull base surgery and endoscopic sinus surgery, and a neurosurgeon trained in open skull base surgery and comfortable with endoscopy. This team approach is not the usual skull base team approach where one surgeon performs one portion and then leaves, and the other surgeon then performs the other part. Rather, the two surgeons operate in parallel, with dynamic endoscopy and team problem solving. Dynamic endoscope movement takes full advantage of the endoscope by providing both close views when needed, mixed rapidly with panoramic views for orientation and instrument introduction. The team also learns to operate seamlessly, knowing what steps the other will take next and anticipating them. Finally, two surgeons working together are much more likely to avoid complications as a result of a single surgeon's error.

Operating Room Setup

Patients with cervicomedullary compression have somatosensory evoked potential (SSEP) monitoring before, during, and after positioning. This may detect a meaningful increase in compression related to positioning. In addition, patients undergoing EEAs for craniocervical junction disease may benefit from electromyographic (EMG) monitoring of the hypoglossal nerves. If relevant, in cases with lateral extension of pathology, EMG monitoring of all lower cranial nerves is useful.

When learning new techniques, especially involving the addition of an endoscope and the complex anatomy of the skull base, neuronavigation is critical. Although MRI can be very helpful with preoperative evaluation and operative planning, CTA guides much of the surgery. Avoiding vascular injury and identifying critical bony landmarks are foremost. This is especially true with the anteromedial corridor provided by an endonasal approach, which is chosen to avoid crossing critical neural structures.

We operate with both members of the team on the patient's right side. We find this to be the easiest for right-handed surgeons, allowing their dominant hand the greatest freedom of movement. We prepare the midface and abdomen (in case of fat graft) with a Betadine solution, taking care to avoid the eyes. All patients are given a third- or fourth-generation cephalosporin or equivalent with good cerebrospinal fluid (CSF) penetration and broad-spectrum coverage.

Odontoid Approach

Accessing the foramen magnum, ring of the atlas, and odontoid process is relatively simple. It is important to identify the middle and inferior turbinates and eustachian tubes. To widen the corridor, the inferior turbinates can be lateralized. As long as there are not anomalous ICAs, there are only mucosa, longus capitis muscle, and ligamentous attachments to address. Monopolar electrocautery can be used very effectively to remove these attachments between the eustachian tubes, which are typically medial to the parapharyngeal ICAs. We do not attempt a mucosal or muscle flap, as this is not necessary in the nasopharynx, which is not exposed to the forces of swallowing. In addition, preserving a flap limits the exposure either laterally or inferiorly.

The width of exposure should be maximized prior to bony resection. There is a tendency with endoscopic approaches to funnel the exposure. The superficial exposure determines deep access. The ring of C1 is typically at the most caudal extent of reach via an EEA (**Fig. 43.2**). This can be confirmed with image guidance prior to soft tissue removal. The caudal reach can be improved slightly by drilling the maxillary crest flush with the hard palate. The hard palate itself can even be drilled posteriorly, but care must be taken to preserve the oral mucosa or many of the advantages of the endonasal approach are obviated. Curved drills or instruments may also improve caudal access. In general, angled endoscopes are not used, as it is instrumentation that is the limitation, not the view.

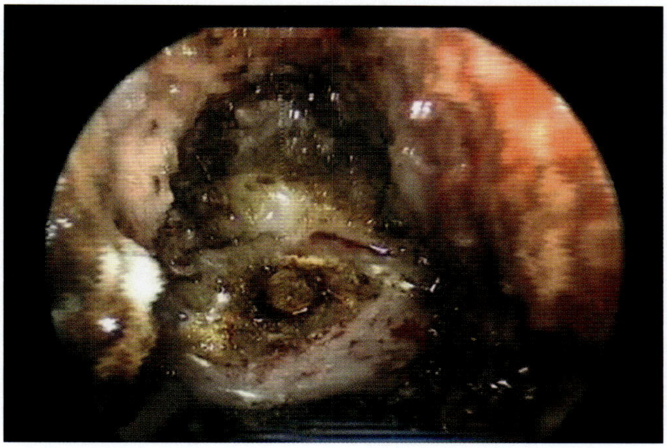

Fig. 43.2 Endoscopic view of the exposure of the ring of C1 at the caudal extent of endonasal access.

The ring of C1 can be resected with a high-speed drill or Kerrison rongeur. The minimum that should be removed is up to the lateral masses immediately adjacent to the odontoid process. This allows complete exposure of and access to the dens (**Fig. 43.3**). The tip of the dens may be obscured by the remaining atlanto-occipital membrane. This tissue can be resected with care to avoid durotomy. The dens should be removed from the tip downward to avoid disconnecting the tip from the body of C2, thereby leaving a free-floating bony fragment to be detached from the apical and transverse ligaments. Using a drill to thin the bone at the point of maximal compression, followed by careful dissection of the ligamentous attachments to fracture the remaining cortical bone is a safe way to perform this decompression (**Fig. 43.4**). The remainder of the dens can then be removed with a drill

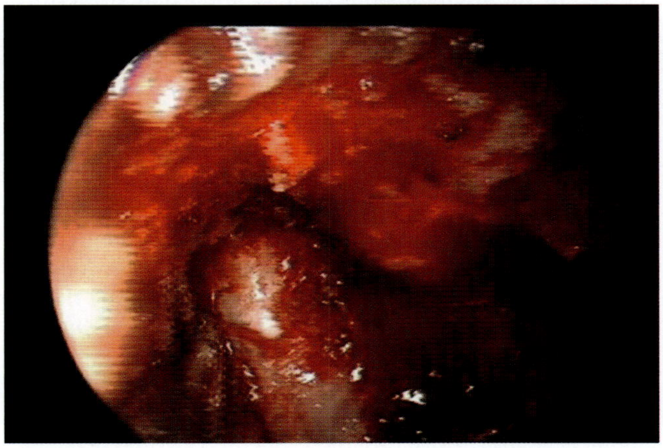

Fig. 43.3 Endoscopic view of the odontoid process following removal of the anterior ring of C1.

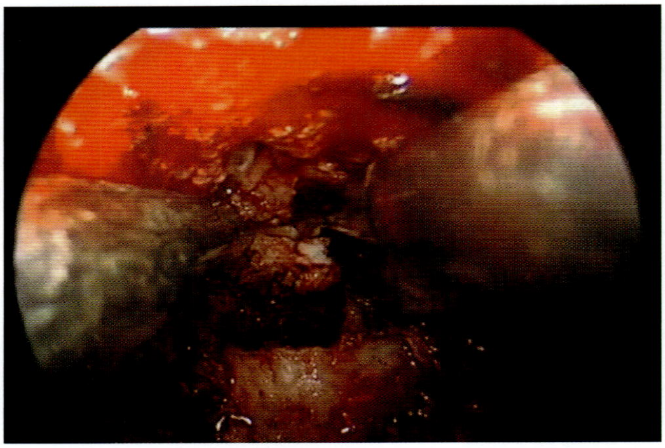

Fig. 43.4 Endoscopic view of dissection of the thinned, deep cortical bone of the dens following drilling.

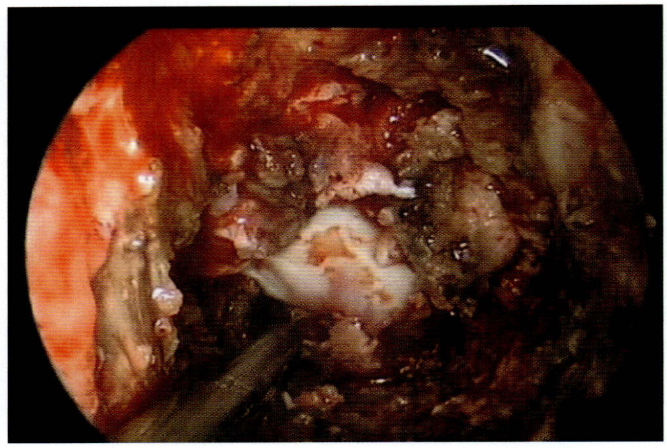

Fig. 43.5 Endoscopic view of the tectorial membrane following resection of the dens and associated ligaments.

or even rongeur if it is deemed safe to insert the rongeur footplate between the posterior cortical bone and cervicomedullary junction. The tectorial membrane is present in many cases (**Fig. 43.5**), but may be replaced or obscured by pannus in degenerative disease. If there is pannus present, this should be resected until the underlying dura is observed to be pulsatile, confirming decompression.

Simple odontoid resections are reconstructed by merely applying fibrin glue to the defect. The defect heals very nicely by mucosal regrowth without sequelae. If there is a dural defect, vascularized tissue provides the lowest rates of postoperative CSF leak.[3] However, the depth and caudal location of defects in this area often require packing of the defect with fat prior to placement of a mucosal flap for coverage.

Far Medial Approach

There are situations in which a lateral exposure at the level of the foramen magnum is necessary. This is frequently the case in foramen magnum meningiomas that are often eccentric. In these circumstances it is important to perform further lateral exposure at the side with major tumor involvement. This maneuver is particularly important to allow proximal vertebral control. To expand the approach laterally, the medial aspect of the occipital condyle is drilled. The drilling process can be extended up to the hypoglossal canal, which limits the exposure laterally. Neurophysiology can be extremely helpful when drilling the occipital condyle to preserve cranial nerve XII function. However, avoiding cranial nerve injury is dependent on the surgeon's knowledge of anatomy. The presence of cortical bone surrounding the hypoglossal canal is a very important landmark to prevent cranial nerve XII damage.

Once the medial condyle is removed, the foramen magnum ventral dura is exposed and can be opened laterally, allowing vertebral artery proximal control. The dura is opened carefully and the subarachnoid space is reached. While the ventral branch of the C1 nerve is seen medially, the hypoglossal nerves are located lateral to the vertebral arteries. The dentate ligaments are also seen laterally in the depth.

Our experience shows that if the medial condylectomy is performed on only one of the sides without disrupting the contralateral alar ligament, then the craniocervical junction can be considered stable. The reconstruction is similar to that described above in the section on the odontoid approach, above.

Functional Outcomes

Between May 2004 and October 2008, 24 patients (13 females and 11 males) underwent endoscopic endonasal approach for craniocervical junction pathology at the University of Pittsburgh Medical Center. The average age of our patients was 68 years old (range 11–96). The majority (n = 19) were for irreducible compression related to degenerative (osteo- or rheumatoid) arthritis. Other pathologies included clival meningioma (n = 1), chondrosarcoma (n = 1), metastasis from breast cancer (n = 1), and Chiari malformation with cranial settling (n = 2). The majority of these patients (n = 15) presented with myelopathy. Posterior fusion was employed in 22 patients, with 21 fusions including the occiput.

No patient developed new or worsened neurological deficit postoperatively. The Nurick and Neck Disability Index (NDI) data were available for 12 patients who had a mean follow-up of 28.6 months (range 3–57). The mean Nurick score postoperatively was 0.9, and no patient received a score of 5. The mean NDI score was 9.1 (range 0–32); 75% of patients had a NDI score of less than 15.

Complications

Two patients required intraoperative repair of CSF leaks. Both patients were treated with lumbar drainage for 5 days and suffered no sequelae. There were no instances of new postoperative dysphagia or permanent palatal insufficiency.

Three patients experienced respiratory failure secondary to pneumonia and required temporary tracheostomy. One patient was anticoagulated successfully for a deep venous thrombosis without evidence of pulmonary embolism. There were no intraoperative deaths in this series. One patient died on postoperative day 11 of unknown cause after successful recovery from surgery.

Conclusion

The endoscopic endonasal approach provides a low-morbidity approach to anteromedial pathology at the craniocervical junction. It avoids many of the morbidities associated with a transoral approach. A team approach to the surgery allows dynamic visualization and cross-fertilization of anatomic and functional knowledge related to the approach. Vascularized reconstruction provides the lowest postoperative CSF leak rates, but is not necessary for extradural pathologies.

References

1. Hull MW, Chow AW. Indigenous microflora and innate immunity of the head and neck. Infect Dis Clin North Am 2007;21:265–282, v
2. de Almeida JR, Zanation AM, Snyderman CH, et al. Defining the nasopalatine line: the limit for endonasal surgery of the spine. Laryngoscope 2009;119:239–244
3. Kassam AB, Thomas A, Carrau RL, et al. Endoscopic reconstruction of the cranial base using a pedicled nasoseptal flap. Neurosurgery 2008;63(1, Suppl 1):ONS44–ONS52, discussion ONS52–ONS53

XII Tips and Pearls in Complications of Endoscopic Skull Base and Brain Surgery

44 Management of Skull Base Defects After Extended Endoscopic Skull Base Surgery: From Free Grafts to Vascularized Flaps

Gustavo Hadad, Luis Bassagaisteguy, Daniel Timperley, and Aldo Cassol Stamm

Tips and Pearls

- The Hadad–Bassagaisteguy flap (HBF) is the gold standard" for the closure of skull base defects after endoscopic transnasal craniectomy.
- This flap is reliable and robust because it is a vascularized graft.
- The nasoseptal flap has the ability to close skull base defects in an anteroposterior direction from the cribriform region to the craniocervical junction and in a horizontal plane from orbit to orbit.
- The surgical technique for the nasoseptal flap is simple and can be performed by any endoscopic sinus surgeon.
- The HBF has a high rate of success in closing small and large skull base defects as it is vascularized by the sphenopalatine bundle.
- The HBF vascular branches lie within mucosal tissue. This protects them from exposure to drying by nasal air flow.
- The HBF can be removed and reused in cases of revision surgery.
- The HBF has a low rate of significant postoperative complications such as nasal obstruction.
- However, the postoperative period is key for potential complications, and nasal cleaning is paramount, because there is more crusting with the use of the HBF.
- Endonasal alternatives to the HBF include the anterolateral nasal flap and the posterolateral (posterior pedicle inferior turbinate) flap

Introduction

During the 1980s a patient who presented with a tumor of the anterior skull base was offered open craniofacial surgery and skull base reconstruction with galea and fixation with metal plates or bone flaps. Moreover, the patient would undergo a prolonged stay in an intensive care unit (ICU) with a lumbar drainage catheter and ran a high risk of infections and other types of postoperative complications.[1]

Twenty years later this patient has the option of minimally invasive endoscopic surgery, with maximal tumor resection by a natural orifice. This is due to the development of endoscopic transnasal craniectomy surgery.

This endoscopic access allows a wide resection of the tumor and a short hospital stay, without external incisions or lumbar drainage. However, morbidity and mortality rates are still ranging from 10 to 40%, mostly because of the inability to deal with large defects created in the skull base.[2]

In an effort to achieve better results, many techniques have been designed to try to reduce these complications, mainly postoperative cerebrospinal fluid (CSF) fistula and its potential infective complications such as meningitis and ventriculitis.

Several techniques have been described, including the use of free grafts and fascia lata or temporalis in an underlay or overlay fashion, with double or triple layers and use of biologic substitutes, among others.[3–7] All these grafts were nonvascularized and the results were variable, depending on whether the graft gained sufficient vascular supply from the adjacent tissues.

The results were worse if there was previous irradiation at the surgical field, and multiple closure surgeries were common, further increasing the risk of infective complications.

Nasoseptal (Hadad–Bassagaisteguy) Flap

History

In 1996, Drs. Gustavo Hadad and Luis Bassagaisteguy, from Argentina, developed their first nasal septal mucoperiosteal flap in the form of a sliding rotation flap that could not cover all skull base defects. Based on the concept of regional flaps in the reconstruction of other parts of the body, these nasal septal flaps also resulted in improved closure and, because they were vascularized, less retraction than with traditional free grafts.

The flaps were harvested at the end of the tumor removal procedure. The relatively simple technique kept a wide pedicle to ensure vascular supply. However, the wide pedicle restricted the range of rotation, limiting the ability to position the flap due to the risk of compromising the vascular supply.

After cadaver studies, the doctors from Argentina designed an axial flap with a narrow pedicle, based on a single artery, which allowed rotation in any direction while protecting the artery and maintaining vascular supply.

The sphenopalatine artery was the vessel with the largest possible vascular territory. Because of the course of its septal branch arching over the posterior choana into the nasal septum, it allowed the creation of large vascularized flaps with a wide arc of rotation.

The Hadad–Bassagaisteguy flap (HBF), pedicled on the sphenopalatine artery, was finally developed in 1999, and, shortly after, the first clinical human studies were successfully performed in patients with iatrogenic CSF leaks after endoscopic sinus surgery.

The generous dimensions of the flap, its versatility, and the ease of design with a robust vascular pedicle enabled surgeons to perform the first procedure in 1999 using the HBF in the closure of a large skull base CSF fistula, after craniofacial surgery for the resection of a meningoencephalocele.

Since 2005, the HBF has been consistently used for skull base closure at the University of Pittsburgh, the Sao Paulo ENT Center, and many other institutions through the world. The short- and long-term complications of CSF fistula, infections, and postoperative morbidity and mortality have decreased dramatically with the use of the HBF.[8–10]

Anatomy and Surgical Technique

The sphenopalatine artery is the terminal branch of the internal maxillary artery, and it enters the nose through the sphenopalatine foramen after traversing the pterygopalatine fossa. At the foramen it then divides into two branches.

The anterior branch runs along the inferior turbinate and nasal lateral wall. The posterior branch (septal artery) runs over the rim of the posterior choana on the sphenoid bone to the apex of the vomer, where it divides into a network of arteries running through the septum from posterior to anterior in the submucosal plane above the periosteum and perichondrium.

This fact allows the flap to be harvested from the nasal septum in a subperichondrial and subperiosteal fashion (**Figs. 44.1, 44.2,** and **44.3**). The creation of the flap starts at the beginning of the surgery. It is limited posteriorly by the posterior choana. Following topical vasoconstriction and local infiltration with adrenalin containing local anesthetic, the middle and superior turbinates are lateralized or resected to expose the nasal septum from cribriform to nasal floor. An inferior horizontal incision is made 0.5 cm above the nasal floor. The anterior limit is at the entrance of the nostril. It is important to remember that this will determine the length of the HBF. If the flap is intended to close a skull base defect of the anterior cribriform, it should be designed as long as possible, because it is pedicled posteriorly. Posteriorly, this incision follows the posterior border of the nasal septum and then arches over the posterior choana just below the front

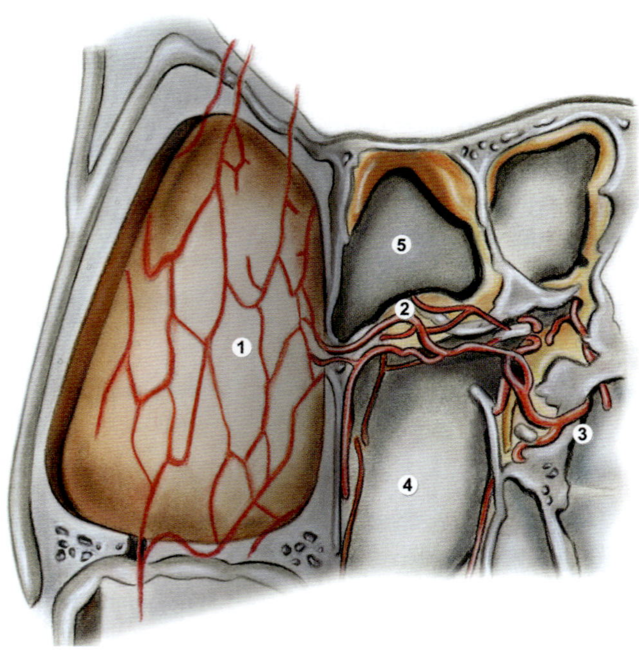

Fig. 44.1 Drawing showing the vascular supply of the Hadad–Bassagaisteguy flap (HBF). 1, donor site for raising the flap from the septal mucosa; 2, area of the nasoseptal artery; 3, sphenopalatine artery; 4, left posterior choana; 5, sphenoid sinus.

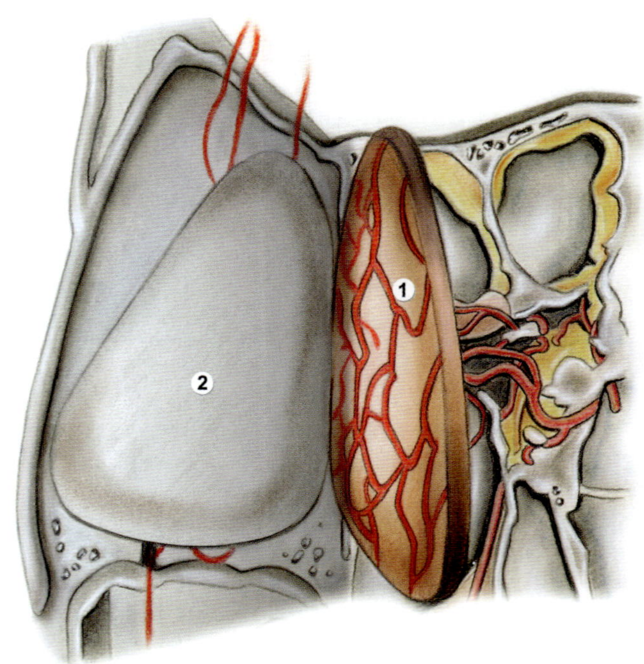

Fig. 44.2 Drawing of the anatomy for the surgical procedure for the HBF (continued). 1, nasoseptal flap separated from the nasal cartilage; 2, denuded septal cartilage.

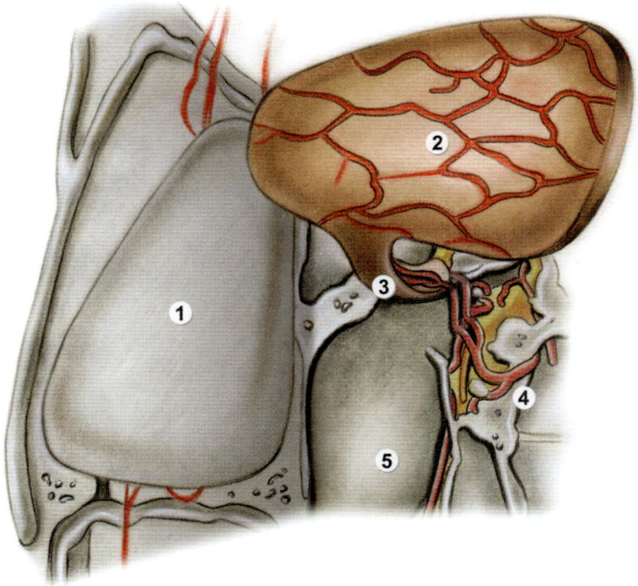

Fig. 44.3 Drawing of the anatomy for the surgical procedure for the HBF (continued). 1, denuded septal cartilage; 2, elevated nasoseptal flap; 3, mucosa and vascular pedicle through which the flap receives blood supply by the nasoseptal artery; 4, sphenopalatine artery; 5, left posterior choana.

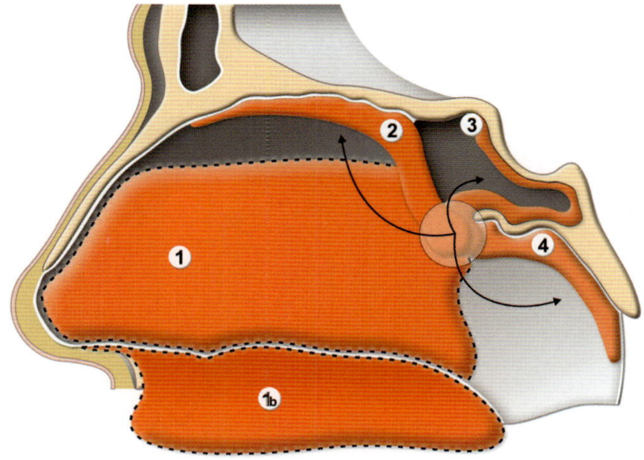

Fig. 44.4 Schema of the right nasal fossa in the sagittal plane. 1, area of origin of the nasoseptal flap (*dotted line*); 1b, area of origin of the extended nasoseptal flap, including the floor of the nasal fossa, and if necessary, the mucosa of the inferior meatus; 2, position of the nasoseptal flap used for repair of the anterior and posterior ethmoid roof and cribriform plate; when bilateral flaps are taken, the anterior skull base can be repaired from orbit to orbit; 3, position of the nasoseptal flap used for repair of the sellar and parasellar regions; 4, position of the nasoseptal flap used for repair of the region of the clivus; the arrows indicate the different ways in which the nasoseptal flap (HBF) can be rotated from the nasal septum for repair of different zones of the cranial base.

face of the sphenoid. The superior horizontal incision is usually performed 1 cm below the cribriform. Posteriorly this incision crosses the sphenoid face at the level of the inferior border of the natural sphenoid ostium. A vertical incision joins the two horizontal incisions anteriorly. The anterior reach of the flap can be improved if required by extending the horizontal incisions onto the lateral nasal wall. The inferior incision is continued forward at the level of the inferior turbinate insertion, and the superior incision is made above the level of the sphenopalatine foramen. The flap can then be elevated as far forward as the sphenopalatine foramen. If necessary, the anterior aspect of the foramen and part of the posterior wall of the maxillary sinus are opened using Kerrison rongeurs, and the vessels are dissected free to further improve the reach of the flap.

The flap is elevated in a submucoperichondrial/mucoperiosteal plane using a Cottle or Freer elevator. The incisions are completed if necessary using endoscopic scissors or other cutting instruments. Elevation of the flap over the choanal rim and anterior sphenoid bone is a key step that ensures that the flap will be freely mobile in all directions.

Once the flap is raised entirely from its bed, it is placed into the nasopharynx or maxillary sinus to protect it during the extirpative phase of the surgery. The harvesting of the flap should be planned prior to resection to maximize its size and protect the pedicle[10] (**Fig. 44.4**).

Furthermore, this flap can be revised if needed. In cases of revision procedures, the surgeon can dissect the HBF and reposition it during the surgery to the nasopharynx or maxillary antrum and re-close the skull base defect with the same HBF. This is possible because the flap is based on the perichondrium-periosteum, which maintains the plane of dissection.[10]

One of the most important features of this flap is that despite being pedicled on vascular branches, those vessels lie within tissue that surrounds and protects them from exposure to drying by the nasal airflow.

The HBF can cover the anterior skull base, including areas that go from the frontal sinus to the craniocervical junction, and from orbit to orbit.[10] A wide flap can be raised simply by extending the incision to include the mucoperiosteum of the nasal floor, or occasionally bilateral flaps are required with sacrifice of part of the nasal septum (**Figs. 44.4, 44.5, 44.6,** and **44.7**).

During surgery it is important to be careful with removal of bone and mucosal tissue to avoid damaging the sphenopalatine artery pedicles.

After the resection of the tumor, we usually perform a multilayer technique for the reconstruction of the skull base defect.

A collagen matrix is placed as a subdural layer. An additional layer can be placed or free abdominal fat used to fill dead space, for example, in clival defects. The HBF can be placed directly on the fat or fascia grafts. Fibrin glue or other biologic glue is also utilized.

A Foley balloon catheter is then placed, which is inflated under endoscopic visualization to support and hold the HBF against the skull base defect.

Inflation of the balloon is always under endoscopic visualization because this inflation can lead to compression of

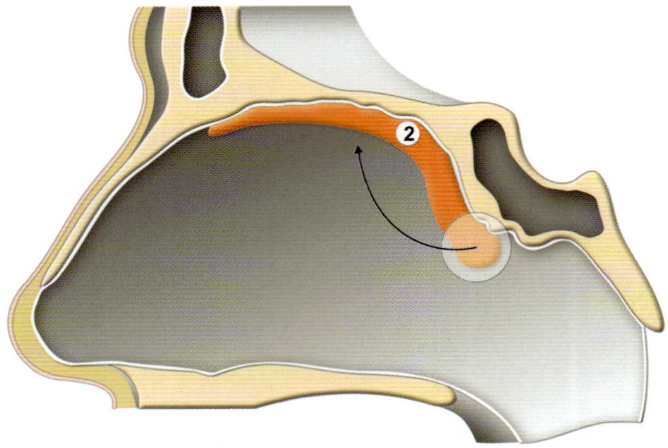

A

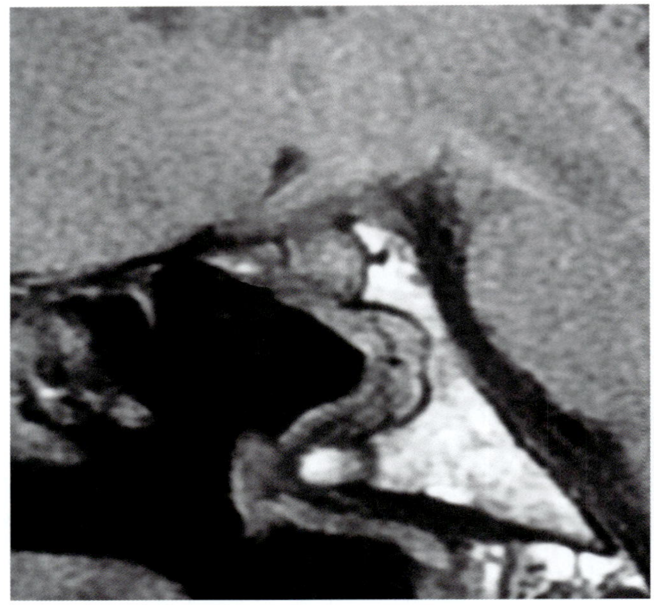

B

Fig. 44.5 (A) Schema of the nasoseptal flap for repair of the anterior skull base. 2, form of the flap projected to the superior and anterior aspect of the roof of the nasal fossa, taking the sphenopalatine artery as the vascular pedicle. **(B)** Postoperative sagittal magnetic resonance imaging (MRI) scan demonstrating the position of the nasoseptal flap used for anterior skull base repair.

intracranial structures or compromise neurovascular pedicles. This catheter is left for 2 or 3 days after the surgery. Spacers or silicone splits are used to protect the nasal septum, and they usually remain in place for 10 to 14 days.[10] Antibiotics and analgesics are given to the patients for 14 days. No lumbar drainage catheter is used.

Anterior Lateral Endonasal Flap

The anterior lateral endonasal flap has been developed by the authors to enable repair of defects when the nasoseptal flap is unsuitable (e.g., posterior table of frontal sinus) or unavailable due to disease or previous surgery. It is a random pattern flap based on the anterior ethmoid supply, allowing the mucoperiosteum of the entire inferior turbinate and inferolateral nasal wall to be utilized (**Fig. 44.8**). Anteriorly based inferior turbinate flaps have been described for use in nasal and septal reconstruction[11,12]; however, these are pedicled at the anterior end of the turbinate and lack the reach to enable large skull base repairs.

Vascular Anatomy

Following its course in the olfactory fossa, the anterior ethmoid artery enters the nasal cavity to run under the nasal bones, supplying branches to the anterior septum and the

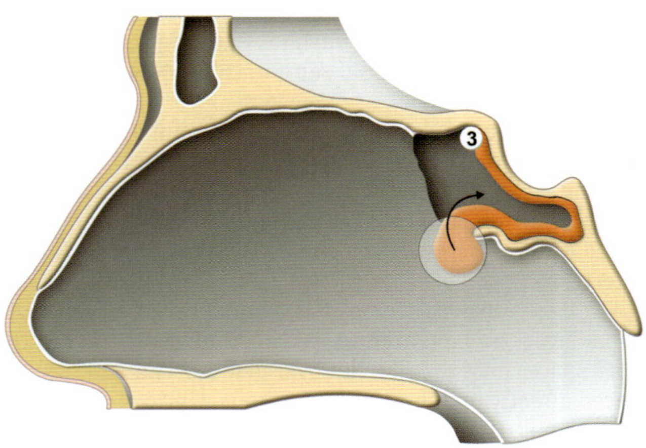

A

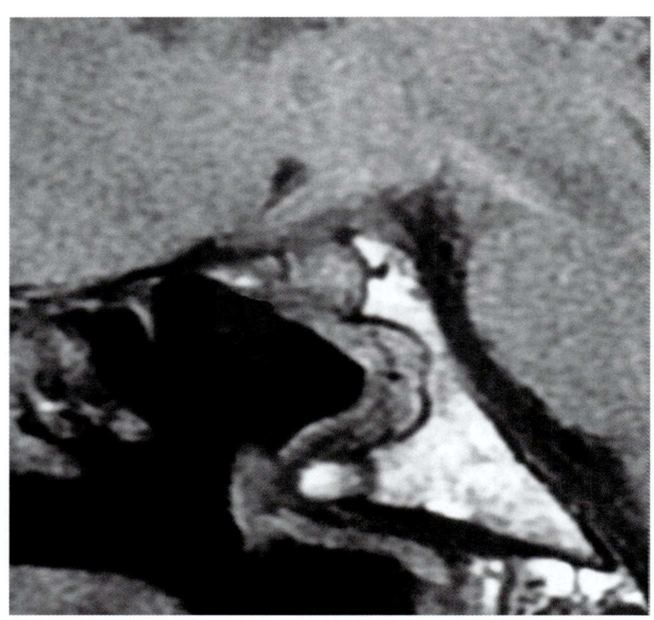

B

Fig. 44.6 (A) Schema of the nasoseptal flap for repair of the anterior skull base. 3, form of the flap projected to the superior and posterior aspect of the roof of the sphenoid sinus, taking the sphenopalatine artery as the vascular pedicle. **(B)** Postoperative sagittal MRI scan demonstrating the position of the nasoseptal flap used for repair of the roof of the sphenoid sinus.

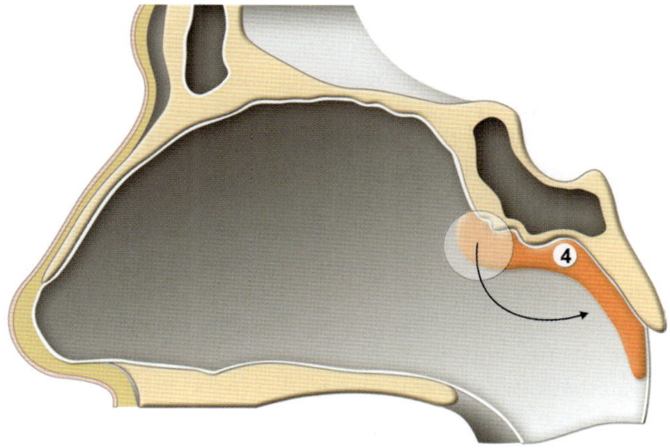

Fig. 44.7 Schema of the nasoseptal flap for repair of the anterior skull base. 4, form of the flap projected posteriorly to reach the zone of the clivus, taking the sphenopalatine artery as the vascular pedicle.

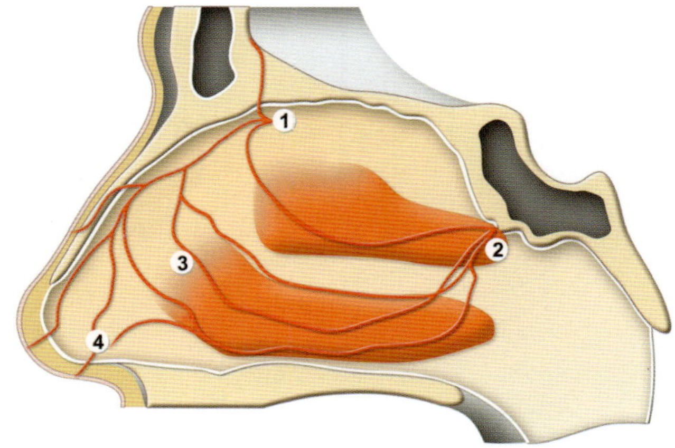

Fig. 44.8 Vascular supply of the inferior turbinate and anterolateral nasal wall. 1, anterior ethmoid artery after its exit from the olfactory fossa; 2, posterior lateral nasal artery giving rise to the middle and inferior conchal arteries; 3, anastomoses between the anterior and posterior vessels; 4, branches of the angular artery.

anterolateral nasal wall. The inferior turbinate has a dual blood supply, from both anteriorly and posteriorly.[13] The posterior supply is via the posterior lateral branch of the sphenopalatine artery, giving rise to the inferior conchal arteries.[13–15] The anterior supply is not well described, and its existence has been disputed.[14] However, the size of the inferior conchal arteries has been observed to increase anteriorly,[13] and measurements of the effects of sphenopalatine artery compression via pterygopalatine fossa injection also suggest the presence of a collateral blood supply.[16] This supply may arise from both branches of the angular artery and the anterior ethmoid via anastomoses between them and the inferior conchal arteries[17] (**Fig. 44.8**). A wide pedicle is therefore necessary to ensure sufficient vascular supply to the flap.

Surgical Technique

The anterior/inferior incision is made on the lateral nasal wall from under the nasal bones to the head of the inferior turbinate (**Fig. 44.9**). The incision forks at this point. One incision runs down the head of the inferior turbinate, giving access to the anterior edge of the turbinate bone. The inferior incision continues into the inferior meatus and may include the nasal floor.

The posterior/superior incision begins 1 cm above the axilla of the middle turbinate and then continues down over the frontal process of the maxilla and lacrimal bone to reach the superior border of the inferior turbinate. At this point the incision joins the middle meatal antrostomy (if performed) or is continued posteriorly along the inferior turbinate attachment. The flap is then elevated in a subperiosteal plane beginning at the anterior incision to expose the nasal bone, the frontal process of maxilla, and the lacrimal bones. The mucoperiosteum of the inferior turbinate is elevated on the medial and lateral aspects to form tunnels over the entire length of the turbinate bone. Fracturing the turbinate bone medially aids dissection in the inferior meatus. The bone can then be removed via the anterior incision, and the mucosa of the inferior meatus, and the nasal floor, if required, can be elevated. A silicone stent may be placed into Hasner's valve, or the sac opened with or without a formal dacryocystorhinostomy (DCR). A large middle meatal antrostomy is performed with the inferior edge of the antrostomy forming the superior border of this part of the flap. The final step is to release the flap posteriorly and cauterize the inferior conchal arteries entering 1 to 1.5 cm anterior to the posterior end of the turbinate. The flap can then be positioned to cover anterior skull base defects (**Fig. 44.10**).

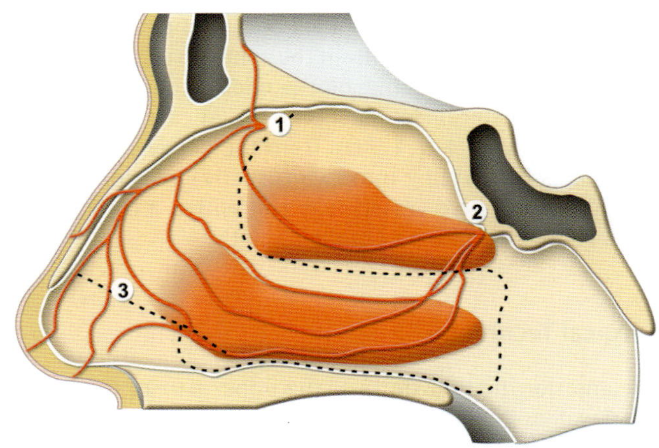

Fig. 44.9 Incisions for the anterolateral endonasal flap. 1, incision from above the axilla of the middle turbinate, running inferiorly just anterior to the uncinate attachment, and then to the inferior edge of the middle meatal antrostomy; 2, posterior lateral nasal artery emerging from the sphenopalatine foramen; 3, incision from under the nasal bones to the insertion of the inferior turbinate; the incision forks, with one arm running on the anterior aspect of the bone of the inferior turbinate and the other running into the inferior meatus.

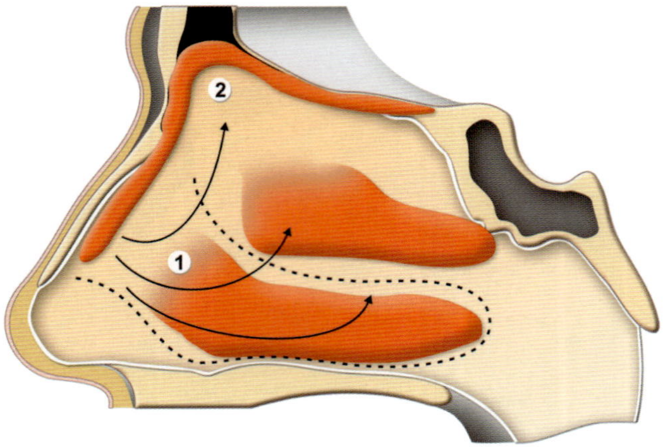

Fig. 44.10 Positioning of the anterolateral endonasal flap. 1, the flap in situ; 2, the flap has been rotated superiorly, where it can cover defects of the anterior skull base including the posterior wall of the frontal sinus.

Posterior Lateral (Extended Posterior Pedicle Inferior Turbinate) Endonasal Flap

The posterior pedicle inferior turbinate flap is an axial flap based on the posterior supply via the inferior conchal arteries. It is an alternative to the HBF for skull base repair where the HBF is unavailable.[18] It has excellent coverage for posterior fossa defects; however, its anterior reach is limited.[19] The authors' modification is to raise an extended flap by including the mucosa of the entire lateral nasal wall anterior to the uncinate insertion to increase flap coverage where necessary.

Vascular Anatomy

The posterior lateral nasal branch of the sphenopalatine artery arises prior to its exit from the sphenopalatine foramen and passes inferiorly, giving off the middle conchal artery. It crosses the posterior fontanelle in 38% of cases, enters the inferior turbinate 1 to 1.5 cm from the posterior end, and terminates by dividing into two (usually) inferior conchal arteries.[13,15,17] These vessels may run within a complete or partial bony canal for part of their length.[13,14]

Surgical Technique

The anterior incision starts at the upper part of the lateral nasal wall as far anteriorly as possible under the nasal bone. It then runs down to the inferior turbinate insertion where it forks. One incision runs over the head of the inferior turbinate to expose the anterior edge of the turbinate bone. The other runs down into the anterior aspect of the inferior meatus, and, if necessary, onto the nasal floor. A second incision is made 1 cm above the axilla of the middle turbinate running anteriorly to join the first incision. The next incision runs from above the axilla vertically downward to reach the superior border of the inferior turbinate just anterior to the insertion of the uncinate process. The flap is then elevated in a subperiosteal plane beginning anteriorly, exposing the nasal bone, the frontal process of maxilla, and the lacrimal bone. Elevation of the mucoperiosteum of the head of the inferior turbinate is then performed, and may be facilitated by medial displacement of the turbinate. The flap is elevated to create tunnels over the full length of the bone medially and laterally. The bone is detached from the nasal wall and from the soft tissue inferiorly and then removed via the anterior incision. Once this is complete, the mucosa of the inferior meatus, and the floor of the nose, if required, can be elevated. Hasner's valve is managed as in the anteriorly based flap. A large middle meatal antrostomy defines the superior boundary of this part of the flap; the surgeon must keep in mind that the feeding vessels may cross the posterior part of the fontanelle. Finally, the flap is checked to ensure it is free of attachments to the nasal floor and inferior meatus and is freely mobile about the arterial pedicle.

■ Conclusion

The development of pedicled flaps has marked a new era and has been a turning point in endoscopic skull base surgery. The use of these pedicled flaps has led to the development of several other endoscopic approaches to the skull base, mainly because they provide a very robust and reliable method for closure of large skull base defects.

References

1. Carrau RL, Snyderman CH, Kassam AB. The management of cerebrospinal fluid leaks in patients at risk for high-pressure hydrocephalus. Laryngoscope 2005;115:205–212
2. Carrau RL, Kassam AB, Snyderman CH, Duvvuri U, Mintz A, Gardner P. Endoscopic transnasal anterior skull base resection for the treatment of sinonasal malignancies. Operative Techniques in Otolaryngology 2006;17:102–110
3. McMains KC, Gross CW, Kountakis SE. Endoscopic management of cerebrospinal fluid rhinorrhea. Laryngoscope 2004;114:1833–1837
4. Kirtane MV, Gautham K, Upadhyaya SR. Endoscopic CSF rhinorrhea closure: our experience in 267 cases. Otolaryngol Head Neck Surg 2005;132:208–212
5. Locatelli D, Rampa F, Acchiardi I, Bignami M, Pistochini A, Castelnuovo P. Endoscopic endonasal approaches to anterior skull base defects in pediatric patients. Childs Nerv Syst 2006;22:1411–1418
6. Casiano RR, Livingston JA. Endoscopic Lothrop procedure: the University of Miami experience. Am J Rhinol 1998;12:335–339
7. Shah AR, Pearlman AN, O'Grady KM, Bhattacharyya TK, Toriumi DM. Combined use of fibrin tissue adhesive and acellular dermis in dural repair. Am J Rhinol 2007;21:619–621
8. Harvey RJ, Smith JE, Wise SK, Patel SJ, Frankel BM, Schlosser RJ. Intracranial complications before and after endoscopic skull base reconstruction. Am J Rhinol 2008;22:516–521
9. Harvey RJ, Nogueira JF Jr, Schlosser RJ, Patel SJ, Vellutini E, Stamm AC. Closure of large skull base defects after endoscopic transnasal craniotomy. Clinical article. J Neurosurg 2009;111:371–379
10. Hadad G, Bassagaisteguy L, Carrau RL, et al. A novel reconstructive technique after endoscopic expanded endonasal approaches: vascular pedicle nasoseptal flap. Laryngoscope 2006;116:1882–1886

11. Murakami CS, Kriet JD, Ierokomos AP. Nasal reconstruction using the inferior turbinate mucosal flap. Arch Facial Plast Surg 1999;1:97–100

12. Friedman M, Ibrahim H, Ramakrishnan V. Inferior turbinate flap for repair of nasal septal perforation. Laryngoscope 2003;113:1425–1428

13. Padgham N, Vaughan-Jones R. Cadaver studies of the anatomy of arterial supply to the inferior turbinates. J R Soc Med 1991;84:728–730

14. Hadar T, Ophir D, Yaniv E, Berger G. Inferior turbinate arterial supply: histologic analysis and clinical implications. J Otolaryngol 2005;34: 46–50

15. Lee HY, Kim HU, Kim SS, et al. Surgical anatomy of the sphenopalatine artery in lateral nasal wall. Laryngoscope 2002;112:1813–1818

16. Gurr P, Callanan V, Baldwin D. Laser-Doppler blood flowmetry measurement of nasal mucosa blood flow after injection of the greater palatine canal. J Laryngol Otol 1996;110:124–128

17. Babin E, Moreau S, de Rugy MG, Delmas P, Valdazo A, Bequignon A. Anatomic variations of the arteries of the nasal fossa. Otolaryngol Head Neck Surg 2003;128:236–239

18. Fortes FSG, Carrau RL, Snyderman CH, et al. The posterior pedicle inferior turbinate flap: a new vascularized flap for skull base reconstruction. Laryngoscope 2007;117:1329–1332

19. Harvey RJ, Sheahan PO, Schlosser RJ. Inferior turbinate pedicle flap for endoscopic skull base defect repair. Am J Rhinol Allergy 2009;23: 522–526

45 Management of Vascular Complications During Endoscopic Skull Base Surgery

Ricardo L. Carrau, Juan C. Fernandez-Miranda, Daniel M. Prevedello, Paul A. Gardner, Carl H. Snyderman, and Amin B. Kassam

Tips and Pearls

- Inexperience and lack of proper training with new instruments or techniques, and disorientation with the endoscopic anatomical perspective can result in catastrophic vascular injuries.
- A co-surgeon improves visualization of the surgical field and surveillance of its periphery, increases efficiency, assists with problem solving, provides a continuous second opinion, and counterbalances individual biases.
- Computed tomographic angiography (CTA) is recommended for image guidance, as it highlights the vascular anatomy.
- Intraoperative computed tomography can be used to provide updated information for image guidance and to detect vascular complications such as brain hemorrhage.
- Bimanual dissection and minimal traction on intracranial tumors are recommended to avoid inadvertent avulsion of the surrounding vessels.
- Small perforating vessels to the brainstem and optic chiasm provide important contribution to their blood supply, and sacrificing or injuring them often leads to ischemic deficits.
- Control of small arteries is best achieved using bipolar electrocauterization or by irrigating warm water (40°C) for several minutes.
- If large vessels are injured, hypotensive anesthesia as an attempt to control the bleeding is contraindicated because it results in cerebral hypoperfusion. Neurophysiologic monitoring is critical, as it reflects cerebral perfusion.
- Options for a large-vessel injury include bipolar electrocauterization of the vessel to weld the tear shut or to induce thrombosis of the vessel, direct compression, compressive packing, suture repair, reconstruction using aneurysm clips, and circumferential ligation or clipping of the vessel.
- A follow-up angiography is also recommended after any intraoperative vascular injury. These patients are at risk for a delayed pseudoaneurysm and rupture that can present weeks to years after the event.
- Prevention of serious complications requires a proper selection of cases, and a surgeon who has mastered the skull base anatomy from an endoscopic perspective, with training in endoscopic techniques, and who can perform meticulous dissection and deliver perioperative care with the utmost attention to detail.

Introduction

Prevention and management of complications is an important cornerstone of surgery and directly relates to the first tenet of "do no harm." As different surgical specialties evolved into minimally invasive approaches, using new technique or technologies, they universally encountered a higher frequency of surgical complications. Even the most experienced surgeons are not immune to complications, but they can be ameliorated by proper training and mentorship that promotes and facilitates sequential and progressive learning. Despite its minimally invasive approach, endoscopic skull base surgery presents many of the risks and the potential for major complications that are associated with traditional approaches. Inexperience and lack of proper training with new instruments or techniques, and disorientation with the endoscopic anatomical perspective are important factors leading to catastrophic vascular injuries.

In our experience (which includes over 1400 endoscopic endonasal skull base surgeries), the incidence and morbidity of catastrophic vascular complications compare favorably to that of traditional approaches. However, in our practice endoscopic and traditional approaches are complementary, and therefore their indications and limitations preclude a direct comparison. This chapter summarizes our experience and presents guidelines for the prevention and management of vascular complications during endoscopic skull base surgery.

Incidence of Complications

Vascular complications may be classified by the type of vessel (capillary, venous, or arterial), size of the vessel (minor or major), flow of the vessel (low flow or high flow), severity of the complication (major or minor), location (intra- or extracranial), and timing (intraoperative or postoperative). **Table 45.1** summarizes the vascular complications of our

Table 45.1 Vascular Complications in the First 800 Patients Who Underwent Expanded Endonasal Approaches

Type of Lesion and/or Deficit	
No case	Death (0%)
• P1 perforator (aphasia)	Transient deficit (0.1%)
• Pontine bleed (quadriplegic) • Maxillary artery laceration (hemiplegic) • Frontopolar avulsion (right lower limb paresis)	Permanent deficit (0.4%)
• 1 Ophthalmic (already blind) • 2 ICA lacerations	No deficit (0.4%)

first 800 endoscopic endonasal skull base surgeries.[1–3] It comprises a 10-year experience including a wide variety of diagnoses and endonasal surgical approaches. Interestingly, we did not encounter any vascular injury during our early experience. We believe that this may be due to the progressive evolution in our technique and indications. Stated differently, we did not tackle complex or high-risk cases until we had matured as a team and until we had developed and mastered hemostatic and reconstructive techniques.

Prevention of Complications

Prevention of complications starts with a clear understanding of the skull base and vascular anatomy from the endoscopic perspective. The skull base is a relay station where all the cranial nerves and vessels are distributed to their corresponding areas. Our modular endoscopic approaches are based on the identification and control of critical neurovascular structures, especially the internal carotid artery (ICA). From the ventral standpoint the ICAs are brackets that define the lateral limits of the coronal plane. They define the surgical field, which narrows as the ICAs move from proximal to distal (**Fig. 45.1**). From the endoscopic view, the ICA can be divided into five segments marked by distinct anatomical points (**Table 45.2**): the parapharyngeal or extracranial segment, the petrous or horizontal segment, the paraclival or vertical segment, the parasellar or cavernous segment, and the supraclinoid segment. Anatomical variations, space-occupying lesions, prior surgery, and varying degrees of pneumatization of the sinonasal tract also influence the position and approach to each segment.

Proper training is also critical for the prevention and management of surgical complications.[4] We have proposed guidelines to train endoscopic skull base surgeons, regardless of the specialty, who have to progress through sequential and incremental modules (see Chapter 9). Levels of training are defined by the complexity of the involved anatomy, the technical difficulty associated with the surgery, the potential risk of neurovascular complications, the extent of intradural dissection, and the type of pathology. Proficiency in one level has to be acquired before the surgeon advances to the next. We also developed an animal model for training on endoscopic hemostatic and dissection techniques. This chapter presents the key points regarding vascular control and management of vascular injuries.

Intraoperative Considerations

Interdisciplinary cooperation leading to team surgery is one of the most remarkable advances in skull base surgery. A co-surgeon improves visualization of the surgical field and surveillance of its periphery, increases efficiency, assists with problem solving, provides a continuous second opinion, and counterbalances individual biases.

Neurophysiologic monitoring of cortical and brainstem function is routinely performed. Electromyographic monitoring of cranial nerves is also performed according to the position of the lesion and the required dissection. We advocate using computerized tomographic angiography (CTA) for image guidance, as it highlights the vascular anatomy (except for sellar lesions where we advocate magnetic resonance imaging [MRI]).[5] Intraoperative computed tomography (CT) can be used to provide updated information for image guidance and to detect vascular complications such as brain hemorrhage.

Proper surgical technique avoids complications, especially vascular injuries. We strongly advocate bimanual dissection and minimal traction on intracranial tumors to avoid inadvertent avulsion of the surrounding vessels. Following microsurgical principles, the tumor is debulked in a centrifugal direction to allow extracapsular dissection of adjacent neurovascular structures. Hemostasis is achieved using a combination of strategies that include clipping or cauterization of feeding vessels, use of a diamond drill bit for bone removal, application of hemostatic materials, and warm water irrigation.[6] Bipolar electrocautery should be used for any intracranial cauterization and whenever a critical nerve or vessel is adjacent to the bleeding site.

Catastrophic bleeding is better prevented than treated. Its potential increases exponentially in the presence of prior surgery, prior radiation therapy, and tumor encasement. Every team should have a plan to follow in case of such occurrence. It is difficult to formulate and execute a plan of action in the middle of a crisis. Significant bleeding from the cavernous

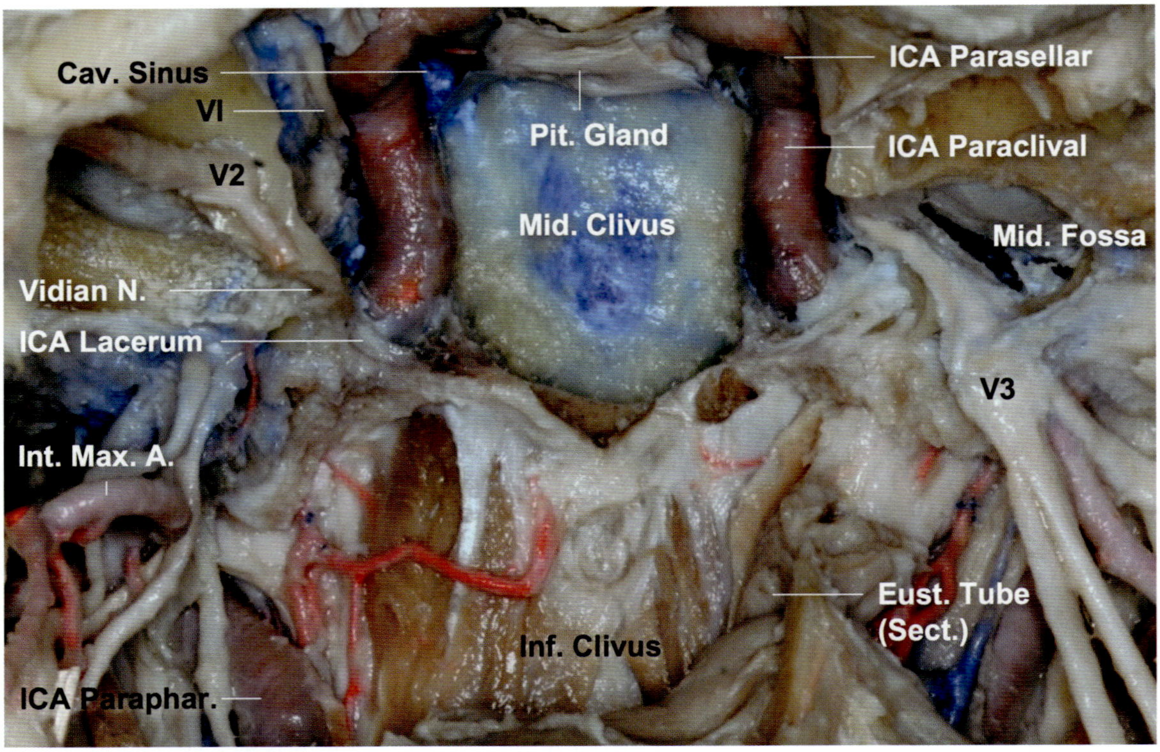

Fig. 45.1 Internal carotid artery (ICA) classification. The ICA can be divided into five segments marked by distinct anatomical points: the parapharyngeal or extracranial segment, the petrous or horizontal segment, the paraclival or vertical segment, the parasellar or cavernous segment, and the supraclinoid segment. The transitional segment between the paraclival and petrosal segments is also called the lacerum segment, as it occupies the upper portion of the foramen lacerum. For communication purposes we consider that the endonasal approaches to expose the area between the ICAs belong to the sagittal plane, and the approaches around the ICA define the coronal plane modules. The latter are anatomically and technically more demanding and carry an increased risk of vascular injury. A.: artery; Cav.: cavernous; Eust.: eustachian; Inf.: inferior; Int.: internal; Max.: maxillary; Mid.: middle; N.: nerve; Paraphar.: parapharyngeal segment; Pit.: pituitary; Sect.: sectioned.

sinus and basilar plexus should be anticipated and its management effected by direct application of hemostatic materials and gentle pressure. Staging of a procedure is occasionally warranted for lesions requiring a transclival approach in which the surgeon encounters significant bleeding from the basilar plexus. During the first stage the bone is removed to expose the dura of the posterior fossa, which is then cauterized (bipolar electrocautery) and the basilar plexus is thrombosed with any of the commercially available paste-like hemostatic agents. At this point the surgery can be aborted to stabilize the patient and a second stage is performed 1 to 2 days later.

Table 45.2 Anatomical Landmarks of the Internal Carotid Artery (ICA)

Segment	Anatomical Landmark
Parasellar	mOCR
Vertical ICA	Medial pterygoid
Horizontal ICA	Vidian nerve
Carotid canal	Eustachian tube
Ascending ICA	Eustachian tube

mOCR: medial optic carotid recess.

Injury to small and large arteries produce bleeding that is proportional to the size of the vessel and injury. Nonetheless, the consequences of such an injury may lead to consequences that are not necessarily proportional to the size of the vessel. Small perforating vessels to the brainstem and optic chiasm provide important contribution to their blood supply, and sacrifice or injury often lead to ischemic deficits. Control of small arteries, however, is best achieved using bipolar electrocauterization or by irrigating warm water (40°C) for several minutes. Alternatively, a hemostatic material can be gently applied using cottonoids. This is repeated as needed until the bleeding stops.

Injury to the ICAs is usually accompanied by catastrophic bleeding that has to be controlled while maintaining cerebral perfusion (**Fig. 45.2**). During the crisis, neurophysiologic monitoring is critical as it reflects cerebral perfusion. Hypotensive anesthesia as an attempt to control the bleeding is contraindicated because it results in cerebral hypoperfusion. Digital compression of the cervical carotid may diminish its flow. Another measure that may be counterintuitive is the administration of heparin to avoid embolic phenomena. A

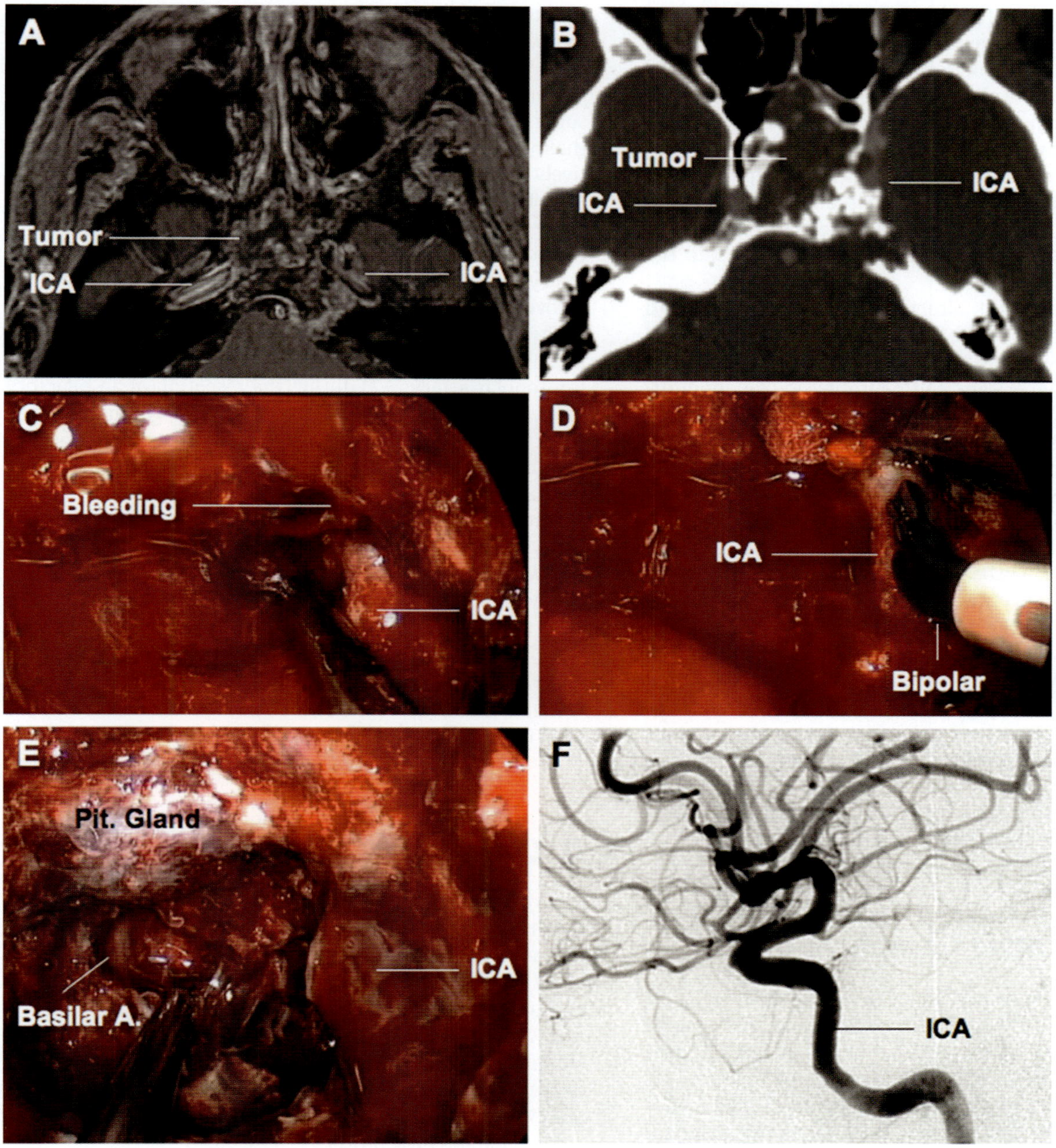

Fig. 45.2 An example of a vascular injury. **(A)** Axial T1-weighted magnetic resonance imaging showing a skull base tumor (chondrosarcoma) that invades the clival and petrous bone, particularly on the left side. Note the tumor encasement and anterolateral displacement of the left ICA at the petrous segment. **(B)** Computed tomographic angiogram on the same patient. Note the encasement and displacement of the left paraclival ICA. The intraluminal diameter of the ICA appears diminished and irregular in comparison to the contralateral ICA, suggesting invasion of the vessel. **(C)** While removing tumor that encased the left paraclival ICA, brisk arterial bleeding was encountered despite a careful dissection. The bleeding was controlled by gentle compression with a small cottonoid, but upon release of the pressure the bleeding was copious. **(D)** Digital compression to the cervical segment of the ICA to diminish its flow and allow for the accurate identification of a pinhole in the carotid wall. Selective bipolar electrocauterization of the tear was successfully accomplished, with immediate cessation of bleeding. Vital signs and neurophysiologic monitoring remained stable throughout the procedure. **(E)** The carotid wall was reinforced with fibrin glue, and the remaining tumor was subtotally resected. The tumor eroded the clival dura, enabling identification of the basilar artery. **(F)** Immediate postoperative angiogram was performed showing a patent and completely normal ICA. Follow-up angiogram was performed 1 month after the injury, with similar results. A close follow-up is needed to rule out the development of a carotid pseudoaneurysm. A.: artery; Pit.: pituitary.

two-surgeon, four-hand technique with dynamic handling of the endoscope to preserve an adequate view of the surgical field and the use of two suctions offers the best opportunity to identify and control the site of bleeding. Options at that point include bipolar electrocauterization of the vessel to weld the tear shut or to induce thrombosis of the vessel, direct compression, compressive packing, suture repair, reconstruction using aneurysm clips, and circumferential ligation or clipping of the vessel. Compressive packing is not an option if the dura is opened, as the blood will track into the subdural space.

Initially the bleeding is directed into the suction tips to maintain visualization while focal pressure is applied with a cottonoid. If the hemostasis and resuscitation are successful and the patient's vital signs and neurophysiologic monitoring are stable, additional packing can be placed and the patient may be transported to an angiography suite for definitive management. If packing is inadequate or not feasible, the ICA is better exposed to obtain control of the vessel proximal and distal to the injury. Suture repair is possible, albeit technically difficult and in most instances impractical. Preservation of the vessel may be better achieved by reconstructing the vessel with aneurysm clips or using Sundt-Keyes clips. Sacrifice of the ICA is the most commonly used alternative.

Ideally, the endovascular surgeon should preserve the patency of the ICA by using a covered stent; however, a covered stent may not be available for intracranial use in all institutions. Insertion of a covered stent into the cavernous sinus segment of ICA is technically challenging; therefore, in most cases, permanent occlusion is performed. Assessment of collateral blood flow with a balloon occlusion test identifies the risk of ischemic stroke and the need for a bypass.

Postoperative Complications

A postoperative CT scan, performed in the first 24 hours after surgery, provides early detection of complications such as cerebral hemorrhage or intracranial hematoma. A CT scanner that is in the operating room offers the opportunity for intraoperative and immediate postoperative evaluation. We have encountered two unexpected complications: a subdural hematoma due to cerebrospinal fluid (CSF) loss in an elderly man, and an epidural hematoma from improper placement of a three-pin head fixation system in a pediatric patient. Early identification and immediate surgical treatment resulted in the best outcome.

Any significant postoperative epistaxis mandates endoscopic examination of the nasal cavity. Similarly, an immediate angiography is recommended if the patient is at risk for a carotid blowout or bleed. A follow-up angiography is also recommended after any intraoperative vascular injury. These patients are at risk for a delayed pseudoaneurysm and rupture that can present weeks to years after the event.[7]

We reviewed all perioperative complications associated with endoscopic endonasal skull base surgeries in our first 800 patients at the University of Pittsburgh Medical Center. Intraoperative complications such as vascular or neural injuries were rare and included seven major vascular complications (0.9%). One patient suffered an avulsion of a P1 perforator during the resection of a craniopharyngioma. Two patients suffered an ICA injury, and one suffered avulsion of the ophthalmic artery; all three injuries were controlled intraoperatively before transferring the patients to the endovascular suite for additional control or sacrifice of the vessel. None of these four patients suffered a new permanent deficit, though the patient with a posterior cerebral artery (PCA) branch injury suffered a stroke with a severe aphasia that eventually recovered completely.

The remaining three patients suffered permanent neurologic deficits (0.4%). One patient suffered an avulsion of a frontopolar artery (A2) during the resection of an olfactory groove meningioma. About 2 weeks later, the patient suffered a frontal lobe hemorrhage from a pseudoaneurysm. This required sacrifice of the A2 and the recurrent artery of Huebner, leading to a permanent right hemiparesis and cognitive deficit. Another patient suffered a delayed postoperative pontine hemorrhage after an episode of hypertension following the resection of a clival chordoma with brainstem involvement. This produced a permanent quadriplegia. The third patient suffered an injury of the internal maxillary artery during the dissection of an infratemporal fossa encephalocele, resulting in an acute subdural hematoma that required multiple craniotomies. This patient has a permanent, mild weakness (4/5) of the left upper limb.

Conclusion

Risks of complications associated with endoscopic endonasal skull base surgery including large vessel injury compare favorably with those of traditional skull base surgery. Prevention of serious complications requires a proper selection of cases, and a surgeon who has mastered the skull base anatomy from an endoscopic perspective, with training in endoscopic techniques, and who can perform meticulous dissection and deliver perioperative care with the utmost attention to detail. Progressive acquisition of skills and experience leads to an acceptable safety profile.

References

1. Kassam A, Snyderman CH, Mintz A, Gardner P, Carrau RL. Expanded endonasal approach: the rostrocaudal axis. Part I. Crista galli to the sella turcica. Neurosurg Focus 2005;19:E3
2. Kassam A, Snyderman CH, Mintz A, Gardner P, Carrau RL. Expanded endonasal approach: the rostrocaudal axis. Part II. Posterior clinoids to the foramen magnum. Neurosurg Focus 2005;19:E4
3. Kassam AB, Gardner P, Snyderman C, Mintz A, Carrau R. Expanded endonasal approach: fully endoscopic, completely transnasal approach to the middle third of the clivus, petrous bone, middle cranial fossa, and infratemporal fossa. Neurosurg Focus 2005;19:E6
4. Snyderman C, Kassam A, Carrau R, Mintz A, Gardner P, Prevedello DM. Acquisition of surgical skills for endonasal skull base surgery: a training program. Laryngoscope 2007;117:699–705

5. Gardner PA, Kassam AB, Rothfus WE, Snyderman CH, Carrau RL. Preoperative and intraoperative imaging for endoscopic endonasal approaches to the skull base. Otolaryngol Clin North Am 2008;41:215–230, vii

6. Kassam A, Snyderman CH, Carrau RL, Gardner P, Mintz A. Endoneurosurgical hemostasis techniques: lessons learned from 400 cases. Neurosurg Focus 2005;19:E7

7. Biswas D, Daudia A, Jones NS, McConachie NS. Profuse epistaxis following sphenoid surgery: a ruptured carotid artery pseudoaneurysm and its management. J Laryngol Otol 2009;123:692–694

46 Endocrine Complications After Endoscopic Skull Base Surgery

Zachary M. Bush, Mary Lee Vance, and John A. Jane Jr.

Tips and Pearls

- Optimal perioperative management of patients undergoing endoscopic transsphenoidal surgery requires an experienced multidisciplinary team including specialists from neurosurgery and endocrinology.
- Postoperative hormone deficiencies are the most common complication of modern transsphenoidal surgery, and can cause significant morbidity and mortality if unrecognized and untreated.
- Preoperative evaluation of pituitary function in patients undergoing transsphenoidal surgery is critical in surgical and postoperative care planning.
- Preoperative high-resolution magnetic resonance imaging (MRI) of the sella to localize normal pituitary is important in surgical planning.
- Postoperative management is individualized according to the type of pituitary or sellar lesion, especially in secretory pituitary adenomas.
- Non-Cushing's patients with any preoperative pituitary dysfunction are often given empiric stress dose steroids for 24 hours after surgery as a safety measure.
- Hormone deficiencies noted in preoperative evaluation are not expected to resolve rapidly, and empiric treatment for central hypothyroidism, adrenal insufficiency, and diabetes insipidus should be continued until the first follow-up visit 8 to 10 weeks after surgery.
- Posterior pituitary dysfunction is common following pituitary surgery, with diabetes insipidus often occurring in the first 72 hours, and a delayed risk of the syndrome of inappropriate antidiuretic hormone secretion (SIADH) and symptomatic hyponatremia occurring 5 to 14 days postoperative.
- Patients who are not on steroid replacement therapy, must be evaluated for iatrogenic adrenal insufficiency with an early-morning plasma cortisol level before the patient leaves the hospital. Physiologic glucocorticoid replacement should be instituted upon discharge if the morning cortisol is low (<10 μg/dL).
- Detailed discharge instructions should include a description of the symptoms of adrenal insufficiency (AI), diabetes insipidus, and hyponatremia (SIADH). Patients should be asked to report to the nearest emergency room if symptoms of AI or hyponatremia occur, with instructions to have a cortisol and sodium level measured.
- Reevaluation of all anterior pituitary hormones should be performed at the first postoperative visit.

Introduction

The endonasal surgical approach to the sella was first described by Hirsch and subsequently modified by Halstead[1] in 1910. By 1912 Cushing[2] adopted a sublabial variation of Halstead's procedure to perform over 200 pituitary operations with a perioperative mortality rate of 5.2%. The poorly illuminated and limited surgical field, along with high rates of meningitis delayed the widespread use of the surgical technique; not until the advent of the antibiotic era and the development of the operating microscope during the 1950s and 1960s was the renaissance of transsphenoidal surgery possible.[3] Over the last four decades transsphenoidal surgery has become the principal technique for approaching sellar and parasellar lesions, and advances in medical and surgical practice have improved the safety of the procedure, with most authors reporting mortality rates of 0 to 1%.[4–7] The pure endoscopic transsphenoidal surgery was popularized by Jho and Carrau[4] in the 1990s, and has now either replaced surgical microscopes or is serving as an important adjuvant technique at many medical centers around the world.[8]

As rates of iatrogenic complications such as infection, cerebrospinal fluid (CSF) leaks, hemorrhage, and neuronal injury, have declined, endocrine complications have become the most common cause of postoperative morbidity following skull base surgery.[9] Published complication rates are generally reported only by experienced surgeons, thus underestimating the actual rate of complications in the community. A large survey published in 1997 by Ciric et al[9] offers a more realistic look at complication rates through self-reported data from 958 American neurosurgeons with a wide range of skull base surgery experience; the cohort as a whole reported anterior pituitary insufficiency in 19.4% and diabetes insipidus in 17.8% (7.6–19%) of transsphenoidal cases.

Expertise of the Surgeon Predicts Endocrine Complication Rates

Not surprisingly, the experience of the surgeon is a critical determinant in predicting perioperative complications from transsphenoidal skull base surgery. Ciric et al's[9] published survey shows at lease a threefold increase in complication rates in the least experienced tertile (87.3% of respondents with <200 operations) compared with the most experienced tertile (3% of respondents with >500 operations). Rates of anterior pituitary insufficiency in the two groups were 20.6% versus 7.2%, rates of diabetes insipidus were 19% versus 7.6%, and mortality rates were 1.2% versus 0.2%, respectively.

The Multidisciplinary Team

Coordinated preoperative evaluation by neurosurgeons and endocrinologists ensures optimal perioperative hormone management. At least 50% of the hormone deficits present in the preoperative state will persist following surgery, and appropriate preoperative hormone replacement to address adrenal insufficiency, diabetes insipidus, or central hypothyroidism is necessary and can reduce anesthesia and surgical complications and speed recovery in the immediate postoperative period.[10] It is imperative to identify patients who have adrenal insufficiency prior to initiating thyroid replacement to avoid an adrenal crisis.[11] Accurate analysis of thyroid and gonadal function is best done in the preoperative outpatient setting because the stress of surgery and administration of corticosteroids can transiently suppress these hormone axes. Furthermore, accurate characterization of functional pituitary lesions can prevent the need for surgery (prolactinomas), or identify patients at high risk for respiratory failure after anesthesia (acromegaly) or perioperative thromboembolism (Cushing's disease).[12,13]

The Role of Preoperative Imaging

High-resolution magnetic resonance imaging (MRI) of the sella is a critical component of preoperative planning. The size and the type of sellar lesion are important predictors of postoperative hormone deficiencies.[10] As a result of differential uptake of gadolinium contrast, MRI can also help to differentiate mass lesions from regions of normal pituitary tissue, thus minimizing intraoperative exploration or unnecessary resection of the normal pituitary gland. Preservation of 30 to 40% of the normal anterior pituitary is usually adequate to preserve postoperative hormone function; however, pituitary glands that have been compressed by very large macroadenomas are often less resilient to surgical resection, and rates of postoperative hormone deficiency are more common.

Surgical Techniques to Minimize Endocrine Dysfunction

Careful anatomical analysis with preoperative MRI studies is essential in maintaining the midline approach.[8] The preservation of midline structures and careful hemostasis allow the surgeon to maintain anatomical orientation until the sella is opened, and once in the sella, careful hemostasis is necessary to allow the surgeon to identify the subtle tissue characteristics that differentiate the anterior and posterior pituitary as well as the tumor capsule and parenchyma. To further guide the surgical approach, lateral-view x-ray control or frameless stereotactic image guidance can be used. Diabetes insipidus can best be prevented by avoiding traction on the pituitary stalk and manipulation of the posterior pituitary. If an individual case necessitates exposure of the posterior pituitary or perturbation of the pituitary stalk, the postoperative care team should be made aware of the increased likelihood of iatrogenic diabetes insipidus. Preservation of the normal pituitary gland depends on the ability of the surgeon to recognize remnants of the normal pituitary, which can be fibrous in character when tumor compression has occurred.[6]

Immediate Postoperative Management

In the first 24 hours after surgery, clinical attention should focus on the potential for acute adrenal insufficiency or diabetes insipidus. Aside from surgical remission of Cushing's disease, acute adrenal insufficiency is an uncommon complication of endoscopic skull base surgery, but failure to recognize the condition can lead to untoward morbidity and mortality. For this reason, many centers empirically treat non-Cushing's patients with stress-dose glucocorticoids for 24 hours, with the first dose given before the patient leaves the operating room. Intravenous hydrocortisone 50 mg every 6 hours or 100 mg every 8 hours for 24 hours are common regimens.[10,14] The short half-life of hydrocortisone ($t_{½}$ = 90–120 minutes) leads to rapid clearance so that the exogenous glucocorticoid does not interfere with the necessary evaluation of the patient's endogenous cortisol production before discharge from the hospital. Another reasonable practice is to give stress-dose glucocorticoids only to patients who are found to have adrenal insufficiency preoperatively. In these patients it is reasonable to begin stress-dose steroids and then taper them to a standing oral glucocorticoid regimen after discharge from the hospital. All other patients can be monitored clinically and biochemically for signs of adrenal insufficiency.

Symptoms of acute adrenal insufficiency usually develop within 24 to 72 hours of surgery (e.g., lethargy, headache, nausea/abdominal pain, and orthostatic hypotension). A morning serum cortisol of less than 10 µg/dL in a symptomatic postoperative patient establishes the diagnosis, and should be treated with moderate stress-dose steroids until stable for discharge (intravenous [IV] hydrocortisone 50 mg every 6 hours in the first 48 hours after surgery, or hydrocortisone PO 40 mg in the a.m./20 mg in the p.m. in the stable patient approaching discharge) before transitioning to physiologic doses. Asymptomatic patients should be evaluated for relative adrenal insufficiency with a plasma cortisol between 6 a.m. and 8 a.m. on the day of discharge. A value of less than 10 µg/dL is suggestive of relative adrenal insufficiency, and patients should be treated with physiologic glucocorticoid replacement upon discharge (prednisone 5 mg daily, or hydrocortisone 20 mg daily in divided doses).

Diabetes insipidus (DI) occurs in 5 to 20% of patients and is often the earliest endocrinopathy to develop after surgical manipulation of the pituitary gland, usually within the first 12 to 24 hours of surgery. It is important to note that an avid postoperative diuresis is not adequate to establish the diagnosis. Patients with acromegaly who achieve surgical remission are expected to have a 3- to 10-L diuresis as the sodium and water retention effects of excess growth hormone resolves. Furthermore, polydipsia is common in patients undergoing transsphenoidal surgery because nasal packing and sinonasal congestion necessitate mouth-breathing. The accurate diagnosis of postoperative DI is established by routine serial measurements of urine specific gravity every 6 hours, daily or twice daily measurements of plasma sodium, and strict recording of daily fluid intake and output. Once again, multidisciplinary postoperative management is important in reducing complications.

Endocrine Complications After Discharge from the Hospital

After leaving the hospital, the most common endocrinopathy is transient posterior pituitary dysfunction resulting in a syndrome of inappropriate antidiuretic hormone secretion (SIADH). This occurs in 9% or more of patients undergoing transsphenoidal pituitary surgery, and may occur more often in patients who have transient diabetes insipidus during postoperative hospitalization.[15] Nearly all postoperative SIADH spontaneously resolves within 72 hours of onset, and is often mild and clinically unrecognized. The occurrence of symptomatic hyponatremia can be minimized by instructing patients to regulate fluid intake only in response to symptomatic thirst during the first 7 to 10 days at home. The symptoms of hyponatremia are very similar to adrenal insufficiency: lethargy, confusion, headache, nausea, and generalized weakness (very severe hyponatremia can result in seizures). Patients should be educated about these symptoms before discharge and their onset should prompt an urgent visit to the nearest hospital center for measurement of serum sodium (sodium levels of 116–126 mmol/L are common in symptomatic patients). Prompt treatment should be implemented with inpatient observation and strict fluid restriction (500 mL/day).[10] Because the clinical presentation can mimic adrenal insufficiency, serum cortisol should also be measured at the time of presentation if the patient is not receiving glucocorticoid replacement; a random cortisol <10 µg/dL in a symptomatic patient should prompt stress-dose glucocorticoid treatment for at least 24 hours followed by physiologic replacement until outpatient endocrinology follow-up occurs.

Outpatient Postoperative Follow-Up

A postoperative follow-up visit with a multidisciplinary team should be scheduled 8 to 10 weeks after surgery to allow time for potential recovery of preexisting or iatrogenic hormone deficiencies. Those patients requiring glucocorticoid replacement should stop treatment 24 hours before the first follow-up visit to allow measurement of the endogenous hypothalamic-pituitary-adrenal axis with a serum cortisol, and adrenocorticotropic hormone (ACTH). Similarly, patients receiving desmopressin treatment for DI should hold at least one dose before follow-up to evaluate for recurrence of polydipsia and polyuria.

A full clinical assessment and physical examination in all patients at the follow-up visit should be augmented by measurement of serum cortisol, free thyroxine (T_4), insulin-like growth factor 1 (IGF-1), and prolactin.[10] Measurement of gonadotropins and estradiol in female patients with reproductive capacity may be unnecessary if return of normal menstrual function occurs (this is the most sensitive and accurate sign of normal gonadotropin function). In women with amenorrhea, gonadotropins and estradiol should be measured. A total testosterone, or a free testosterone, level should be measured in men.

If morning cortisol remains below 10 µg/dL, long-term physiologic steroid replacement is indicated and patients should wear a medical alert bracelet or necklace indicating adrenal insufficiency. Repeat testing should be performed at 6 and 12 months after surgery. Free T_4, not a thyroid-stimulating hormone (TSH) level, should be used to guide thyroid hormone replacement. Replacement of estrogen and progesterone in hypogonadotropic premenopausal women is appropriate. Testosterone replacement in hypogonadotropic hypogonadal men should be initiated only after age-appropriate screening for prostrate cancer (digital rectal exam, measurement of prostate-specific antigen). Growth hormone (GH) replacement may require an insulin tolerance test to confirm GH deficiency. If diabetes insipidus is persistent, the lowest therapeutic dose of desmopressin should be determined; once-daily dosing at bedtime can often ameliorate symptoms and reduce the risk of treatment related hyponatremia.

Recurrence of skull base tumors is common, and long-term clinical follow-up requires serial MRIs and biochemical evaluation. Successful long-term management of these patients demands involvement of specialists from neurosurgery (including radiosurgery), pathology, radiology, and endocrinology.

References

1. Halstead AE. Remarks on the operative treatment of the tumors of the hypophysis. Surg Gynecol Obstet 1910;10:494–502
2. Cushing H. Transsphenoidal methods of access. In: Cushing H, ed. The Pituitary Body and Its Disorders. Philadelphia: JB Lippincott; 1912: 296–303
3. Hardy J. [Excision of pituitary adenomas by trans-sphenoidal approach.]. Union Med Can 1962;91:933–945

4. Jho HD, Carrau RL. Endoscopic endonasal transsphenoidal surgery: experience with 50 patients. J Neurosurg 1997;87:44–51

5. Cappabianca P, Cavallo LM, Colao AM, de Divitiis E. Surgical complications associated with the endoscopic endonasal transsphenoidal approach for pituitary adenomas. J Neurosurg 2002;97:293–298

6. Laws ER Jr, Kern EB. Complications of transsphenoidal surgery. In: Laws ER, Randall RV, Kern EB, eds. Management of Pituitary Adenomas and Related Lesions. New York: Appleton-Century-Crofts; 1982:329–346

7. McCormick P, ed. Postoperative Complications in Intracranial Neurosurgery. Chicago: Thieme Medical Publishers; 1993:61–73

8. Jane JA Jr, Han J, Prevedello DM, Jagannathan J, Dumont AS, Laws ER Jr. Perspectives on endoscopic transsphenoidal surgery. Neurosurg Focus 2005;19:E2

9. Ciric I, Ragin A, Baumgartner C, Pierce D. Complications of transsphenoidal surgery: results of a national survey, review of the literature, and personal experience. Neurosurgery 1997;40:225–236, discussion 236–237

10. Vance ML. Perioperative management of patients undergoing pituitary surgery. Endocrinol Metab Clin North Am 2003;32:355–365

11. Fonseca V, Brown R, Hochhauser D, Ginsburg J, Havard CW. Acute adrenal crisis precipitated by thyroxine. Br Med J (Clin Res Ed) 1986;292: 1185–1186

12. Goldhill DR, Dalgleish JG, Lake RHN. Respiratory problems and acromegaly. An acromegalic with hypersomnia, acute upper airway obstruction and pulmonary oedema. Anaesthesia 1982;37:1200–1203

13. Messick JM Jr, Laws ER Jr, Abboud CF. Anesthesia for transsphenoidal surgery of the hypophyseal region. Anesth Analg 1978;57:206–215

14. Laws ER Jr, Abboud CF, Kern EB. Perioperative management of patients with pituitary microadenoma. Neurosurgery 1980;7:566–570

15. Cusick JF, Hagen TC, Findling JW. Inappropriate secretion of antidiuretic hormone after transsphenoidal surgery for pituitary tumors. N Engl J Med 1984;311:36–38

47 Successful Management of Endoscopic Skull Base Surgery Complications

Ameet Singh, Vijay K. Anand, and Theodore H. Schwartz

Tips and Pearls

- Meticulous surgical dissection to preserve the pituitary stalk, and supporting vasculature is important to prevent postoperative diabetes insipidus.
- Careful study of neurovascular anatomy on preoperative imaging studies is imperative to prevent intraoperative catastrophic neurovascular injuries.
- Careful study of sphenoid septations can identify the course of the carotid.
- Characteristics of the defect, type of tumor pathology, and volume of cerebrospinal fluid leak influence the type of skull base reconstruction.
- Intrathecal fluorescein can identify subtle cerebrospinal fluid leaks and help improve skull base reconstruction, thereby preventing postoperative morbidity.
- Lumbar drainage, bed rest, and stool softeners can successfully treat the majority of postoperative cerebrospinal fluid leaks in the absence of pneumocephalus, assuming a meticulous closure of the skull base has been performed.
- Infectious complications are rare in endoscopic skull base surgery. These may be reduced with 24 to 48 hours of antibiotics delivered in the perioperative period.
- Mucosal-sparing surgery followed by meticulous postoperative care (topical nasal therapy, postoperative debridement) can significantly decrease sinonasal complications after endoscopic pituitary and skull base surgery.
- Preserve a stump of the middle turbinate or the entire middle turbinate to prevent postoperative sinusitis.

Introduction

Endoscopic skull base surgery offers a new paradigm for the management of anterior midline skull base lesions. Its advantages over traditional open transcranial or transfacial approaches include superior visualization of lesions and surrounding neurovasculature, decreased retraction and manipulation of brain and cranial nerves, and potential improvements in surgical outcomes. Complications are an inherent part of any surgical management strategy, and endoscopic skull base procedures are no different. Preventing, minimizing, and successfully managing complications with minimal morbidity and mortality remain the goals in endoscopic skull base surgery. The management of many potential complications (e.g., endocrinologic, neurologic) in endoscopic skull base surgery is similar to transcranial surgery. Management of other complications (e.g., vascular, cerebrospinal fluid [CSF] leaks, sinonasal) differs in some respects from transcranial surgery.

Complications

Endocrinologic

Diabetes insipidus (DI) is one of the more frequently encountered complications in transsphenoidal pituitary and craniopharyngioma surgery. Disturbance of the posterior pituitary, pituitary stalk, and neurons from the hypothalamus may lead to temporary or permanent imbalance of antidiuretic hormone–regulated water homeostasis. The overall incidence of transient and permanent postoperative DI in transsphenoidal pituitary surgery has been reported to range from 4 to 20% (transient) and 0 to 5% (permanent)[1] but may be as high as 68% for transsphenoidal craniopharyngioma.[2] In our series, transient DI was experienced in 10% of endoscopic pituitary and anterior skull base approaches for a variety of tumor pathologies, with permanent DI in less than 2% of cases. Craniopharyngiomas had the highest rate (40%) of postoperative DI (unpublished data).

The recent literature has shown that patients with microadenomas, craniopharyngiomas, Rathke's cleft cysts, and intraoperative CSF leak have an increased incidence of postoperative DI. In addition, transitioning from a microscopic to endoscopic pituitary surgery can be accomplished with a low incidence of DI.[3] Theoretically, improved visualization, magnification, angled endoscopes, and enhanced surgical instrumentation should enable surgeons to better preserve the posterior pituitary, pituitary stalk, hypothalamic nuclei, and supporting vasculature. Preservation of the hypothalamic-pituitary axis and supporting vasculature through meticulous surgical dissection is paramount to preventing postoperative transient or permanent DI.

Vascular

Vascular complications include hemorrhage and stroke. Bleeding can entail nasal mucosal bleeding from a traumatic opening, troublesome slow oozing at the tumor bed, brisk venous bleeding from the cavernous sinus, pulsatile arterial bleeding from a small intracranial perforator, arterial bleeding

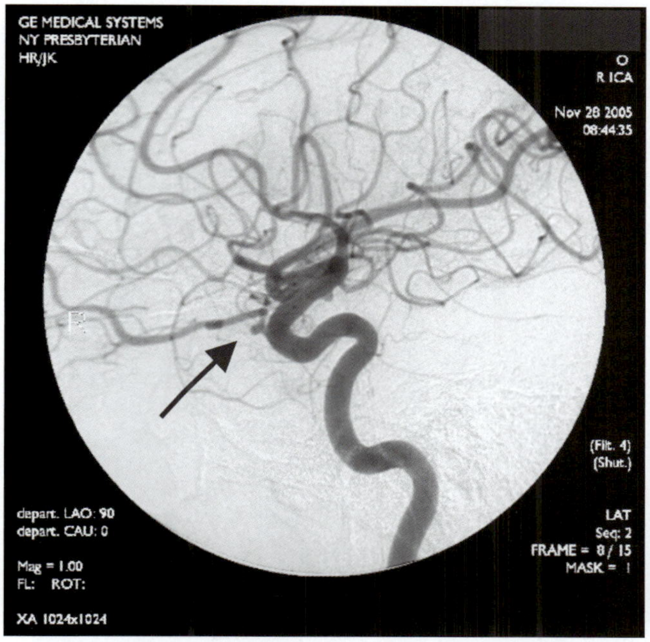

A

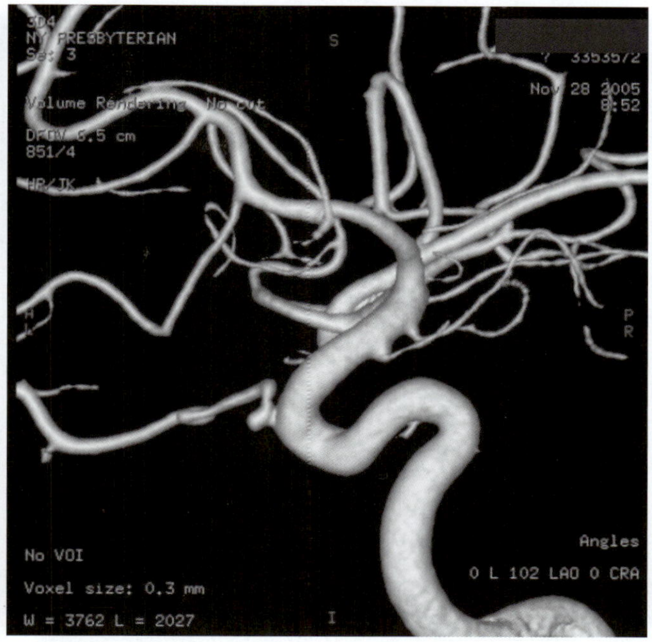

B

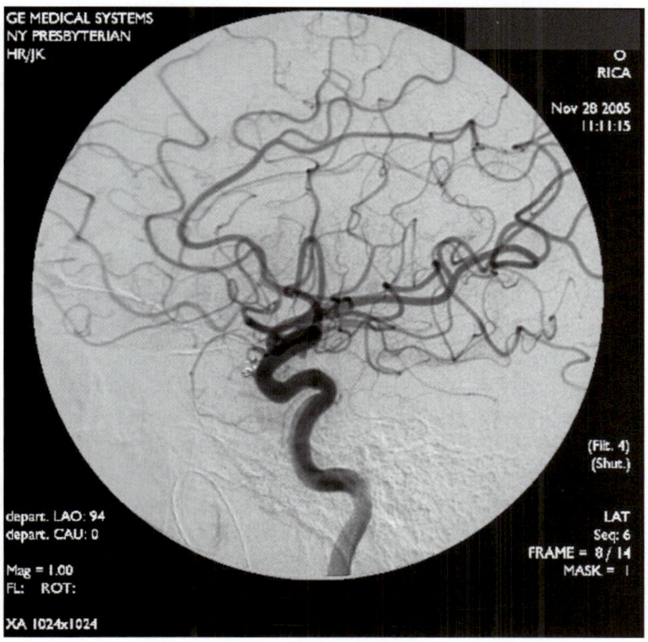

C

Fig. 47.1 Pseudoaneurysm at the origin of the ophthalmic artery demonstrated on angiogram **(A)** and three-dimensional (3D) reconstruction **(B)**. **(C)** Definitive treatment consists of occlusion of the ophthalmic artery at its origin. There were extensive collaterals feeding the artery through the external circulation and ethmoidal arteries, so vision was preserved.

within the nose from branches of the sphenopalatine artery, or more devastating arterial injuries to the internal carotid artery. Each of these vascular injuries can be managed in a variety of ways. Meticulous intraoperative hemostasis is essential for the approach to and resection and reconstruction of the skull base. Nasal mucosal bleeding can be managed with injection of epinephrine, direct cautery, or application of hemostatic agents such as FloSeal (Baxter, Deerfield, IL). Bleeding from the sphenopalatine artery usually requires direct cautery or ligation. Control of venous ooze within the brain can be managed with warm saline irrigation, thrombin-soaked Gelfoam, gentle pressure, FloSeal, and bipolar electrocautery. Arterial bleeding from small intracranial vessels is quite tricky because the parent artery must often be preserved to prevent stroke. Direct cautery to "weld" the opening closed is ideal. Pressure with FloSeal may work in some circumstances, and sacrifice of the parent artery is a last resort (**Fig. 47.1**). Internal carotid artery (ICA) injury is best avoided by thoroughly studying the neurovascular anatomy on preoperative imaging, and utilizing image guidance and Doppler intraoperatively. These techniques are imperative to confirm anatomical landmarks and avoid a vascular injury.

In the event of a major vascular injury (<1% in our series of 250 patients), direct pressure with packing and placement of a Foley balloon will usually be suitable for temporary control. Once the acute bleeding is managed, immediate transfer

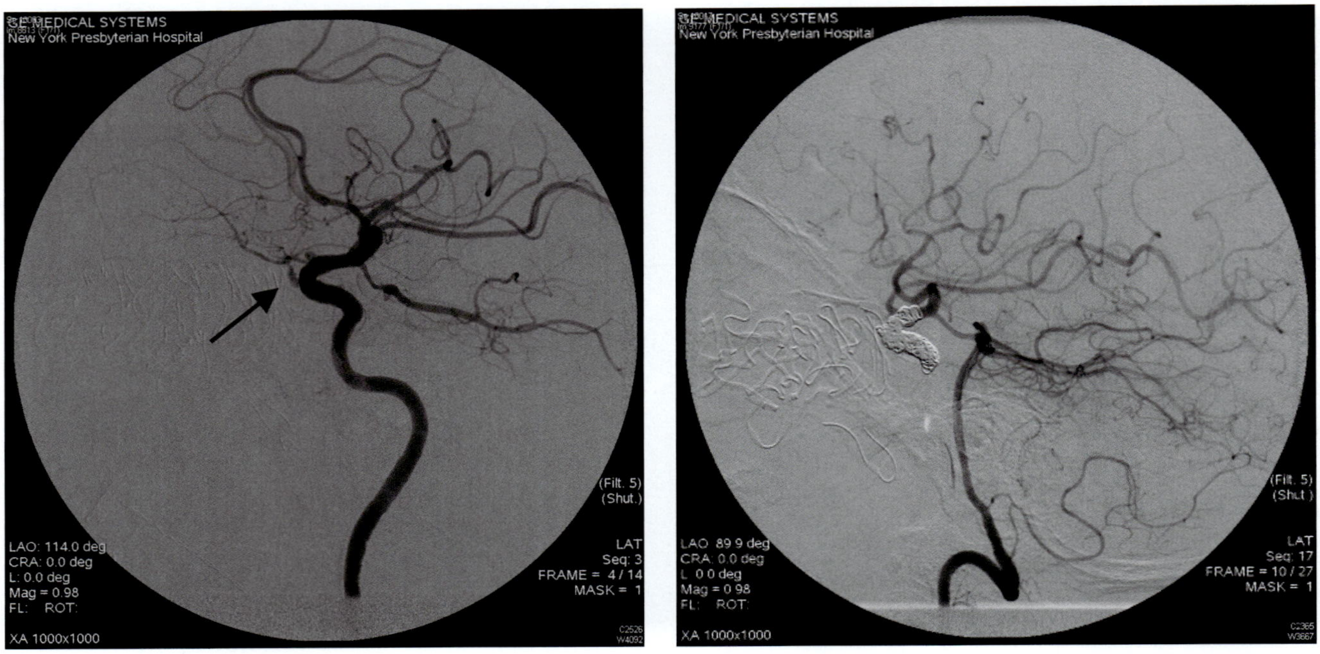

A B

Fig. 47.2 **(A)** Internal carotid artery injury (*arrow*) within the sphenoid sinus is demonstrated with the extravasation of contrast material from the internal carotid artery (ICA) into the sphenoid sinus. **(B)** Definitive repair in this case included occlusion of the ICA. Notice that the anterior circulation fills through the posterior communicating artery.

to interventional neuroradiology for angiography is optimal. A perforation in the carotid can be managed by stenting or occlusion (**Fig. 47.2**). A balloon occlusion test is advisable prior to sacrificing the artery, to assess the presence of collateral flow and the patient's ability to tolerate occlusion. Stenting may be performed but requires anticoagulation and is currently not Food and Drug Administration (FDA) approved for treating these injuries. If a stent is placed, repeat endonasal surgery can be performed to further cover the defect in the artery with tissue sealant.

Significant postoperative epistaxis is uncommon, especially if meticulous hemostasis is maintained intraoperatively. Perioperative local infiltration of the sphenopalatine foramen can reduce bleeding in the operative field, enabling superior visualization of vessels.[4] Superior visualization with straight and angled endoscopes providing excellent illumination, and magnification may be another reason for a low incidence of postoperative epistaxis. Finally, an otolaryngologist with intimate knowledge of nasal and paranasal anatomical variations is an asset for avoiding postoperative vascular complications.

Cerebrospinal Fluid Leaks

Separation of the intracranial and sinonasal cavities after skull base surgery to prevent CSF leaks is of paramount importance to avoid morbidities such as meningitis and pneumocephalus (**Fig. 47.3**). Postoperative CSF leaks have been the Achilles heel for extended endoscopic approaches to the anterior skull base. Initial reports after extended endonasal approaches revealed a CSF leak rate as high as 40%.[5] Utilization of the vascularized nasoseptal flap reduced the CSF rate to a little over 10% in subsequent series.[6,7] The introduction of the gasket-seal closure also significantly reduced the postoperative CSF leak rate to 0% in a small series of patients with extended skull base defects.[8] This technique requires countersinking a rigid buttress into an onlay fascial graft that overlaps the margins of bony defect, thereby creating a watertight seal (**Fig. 47.4**). Subsequent use of the gasket seal in combination with the nasoseptal flap has further reduced the postoperative CSF leak rate to 0 to 5% (unpublished data). The leak rate in our most recent 150 cases was reduced to 2.3%, most likely attributable to technical advances and our greater experience. Vascularized flaps such as the temporoparietal, turbinate, palatal, and endoscopic pericranial have enhanced reconstructive options available in primary and revision endoscopic skull base cases.[9,10]

Multilayered closure with or without a vascularized flap remains the mainstay in endoscopic skull base reconstruction. An algorithmic approach to skull base repair is employed after evaluating the size and location of the skull base defect, type of pathology, and volume of CSF leak.[11] Small sellar defects with CSF leaks may be reconstructed with fat, and a rigid buttress to reconstruct the floor of the sella followed by a tissue sealant. Larger defects in the skull base created for the removal of intracranial pathology can be sealed with a multilayered reconstruction, or preferably the gasket-seal closure with or without a vascularized pedicle flap. Some authors recommend placement of a Foley balloon in the sphenoid after the closure to keep everything in place.[7]

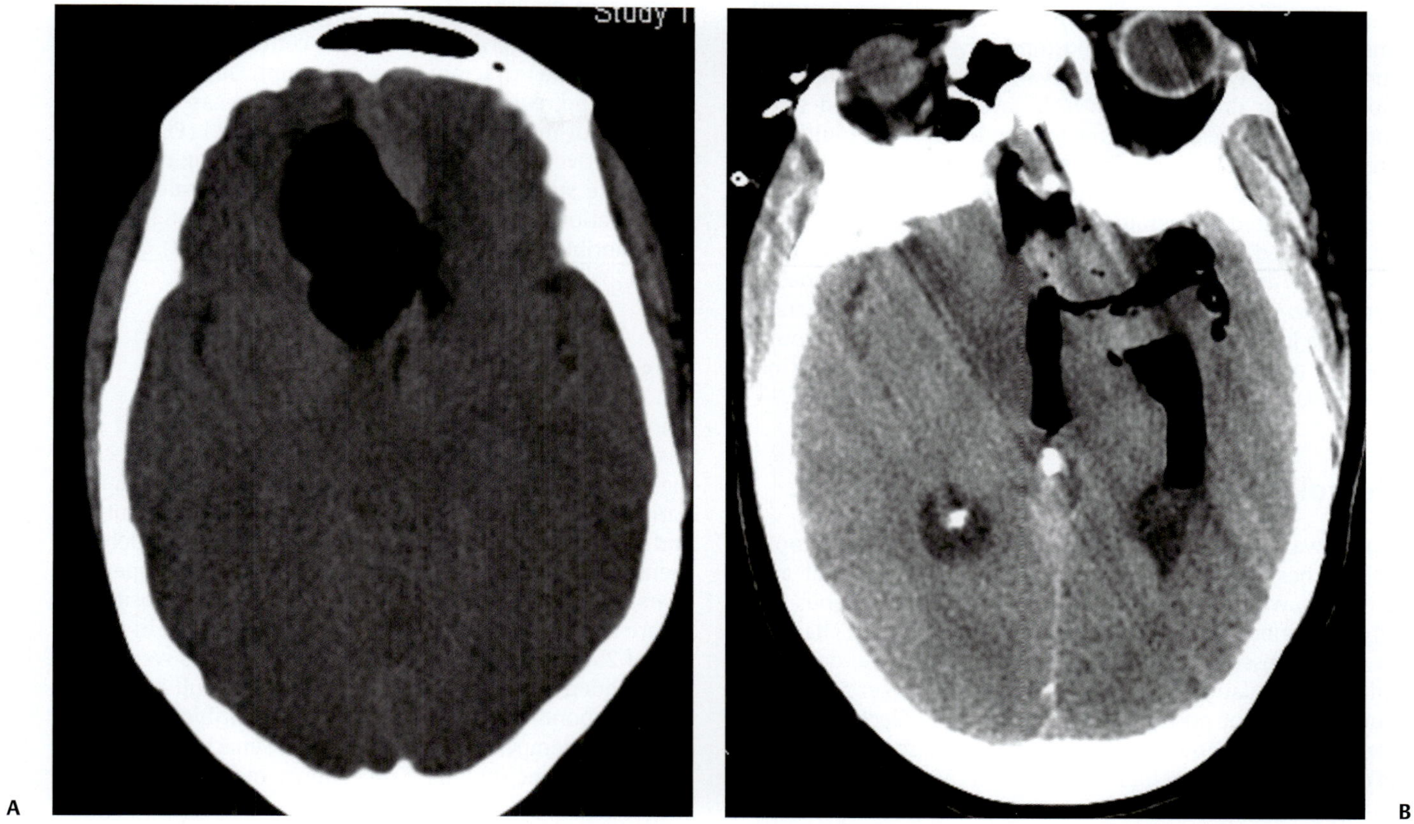

Fig. 47.3 Examples of intracranial pneumocephalus after endoscopic skull base surgery. **(A)** Air under tension introduced at the base of the frontal lobe can extend intraparenchymally. **(B)** Air can enter in the subarachnoid space and intraventricularly.

Intrathecal fluorescein is an invaluable agent to identify intraoperative CSF leaks. Our experience has demonstrated the safety and utility of intrathecal fluorescein for the detection and repair of intraoperative CSF leaks.[12,13] Fluorescein, a green fluorescent dye, can help identify small and subtle CSF leaks that may be overlooked when surrounded with mucus, blood, and irrigation fluid. Another surgical adjunct utilized to decrease postoperative CSF leaks is the lumbar drain. Lumbar drainage serves as a temporary diversion of CSF, thereby decreasing pooling and resultant pressure on the skull base reconstruction. Contemporary indications for lumbar drainage include anticipated large skull base defects, large tumors, preoperative CSF leaks, high-flow intraoperative CSF leak, and increased intracranial pressure. In addition,

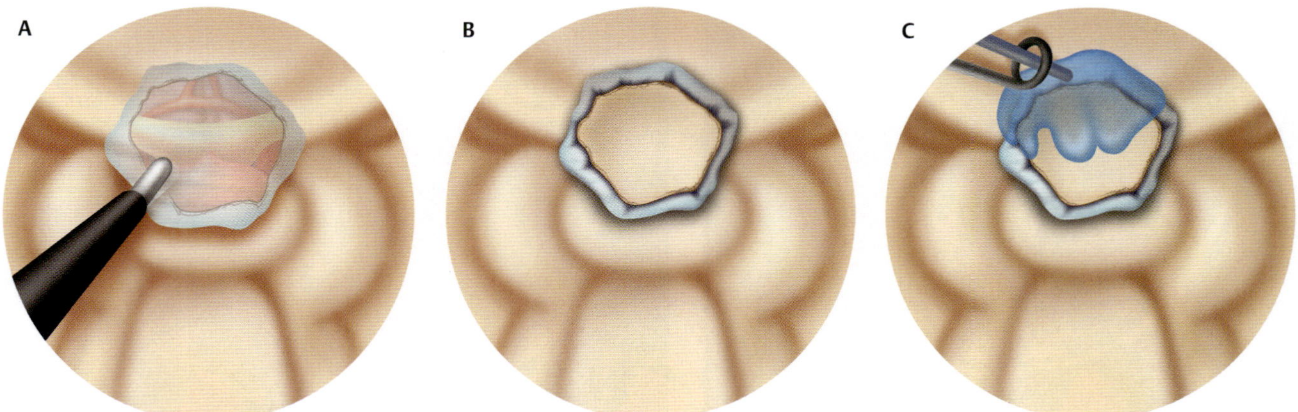

Fig. 47.4 **(A)** Placement of a large fascial graft over a bony skull base defect. **(B)** Countersinking of rigid buttress over fascial graft into bony defect. **(C)** Placement of tissue glue.

results in our series of 250 endoscopic skull base cases demonstrate that the majority of postoperative CSF leaks may be successfully treated with conservative measures, which include lumbar drainage for 2 to 5 days, bed rest, and stool softeners. This technique is recommended only if a multilayered closure has been performed and a low rate of drainage (5 cc/hr) is used; otherwise, there is risk of pneumocephalus. Serial computed tomography (CT) imaging of the brain should be performed to rule out the development of pneumocephalus. Some authors advocate immediate repeat endonasal surgery to close CSF leaks, which is another possible strategy. As a last resort, one can perform a bifrontal craniotomy and use a pericranial flap to close the skull base defect or place a ventriculoperitoneal shunt.

Neurologic

Cerebrovascular accidents and hemorrhages in endoscopic approaches have similar etiologies to the traditional approaches, which include injury to blood vessels, venous infarction, embolic strokes, or significant intraoperative changes in blood pressure. Meticulous hemostasis and the delay of full anticoagulation for several weeks after surgery will reduce the risk of postoperative hemorrhage. Electrophysiologic monitoring in the operating room may reduce the risk of cranial nerve injury for cases in which these structures are at high risk.

Infectious

Central nervous system (CNS) infectious complications of endoscopic skull base surgery are rare. This is intriguing, given the frequent passage of surgical instruments and reconstruction materials through the contaminated sinonasal cavity into the intracranial compartment. Our review of 250 primary and revision endoscopic skull base cases revealed a 0.7% risk of infection (meningitis or abscess) (**Fig. 47.5**). A retrospective review of 90 patients undergoing endoscopic skull base surgery for benign pathologies revealed no CNS complications. All these patients received 24 to 48 hours of a single antibiotic: cefazolin (87%), vancomycin (10%), or clindamycin (3%).[14]

Nasal and Sinus Complications

Sinonasal complications of endoscopic pituitary and skull base surgery include acute and chronic rhinosinusitis, crusting, and synechiae. Postoperative crusting is common in all patients after endoscopic pituitary and skull base surgery, and requires nasal hygiene, topical therapy, and debridements. Crusting is rarely noted after the first postoperative visits in endoscopic pituitary patients. Acute rhinosinusitis is rare and was limited to less than 5% of patients in our series of 250 patients. The majority of these cases were noted in extended endoscopic approaches to the skull base. Most cases respond to culture-directed oral antibiotics, topical antibiotic therapy, and irrigation. Nasal synechiae may occur after endoscopic skull base procedures, most commonly between the nasal septum and turbinates. Soft, immature synechiae may be easily lysed during nasal endoscopy in the acute postoperative period. Mucosal-sparing surgery, followed by meticulous postoperative care, which includes topical nasal therapy and debridement, can significantly decrease sinonasal complications after endoscopic pituitary and skull base surgery.

A 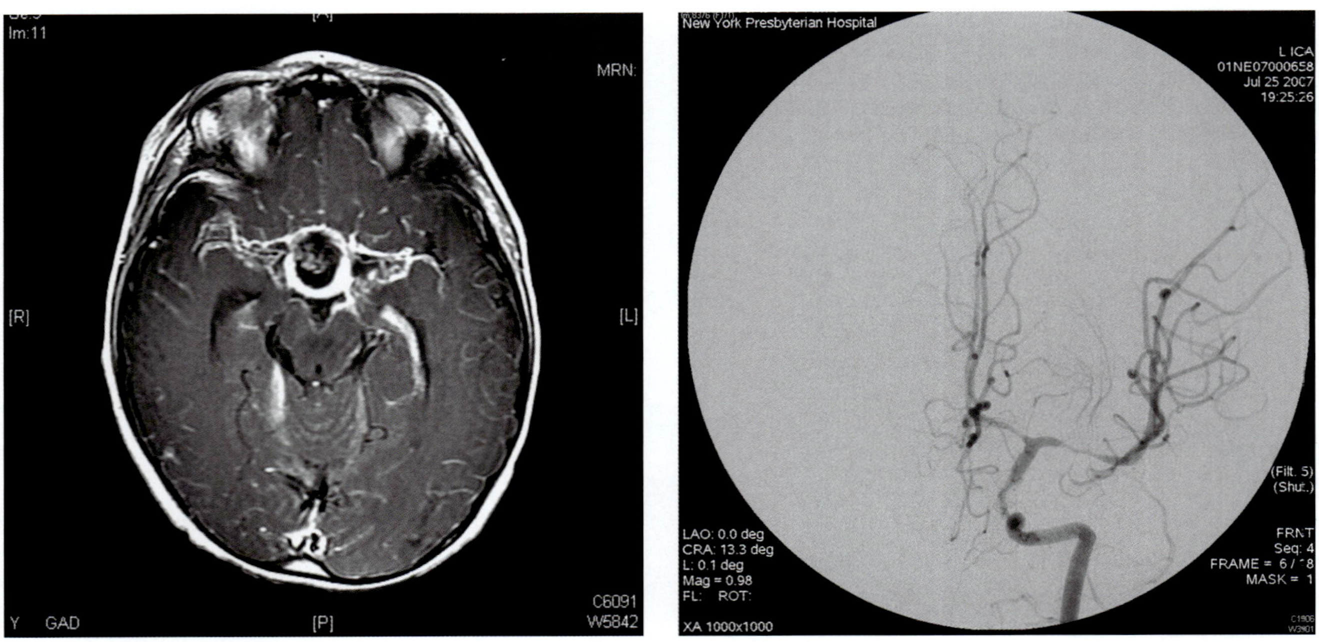 B

Fig. 47.5 **(A)** Intracranial abscess formed around a fat graft seen on a diffusion-weighted image showing increased signal. **(B)** Arteriogram shows a vasospasm as a result of the infection in the suprasellar cistern, which led to a stroke.

Deep Venous Thrombosis

Deep venous thrombosis (DVT) is a risk of any long surgery, whether the approach is transcranial or endonasal. In addition, prolonged bed rest after surgery predisposes patients to DVT. Hence, the use of lumbar drainage should be limited if possible. Use of venous compression stockings during and after surgery as well as prophylactic anticoagulation and early mobilization decrease the risk of DVT. In patients with a prior history of DVT, we sometimes recommend placement of a prophylactic vena cava filter prior to surgery. In our series the risk of DVT is <2%.

■ Conclusion

Complications are inherent in any surgical approach. Careful patient selection, systematic preoperative planning, meticulous surgical dissection, constant communication with all members of the operative team, and vigilant postoperative care can minimize intraoperative and postoperative complications. Adequate surgical instrumentation, neuronavigation, and extensive training of personnel are critical for surgical success and management of potential complications. In addition, a team approach consisting of otolaryngologists and neurosurgeons is paramount to achieving an excellent surgical result and successful management of complications.

References

1. Tabaee A, Anand VK, Barrón Y, et al. Predictors of short-term outcomes following endoscopic pituitary surgery. Clin Neurol Neurosurg 2009; 111:119–122
2. Honegger J, Buchfelder M, Fahlbusch R, Däubler B, Dörr HG. Transsphenoidal microsurgery for craniopharyngioma. Surg Neurol 1992; 37:189–196
3. Sigounas DG, Sharpless JL, Cheng DM, Johnson TG, Senior BA, Ewend MG. Predictors and incidence of central diabetes insipidus after endoscopic pituitary surgery. Neurosurgery 2008;62:71–78, discussion 78–79
4. Wormald PJ, Athanasiadis T, Rees G, Robinson S. An evaluation of effect of pterygopalatine fossa injection with local anesthetic and adrenalin in the control of nasal bleeding during endoscopic sinus surgery. Am J Rhinol 2005;19:288–292
5. Gardner PA, Kassam AB, Thomas A, et al. Endoscopic endonasal resection of anterior cranial base meningiomas. Neurosurgery 2008;63:36–52, discussion 52–54
6. Hadad G, Bassagasteguy L, Carrau RL, et al. A novel reconstructive technique after endoscopic expanded endonasal approaches: vascular pedicle nasoseptal flap. Laryngoscope 2006;116:1882–1886
7. Kassam AB, Thomas A, Carrau RL, et al. Endoscopic reconstruction of the cranial base using a pedicled nasoseptal flap. Neurosurgery 2008; 63(1, Suppl 1):ONS44–ONS52, discussion ONS52–ONS53
8. Leng LZ, Brown S, Anand VK, Schwartz TH. "Gasket-seal" watertight closure in minimal-access endoscopic cranial base surgery. Neurosurgery 2008;62(5, Suppl 2):E342–E343, discussion E343
9. Oliver CL, Hackman TG, Carrau RL, et al. Palatal flap modifications allow pedicled reconstruction of the skull base. Laryngoscope 2008; 118:2102–2106
10. Zanation AM, Snyderman CH, Carrau RL, Kassam AB, Gardner PA, Prevedello DM. Minimally invasive endoscopic pericranial flap: a new method for endonasal skull base reconstruction. Laryngoscope 2009; 119:13–18
11. Tabaee A, Anand VK, Brown SM, Lin JW, Schwartz TH. Algorithm for reconstruction after endoscopic pituitary and skull base surgery. Laryngoscope 2007;117:1133–1137
12. Placantonakis DG, Tabaee A, Anand VK, Hiltzik D, Schwartz TH. Safety of low-dose intrathecal fluorescein in endoscopic cranial base surgery. Neurosurgery 2007;61(3, Suppl):161–165, discussion 165–166
13. Tabaee A, Placantonakis DG, Schwartz TH, Anand VK. Intrathecal fluorescein in endoscopic skull base surgery. Otolaryngol Head Neck Surg 2007;137:316–320
14. Brown SM, Anand VK, Tabaee A, Schwartz TH. Role of perioperative antibiotics in endoscopic skull base surgery. Laryngoscope 2007;117: 1528–1532

48 The History and Future of Endoscopic Skull Base Surgery

Wolfgang Draf

In all specialties dealing with the sinuses located deep in the body, tubes and cavities have been needed from the very beginning of modern practical medicine for transmitting light into these hollow spaces. This common necessity was the reason why otology, deriving originally from general surgery, as the complications of otitis media frequently required surgery, rhinology, and laryngology, originating in internal medicine for diagnosis and treatment of tuberculosis, have been united as the field of otorhinolaryngology. The first specialty in which endoscopy was developed was urology, where it was used to examine the urethra and the bladder.[1]

Very early endoscopic diagnostic and therapeutic procedures have been used by several disciplines, of which otorhinolaryngology was one of the first. In neurosurgery it took much more time until the endoscope was introduced as a surgical tool, mostly in interdisciplinary cooperation with otorhinolaryngologists interested in skull base surgery. There are several historical reviews of endoscopic skull base surgery,[2–4] some of which discuss the development of endoscopic pituitary surgery.[4,5,6]

The advances in endoscopic skull base surgery demanded a new, much more detailed description of anatomy. We have to be grateful for the immense work and cooperation of three outstanding clinically oriented anatomists: Johannes Lang (**Fig. 48.1**), the founder of microanatomy; Albert L. Rhoton (**Fig. 48.2**), who developed surgical microanatomy; and Manfred Tschabitscher (**Fig. 48.3**), who taught the endoscopic anatomy of the skull base.

I became interested in the Hopkins telescopes in the late 1960s, after having been disappointed with the older generation of telescopes. The main stimulus for developing the Hopkins telescopes was the idea that nasal and paranasal sinus endoscopy is needed not only for improving diagnostics but also for therapy.

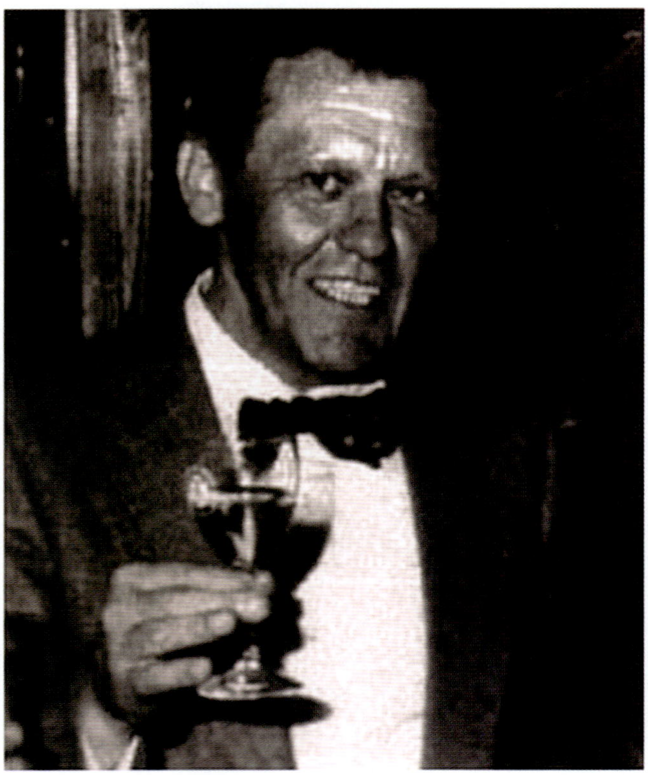

Fig. 48.1 Johannes Lang (1923–2003), Wurzburg, Germany; anatomist, and founder of microanatomy.

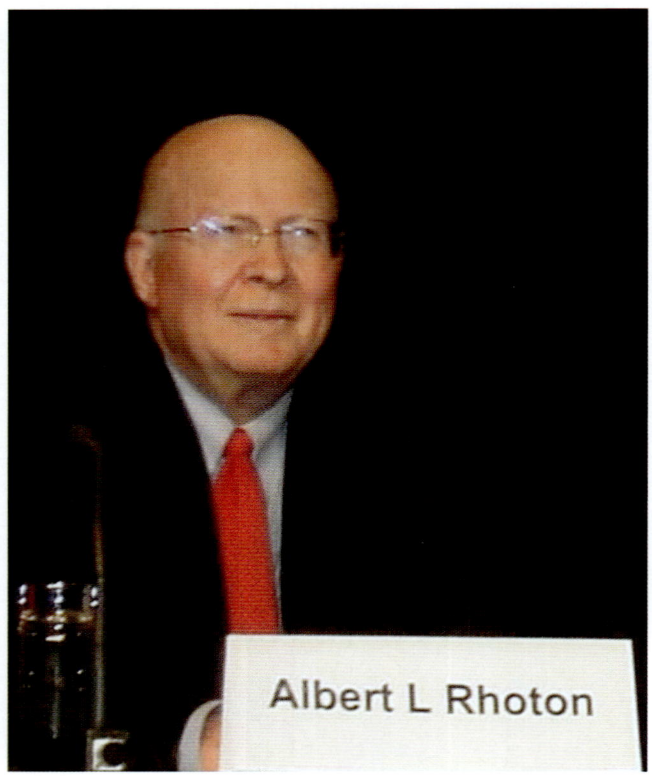

Fig. 48.2 Albert L. Rhoton, Gainesville, Florida; neurosurgeon and neurosurgical microanatomist.

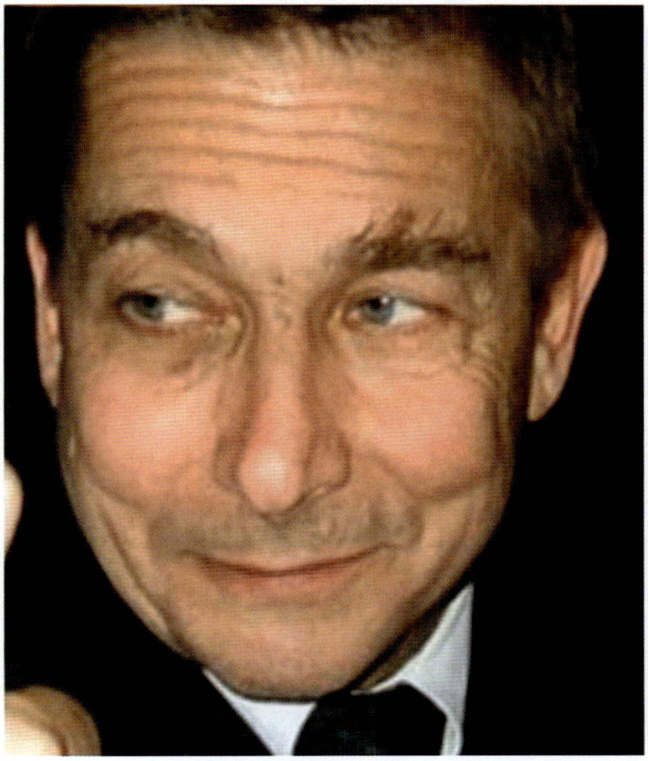

Fig. 48.3 Manfred Tschabitscher, Vienna, Austria; founder of endoscopic anatomy.

This chapter is my somewhat personal comprehensive overview of the history of endoscopic skull base surgery.

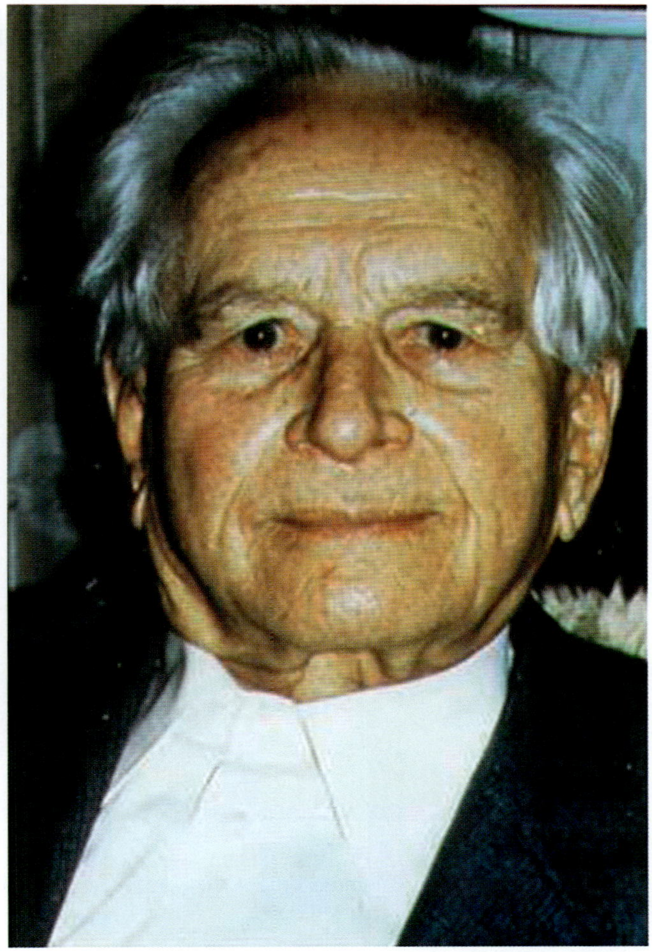

Fig. 48.4 Hans Heermann (1933–1967), Essen, Germany; originated microscopic endonasal surgery.

Development of Endonasal Surgery

Endonasal surgery using just a head light and the naked eye was developed at the turn of the 20th century.[7] Endonasal drainage of the frontal sinus was already being successfully performed.[8] Because visual tools such as the microscope and endoscope had not yet become available, and anesthesia had not reached the level of providing a surgical field with minimal bleeding, it was difficult for the average surgeon to perform endonasal sinus operations and in particular to reach the frontal sinus through the nose. Many complications had been reported. Mosher[9] stated that endonasal ethmoidectomy was the easiest operation with which to kill a patient. Therefore, between 1920 and 1980, endonasal surgery was abandoned at most centers worldwide, with only a few exceptions.[10–15]

The real revival of endonasal surgery started when H. Heermann began to use the operating microscope, primarily introduced for microsurgery of the ear,[16–19] for various operations through the nose, such as for sinus surgery of inflammatory diseases, but also for pituitary operations and others (**Figs. 48.4, 48.5, 48.6,** and **48.7**).

Evolution of Endonasal Endoscopic Surgery

Early attempts to look into the maxillary sinus were reported by Hirschmann[20] (**Fig. 48.8**). Nitze[21] used the cystoscope for naso- and antroscopy. Various attempts to look into the maxillary sinus were reported by Reichert[22] in 1902 and by others.[23–25] The following decades witnessed the ups and downs of sinus endoscopy, which was also called antroscopy, engendered by a succession of technical improvements.

The real breakthrough to endoscopic[26,27] and microendoscopic (which I reported in 1982) surgery in otorhinolaryngology is attributed to the ingenuity of Harold Horace Hopkins (**Fig. 48.9**), a professor of physics at the University of Reading, United Kingdom.[28–30] It was his idea in 1954 to construct a flexible endoscope,[31] which was developed into a useful prototype by the American gastroenterologist Basil Hirschowitz together with the physicist Larry Curtis. They presented it for the first time in 1957.[32,33]

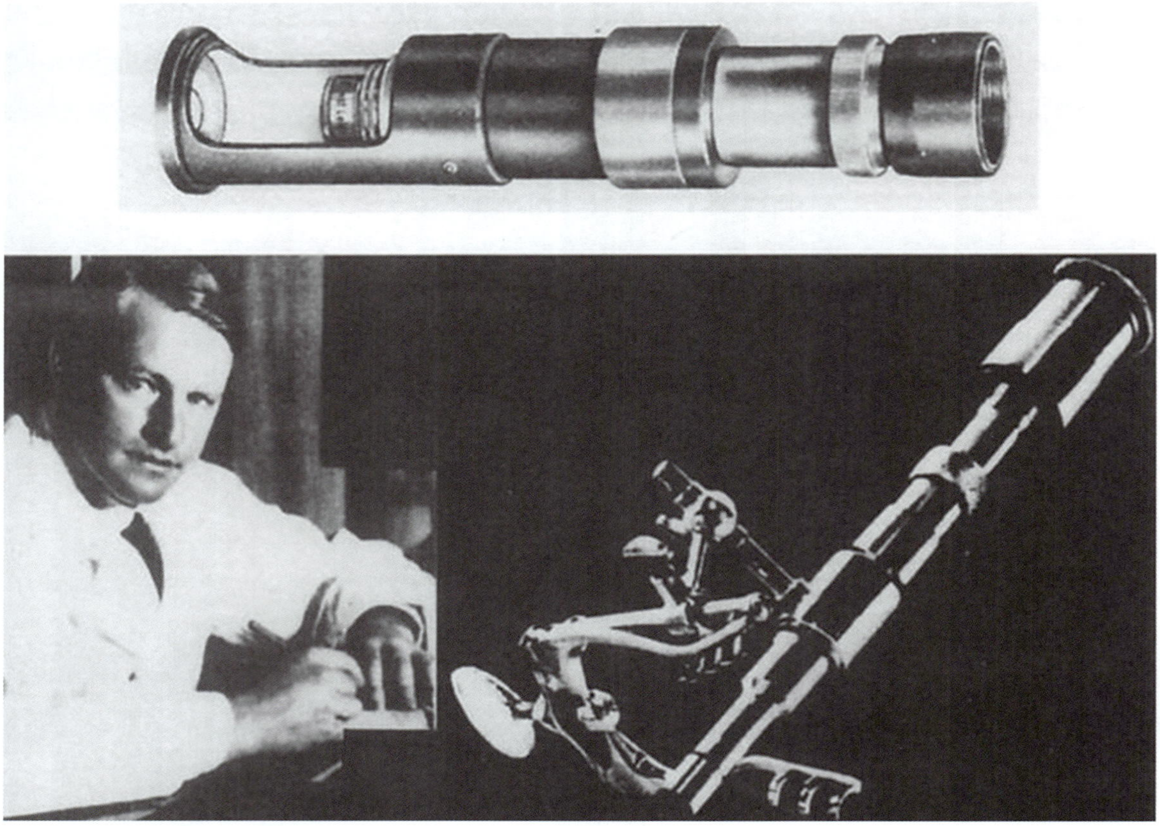

Fig. 48.5 C.O. Nylen (1892–1978), Stockholm, Sweden; introduced the operating microscope to otology. From Miehlke A. Geschichte der Mikrochirurgie. Munich, Vienna, Baltimore: Urban & Schwarzenberg; 1996. Reprinted by permission.

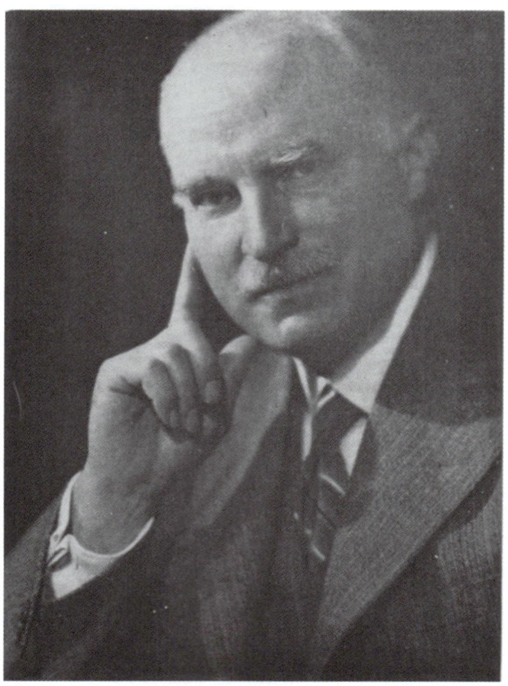

Fig. 48.6 Gunnar Holmgren (1875-1954), Stockholm, Sweden; eminent figure in otology, originated the use of a binocular microscope for fenestration surgery in otosclerosis. From Shambaugh GE Jr. Surgery of the Ear, 2nd ed. Philadelphia: Saunders, 1967. Reprinted by permission.

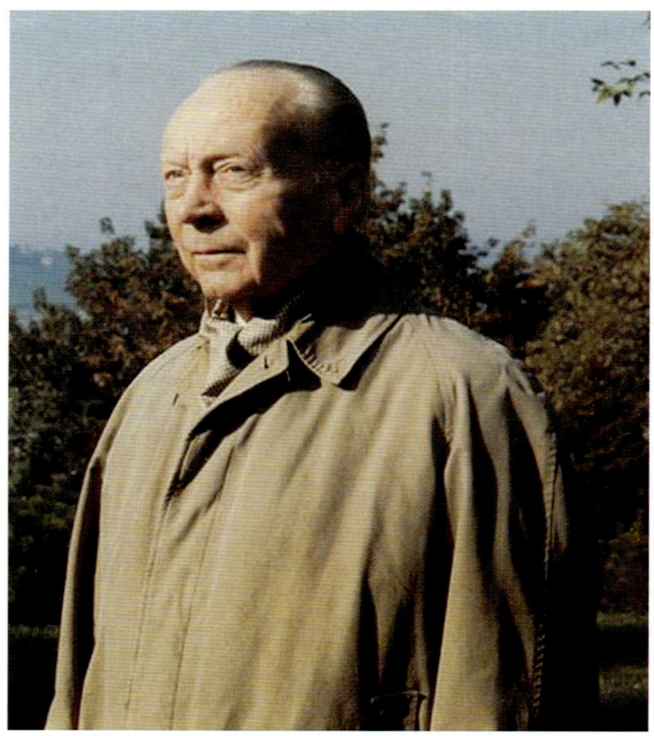

Fig. 48.7 Horst Ludwig Wullstein (1906–1987); built the first modern binocular operating microscope with the Zeiss Company.

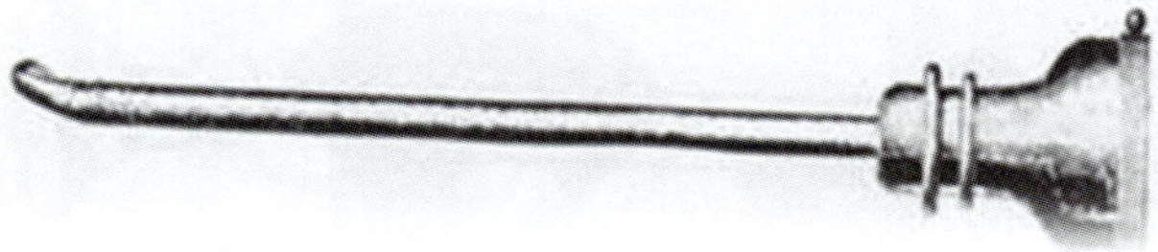

Fig. 48.8 Nasendoscope of A. Hirschmann. From Buiter CT. Endoscopy of the Upper Airways. Excerpta Med. Amsterdam, New York: American Elsevier; 1976. Reprinted by permission.

Although Hopkins was disappointed by the lack of support for the development of the flexible endoscope, he also recognized the legitimacy of the complaints of the British urologist J.G. Gow about the poor quality of the rigid endoscopes that were available on the market at that time. After he received a small grant of about 3000 British pounds, he began work to revolutionize the existing optics technique for constructing endoscopes[28,34]; he replaced the relay of lenses with interspaces of air and glass inside the shaft. The higher refractive index of glass in comparison to air increased the viewing angle and thus led to the very welcomed decrease of the diameter of the instrument. This ingenious invention increased light transmission by a factor of nine, which meant an approximately 80-fold better illumination. The image quality improved dramatically with regard to brightness, contrast resolution, and color fidelity.

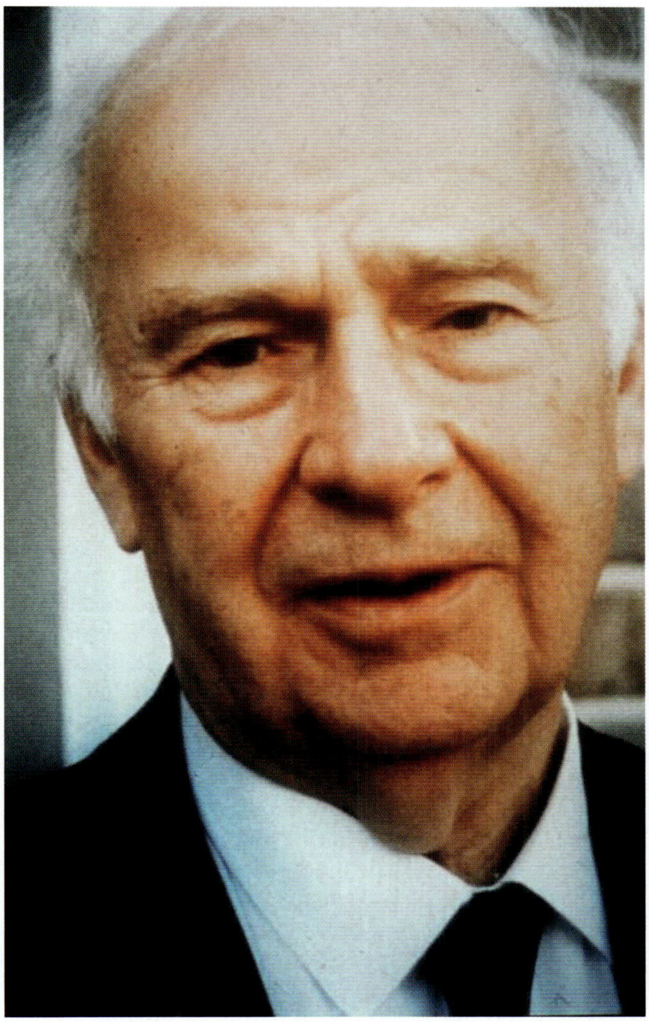

Fig. 48.9 Harold Horace Hopkins (1918–1994), Reading, United Kingdom; physicist and inventor of the rod-lens rigid telescope system and the flexible endoscope.

As frequently is the case in such situations, the brilliance of this invention was not recognized immediately. The first presentation of the new telescope at a urology meeting in Rio de Janeiro in 1961 was mostly ignored. It was Dr. George Berci (personal communication, 2005, 2009) (**Fig. 48.10**) of the United States who brought together the genius physicist Hopkins and the no less ingenious instrument maker Karl Storz from Tuttlingen (**Fig. 48.11**). Hopkins had given Berci a demonstration of the new invention of the rod lens system in London. Then Berci went to Tuttlingen and urged Storz to visit Hopkins in England. Storz realized immediately the importance of Hopkins's invention. He and Hopkins got along well and worked well together, and thus construction of the telescope began. Storz constructed the first practical rigid Hopkins telescope that was stable enough for daily use; it separated the light source from the telescope (so-called cold

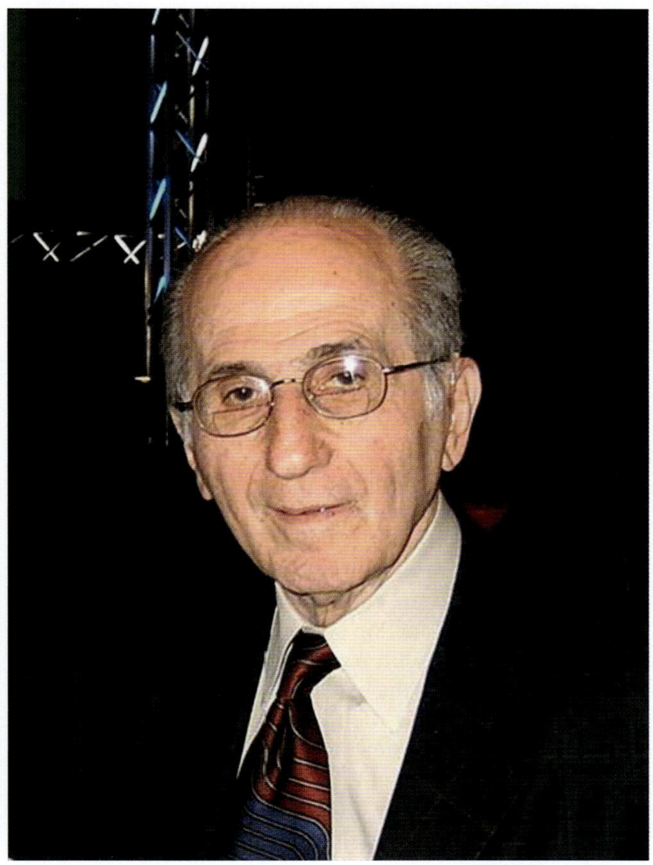

Fig. 48.10 George Berci, Hollywood, California; surgical endoscopic pioneer who introduced Harold Hopkins to Karl Storz.

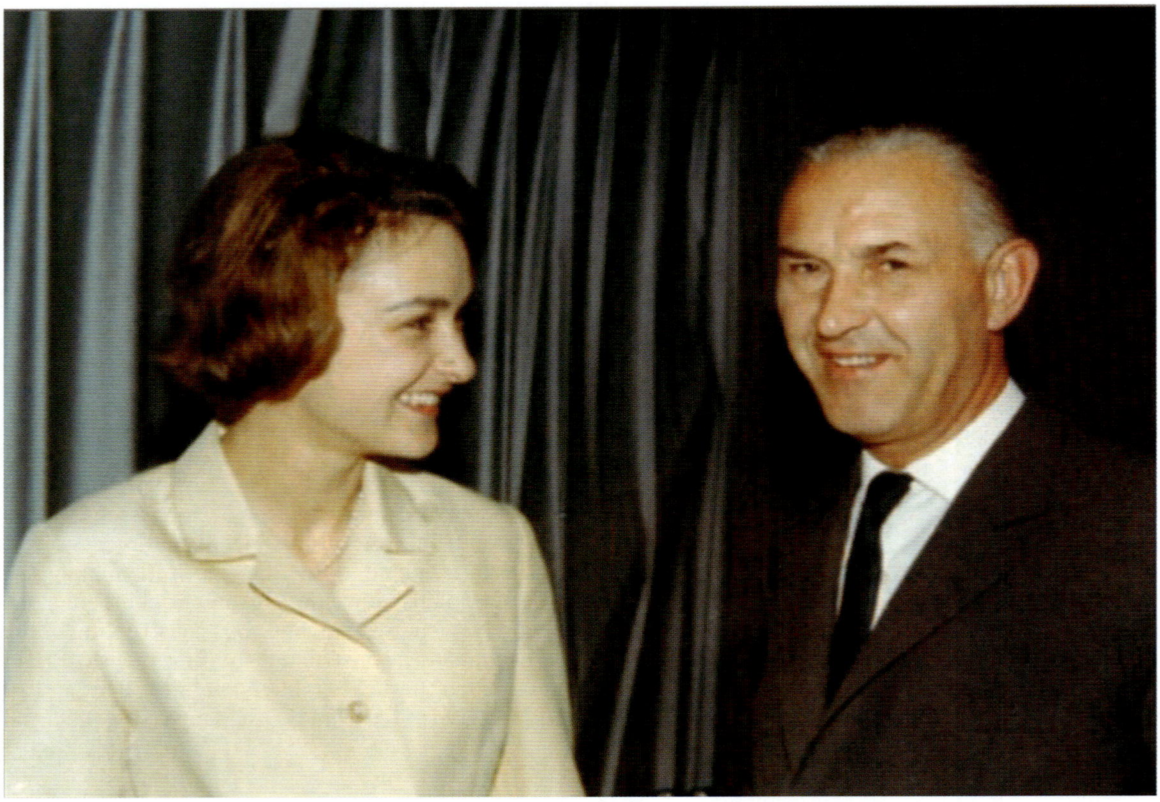

Fig. 48.11 Karl Storz (1911–1996), shown with his daughter Sybill Storz, Tuttlingen, Germany; genius instrument inventor and developer, founder of the worldwide Karl Storz Company. Sybill Storz followed her father in the leadership of the company, which she continues to lead with great success.

light[28]). Since 1969, rod-lens endoscopes have also been produced by Richard Wolf in Knittlingen, Germany.[28] Since then, the rigid telescopes have continually improved, so that today we have, for example, a 5-mm Storz endoscope for tumor surgery in the central skull base, which was initiated by Aldo C. Stamm of Sao Paulo, Brazil (**Fig. 48.12**). Further construction is already underway of a telescope that will enable not only three-dimensional (3D) visualization but also 3D recording of endoscopic surgery without increasing the diameter of the telescopes.

It is not an overestimation to say that with these telescopes, a new era in endoscopic surgery began for many medical disciplines and for veterinary medicine. In otorhinolaryngology it was Messerklinger (**Fig. 48.13**) who in the late 1960s began to use an endoscope as a visual tool, having already studied the function of nasal and paranasal sinus mucosa for many years with a microscope. The small diameter of the new telescopes, the high light intensity, the wide angle view, and the magnification, which brings the endoscope near to the object of interest, gave him a new inside view, without the need of major procedures to expose these areas, for recognizing the importance of minor pathologies in the ostiomeatal complex and for recognizing the pathogenesis of inflammatory diseases in the paranasal sinuses. He noted that most of these sinuses drained into the middle nasal meatus.[35] His student Heinz Stammberger (**Fig. 48.14**) disseminated Messerklinger's work throughout the world and is an important contributor to the continual evolution in this field.

All of this work paved the way for doing surgical procedures in smaller anatomical areas, as I began doing in 1973, culminating in the concept of functional endoscopic sinus surgery for the treatment of inflammatory diseases (**Fig. 48.15**).[36] The International Functional Endoscopic Sinus Surgery (FESS) courses in Graz and in Fulda began at about the same time in 1985–86. At first these courses were competitive, but a few years later a fruitful exchange of philosophies and practical techniques originated when Stammberger was teaching and operating at the course in Fulda and I was lecturing at the course in Graz.

At that time, in the 1970s, I believed that too many radical procedures were being done to treat inflammatory diseases of the paranasal sinuses, resulting in too many negative side effects. After Caldwell–Luc procedures were performed, we saw about 20 to 30% of our patients develop infraorbital nerve neuralgia because of surgical irritation of this nerve and because imaging was limited to plain x-ray. For exceptional situations, such as the suspicion of a tumor, conventional tomography was available. By comparing endoscopic examinations of the maxillary sinus with diagnosis based on plain x-ray images, we found that in 30% of our patients an incorrect diagnosis was made on the basis of plain x-ray. The goal

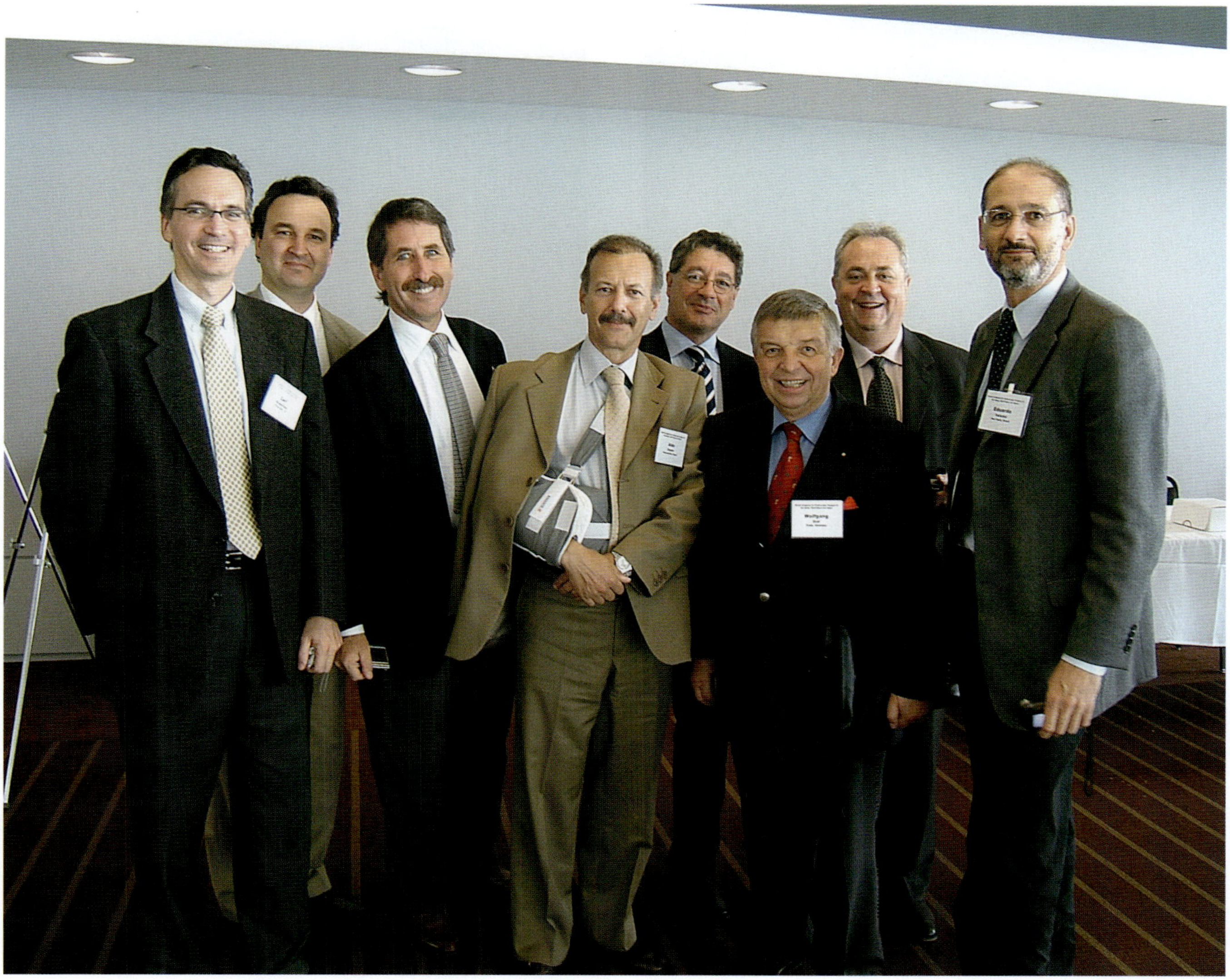

Fig. 48.12 An international group of endoscopic skull base surgeons at the First World Congress of Endoscopic Surgery of the Brain, Skull Base, and the Spine, in Pittsburgh, Pennsylvania, in 2005. From left to right: Carl Snyderman, Pittsburgh, Pennsylvania; David Holzmann, Zurich, Switzerland; Paolo Cappabianca, Naples, Italy; Aldo C. Stamm, Sao Paulo, Brazil; Davide Locatelli, Pavia, Italy; Wolfgang Draf, Fulda, Germany; Paolo Castelnuovo, Varese, Italy; and Eduardo Velutini, Sao Paulo, Brazil.

of systematic endoscopic evaluation of the paranasal sinuses was different: I wanted to improve the diagnosis and treatment of sinus diseases.

The Messerklinger School from the very beginning exclusively used the endoscope for surgical treatment of inflammatory diseases, working under local anesthesia for rather limited and mucosa-preserving operations. The main argument was that under local anesthesia patients were able to warn the surgeon that they were feeling pain if dangerous areas such as the periorbit and dura were touched.

The Fulda (beginning in 1979) and the Wigand et al (**Fig. 48.16**)[37] schools of endoscope-assisted endonasal surgery in Erlangen preferred general anesthesia so that they could perform more extended procedures if necessary. Wigand used for the endonasal ethmoidectomy head light and endoscope, and coined the term *isthmus surgery* because diseases in the ethmoid, which represents the isthmus in the middle nasal meatus, frequently result in a blockage of the paranasal sinuses that were draining into the middle nasal meatus.[38] Wigand was a visionary who realized very early that this type of intervention should be a part of skull base surgery.[39]

Developing a system of endonasal drainage procedures for the frontal and sphenoid sinuses began between 1980 and 1984 when the Fulda school combined the use of the microscope and the endoscope, making the work with the available drills easier and faster. I waited 7 years before publishing the concept of endonasal surgery for the frontal sinus because I wanted to have evidence of its success.[40] The new shaver drills had been available for several years, which led me and many others to use the telescopes almost exclusively as visual aids, although the microscope was needed in cases of severe bleeding.

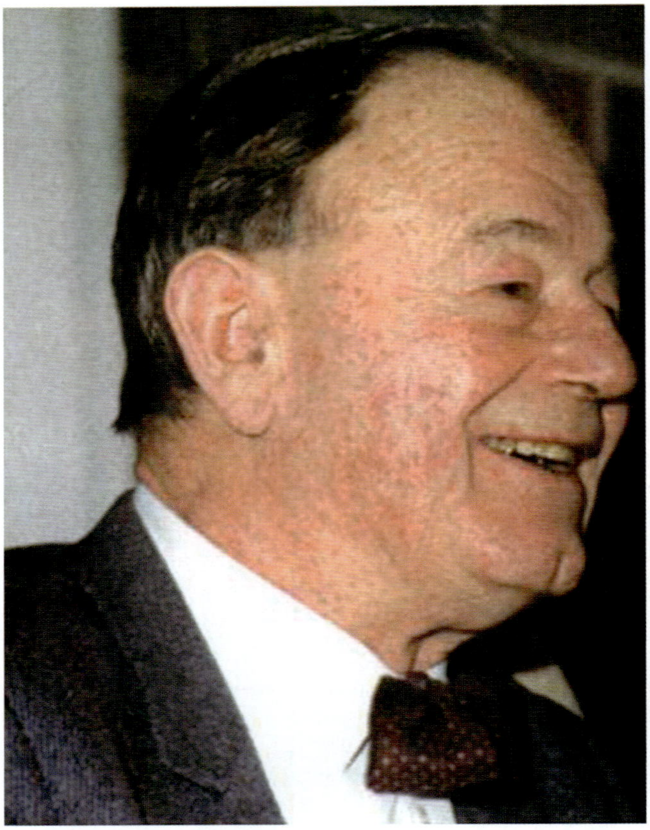

Fig. 48.13 Walter Messerklinger (1920–2001), Graz, Austria; developed the Messerklinger technique of endoscopic sinus surgery.

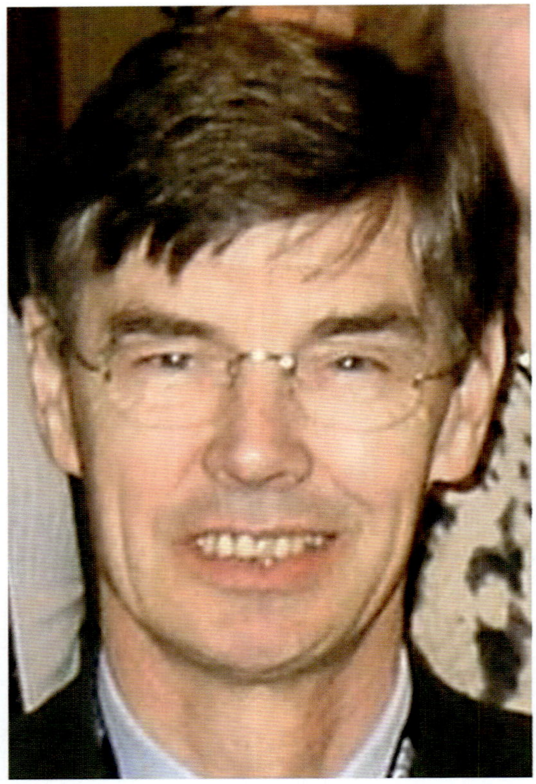

Fig. 48.14 Heinz Stammberger, former student of Walter Messerklinger, who disseminated the Messerklinger functional endoscopic sinus surgery throughout the world and has a worldwide reputation as he continues to develop the technique.

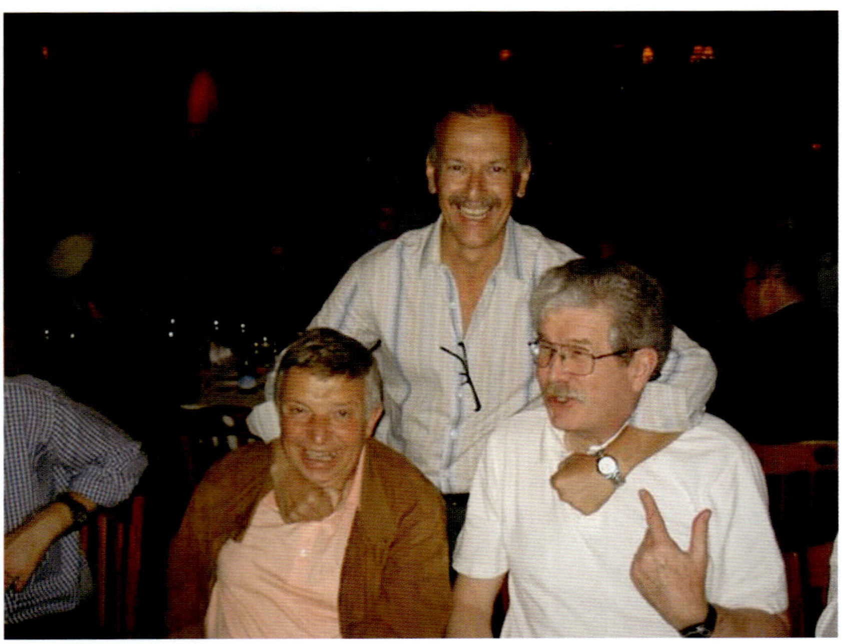

Fig. 48.15 Three promoters of endoscopic skull base surgery at the Third World Congress of Endoscopic Surgery of the Brain, Skull Base, and Spine, May 2008, in Sao Paulo. From left to right: Wolfgang Draf, Hannover, Germany; Aldo C. Stamm, Sao Paulo, Brazil; David Kennedy, Philadelphia, Pennsylvania.

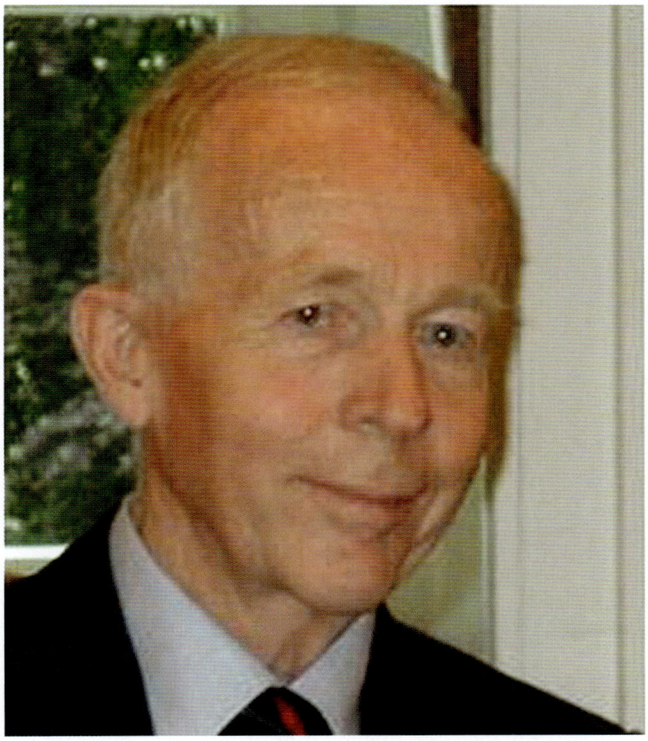

Fig. 48.16 Malte Erik Wigand, Erlangen, Germany; in 1977 he founded the Erlangen school of endoscope-assisted sinus surgery.

From Advanced Endonasal Endoscopic Surgery to Endonasal Endoscopic Tumor and Skull Base Surgery

Endoscopic endonasal surgery started treating inflammatory diseases of the nose and paranasal sinuses, and continued with surgery for disease and for related orbital and endocranial complications, such as dural defects created by the surgeon or as part of a skull base malformation. I along with Wigand started doing surgery for benign tumors in the late 1980s,[41,42] and I operated on the first malignant space-occupying lesion in 1991. This surgery was at that time strongly attacked, but now it has become routine.[43–47] Several groups demonstrated this less mutilating technique, using multiple frozen sections and different techniques of tumor removal, such as en-bloc resection in smaller lesions. Piecemeal and enucleation techniques gave even better results than the classic external procedures such as lateral rhinotomy, midfacial degloving, and subcranial operations. This does not mean that these surgical techniques are obsolete. They are still needed for larger tumors; for example, the lateral rhinotomy with the Weber–Fergusson incision is needed if orbital exenteration cannot be avoided.

Soon endonasal dacryocystorhinostomy, orbital surgery, optic nerve decompression, and difficult biopsies became part of advanced endoscopic endonasal surgery. These very different types of endoscopic surgical measures have been used frequently in the skull base and have led in an evolutionary process to systematic interdisciplinary surgery of the skull base, brain, and vertebral spine.

Independently, in the 1980s and early 1990s, several groups of European neurosurgeons created minimally invasive endoscopic neurosurgery,[48] which underwent further development and is now known as neuroendoscopy.[28,49] It is in fact intraventricular neuroendoscopy applied with a frameless approach or as stereotactic endoscopy using rigid rod-lens endoscopes or flexible steerable telescopes. Because this technique is not part of skull base surgery, it will not be discussed in detail here.

In 1979, for the first time, the neurosurgeons Halves and Bushe[50] in Wurzburg reported on the advantage of the operating endoscope for transsphenoidal surgery in cases of extrasellar extension of craniopharyngioma. Early multidisciplinary groups have performed endoscopic skull base surgery based on the initiatives of Sethi and Pillay[51] in Singapore. Jho et al[52,53] in Pittsburgh started routinely performing endoscopic endonasal pituitary surgery. The first Interdisciplinary Congress of Endoscopic Surgery of the Skull Base, Brain, and Spine took place in Pittsburgh in 2005 due to the efforts of Ricardo Carrau, Amin Kassam, and Carl H. Snyderman (**Fig. 48.17**).

The meeting in Pittsburgh brought together many pioneers of endonasal endoscopic surgery. In addition to the Pittsburgh group, most of the advanced interdisciplinary groups from around the world attended, such as Paolo Castelnuovo and Piero Nicolai from Varese/Brescia and their neurosurgical partner Davide Locatelli; me and my neurosurgeon Robert Behr from Fulda; the neurosurgeon Georgio Frank and the otorhinolaryngologist Ernesto Pasquini from Bologna; Paolo Cappabianca from Naples; Aldo C. Stamm from Sao Paulo and his neurosurgeons, in particular Eduardo Velutini (**Fig. 48.12**); Heinz Stammberger and Michael Mokry from Graz; the otorhinolaryngologist Vijay Anand the neurosurgeon Theodore Schwartz from New York; Alfredo Herrera from Bogota and his neurosurgeon; and many others. It was a most stimulating event, and the participants decided to continue this exchange in different cities around the world.

Endonasal Endoscopic Skull Base Surgery: Update and Future Aspects

Endonasal endoscopic surgery expanded from extra- to intracranial and extra- to intradural procedures, and from surgery of the anterior and middle to surgery of the posterior fossa. The Pittsburgh group and others performed progressive, innovative, and spectacular operations, and dealt with complications such as a high rate of cerebrospinal fluid (CSF) fistulas. Intensive and honest discussion clarified the need to improve the methodology of performing duraplasties. In addition to a great variety of proven techniques for duraplasty using free autogenic and preserved allografts, Hadad

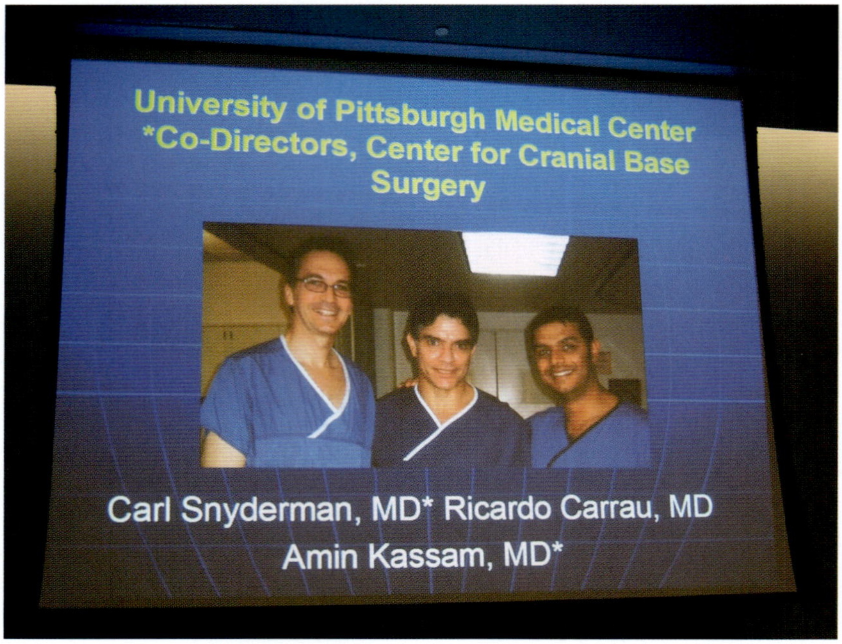

Fig. 48.17 The Pittsburgh Group. From left to right: Carl H. Snyderman, Ricardo Carrau, and Amin Kassam. Courtesy of Carl H. Snyderman.

and Bassagasteguy[54] (**Fig. 48.18**) introduced a large pedicled septal mucosal flap that was brought up to close dural defects after extended clivus surgery. Carrau and many other groups helped to reduce considerably the number of CSF leaks even after major operations. It was recognized that the three parts of a major tumor operation—exposure, resection, and reconstruction—need to be of the highest possible quality.

Whereas at the beginning of interdisciplinary endonasal endoscopic surgery of the brain, skull base, and spine the range of indications was perhaps too great, now the trend is to allow only well-established indications. Amin Kassam recently stated, "Don't cross intradurally vital neural and vascular structures." It will take time to balance the indications for endonasal endoscopic extra- and intradural surgery with well-established classic microsurgical procedures with regard to the time needed, the frequency of complications, and the availability of appropriate surgical facilities. There is no doubt that endoscopic surgery has led to a remarkable widening of the armamentarium in skull base surgery, and the patient benefits from the reduction of surgical side effects.

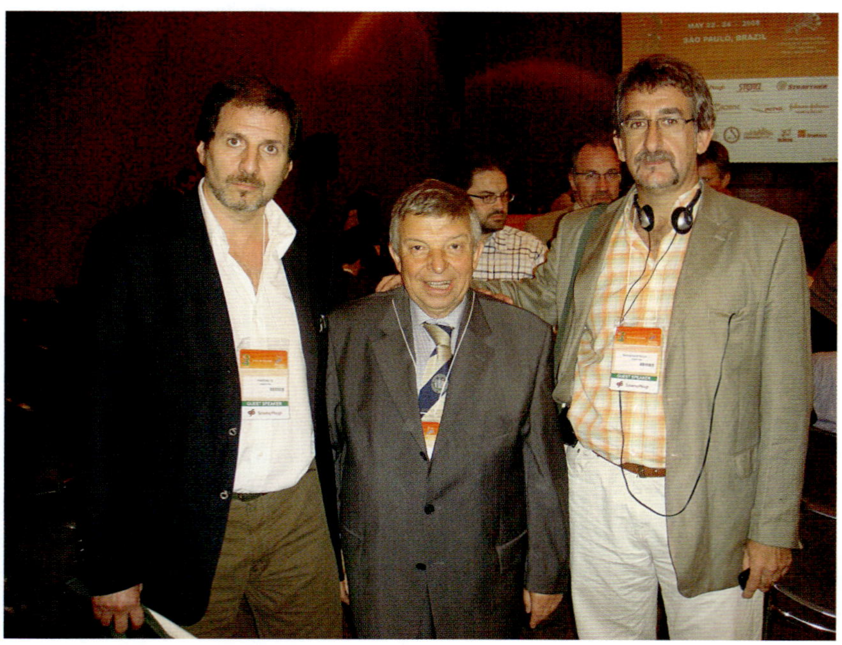

Fig. 48.18 The inventors of the large sphenopalatine artery pedicled septal flap: G. Hadad (*left*) and L. Bassagasteguy (*right*), together with the chapter author in Sao Paulo, 2008.

The term *minimally invasive surgery*[55] is misleading and should be avoided. This is invasive surgery via a smaller approach, and sometimes it is aggressive. The term *cold light* also is misleading and should be avoided because the tip of the endoscope becomes quite hot. Therefore, the tip should never touch important structures to avoid thermal lesions.

■ Conclusion

The history and evolution of endoscopic skull base surgery is fascinating. The tremendous recent advances are due to fundamental technical innovations of endoscopes and other new instruments, imaging, navigation, nerve monitoring, and video documentation as result of clinical and technical cooperation, interdisciplinary discussion, and the multidisciplinary teamwork of highly qualified surgeons.

Endoscopic skull base surgery will continue to evolve, and new advances will continue to be made.

References

1. Reuter HJ, Reuter MA. Philipp Bozzini and Endoscopy in the 19th Century. Stuttgart: Max Nitze Museum; 1988
2. Doglietto F, Prevedello DM, Jane JA Jr, Han J, Laws ER Jr. Brief history of endoscopic transsphenoidal surgery—from Philipp Bozzini to the First World Congress of Endoscopic Skull Base Surgery. Neurosurg Focus 2005;19:E3
3. Maroon JC. Skull base surgery: past, present, and future trends. Neurosurg Focus 2005;19:E1
4. Prevedello DM, Doglietto F, Jane JA Jr, Jagannathan J, Han J, Laws ER Jr. History of endoscopic skull base surgery: its evolution and current reality. J Neurosurg 2007;107:206–213
5. Gandhi CD, Post KD. Historical movements in transsphenoidal surgery. Neurosurg Focus 2001;11:E7
6. Cappabianca P, de Divitiis E. Endoscopy and transsphenoidal surgery. Neurosurgery 2004;54:1043–1048, 1048–1050
7. Draf W. Surgical treatment of the inflammatory diseases of the paranasal sinuses: indication, surgical technique, risks, mismanagement, and complications, revision surgery. [Die chirurgische Behandlung entzündlicher Erkrankungen der Nasennebenhoehlen. Indikation, Operationsverfahren, Gefahren, Fehler und Komplikationen, Revisionschirurgie]. Arch Otorhinolaryngol 1982;235:133–205 (Kongressbericht 1982)
8. Halle M. Externe und interne Operation der Nebenhoehleneiterungen. Berl Klin Wschr 1906;43:1369–1372
9. Mosher HP. The surgical anatomy of the ethmoid labyrinth. Ann Otol Rhinol Laryngol 1929;38:869–901
10. Van Alyea OE. Management of chronic sinus disease. A critical analysis of modern therapeutic measures. Ann Otol Rhinol Laryngol 1945;54: 443–457
11. Eichel BS. The intranasal ethmoidectomy procedure: historical, technical and clinical considerations. Laryngoscope 1972;82:1806–1821
12. Eichel BS. Revision sphenoidethmoidectomy. Laryngoscope 1985;95: 300–304
13. Friedman WH. Surgery for chronic hyperplastic rhinosinusitis. Laryngoscope 1975;85(12 pt 1):1999–2011
14. Heermann H. [Endonasal surgery with utilization of the binocular microscope.]. Arch Ohren Nasen Kehlkopfheilkd 1958;171:295–297
15. Kidder TM, Toohill RJ, Unger JD, Lehman RH. Ethmoid sinus surgery. Laryngoscope 1974;84:1525–1534
16. Miehlke A. Geschichte der Mikrochirurgie. Munich, Vienna, Baltimore: Urban & Schwarzenberg; 1996
17. Nylen CO. An oto-microscope. Acta Otolaryngol 1923;5:414–417
18. Nylen CO. The microscope in aural surgery, its first use and later development. Acta Otolaryngol Suppl 1954;116:226–240 Suppl
19. Wullstein H. [Prognosis and results in tympanoplasty.]. Acta Otolaryngol 1955;45:440–454
20. Hirschmann A. Über die Endoskopie der Nase und deren Nebenhöhlen. Eine neue Untersuchungsmethode. Arch Laryng Rhinol (Berl) 1903;14: 1903
21. Nitze M. Über eine neue Beleuchtungsmethode der Höhlen des menschlichen Körpers. Wien Med Presse, 1879;851–858
22. Reichert M. Über eine neue Untersuchungsmethode der Oberkieferhöhle mittels des Antroskopes. Berl Klin Wschr 1902:401
23. Buiter CT. Endoscopy of the Upper Airways. Excerpta Med. Amsterdam, New York: American Elsevier; 1976
24. Draf W. [Clinical value of sinus endoscopy (author's transl)]. Z Laryngol Rhinol Otol 1973;52:890–896
25. Draf W. Endoscopy of the Paranasal Sinuses. Heidelberg, New York: Springer; 1978 (German), 1983 (English)
26. Messerklinger W. Endoscopy of the Nose. Baltimore, Munich: Urban & Schwarzenberg; 1978
27. Stammberger H. Functional Endoscopic Sinus Surgery: the Messerklinger Technique. Philadelphia: BC Decker; 1991
28. Grunert P, Gaab MR, Hellwig D, Oertel JM. German neuroendoscopy above the skull base. Neurosurg Focus 2009;27:E7
29. McCombie CW, Smith JC. Harold Horace Hopkins, 6 December 1918–22 October 1994. In: Biographical Memoirs of the Fellow of the Royal Society. 1998;44:239–252
30. Shah J. Endoscopy through the ages. BJU Int 2002;89:645–652
31. Hopkins HH, Kapany NS. A flexible fiberscope using static scanning. Nature 1954;173:39–41
32. Hirschowitz BI, Curtiss LE, Peters CW, Pollard HM. Demonstration of a new gastroscope, the fiberscope. Gastroenterology 1958;35:50–53, discussion 51–53
33. Hirschowitz BI. Endoscopy—40 years since fiber optics. Any light at the end of the tunnel? Dig Surg 2000;17:115–117
34. Kieser CW. [Introduction of cold light to endoscopy]. Aktuelle Urol 2008;39:130–134
35. Messerklinger W. [Technics and possibilities of nasal endoscopy]. HNO 1972;20:133–135
36. Kennedy DW. Functional endoscopic sinus surgery. Technique. Arch Otolaryngol 1985;111:643–649
37. Wigand ME, Steiner W, Jaumann MP. Endonasal sinus surgery with endoscopical control: from radical operation to rehabilitation of the mucosa. Endoscopy 1978;10:255–260
38. Wigand ME. Transnasal ethmoidectomy under endoscopical control. Rhinology 1981 a;19:7–15
39. Wigand ME. Transnasal endoscopical surgery of the anterior skull base. Proceedings of the Twelfth Otorhinolaryngology World Congress. Budapest: Hungarian Academy of Sciences; 1981:137–140
40. Draf W. Endonasal micro-endoscopic frontal sinus surgery. The Fulda concept. Oper Tech Otolaryngol--Head Neck Surg 1991;2:234–240
41. Schick B, Steigerwald C, el Rahman el Tahan A, Draf W. The role of endonasal surgery in the management of frontoethmoidal osteomas. Rhinology 2001;39:66–70
42. Wigand ME. Micro-Endoscopic Surgery of the Paranasal Sinuses and the Skull Base. Stuttgart, New York: Thieme; 1989
43. Bockmühl U, Minovi A, Kratzsch B, Hendus J, Draf W. [Endonasal microendoscopic tumor surgery: state of the art]. Laryngorhinootologie 2005;84:884–891
44. Casiano RR, Numa WA, Falquez AM. Endoscopic resection of esthesioneuroblastoma. Am J Rhinol 2001;15:271–279
45. Stammberger H, Köle W, Anderhuber W. Skull base tumors: can you safely remove them with endoscopes? Am J Rhinol 2000;(Special Issue): A-177
46. Stamm AC, Draf W. Micro-Endoscopic Surgery of the Paranasal Sinuses and the Skull Base. Berlin, Heidelberg, New York: Springer; 2000

47. Wigand ME. Endoscopic Surgery of the Paranasal Sinuses and Anterior Skull Base. Stuttgart, New York: Thieme, 2008

48. Bauer BL, Hellwig D. Minimally invasive endoscopic neurosurgery—a survey. Acta Neurochir Suppl (Wien) 1994;61:1–12

49. Cappabianca P, Cinalli G, Gangemi M, et al. Application of neuroendoscopy to intraventricular lesions. Neurosurgery 2008;62(Suppl 2):575–597, discussion 597–598

50. Halves E, Bushe KA. Transsphenoidal operation on craniopharyngiomas with extrasellar extensions. The advantage of the operating endoscope [proceedings]. Acta Neurochir Suppl (Wien) 1979;28:362 (Proceedings)

51. Sethi DS, Pillay PK. Endoscopic management of lesions of the sella turcica. J Laryngol Otol 1995;109:956–962

52. Jho HD, Carrau RL, Ko Y, Daly MA. Endoscopic pituitary surgery: an early experience. Surg Neurol 1997 a;47:213–222, discussion 222–223

53. Jho HD, Carrau RL. Endoscopic endonasal transsphenoidal surgery: experience with 50 patients. J Neurosurg 1997 b;87:44–51

54. Hadad G, Bassagasteguy L, Carrau RL, et al. A novel reconstructive technique after endoscopic expanded endonasal approaches: vascular pedicle nasoseptal flap. Laryngoscope 2006;116:1882–1886

55. Wickham JEA. Endoscopic surgery. Br Med Bull 1986;42:221–339

Index

Note: Page references followed by *f* indicate figures; page references followed by *t* indicate tables.

R

S

U

V